Pathogenesis of Bacterial Infections in Animals

Pathogenesis of Bacterial Infections in Animals

Editor and Author
Dr. S.K. SRIVASTAVA
Former Head, Division of Bacteriology & Mycology
Indian Veterinary Research Institute, Izatnagar-243122
Bareilly (U.P.)

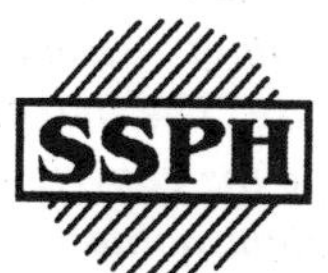

SATISH SERIAL PUBLISHING HOUSE
403, Express Tower, Commercial Complex, Azadpur, Delhi-110033 (India)
Phone : 011-27672852, Fax : 91-11-27672046
E-mail : info@satishserial.com, hkjain1975@yahoo.com
Website : www.satishserial.com

Published by :

SATISH SERIAL PUBLISHING HOUSE
403, Express Tower, Commercial Complex, Azadpur, Delhi-110033 (INDIA)
Phone : 011-27672852 Fax : 91-11-27672046
E-mail : info@satishserial.com, hkjain1975@yahoo.com

ISBN 978-93-81226-34-6

This book contains information obtained from authentic and highly regarded sources. Reasonable efforts have been made to publish reliable data and information, but the authors/editor(s)/contributors and publisher cannot assume responsibility for the validity of all materials or the consequences of their use. The authors/editor(s)/contributors and publisher have attempted to trace and acknowledge the copyright holders of all material reproduced in this publication and apologize to copyright holders if permission and acknowledgements to publish in this form have not been given. If any copyright material has not been acknowledged please write and let us know so we may rectify it.

Typeset at: Harminder Kharb *for* Laxmi Art Creation # 9971212252
Printed at: Salasar Imaging Systems, Delhi-110035

Catalyzed and Supported by the

Department of Science and Technology

Under its Utilization of Scientific Expertise of Retired Scientist Scheme

Contents

Dedication v

Introduction ix

Chapter 1 Staphylococcal Infections 1

Chapter 2 Listeriosis 29

Chapter 3 Diseases Caused by Clostridium spp. 47

Chapter 4 Diseases Caused by *Corynebacterium* spp. 89

Chapter 5 Arcanobacterium Pyogenes (Actinomyces Pyogenes) Infection 115

Chapter 6 Disease Caused by *Streptococcus* spp. 141

Chapter 7 Disease Caused by *Shigella* spp. 201

Chapter 8 Anthrax 223

Chapter 9 Leptospirosis 241

Chapter 10 Diseases Caused by *Actinobacillus* spp. 275

Chapter 11 Pseudomonas Infections 307

Chapter 12 Yersinia Infections 333

Chapter 13 Mycobacterium avium Subsp. Paratuberculosis 361

Chapter 14 Dichelobactor nodosus 381

Chapter 15 Helicobacter 399

Chapter 16 Erysipelothrix rhusiopathiae 419

Chapter 17 Bordetella Infection 437

Chapter 18 Moraxella Infection 457

Chapter 19 Haemophilus 471

Chapter 20 Fusobacterium necrophorum 495

Chapter 21 Pathogenic Actinomycetes (Nacardia and Actinomyces) .. 505

Chapter 22 Chlamydia 521

Chapter 23 Q Fever 533

Chapter 24 Glanders : A Fatal Zoonotic Disease 547

Chapter 25 Campylobacter 567

Chapter 26 Salmonella 581

Chapter 27 Haemorrhagic Septicaemia (HS) 597

Chapter 28 Brucellosis 615

Chapter 29 Bovine Tuberculosis 639

Chapter 30 Animal Mycoplasmas 667

Chapter 31 Escherichia coli 679

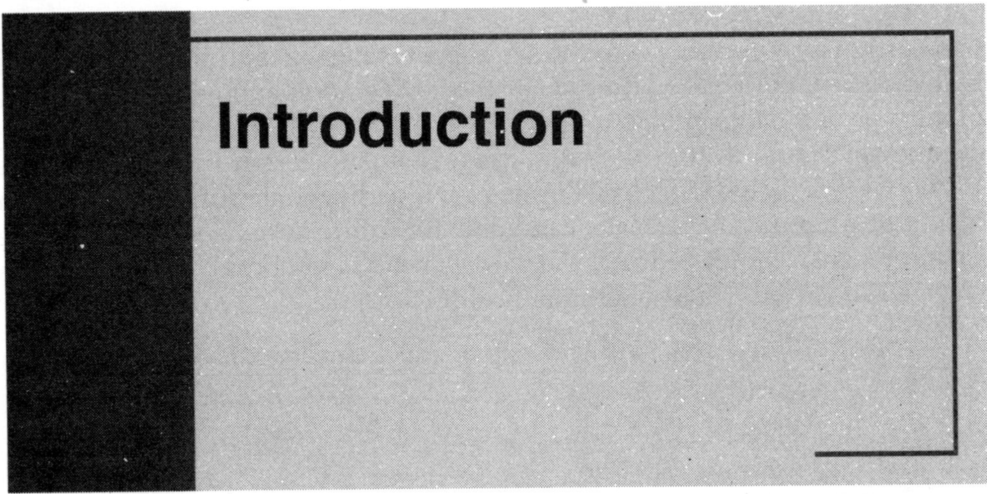

Introduction

Bacterial Pathogenesis

The basic Aims and Objectives of the study of pathogenesis of diseases is to describe the complex interaction between bacteria and the animal host leading to the production of disease. It provides a knowledge of mechanisms of establishment of infection or disease in a host by a pathogen. It is an intricate mechanism which requires involvement of several pathogen and host related factors. This also includes the modes of transmission, progression and outcome of infection. Through the knowledge of the pathogenesis one should be able to define the various terms relevant to host –parasite relationships, such as, commensalisms, symbiosis, parasitism, saprophytism, opportunistic infection and nosocomial infection. An understanding of the spectrum of virulence mechanisms employed by micro-organisms for establishment of the disease is also possible through the study of pathogenesis. Bacterial strains are known to vary in their virulence attributes subsequently the pathogenesis of the disease caused also show some variation. However, the immune status of the animal host has a significant bearing on the outcome of the exposure to the infectious agent.

Pathogenesis is often considered by the microbiologists a topic of secondary importance as its study is not directly applicable for achieving diagnosis, treatment or immunoprophylaxis of a disease. Nevertheless, the knowledge is useful in devising improved diagnostic procedures, treatment protocols and vaccines in several ways. The selection of a right clinical specimen for microbiological processing requires the knowledge about the spread and multiplication of the pathogen in the host particularly in various organs and tissues. Similarly the choice of the serodiagnostic assay and the suitable time of collection of the sera and fluids from the host requires a complete knowledge of the type of the infection in terms of the severity of the infection and various events which follow after the organisms have gained entry in the host. The knowledge of various virulence traits of the pathogen is extremely useful in identifying a most appropriate candidate for future vaccine work. Therefore a comprehensive knowledge of the pathogenesis is important to the scientists engaged in various areas of animal health.

While studying the pathogenesis acquaintance with various terms is essential:

Infection

When an organism enters the body and increases in number as a result of multiplication.

Disease

When an microorganism is able to cause tissue damage in host. It is a state of harmful alteration to the host physiological or metabolic state.

A pathogen

An organism that is able to evade the various normal defenses of the animal host to cause infection. Literally, a pathogen can cause disease in animal, man, insects as well as plants.

Pathogenicity

The ability of a pathogen to cause disease in a host. Pathogens express their pathogenicity by means of their virulence.

Virulence

Virulence is the measure of the degree of pathogenicity of an organism. The degree of virulence is related directly to the ability of the organism to cause disease irrespective of host resistance mechanisms. It is affected by numerous variables such as the number of infecting bacteria, route of entry into the body, specific and nonspecific host defense mechanisms, climatic factors affecting immune status of the host and virulence factors of the bacterium. Virulence can be measured experimentally by determining the number of bacteria required to cause animal death, illness, or lesions in a defined period after the bacteria are administered by a designated route. Consequently, calculations of a lethal dose affecting 50 percent of a population of animals (LD_{50}) or an effective dose causing a disease symptom in 50 percent of a population of animals (ED_{50}) are useful in comparing the relative virulence of different bacteria.It should be understood that the pathogenic mechanisms of many bacterial diseases are poorly understood, while those of others have been probed at the molecular level.

Pathogenesis

Mechanisms involved in causation of a disease in a host

Bacterial pathogenesis

Pathogenesis of a disease caused by a bacterial pathogen

Molecular pathogenesis

Study of genes involved in expression of virulence factors of a pathogen that determine the course of infection or pathogenesis. For example plasmids pX01 and pX02 of B.anthracis encode, respectively, the anthrax toxin and capsule. Curing the bacteria of pX01 produces an encapsulated, nontoxigenic strain that is nonprotective. Curing of pX02 produces a toxigenic nonencapsulating strain that can be used as a protective vaccine.Both mutants are non-infective.

Host-Mediated Pathogenesis

The pathogenesis of many bacterial infections cannot be separated from the host immune response, for much of the tissue damage is caused by the host response rather than by bacterial factors. Classic examples of host response-mediated pathogenesis are seen in diseases such as Gram-negative bacterial sepsis, tuberculosis, and tuberculoid leprosy. The tissue damage in these infections is caused by toxic factors released from the lymphocytes, macrophages, and polymorphonuclear neutrophils infiltrating the site of infection (Fig. 7-3). Often the host response is so intense that host tissues are destroyed, allowing resistant bacteria to proliferate. In lepromatous leprosy, in contrast, the absence of a cellular response to Mycobacterium leprae allows the bacteria to multiply to such large numbers in the skin that they become tightly packed and replace healthy tissue. The molecular basis for this specific immune anergy is poorly understood.

Bacterial Infectivity

Bacterial infectivity results from a disturbance in the balance between bacterial virulence and host resistance. The "objective" of bacteria is to multiply rather than to cause disease; it is in the best interest of the bacteria not to kill the host.

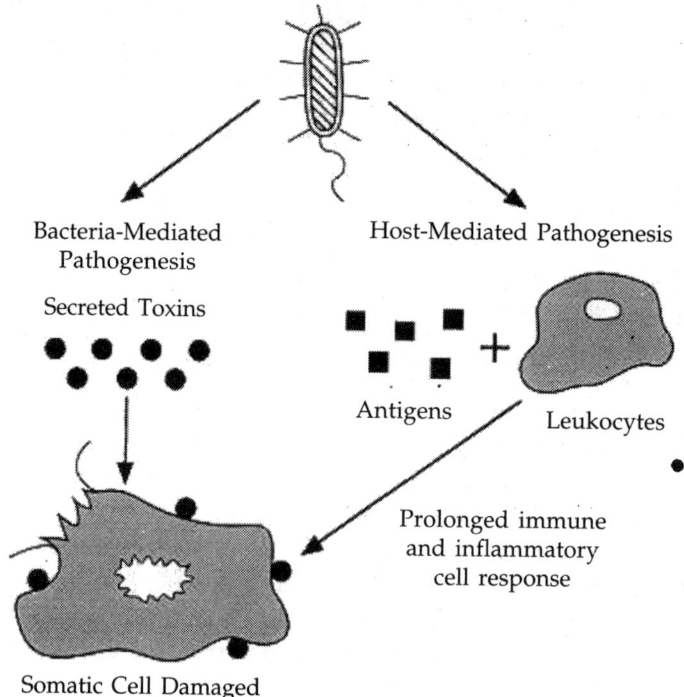

Figure : Generalized mechanisms of bacterial pathogenesis: bacteria-induced toxicity or host-mediated damage.

Terms applicable to describe host-parasite relationships

Commensalism: Literally 'eating at the same table'! This refers to a neutral situation where the host and bacteria live together, but have no effect on each other's life cycle - either positive or negative. Some authors broaden the definition to allow benefit to occur to one group through the association, providing no damage is caused to the other. Overall, this is just about the best way to describe the relationship that humans have with most of the normal bacterial flora of the skin and mucus membranes, including the upper respiratory tract, the lower gastrointestinal tract and the vagina. These bacteria are often described as non-pathogenic or commensal.

Symbiosis: This describes a situation where species live together for their mutual benefit, with each receiving a valuable contribution from the other. There is an element of symbiosis in the relationship between the human host and the gut flora; humans provide the bacteria with a warm, moist, protected environment and, in return, the gut flora uses up all the available nutrients and so makes it difficult for more pathogenic species to become established and initiate infection.

Parasitism: This describes an unequal relationship where one organism clearly benefits from an association to the detriment of another. To some extent this happens in all infections, but the word is often reserved for situations where the invading pathogen has quite clearly hijacked host processes for its own benefit, such as in viral infections.

Saprophytism: This refers to the situation where one organism lives on the dead tissues of another. Fungi often display this ability.

Opportunistic infection: This occurs when the normal human defenses are so weakened that it allows infection to take place by organisms that would not generally be able to cause infection in a healthy human. Examples of these include the many infections that are seen in AIDS patients, including Pneumocystis carinii pneumonia, Toxoplasma gondii brain abscesses and systemic infections with Candida sp. and atypical Mycobacterium sp.

Nosocomial infection: These are infections that are transmitted in hospitals. Some of these may be opportunistic infections mentioned above affecting seriously ill patients, others, for example infections with Methicillin-Resistant Staphylococcus aureus (MRSA), may occur because of the condusive nature of the hospital environment.

As a matter of fact, the relationship between a host and a pathogen is dynamic, since each modifies the activities and function of the other. The outcome of an infection depends on the virulence of the pathogen and the relative degree of resistance or susceptibility of the host, whether acquired or innate.

The underlying mechanisms of bacterial pathogenicity can be attributed to the following properties:

1. *Invasiveness*: It is the mechanism to overcome host defences and the production of extra cellular which facilitate invasion.
2. *Toxigenicity*: The ability to produce toxins; endotoxins and exotoxin, both helping the bacteria to produce various pathological changes in the host leading to the disease. The properties of each have been described in latter chapters in this book.

To produce the disease the pathogen must be able to metabolize or multiply in or upon host tissues i.e., the temperature, gaseous environment and nutrition must be suitable for the growth. Many bacteria can thus colonize over the mucosal surface and cause damage or enter in the host without causing any local damage.

Types of Bacterial Infections

Infection type	Description	Example
Clinical infection	Infection with apparent clinical symptoms	H.S. in cattle
Sub-clinical infection	No detectable clinical symptoms of infection	Sub-clinical mastitis
Latent infection	Carrier state	Carrier of Salmonella
Primary	Clinically apparent	Anthrax
Secondary	Microbial invasion and disease subsequent to Primary infection	H.S. in cattle following F.M.D.
Opportunist	Infection caused by normal flora or transient bacteria when the host is immunocompromised	Candida infection
Mixed	Two pathogens are causing the infection	Foot rot in sheep
Acute	Rapid onset(hours or days) and short duration(days or weeks)	Calf diphtheria
Chronic	Prolonged duration(months or Years)	Mycobacterial infections
Localized	Confined to a local area or to an organ	Keratoconjunctivitis in cattle
Generalized	Disseminated to various body organs	Leptospirosis, H.S.
Ascending	Pathogens ascending in a duct against the secretions or excretions	E.coli urinary tract infection
Endogenous	Pathogen is usually present in the host as a normal flora	Enterotoxaemia in sheep
Exogenous	Pathogen is acquired from the environment	Many; Anthrax as an example

Most endogenous bacterial diseases are opportunistic infections, meaning that the organism must have a special opportunity of weakness or let-down in the host defenses in order to cause infection.

Patterns of Infectious Disease

Infective disease can manifest in many different ways. These depend on the properties of the organsim(s) involved, the patient and the way the two meet.

Three general patterns can be discerned

1. Acute pyogenic infections

- Generally rapid growing organisms
- Interaction with innate immune system and acute inflammation predominate.
- Blood neutrophil count increases
- Where immune damage occurs it is often "post-infective"

Examples

- All *S. aureus* infections except group 4 (toxin mediated) and endocaditis.
- *E. coli* urinary tract infections

2. Chronic (granulomatous)

- Bacterial growth rate often moderate or slow
- Organisms often survive and grow intracellularly
- Immune damage occurs with infection - predominantly cell-mediated

Example: Tuberculosis caused by *Mycobacterium tuberculosis*

- *Streptococcus pneumoniae* infections (Gram positive coccus) - lobar pneumonia and meningitis
- Acute pyogenic with immune damage: *Streptococcus pyogenes* (Gram positive coccus) - acute pharyngitis followed by nephritis or rheumatic fever

1 & 3 often occur together

Stage	Acute pyogenic	Chronic granulomatous
Encounter	Often with symptomatic patient or after trauma.	Often impossible to pin down.
Entry/ Establishment	Obvious if associated with trauma. Adhesins and entry mechanisms well-studied.	Not well understood but uptake into macrophages a common feature.
Spread	Often associated with damage.	Usually imperceptible.
Multiplication	Rapid.	Slow.
Damage	Acute inflammation, toxins.	Cell mediated immunity.
Outcome	Easy to treat with antibiotics.	Difficult

3. Toxin-mediated disease

- Pathology often distant from site of bacterial growth.
- Protective immunity may be mediated by anti-toxin antibodies alone
- Disease may be fully reproduced by administering the toxin alone

Stages of Infection

The time between the exposure to an agent and the first appearance of clinical symptoms is called the incubation period and, although there are no symptoms, the organism may be causing substantial damage during this interval. There may follow a period known as the prodrome, where non-specific signs and symptoms such as headache, fever and lethargy are noted, before the development of a specific symptom complex suggestive of a classical infectious disease such as pneumonia, meningitis or diarrhoea. Once the acute stage has passed, a period of resolution occurs, where the severity of the symptoms gradually decreases, and finally convalescence where the symptoms have largely gone, but the body is still recovering.

The time course and severity of the disease depends upon the balance between the virulence of the infecting agent and the success with which the immune system combats the organism. Some infections may occur which are not sufficiently severe to produce clinical symptoms (asymptomatic or subclinical infections). Clinical infection has a number of outcomes covering the spectrum between death and complete recovery. The term chronic infection is self-explanatory, but carriage is a term that has been used rather loosely. In bacteriology, it is often used to describe the situation where a person continues to harbour a pathogenic organism but suffer no ill-effects themselves, examples being Salmonella typhimurium in the gut and Corynebacterium diphtheriae in the respiratory tract Latency refers to a situation where an agent persists in a dormant, inactive form without causing damage, but which may reactivate to cause problems at a later date; an example is Clostridium perfringens in sheep.

Some of the earliest and most influential work in this area was performed by the German microbiologist, Robert Koch, in the late nineteenth century. In identifying the bacteria responsible for diseases such as anthrax and tuberculosis, he described a number of requirements that must be satisfied before an organism can definitely be regarded as the cause of the disease. These conditions have become known as Koch's postulates and they can be summarised as follows:

1. The organism occurs in every case of the disease and under circumstances which account for the pathological changes and clinical course of the disease.

2. The organism occurs in no other disease as a fortuitous and non-pathogenic finding.
3. After being isolated from the body and grown in pure culture, the organism will repeatedly produce exactly the same clinical disease when inoculated into a new host.

These ideas have formed the foundation for all our ideas about infectious diseases, although it is now becoming increasingly clear that they can no longer be applied in all situations. For example, they do not take account of advances in serological diagnosis nor the recent developments in molecular biology looking at agents that cannot be cultured in the laboratory. They also seem less appropriate when considering infections by commensal organisms in immunosuppressed patients, a group that has become much more important as a result of the advances in modern medical care. Our current medical ethics would prevent many of the human challenge studies that were carried out in the past and for many infections there is no acceptable animal model of infection. However, we should not forget that Koch's postulates have been an extremely valuable tool over the years because they have provided a firm scientific basis to studies of bacterial pathogenesis. This work has revealed a number of steps in the development of infection which are still very relevant to all of today's infections.

In the molecular biological terms the Koch's Postulates could be explained as follows:

1. The phenotype or property under investigation should be associated with pathogenic members of a genus or pathogenic strains of a species.
2. Specific inactivation of the gene(s) associated with the suspected virulence trait should lead to a measurable loss in virulence in a appropriate model system. In-frame deletions or point mutations are best.
3. Complementation of the mutation either on a plasmid or by allelic replacement of the mutated gene should lead to restoration of pathogenicity.

More explicitly these can be further expanded as:

- Identify gene (or gene product) responsible for virulence determinant
- Show gene present in strains of bacteria that cause the disease
- Not present in avirulent strains
- Disrupting the gene reduces virulence

- Introduction of cloned gene into avirulent strain confers virulence.
- The gene is expressed in vivo
- Specific immune response to gene protects.

Contact with the Host

Transmission

Clearly the commensal flora is already in intimate contact with the host, but these organisms are of low pathogenicity and are usually held in check by the immune mechanisms described below. More pathogenic organisms, that are not normal parts of the commensal flora, have developed numerous strategies that allow them to move from a source or reservoir to the susceptible host in a viable state. The spores that are produced by some bacteria and fungi, and bacteria such as Mycobacterium tuberculosis, are very resistant to the effect of drying in the environment. Gram positive organisms such as Staphylococcus aureus seem to be very well adapted to surviving on skin surfaces such as the hands and this is a very important route of transmission within hospitals. Gram negative organisms can be adept at surviving in fluids; contaminated water supplies are usually responsible for infection with Vibrio cholerae whilst major outbreaks of infection have occurred in hospitals due to contamination of fluids used in medicine by bacteria such as Klebsiella. Other bacteria, such as Salmonella and Shigella, thrive under conditions of poor hygiene and are transmitted by faecal-oral spread, whilst more fragile organisms, such as Neisseria gonorrhoeae, may require the most intimate contact of all.

Protection of External Surfaces

The skin normally represents an impenetrable barrier to micro-organisms and mucosal surfaces, such as those of the respiratory tract and the gut, are protected by a number of factors including the secretion of mucus, powerful proteolytic enzymes, antibodies (particularly IgA) and the high turnover of surface cells.

Injections, vascular lines, accidental trauma, surgery and conditions such as eczema, all breakdown the integrity of the skin and increase the chance of infection. Increased risks of infections are also seen when the mucosal defences are disturbed: this includes alterations in mucus distribution in long term smokers; production of specific IgA proteases by bacteria such as Haemophilus influenzae, Neisseria meningitidis and Streptococcus pneumoniae; and the loss of mucosal endothelial integrity as a side effect of modern cytotoxic therapy.

Adherence

Many of the body surfaces are washed by fluids, including mucus in the upper respiratory tract and the gut, peristalsis of gut contents throughout the bowel and the movement of urine in the urinary tract. If a bacterium is to multiply and cause infection it must have some way of fixing its position and becoming established.

This adherence is produced by bacterial adhesins or ligands that bind specifically to host molecules known as receptors. These adhesins can be proteins found on the bacterial cell wall / membrane or they can be collected together on structures that project from the cell surface, for example fimbriae and pili, which seem to be expressly aimed at increasing the chance of adherence. A huge number of bacterial adhesins and their associated host cell receptors have been described, but one of the most well-studied concerns the ability of certain strains of Escherichia coli to cause urinary tract infection. Studies of E. coli isolates have shown that only a relatively small number of types are found in urinary tract infections, although there are many more types to be found nearby colonising the human gut. The reason seems to be that strains that express the type 1 pilus can attach to the Tamm-Horsfall protein in the mucus of the lower urinary tract and this prevents them being flushed away by the flow of urine; if they do manage to ascend the urethra into the bladder, strains of E. coli that do not express this pilus cannot adhere and are immediately washed out. However, when the isolates from upper urinary tract infections are examined, a different pattern is seen. It appears that these E. coli strains that have swam up against the flow of urine in the ureters may change their cell surface such that they now express P pili that allows them to attach to the P blood group antigen that is found on the cells in the renal pelvis.

The adhesins of *E. coli* are their common pili or fimbriae. A single strain of *E. coli* is known to be able to express several distinct types of fimbriae encoded by distinct regions of the chromosome or plasmids. This genetic diversity permits an organism to adapt to its changing environment and exploit new opportunities presented by different host surfaces. Many of the adhesive fimbriae of *E. coli* have probably evolved from fimbrial ancestors resembling Type-I and Type IV fimbriae.

Type-I fimbriae enable *E. coli* to bind to D-mannose residues on eucaryotic cell surfaces. Type-I fimbriae are said to be "mannose-sensitive" since exogenous mannose blocks binding to receptors on red blood cells. Although the primary 17kDa fimbrial subunit is the major protein component of Type-1 fimbriae, the mannose-binding site is not located here, but resides in a minor protein (28-31kDa) located at the tips or inserted along the length of the fimbriae. By genetically varying the minor "tip protein" adhesin, the organisms can gain ability to adhere to different receptors. For example, tip proteins on pyelonephritis-associated (pap) pili recognize a galactose-galactose disaccharide, while tip proteins on S-fimbriae recognize sialic acid.

Pseudomonas, Vibrio and *Neisseria* possess Type IV pili that contain protein subunit with a methylated amino acid, often phenylalanine, at or near its amino terminus. These "N-methylphenylalanine pili" have been established as virulence determinants in pathogenesis of *Pseudomonas aeruginosa* lung infection in cystic fibrosis patients. These type of fimbriae occur in *Neisseria gonorrhoeae* and their receptor is thought to be an oligosaccharide. Type IV pili are the tcp (toxin coregulated pili) fimbriae used in attachment of Vibrio cholerae to the gastrointestinal epithelium.

Table : Examples of specific attachments of bacteria to host cell or tissue surfaces

Bacterium	Adhesin	Receptor	Attachment site	Disease
Streptococcus pyogenes	Protein F	Amino terminus of fibronectin	Pharyngeal epithelium	Sore throat
Streptococcus equi	M protein		Pharyngeal attachment	Strangles in horses
Staphylococcus aureus	Cell-bound protein	Amino terminus of fibronectin	Mucosal epithelium	Various
Enterotoxigenic E. coli	Type-I fimbriae	Species-specific carbohydrate(s)	Intestinal epithelium	Diarrhea
Uropathogenic *E. coli*	Type I fimbriae	Complex carbohydrate	Urethral epithelium	Urethritis
Uropathogenic *E. coli*	P-pili (pap)	Globobiose linked to ceramide lipid	Upper urinary tract	Pyelonephritis
Mycoplasma	Membrane protein	Sialic acid	Respiratory epithelium	Pneumonia
Chlamydia	Unknown	Sialic acid	Conjunctival or urethral epithelium	Conjunctivitis or abortions

The adhesins of *Streptococcus pyogenes* are M protein and teichoic acids. It has been suggested that LTA loosely tethers streptococci to epithelial cells, and then M protein secures a firmer, irreversible association. Later protein F was discovered and found to be a fibronectin binding protein. More recently M proteins M1 and M3 have been found to bind to Fibronectin thus promoting association between host epithelium and bacterium.

Bacteria may also secrete viscous substances onto their surface which increase adherence in a non-specific fashion. This would include alginate capsule production by Pseudomonas aeruginosa in the lungs of cystic fibrosis patients and the production of polysaccharide slime by Staphylococcus epidermidis when it colonises intravenous lines.

The Ability to Compete for Iron and other Nutrients

Often the ability to be pathogenic is directly related to the bacterial ability to compete successfully with host tissue and normal flora for limited nutrients. One reason the generation time of bacteria growing in the body is substantially slower than in lab culture is because essential nutrients are limited. In fact this is a major reason why the overwhelming majority of bacteria found in nature are not harmful to humans.

To be pathogenic, a bacterium must be able to multiply in host tissue.The more rapid the rate of replication, the more likely an infection may be established. Pathogens, therefore, are able to compete successfully for limited nutrients in the body. Generally bacteria compete for nutrients by synthesizing specific transport systems or cell wall components capable of binding limiting substrates and transporting them into the cell. A good example of this is the ability of bacteria to compete for iron.

The body makes considerable metabolic adjustment during infection to deprive microorganisms of iron. Iron is essential for both bacterial growth and human cell growth. Animals have evolved mechanisms of "withholding" iron from tissue fluids in an attempt to limit the growth of invading bacteria. Most of the iron in blood is bound either to hemoglobin in erythrocytes or to transferrin in plasma. Similarly, the iron in milk and other secretions (e.g., tears, saliva, bronchial mucus, bile, and gastrointestinal fluid) is bound to lactoferrin. Bacteria on the other hand, synthesize iron chelators (compounds capable of binding iron) called siderophores. Many siderophores are excreted by the bacterium into the environment, bind iron, and then re-enter the cell. Others are found on the cell wall where they bind iron and transport it into the bacterium. The ability of bacterial iron chelators to compete successfully with the body's iron chelators as well as those of normal flora may be essential to pathogenic bacteria.

Some bacteria produce in addition to their own siderophore, receptors for siderophores of other bacteria in this way take iron from other bacteria. Furthermore, a number of pathogenic bacteria are able to bind human transferrin, lactoferrin, ferritin, and hemin and use that as their iron source. For example, Pasteurella multocida serotypes are able to produce transferrin binding siderophores and enhance their virulence for birds and animals.while pathogenic *Yersinia* species are able to use transferrin and hemin as iron sources. *Borrelia burgdorferi* doesn't even use iron as a cofactor, but instead uses manganese. The absence of iron triggers transcription of the genes coding for the enzymes that synthesize siderophores, as well as for a set of surface protein receptors that recognize siderophores carrying bound iron. The binding constants of the siderophores for iron are so high that even iron bound to transferrin and lactoferrin is confiscated and taken up by the bacterial cells. An example of a bacterial siderophores is enterochelin, which is produced by *Escherichia* and *Salmonella* species. Classic experiments have demonstrated that Salmonella mutants that have lost the capacity to synthesize enterochelin lose virulence in an assay of lethality in mice. Injection of purified enterochelin along with the Salmonella mutants restores virulence to the bacteria. Therefore, siderophores production by many pathogenic bacteria is considered an important virulence mechanism.

Entry into Cells and Tissues

Certain agents take the attachment process a stage further by using adhesins as the first step towards promoting their uptake into the host cell. The entry of Listeria monocytogenes into phagocytic cells following its attachment to the complement receptor CR3 is one example of this amongst bacteria, but all viruses need to use this mechanism to produce infection. Human immunodeficiency virus (HIV) uses a protein on its surface called gp120 to target CD4-bearing T lymphocytes and initiate uptake, whilst influenza virus attaches and enters cells using a protein called haemagglutinin as the adhesin and neuraminic acid on the surface of respiratory epithelium as the receptor.

Entry into cells may lead to an infection that is limited to that cell type, or it may be a first step towards wider dissemination of the infecting agent throughout the body. As an alternative to bypassing the epithelium through intracellular invasion, some bacteria penetrate this barrier by squeezing through the junctions between adjacent epithelial cells and so reach deeper tissues.

Production of Disease

Once a bacterium has entered the body, there are a number of ways in which it can cause disease. It may produce damage to local tissues as well as damage to distant tissues through the action of bacterial toxins, although this distinction may not be clear cut as there is nothing to stop toxins from acting locally too. Bacteria must continue to evade the responses of the immune system and, although it will not be discussed here, it is important to remember that an excessive immune response may itself produce a great deal of damage and be responsible for many of the symptoms of disease.

Local Effects

Certain bacteria cause diffuse infections by producing enzymes that enable them to breakdown the cells and intracellular matrices of host tissues. Streptococcus produce the enzyme hyaluronidase which hydrolyses hyaluronic acid, a polysaccharide component responsible for binding cells together. Clostridium produce a similar enzyme called collagenase and many bacteria produce different kinases, lecithinases and proteases with varying effects upon host tissues. On the other hand, some bacteria produce more localised infections with the production of pus in the affected tissues; bacteria that do this are described as pyogenic. Staphylococcus aureus produces an enzyme coagulase which coagulates fribrinogen and abscesses are particularly likely to develop where infections involving Bacteroides fragilis take place.

Distant Effects

There are over 220 known bacterial toxins and they can be divided up into two groups. Endotoxin is a component of the cell wall of all gram negative bacteria whilst the exotoxins include a huge number of proteins that are secreted from the bacterial cell and which are mostly, but not exclusively, produced by gram positive bacteria.

Endotoxin is the lipid portion of lipopolysaccharide, lipid A, and is a potent inducer of interleukin-1 (IL-1) from macrophages, which resets the hypothalamus to produce fever, and tumour necrosis factor (TNF) from phagocytes, which induces severe shock. The toxin is effective when it is present within the cell walls of living bacteria, but its greatest effect is usually seen when bacteria are killed, lysed and their products released into the systemic circulation.

The biologic effects of endotoxin have been extensively studied. Purified lipid A (conjugated to bovine serum albumin) and endotoxin elicit the same biologic responses. The more pertinent toxic effects include pyrogenicity, leukopenia followed by leukocytosis, complement activation, depression in blood pressure, mitogenicity, induction of prostaglandin synthesis, and hypothermia. These events can culminate in sepsis and lethal shock. However, not all effects of endotoxin are necessarily detrimental; several induce responses potentially beneficial to the host, assuming the stimulation is not excessive. These include:

1. Mitogenic effects on B lymphocytes that increase resistance to viral and bacterial infections
2. Induction of gamma interferon production by T lymphocytes, which may enhance the antiviral state, promote rejection of tumor cells, and activate macrophages and natural killer cells
3. Activation of the complement cascade with the formation of C3a and C5a
4. Induction of the formation of interleukin-1 by macrophages and interleukin-2 and other mediators by T lymphocytes.

Current research focuses on exploiting some of the potential beneficial effects of "nontoxic" endotoxin derivatives and holds promise for development of future treatment regimens for stimulating the immune response. For example, the toxicity of endotoxin is largely attributed to lipid A, attached to a polysaccharide carrier. The toxicity of lipid A is markedly reduced after hydrolysis of a phosphate group or deacylation of one or more fatty acids from the lipid A molecule. Clinical trials are in progress to test a monophosphoryl lipid A for its potential of inducing low dose tolerance to endotoxin. Tolerance to endotoxin can be achieved by pretreatment of an animal with low doses of endotoxin or a detoxified lipid A derivative before challenge with high doses of endotoxin. Experimental studies have demonstrated that induction of tolerance to endotoxin reduces the dangerous effects of endotoxin. It is hoped that these relatively nontoxic lipid A derivatives may be useful in reducing the severity of bacterial sepsis in which bacterial endotoxin produces a life-threatening clinical course.

Endotoxin, which largely accumulates in the liver following injection of a sublethal dose by the intravenous route, can be devastating because of its ability to affect a variety of cell and host proteins. Kupffer cells, granulocytes, macrophages, platelets, and lymphocytes all have a cell receptor on their surface called CD14, which binds endotoxin. Endotoxin binding to the CD14 receptor on macrophages is enhanced by interaction with a host protein made in the liver (i.e., LPS-binding protein). The extent of involvement of each cell type probably depends on the level of endotoxin exposure. The effects of endotoxin on such a wide variety of host cells result in a complex array of host responses that can culminate in the serious condition gram-negative sepsis, which often leads to shock and death. The effects of endotoxin on host cells are known to stimulate prostaglandin synthesis and to activate the kallikrein system, the kinin system, the complement cascade via the alternative pathway, the clotting system, and the fibrinolytic pathways. When these normal host systems are activated and operate out of control, it is not surprising that endotoxin can be lethal. Although it is difficult to comprehend the mechanisms of all the cell responses and the myriad sequelae of the cell mediators released rather indiscriminately in the host following exposure to endotoxin, it does seem clear that the host cellular response to endotoxin, rather than a direct toxic effect of endotoxin, plays the major role in causing tissue damage .

Endotoxin is omnipresent in the environment. It is found in most deionized-water lines in hospitals and laboratories, for example, and affects virtually every biologic assay system ever examined. It tends to be a scapegoat for all biologic problems encountered in the laboratory, and, many times, this reputation is deserved. Because of its pyrogenic and destructive properties, extreme care must be taken to avoid exposing patients to medical solutions containing endotoxin. Even though all supplies should be sterile, solutions for intravenous administration can become contaminated with endotoxin-containing bacteria after sterilization as a result of improper handling. Furthermore, water used in the preparation of such solutions must be filtered through ion exchange resins to remove endotoxin, because it is not removed by either autoclave sterilization or filtration through bacterial membrane filters. If endotoxin-containing solutions were used in such medical procedures as renal dialysis, heart bypass machines, blood transfusions, or surgical lavage, the patient would suffer immediate fever accompanied by a rapid and possibly lethal alterations in blood pressure.

Solutions for human or veterinary use are prepared under carefully controlled conditions to ensure sterility and to remove endotoxin. Representative samples of every manufacturing batch are checked for endotoxin by one of two procedures: the Limulus lysate test or the rabbit pyrogenicity test. The rabbit pyrogenicity test is based on the exquisite sensitivity of rabbits to the pyrogenic effects of endotoxin. A sample of the solution to be tested usually is injected intravenously into the ear veins of adult rabbits while the rectal temperature of the animal is monitored. Careful monitoring of the temperature responses provides a sensitive and reliable indicator of the presence of endotoxin and, importantly, one measure of the safety of the solution for use in patients.

The Limulus lysate test is more common and less expensive. This test, which is based on the ability of endotoxin to induce gelation of lysates of amebocyte cells from the horseshoe crab Limulus polyphemus, is simple, fast, and sensitive (about 1 ng/ml). It is so sensitive, however, that trace quantities of endotoxin in regular deionized water often obscure the results. It can be used for rapid detection of certain Gram-negative infections (e.g., of cerebrospinal fluid); however, blood contains inhibitors that prevent gelation. Test kits are commercially available. The amebocyte is the sole phagocytic immune cell of the horseshoe crab, and the gelation reaction is believed to be involved in sequestering invading Gram-negative bacteria.

Exotoxins

Exotoxins, unlike the lipopolysaccharide endotoxin, are protein toxins released from viable bacteria. They form a class of poisons that is among the most potent, per unit weight, of all toxic substances. Most of the higher molecular-sized exotoxin proteins are heat labile; however, numerous low molecular-sized exotoxins are heat-stable peptides. Unlike endotoxin, which is a structural component of all Gram-negative cells, exotoxins are produced by some members of both Gram-positive and Gram-negative genera. The functions of these exotoxins for the bacteria are usually unknown, and the genes for most can be deleted with no noticeable effect on bacterial growth. In contrast to the extensive systemic and immune-system effects of endotoxin on the host, the site of action of most exotoxins is more localized and is confined to particular cell types or cell receptors. Tetanus toxin, for example, affects only internuncial neurons. In general, exotoxins are excellent antigens that elicit specific antibodies called antitoxins. Not all antibodies to exotoxins are protective, but some react with important binding sites or enzymatic sites on the exotoxin, resulting in complete inhibition of the toxic activity (i.e., neutralization).

Exotoxins can be grouped into several categories (e.g., neurotoxins, cytotoxins, and enterotoxins) based on their biologic effect on host cells. Neurotoxins are best exemplified by the toxins produced by *Clostridium* spp, for example, the botulinum toxin formed by *C botulinum*. This potent neurotoxin acts on motor neurons by preventing the release of acetylcholine at the myoneural junctions, thereby preventing muscle excitation and producing flaccid paralysis. The cytotoxins constitute a larger, more heterogeneous grouping with a wide array of host cell specificities and toxic manifestations. One cytotoxin is diphtheria toxin, which is produced by *Corynebacterium diphtheriae*. This cytotoxin inhibits protein synthesis in many cell types by catalyzing the ADP-ribosylation of elongation factor II, which blocks elongation of the growing peptide chain.

Enterotoxins stimulate hypersecretion of water and electrolytes from the intestinal epithelium and thus produce watery diarrhea. Some enterotoxins are cytotoxic (e.g., shiga-like enterotoxin from *E coli*), while others perturb eukaryotic cell functions and are cytotonic (e.g., cholera toxin). Enterotoxins also can disturb normal smooth muscle contraction, causing abdominal cramping and decrease transit time for water absorption in the intestine.

Enterotoxigenic *E coli* and *V cholerae* produce diarrhea after attaching to the intestinal mucosa, where they elaborate enterotoxins. Neither pathogen invades the body in substantial numbers, except in the case of *E coli* species that have acquired an invasion plasmid. Importantly, cholera toxin and *E coli* heat-labile enterotoxins I and II cause ADP-ribosylation of cell proteins in a manner similar to diphtheria toxin, except that the primary target is the regulatory protein (G_{s}_) of adenylate cyclase, resulting in increased levels of cyclic 3',5'-adenosine monophosphate (cAMP) (see Ch. 25). In contrast, the organisms responsible for shigellosis (*Shigella dysenteriae, S boydii, S flexneri,* and *S sonnei*) penetrate the mucosal surface of the colon and terminal ileum to proliferate and cause ulcerations that bleed into the intestinal lumen. Despite causing extensive ulceration of the mucosa, the pathogens rarely enter the bloodstream. The Shiga enterotoxin produced by *Shigella* species and the Shiga-like enterotoxin elaborated by many isolates of *E coli* inhibit protein synthesis in eukaryotic cells. It is not clear how this cytotoxic enterotoxin causes hypersecretion of water and electrolytes from the intestinal epithelium. These enterotoxins differ from those secreted by *V cholerae* and *E coli* in that the Shiga toxins are cytotoxic and lethal, whereas the cholera toxin-like enterotoxins are not. The latter enterotoxins cause no structural damage to cells, and are described as cytotonic. The ensuing inflammatory response to the invading bacteria and/or their toxins appears to activate neurologic control mechanisms (e.g., prostaglandins, serotonin) that normally regulate water and electrolyte transport.

Evasion of Host Defences

The host tissue is a hostile environment for bacteria and they need to develop strategies for maintaining their nutrition. The acquisition of iron is particularly important, as its availability is tightly controlled by the host. Most pathogenic organisms have developed a number of secretory proteins, called siderophores, which can steal iron from host carrier-proteins and so make it available to bacteria.

Some bacteria, such as Streptococcus pneumoniae, Haemophilus influenzae and Klebsiella pneumoniae, and the fungus Cryptococcus neoformans produce a glycocalyx capsule that inhibits phagocytosis. Mycobacterium tuberculosis accomplishes this by the insertion of waxes into its cell wall and Streptococcus pyogenes has the M protein in its cell wall to decrease phagocytosis. Staphylococcus and Streptococcus use leukocidins to destroy leukocytes and macrophages and haemolysins to disrupt erythrocytes. The parasite Trypanosoma undergoes rapid antigenic variation to evade the host's immune response and some viruses, such as human immunodeficiency virus, actually infect the cells of the immune system themselves.

Several bacterial diseases are affecting animals which are of economic importance. Some of these are categorized as acute infections whereas some are listed as chronic. The capacity of a bacterium to cause disease reflects its relative pathogenicity. This is attributed to the presence of virulence factors which a bacterium possesses.

Bacteria lacking these virulence factors are non-pathogenic.Different strains of a bacterial species may differ in their pathogenicity depending on the expression of the virulence factors based on its molecular behavior. There may occur a variant completely lacking virulence owing to the deletion of the virulence genes as a result of environmental or host related stress. Some other factors responsible for the virulence of bacteria are route of entry of the pathogen into the body and specific and non-specific host defense mechanisms. Pathogenesis of the disease is the net outcome of these intricate mechanisms of pathogenicity involving host and pathogen. It should be understood that in spite of all the advances, the pathogenic mechanisms of many bacterial diseases are poorly understood, while those of others have been proved at the molecular level. The relative importance of an infections disease to the health of animals does not always coincide with the depth of our understanding of its pathogenesis. In such instances more information is required to fully understand the mechanism of pathogenesis.

❑❑❑

Chapter 1

Staphylococcal Infections

Dr. S.K. SRIVASTAVA
Former, Division of Bacteriology & Mycology
Indian Veterinary Research Institute, Izatnagar-243122
Bareilly (U.P.)

Staphylococci are gram positive cocci occurring in short chains, pairs and mostly clusters. In 1884, Rosenbach described the two pigmented colony types of staphylococci and proposed the appropriate nomenclature: *Staphylococcus aureus* (yellow) and *Staphylococcus albus* (white). The latter species is now named *Staphylococcus epidermidis.*They are facultatively anaerobic, non-motile, catalase positive, oxidase negative and fermentative in breakdown of sugars. Although there occur more than 47 species of *Staphylococcus*, the species of greatest veterinary importances are *Staphylococcus aureus, Staphylococcus intermedius, Staphlococcus chromogenes Staphylococcus hyicus* and *Staphylococcus schleiferi* subsp. *Coagulans.* The major domestic animal species, including pets and livestock, may become contaminated, colonized, or infected with methicillin-resistant staphylococci, including MRSA. Dogs and cats are more likely to be colonized/infected with *Staphylococcus pseudintermedius* than *S. aureus*, but this pathogen can acquire genes encoding methicillin resistance (i.e., MRSP). Significant epidemiological, clinical and genetic differences exist between MRSA in humans and the majority of MRSA infections in the different animal species. Staphylococcus aureus has re-emerged as an important human pathogen in recent decades

The ability to produce the enzyme coagalase divides staphylococci into two main groups. Coagulase positive Staphylococci and Coagulase negative Staphylococci. *S. aureus, S. intermedius, S. schleiferi* subsp. *Coagulaus* and another species *S. delphini* arc coagulase positive, whereas other species are coagulase negative. The species *S. hyicus* is variably coagulase positive and has been included in the group coagulase negative Staphylococci. They are present on epithelial surfaces of all warm blooded animals. Staphylococci are associated with a variety of pyogenic infection in animals. Coaglase negative staphylococci are major cause of mastitis in cattle.

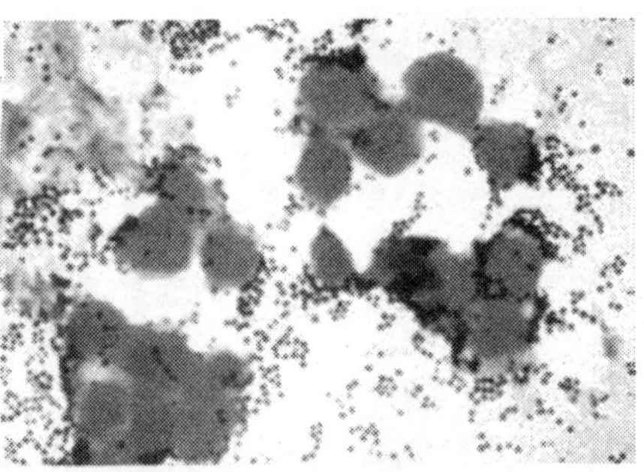
Gram stain of *Staphylococcus aureus* in pustular exudate

S. aureus has five biotypes (Devriese and Oeding 1976). Biotype A strains have been frequently isolated from human beings; biotype B strains from pigs and poultry; biotypes C from cattle and sheep; biotype D strains from horses and biotype E strains from dogs & horses (Hajek 1976). *S. aureus* and *S. intermedius* are phenotypically very similar. *S. epidermidis* is universally present on skin and some mucous membranes but it is rarely pathogenic. The Gram-positive bacteria *Staphylococcus epidermidis* and *Staphylococcus aureus* are the most common pathogens in hospital-acquired infections. The costs related to infections caused by these strains in the hospital setting are enormous and represent a major health care burden. Furthermore, the more recent combination of extraordinary virulence and multiple antibiotic resistance in community-acquired methicillin-resistant strains of *S. aureus* (CA-MRSA) poses an additional severe threat to public health. *S. aureus* may cause a multitude of serious infections, including toxic shock and scalded skin syndromes, endocarditis, and pneumonia, to name a few. In contrast, infections with *S. epidermidis* are usually chronic and less severe. The most important type of disease caused by *S. epidermidis* is the colonization and infection of indwelling medical devices.

Association of coagulase positive Staphylococcus with animal diseases

Coagulase positive species	Host	Major diseases
S. aureus	Bovine	Mastitis, suppurative lesions
	Ovine	Mastitis, tick pyemia
	Porcine	Suppurative lesions, exudation epidermitis
	Equine	Botryomycosis, arthiritis, mastitis
	Canine	Pyoderma, Urinary tract infectious
S. intermedius	Canine	Pyoderma, suppurative lesions, otitis externa
	Equine	Suppurative lesions
S. schleiferi subsp. *coagulans*	Canine	Otitis externa
S. delphini	Dolphin	Suppurative skin lesions

[Source: Jonsson and Wadstrom 1993]

Coagulase negative Staphylococci are sometimes involved in causing arthritis and osteomyelitis in pigs, cattle and poultry.

Virulence factors

Toxins

Various cytolytic toxins and enzymes such as proteases, lipase, hyaluronate lyase and hyaluronidase act together to cause tissue degradation as a source of low-molecuar weight nutrient for bacterial growth. Disease is caused as a result of action of various surface proteins including toxins.

Alpha-toxin (alpha-hemolysin) a 34kDa protein is produced by most of the strains of *S.aureus* and cause lysis of red blood cells (RBC) of most of the animals species. It induces pore formation in the membrane of cells which leads to lysis. This results in release of prostaglandins and other mediators of inflammation. It is dermanecrotic and causes powerful smooth muscle contraction. Beta toxin of *S.aureus* is sphingomyelinase and induces classical hot-cold haemolysis of sheep RBCs. Hot-cold lysis is characterized by partial lysis at 37°C which goes to completion on further incubation at lower temperature. Most *S. aureus* isolate of bovine origin produce beta toxin and may be significant from mastitis point of view. The toxin enhances bacterial growth in the mammary gland (Foster 1992). alpha toxin (alpha-hemolysin) is the best characterized and most potent membrane-damaging toxin of *S. aureus*. It is expressed as a monomer that binds to the membrane of susceptible cells. Subunits then oligomerize to form heptameric rings with a central pore through which cellular contents leak.

In humans, platelets and monocytes are particularly sensitive to alpha toxin. Susceptible cells have a specific receptor for alpha toxin which allows the toxin to bind causing small pores through which monovalent cations can pass. The mode of action of alpha hemolysin is likely by osmotic lysis.

β-toxin is a sphingomyelinase which damages membranes rich in this lipid. The classical test for β-toxin is lysis of sheep erythrocytes. The majority of human isolates of *S. aureus* do not express β-toxin. A lysogenic bacteriophage is known to encode the toxin.

The role of gamma toxin is not known. Its activity is suppressed in agar. Delta toxin behaves like a detergent and damages all types of cells in all host species. It posses the property to bind skin lipids in mice and rabbits and subsequently get neutralized. Its role in pathogenesis is not well understood. The activity of delta toxin is inhibited by serum. All toxins are antigenically distinct RBCs from different species differ in their susceptibility. Delta toxin is a very small peptide toxin produced by most strains of *S. aureus*. It is also produced by *S. epidermidis*.

Leukocidin is produced by some strains of *S. aureus*. It binds to human polymorphonuclear cells (PMN) and cause rapid degranulation. Bovine strains produce a leukocidin which bind the bovine PMN leucocytes. Leukocidin is a multicomponent protein toxin produced as separate components which act together to damage membranes. Leukocidin forms a hetero-oligomeric transmembrane pore composed of four LukF and four LukS subunits, thereby forming an octameric pore in the affected membrane. Leukocidin is hemolytic, but less so than alpha hemolysin.

Only 2% of all of *S. aureus* isolates express leukocidin, but nearly 90% of the strains isolated from severe dermonecrotic lesions express this toxin, which suggests that it is an important factor in necrotizing skin infections.

S. aureus strains also produce 2 types of exfoliative toxins (ETA and ETB) causing blister formation in the skin of infants and adults with under lying immunologic disorders. The exfoliative toxin (ET) is a major virulence factor of Staphylococcus aureus that causes bullous impetigo and its disseminated form, staphylococcal scalded skin syndrome (SSSS). ET selectively digests one of the intracellular adhesion molecules, desmoglein 1, of epidermal keratinocytes; and causes blisters due to intra-epidermal cell-cell dissociation. Most *S. aureus* caused blistering disease produce either ETA or ETB. They are serologically distinct molecules where ETA is encoded on a phage genome; and ETB is on a large plasmid. ETA-producing S. aureus is frequently isolated from impetigo patients and ETB-producing S. aureus is isolated from SSSS. ET-induced blister formation can be reproduced using the neonatal mouse(Kato *et al.*, 2011). In mice, blistering is caused similar to pemphigus or impetigo in humans. They cause cleavage of desmosomes in the stratum granulosum of the epidermis. Both the exfoliatins are approximately 30 kDa but differ antigenically and in their composition. Its significance in animal disease has not been studied.

A 22kDa protein toxin called Toxic Shock Syndrome Toxin (TSST-1) is produced by some strains of *S.aureus* and is responsible for causing a toxin mediated disease. It is similar to enterotoxin F and pyrogenic exotoxin C. It functions as immunomodulator or superantigen. It induces excessive lymphokine production resulting in tissue damage. As the name implies, it can cause fever and toxic shock syndrome in the host. Bovine strains of *S. aureus* produce TSST-1 that is similar in activity to TSST of human strains. A variant is produced by sheep and goat strains. Subinhibitory concentrations of nafcillin induced and prolonged mRNA for Panton-Valentine leukocidin, α-toxin, and toxic-shock syndrome toxin 1 and increased toxin production. In contrast, clindamycin and linezolid markedly suppressed translation, but not transcription, of toxin genes (Stevens *et al.*, 2007).

The staphylococcal enterotoxins (SE) are known as the pyrogenic toxins and this group contains also other staphylococcal toxins (staphylococcal toxic-shock syndrome toxin—TSST-1, A and B exfoliative toxins and streptococcal scarlet fever toxin). Twenty one serological types of staphylococcal enterotoxins are distinguished. All of them are structurally and functionally similar to the toxic shock syndrome toxin (TSST-1). SEs are thermo-stabile proteins, resistant to many proteolytic enzymes (pepsin, trypsine, chymotrypsine, renine and papain), but this resistance depends on the temperature and pH. Staphylococcal enterotoxin-encoding genes are located as well in the chromosomal DNA, as on the pathogenicity island, in phages, transposones and plasmids. Enterotoxins are staphylococcal virulence factors responsible for food poisonings in humans. These proteins are also isolated from cows with mastitis. In various countries, the percentage of enterotoxin-producing S. aureus strains ranges from 5 to 60%, depending on the enterotoxin type. The variability and prevalence of enterotoxins produced by staphylococci isolated from mastitic cows is very important clinical and epidemiological problem (Nawrotek *et al.*, 2005). At least 6 enterotoxins have been identified (A, B, C, C2, D & E). These are heat resistant as boiling for 30 minutes has no effect on their activity. They are composed of a single polypeptide chain of about 30kDa. Clinical signs of human food poisoning caused by enterotoxins are nausea, vomiting and diarrhea with in 1-6 hours of exposure. Vomiting is due to the effect of the toxin on nerve centre in the stomach and intestine, that send a message to the vomiting center in the brain. Enterotoxins are also potent mitogens that induce release of immunomediator such as Interleukin-1 from lymphocytes. They also behave like superantigens. Superantigens stimulate T cells non-specifically without normal antigenic recognition. Up to one in five T cells may be activated, whereas only 1 in 10,000 are stimulated during a usual antigen presentation. Cytokines are released in large amounts, causing the symptoms of enterotoxins. Superantigens bind directly to class II major histocompatibility complexes of antigen-presenting cells outside the conventional antigen-binding grove. This complex recognizes only the Vb element of the T cell receptor. Thus any T cell with the appropriate Vb element can be stimulated, whereas normally, antigen specificity is also required in binding.

Many strains from human and animal infectious produce a membrane damaging polypeptide with amphiphilic properties. It has not been studied for their activity.

Exoenzymes

Out of several extracellular products, coagulase has been studied most. It occurs as a clumping factor (cell bound) or extracellular or free coagulase.

Only the free coagulase is tested in the coagulase test invitro. The latter is responsible for activation of prothrombin to plasma thrombin leading to formation of fibrin from fibrinogen. The fibrin is thus deposited on cell surface and interferes in the phagocytosis being a self molecule. Strains of *S.aureus, S. intermedius, S. sehleiferi* subsp. *Coagulans* and some *S. hyicus* strains produce coagulase. Most strains are positive in test tube method than plate method. However, there is no overwhelming evidence that it is a virulence factor, although it is reasonable to speculate that the bacteria could protect themselves from phagocytic and immune defenses by causing localized clotting.

Virulence determinants of *Staphylococcus aureus*

S.No.	Virulence Determinant	Activity on Host Tissues
1	Capsular polysaccharide	Antiphagocytic
2	Peptidoglycan	Pyrogenic, chemoattractant
3	Teichoic Acid	Released teichoic acid protect against complement
4	Cell surface proteins	
(i)	Protein A	Interacts with Fc region of IgG
(ii)	Fibrinogen blinding protein	Binds fibrinogen
(iii)	Fibronectin binding protein	Binds fibronectin
(iv)	Lamilin, collagen and Vitronectin binding protein	Binds lamilin, collagen and vitronectin respectively
5	Extracellular toxins and Enzymes	
(i)	α–toxin, β-toxin Delta toxin, Gamma toxin	Cytotoxic for tissue cells and leukocytes
(ii)	Toxic shock syndrome toxin	Binds major histocompatibility (Class II) molecule, induces synthesis of cytokines, causes multiple organ dysfunction, diarrheagenic
(iii)	Enterotoxins	Emetic, diarrheagenic
(iv)	Coagulase	Catalyzes conversion of fibrinogen to fibrin
(v)	Lipase	Breakdown lipids
(vi)	Proteases	Degrade a variety of proteins
(vii)	Phospholipases	Degrade phospholipids
(viii)	Staphylokinase	Converts plasminogen to fibrinolytic plasmid
(ix)	Hyaluronidase	Degrades hyaluronic Acid
(x)	Nuclease	Cleaves DNA and RNA

[Source: Jonsson and Wadstrom 1993]

Catalase is another enzyme which is produced by all staphyloccal strains. This enzyme catalyzes the conversion of hydrogen peroxide to water and oxygen. It protects the pathogen from the toxic hydrogen peroxide. It is not produced by streptococci so the catalase test is employed to differentiate Staphylococci from streptococci.

Certain strains of *S.aureus* produce lipases and esterases which degrade lipid present in the skin and causes skin infections. Besides, fatty acids modifying enzymes are also produced by *S.aureus* strains. These fatty acids are antibacterial and their degradation leads to survival of staphylococci and cause abscess efficiently. Coagulase negative staphylococci do not produce these fatty acid modifying enzymes.

Besides, *S. aureus* produces at least four proteases and a specific lesion degrading enzyme (Jonsson and Wadstrom 1993). This enzyme is important in tissue degradation in early infection as well as in degradation of pus in an abscess to release nutrients for utilization by the young cells.

Hyaluronidase, generally referred to as "spreading factor" is produced by staphylococci which degrades hyaluronic acid, the ground substance of connective tissues of host. Lysostaphin is produced by *S. simulans* and is active against staphylococci but not micrococci. It is used in a test to differentiate these genera. Heat stable nucleases cleaves both DNA and RNA and is produced by most strains of *S.aureus, S.hyicus, S.schleiferi* subsp. *caugulans* and *S. intermedius*. Staphylokinase degrade fibrin clot by converting plasminogen to fibrinolytic enzyme plasmin. A leukocidin kills neutrophils and macrophages of some species (rabbit, bovine, human) by altering cell membrane permeability, causing degranulation. It is composed of 2 heat stable interacting proteins.

Many strains of *S. aureus* express a plasminogen activator called staphylokinase. This factor lyses fibrin. The genetic determinant is associated with lysogenic bacteriophages. A complex formed between staphylokinase and plasminogen activates plasmin-like proteolytic activity which causes dissolution of fibrin clots. The mechanism is identical to streptokinase, which is used in medicine to treat patients suffering from coronary thrombosis. As with coagulase, there is no strong evidence that staphylokinase is a virulence factor, although it seems reasonable to imagine that localized fibrinolysis might aid in bacterial spreading.

S. aureus can express proteases, a lipase, a deoxyribonuclease (DNase) and a fatty acid modifying enzyme (FAME). The first three probably provide nutrients for the bacteria, and it is unlikely that they have anything but a minor role in pathogenesis. However, the FAME enzyme may be important in abscesses, where it could modify anti-bacterial lipids and prolong bacterial survival.

The exopolysaccharide PIA contributes to the resistance of *S. epidermidis* to innate host defense. The enzymatic modification of PIA by the IcaB enzyme is a crucial factor in determining the biological function of PIA in biofilm formation, colonization, and immune evasion. *Poly-d--glutamic acid (PGA).* Research has shown that *S. epidermidis* PGA is crucial for survival in the human host during commensal life on the skin and infection. PGA might be a promising antigen for vaccine development against *S. epidermidis* infection.Phenol-soluble modulins (PSM): a novel class of staphylococcal virulence determinants

S. aureus PSMs are key virulence determinants during infection by CA-MRSA strains. These peptides have an extraordinary capacity to lyse human neutrophils. The role of the *agr* and *luxS* quorum-sensing systems during biofilm formation and inflammation has been shown.

Cell surface components

Peptidoglycan is the major cell wall polymer of staphylococci and is a possible virulence factor. It is released in enormous amount in local infections. The peptidoglycan elicits the production of interleukin 1 (IL-1) by phagocytes which eventually reach hypothalamus. The IL-1 then stimulates neuron to produce prostaglandins resulting in pyrexia. In addition IL-1 aids in production of a local inflammatory response leading to further release of cytokines.

Capsule is a major anti-phagocytic factor present on *Staphylococcus aureus* and is associated with virulence of some strains. A thin polysaccharide micro capsule produced by most mastitic isolates and human clinical isolates of *S.aureus* belonging to immunotype 5 or 8 out of a 12 has been identified. In mastitis strain capsule is related with the virulence. It also impedes colonization of damaged heart valves, perhaps by masking adhesins.

Teichoic acid are the entities present on the surface of staphylococcal isolates and are antigenically species specific. These are composed on either polyribitol or polyglycerol phosphates and are probably antiphagocytic factors by interfering in opsonization by activating complement and reducing the complement components in the serum. Another factor responsible for exerting antiphagocytic factor is **Protein A**. It is a major immunoglobulin binding protein through Fc portion of IgG1, IgG2 and IgG4 subclasses. Loss of protein A is related with the reduction in virulence of *S.aureus* strains in subcutaneous and peritoneal infection but no difference in mastitis (Foster, 1992). Similar to Protein A, protein responsible for binding of *S.aureus* to fibronectin of host epithelium are also present. Antibodies against fibronectin binding protein may be protective, however, exact role of this protein is not clear, besides binding to fibronectin. Besides, other proteins identified are fibrinogen binding protein, collagen binding protein and a vitronectin binding protein. Fibrinogen binding protein has been found on at least 95% of both human and animal strains of *S.aureus*. These extra cellular matrix binding proteins are being identified in various coagulase negative staphylococci, which are pathogenic for humans and bovine udder.

Staphylococci, coagulase positive and potentially pathogenic, grow better in iron-restricted conditions as compared to those with less pathogenic potential (Cogulase negative). Under iron-limiting condition, coagulase-positive strains produce a siderophore, *Staphyloferrin B* which is responsible for iron-acquisition from extra cellular sources. This transferrin may be involved with virulence, although the phenomenon is not well understood.

Pathogenesis

For the majority of diseases caused by *S. aureus*, pathogenesis is multifactorial, so it is difficult to determine precisely the role of any given factor. However, there are correlations between strains isolated from particular diseases and expression of particular virulence determinants, which suggests their role in particular diseases. The application of molecular biology has led to advances in unraveling the pathogenesis of staphylococcal diseases. Genes encoding potential virulence factors have been cloned and sequenced, and many protein toxins have been purified. With some staphylococcal toxins, symptoms of human disease can be reproduced in animals with the purified protein toxins, lending an understanding of their mechanism of action.

The adhesion mechanisms mediated by proteins of *S.aureus* with laminin and fibronectin, the extracellular toxins, surface proteins and carbohydrates and enzymes are responsible for a complex interaction leading to the disease. Laminin and fibronectin form the extracellular matrix of epithelial and endothelial surfaces. In addition, most strains express a fibrin/fibrinogen binding protein (**clumping factor**) which promotes attachment to blood clots and traumatized tissue. Most strains of *S. aureus* express both fibronectin and fibrinogen-binding proteins. In addition, an adhesin that promotes attachment to collagen has been found in strains that cause osteomyelitis and septic arthritis. Interaction with collagen may also be important in promoting bacterial attachment to damaged tissue where the underlying layers have been exposed. *Staphylococcus saprophyticus*, a uropathogenic species, has a unique cell wall-anchored protein, uro-adherence factor A (UafA), which shows erythrocyte binding activity. The structure was composed of three domains, designated as the N2, N3, and B domains, arranged in a triangular relative configuration. Hemagglutination inhibition assay with domain-truncated mutants indicated that both N and B domains were necessary for erythrocyte binding. Based on these results, a novel manner of ligand binding in which the B domain acts as a functional domain was proposed as the adhesion mechanism of *S. saprophyticus* (Matsuoka *et al.* 2011). S. saprophyticus does not possess any virulence factors found in S. aureus, such as coagulase, enterotoxins, exoenzymes, and extracellular matrix-binding proteins, although it does have a remarkable expansion of transport systems related to highly variable ion contents in the urinary environment. A further unique feature is that only a single ORF is predictable as a cell wall-anchored protein, and it shows positive hemagglutination and adherence to human bladder cell associated with initial colonization in the urinary tract. It also shows significantly high urease activity in S. saprophyticus. The uropathogenicity of *S. saprophyticus* can be attributed to its genome that is needed for its survival in the human urinary tract by means of novel cell wall-anchored adhesin and redundant uro-adaptive transport systems, together with urease (Kuroda *et al* 2005). Endogenous infections are most frequent but exogenous infection also occur. Transmission is usually by direct contact or by fomites.

Strains of this wide spread commensal have the capacity to invade tissues, producing abscesses, pustules, various other pyogenic infections and on occasion bacteremia and septicaemia. Microcolonies are formed at the site of initial localized infection from which the organisms later spread into surrounding tissues. The presence of a foreign body such as suture material or other, facilitate establishment of staphylococci. *S. aureus*, however, is able to cause disease in unbroken skin. Peptidoglycan and proteases of organisms in damaged tissues will attract neutrophils from the blood due to release of chemotactic compounds. The localized host response to staphylococcal infection is inflammation, characterized by an elevated temperature at the site, swelling, the accumulation of pus, and necrosis of tissue. Around the inflamed area, a fibrin clot may form, walling off the bacteria and leukocytes as a characteristic pus-filled boil or abscess. More serious infections of the skin may occur, such as furuncles or impetigo. Localized infection of the bone is called osteomyelitis. Serious consequences of staphylococcal infections occur when the bacteria invade the blood stream. A resulting septicemia may be rapidly fatal; a bacteremia may result in seeding other internal abscesses, other skin lesions, or infections in the lung, kidney, heart, skeletal muscle or meninges. The abilities of staphylococci to be internalized and form a biofilm can contribute to host immunological defence evasion that subsequently impairs antimicrobial therapy. The invasive capability of six S. aureus field isolates with different biofilmforming profiles was compared in vitro using a bovine mammary epithelial cell line. This was further confirmed in primary cell cultures using fluorescent rRNA probes against S. aureus. The results suggest that S. aureus invasion levels are not related to biofilm formation (Oliviera *et al.*2011).

Typically staphylococci are ingested and killed by neutrophils in which the oxygen dependent antibacterial mechanism appear to be operative besides other factor such as low pH, lysozyme & cationic proteins. Some neutrophils are killed by toxic bacterial products. Mobilization of neutrophils leads to the pyogenic response and later on abscess formation which drain on the surface. Both capsule and Protein A and possibly peptidoglycan of staphylococci are strongly antiphagocytic. The lesions tend to be walled off possibly due to the action of coagulase (Jonsson and Wadstrom 1993). Part of the antiphagocytic effect of capsule and slime is due to their shielding of phagocytic cell from deposited complement component (C3b) that may have bound to peptidoglycan.

Delayed hypersensitivity is considered to play a role in local tissue damage. Extra cellular products may function to permit survival of the organisms on the skin with subsequent tissue invasion.

Pathogenesis of Bovine Mastitis

Mastitis is the most important disease caused by *S.aureus*. At certain farms this is a major cause of the disease followed by *S.agalactiae*. Both coagulase positive and coagulase negative staphylococci (CNS) are capable of causing the disease. In India, the presence of coagulase negative staphylococci in causing mastitis has not been studied however; reports from abroad have shown the prevalence of *S.chromogenes, S.simulans, S.tylosus* and *S.haemolyticus* as the most prevalent species (Hogan etal 1987; Jarp 1991; Birgersson etal 1992; Taponen *et al.*2008). CNS includes various species, but only a few prevail in bovine mastitis. *S. chromogenes* is the major CNS species affecting multiparous and primiparous cows whereas *S. simulans* has been isolated more frequently from older cows. Multiparous cows generally become infected with CNS during later lactation whereas primiparous cows develop infection before or shortly after calving (Pyorala and Taponen,2009). S. aureus can cause clinical mastitis, but often causes sub clinical mastitis, which remains persistent and increases milk somatic cell count. CNS, traditionally regarded as minor pathogens, seem to lack the ability to cause severe mastitis. CNS can, however, persist in the mammary gland and moderately increase milk somatic cell count. Resistance to various antimicrobials is more common in CNS than in S. aureus, but CNS mastitis responds much better to antimicrobial treatment than S. aureus mastitis (Taponen Pyorala (2009).

The route of entrance of the pathogen is via the teat canal. It passes the teat duct into the teat and udder cisterns through propulsion or bacterial growth and subsequently into the milk ducts and may further rise with milk fat. This may aid the bacterium to invade upper parts of the milk ducts and udder. The staphylococci colonize the tip of the healthy teat for a prolonged period of time (du Preez 1985) as distinct micro colonies. Subsequently, staphylococci grow in milk. The organism after passing the barrier of the teat duct binds the epithelial cells through various adhesion factors.

During the course of staphylococcal multiplication chemotactic substances are liberated which cause an infiltration of PMN leukocytes into the mammary glands. However, these PMNs are not fully capable of killing as there have reduced glycogen reserve and a decreased phagocytic capacity in comparison to blood PMNs.

Both acute and chronic form of mastitis may be caused; variation is only in the degree of involvement of mammary tissues. Both are as a result of proliferation of bacteria in the collecting ducts and to a lesser extent in the alveoli. In acute mastitis, the small ducts are quickly blocked by fibrin clots. In the chronic form there are less foci of inflammation and the reaction is milder. This subsides within few days and then the connective tissue proliferation around the ducts takes place leading to blockage and atrophy of drained area (Gudding *et al.* 1984). In chronic mastitis, there is clinical shedding of bacteria from the affected quarter. There is a cyclic variation in the population of PMN cells in the milk and their capacity to phagocytose bacteria. In some cases abscesses occur and botryomycosis is seen. Changes in inflammatory parameters, leukocyte surface markers, functional responses and cytokine mRNA expression of leukocytes from dairy cows with naturally occurring chronic Staphylococcus aureus (S. aureus) mastitis and healthy cows were determined to elucidate the leukocyte responses to S. aureus infection of the mammary gland (Nagahata *et al.* 2011). Increased values in inflammatory parameters and matrix metalloproteinase activities in milk revealed the characteristics of cows with chronic mastitis. Expression of L-selectin and CD18 molecules on neutrophils and proportion of CD8 cells in milk from cows with S. aureus mastitis were significantly ($P<0.05$) increased compared to those found in healthy cows. The FcR-stimulated CL response of blood neutrophils was significantly ($P<0.05$) decreased in cows with S. aureus mastitis. Significantly ($P<0.05$) decreased mitogenic responses of lymphocytes were found in cows with S. aureus mastitis; however, the values were not restored to those of healthy cows when stimulated with both mitogens and the cytokine IL-1β. mRNA expression of the TNF-α, IL-1β and IL-8 on milk leukocytes from cows with S. aureus was found to be increased compared to that of healthy cows. The changes of immune responses found in cows with

S. aureus mastitis appear to be influenced by the severity and duration of inflammation in infected quarters. The down-regulation of the leukocyte functions found in cows with S. aureus mastitis appears to be associated with the progress of the chronic stage of S. aureus mastitis.

Biofilm-forming ability has been increasingly recognized as an important virulence factor in Staphylococci, facilitating their persistence in the host, evading its defences and allowing bacterial survival at high antimicrobial concentrations. Recurrent infections are often attributable to biofilm growth of bacteria . Biofilm formation is accompanied by significant genetic and subsequent physiological changes in the microorganisms resulting, inter alia, in a loss of sensitivity to virtually all classes of antibiotics. Vasudevan *et al* (2003) examined in vitro slime production, biofilm formation, and the presence of the ica gene locus and icaA and icaD genes in S. aureus isolates from bovine mastitis. Thirty-two of the 35 isolates tested produced slime on Congo red agar, whereas only 24 of the isolates were found to produce biofilm in vitro. However, all the 35 isolates possessed the ica locus, icaA and icaD genes. This study indicates a high prevalence of the ica genes among S. aureus mastitis isolates, and their presence is not always associated with in vitro formation of slime or biofilm. A combination of phenotypic and genotypic tests is recommended for investigating biofilm formation in S. aureus. Oliveira *et al.*(2006) aimed at the evaluation of the biofilm-forming ability of Staphylococci field isolates from bovine subclinical mastitis and at the development of a fluorescent in situ hybridisation (FISH) protocol that would allow the direct observation of biofilm formation in milk samples. The analysis of phenotypic expression in Congo Red Agar (CRA) and by FISH, showed that 37.5% of the S. aureus isolates produced biofilm, while by optical density measurement only 18.75% isolates revealed this phenotype. The results showed a fair agreement according to the kappa coefficient test (kappa = 0.259). Regarding S. epidermidis mastitis isolates, 37.5% revealed the ability to produce biofilm, but only four isolates were positive by all methods. This agreement was moderate (kappa = 0.467). The application of FISH to artificially contaminated milk samples allowed the direct observation of biofilm production by 37.5% isolates, showing total agreement with the CRA results. This method better mimics the in vivo conditions, especially in terms of the presence of calcium and iron, which in high concentrations, respectively, are known to inhibit or induce biofilm production.

Kumar *et al.*(2011) elucidated the antibiotic-resistant and virulence gene patterns S. aureus isolates (111) were recovered from intra-mammary infections suffering buffaloes, and characterized using PCR and disk diffusion assays. The pathogenic factors were associated with antibiotic-resistant patterns and analyzed. Molecular and phenotypic characterization of tested isolates showed significantly resistance to tetracycline, macrolides, lincosamides and aminoglycosides. MecA gene was detected in 5.4% of isolates of S. aureus. The isolates showed variation in expression of pathogenic factors. Coagulase genotype VI showed high antibiotics susceptibility while patterns I, III, IV and V belonged to resistant category of tested bacterial population. The prevalence of other virulent genes namely, Ebp, Fib, FnbB, Bbp and Map were present significantly in highly pathogenic isolates. The isolates (41.4%) were found positive for super-antigen enterotoxins Sec, See, Seg and Sei genes only and predominated in methicillin-susceptible compared to resistant ones. The allelic variants of Agr-1 and 3 were considerably associated with coagulase genotypes and other virulence factors, while the enterotoxins were found considerably associated with Agr-1 and 2. Distribution of virulent genes between methicillin-susceptible and resistant isolates was uneven. The distribution of high pathogenic characteristic in antibiotic-susceptible isolates indicated that these were equally responsible in maintaining the intra-mammary infections in animals and cannot be overlooked. The surveillance of pathogenic and antibiotics resistance factors of isolates revealed that certain genetic elements were over producing (Ebp, Fib, FnbB, Bbp, Map, TetK, MsrB, AacA-D) in mastitic S. aureus isolates especially from clinical cases.

Tick Pyemia of lambs

It is a staphylococcal infection of lambs manifested by septicaemia or bacteremia with subsequent localization in many organs. The disease in enzootic in areas where Ixodes ricinus ticks persists. Lambs aged 5 to 10 weeks are affected. They may die quickly of septicaemia and on post mortem abscesses are found on every organ including skin, muscle, tendon sheaths, joints, viscera and meningis. It was previously thought that ticks are required for the disease because through the tick bite the *S.aureus* enters the body. It is now believed that ticks transmit the tick born fever which predisposes lambs to *S.aureus* infection. The organism gain entry in the host through a variety of sources. There is profound immunosuppression in tick infection that predisposes animals to *S.aureus* infection because there is marked lymphocytopenia affecting T&B lymphocytes subsets and also a prolonged neutropenia lasting for 2-3 weeks combined with thrombocytopenia.

Exudative epidermitis (Greasy Pig Disease)

Greasy pig disease in animals is caused by *Staphylococcus hyicus*. It occurs in various countries of the world. Occasionally pigs up to 3 months of age suffer from the disease. Within litters all animals may be affected. Nofrarias *et al* (2006) suggested that the generalized cutaneous infection with Staphylococcus hyicus is severe enough to induce a systemic inflammatory and immune responses in pigs.

The organisms are carried by gilt or sow on their skin. It has also been found on skin of cattle, and also cause disease in horses. Experimentally, the organisms can cause similar lesions in horses. Environmental stress plays an important role in establishment of the disease.

Certain strains of *Staphylococcus hyicus* can cause the skin disease exudative epidermitis in pigs. Exudative epidermitis is characterized by separation of the cells in the epidermis in the upper stratum spinosum, exfoliation of the skin, erythema, and serous exudation. Spontaneous exudative epidermitis in pigs is a generalized infection of the skin caused by strains of *S. hyicus*, which are able to produce a disease-causing factor designated exfoliative toxin. The exfoliative toxins responsible for the characteristic lesion of exudative epidermitis have been identified and purified from strains in Japan and Denmark. These toxins have been characterized as exoproteins of approximately 27 kDa or 30 kDa . The complex of skin lesions called the staphylococcal scalded skin syndrome in humans has several aspects in common with exudative epidermitis in pigs. Staphylococcal scalded skin syndrome is caused by infection with *Staphylococcus aureus* strains that produce exfoliative toxin ETA, ETB, or both.

The virulence factors of *S.hyicus* have not been well defined. It probably produces a cytotoxin which has affect on porcine keratinocytes in culture. Experimental infection leads to a systemic disease suggesting that *S.hyicus* does not cause a local disease. The disease is characterized by excess sebaceous secretion, exfoliation and exudation. These changes result in loss of skin infection. The organisms appear to enter the body through skin wound. Subcutaneous inoculation also results in the infection. Exfoliatin may be responsible for enhancing clinical signs of exudative dermatitis. During the outbreaks mortality as high as 90% has been recorded. Virulence factors of staphylococci such as Exfoliative Toxin are accessory proteins which are not essential for cell growth or division. Genetic determinants for these factors are often associated with mobile genetic elements such as phages, plasmids, and pathogenicity islands For instance, genes for ETA (*eta*) and enterotoxins A and E are encoded on prophage genomes in the *S. aureus* chromosome, and genes for enterotoxin D , ETB (*etb*), and EDIN-C have been shown to exist on plasmids. The term "pathogenicity island" was first coined to describe large chromosomal virulence-associated segments in uropathogenic *Escherichia coli*. Since then, the definition has been broadened to indicate regions, ranging in size from an island of less than 2 kb with a single gene up to a 200-kb island of multigene elements, which have been identified in many species. In staphylococcal species, at least three types of pathogenicity islands have been reported. Yamaguchi *et al* (2002) identified a novel pathogenicity island in Staphylococcus aureus which contains open reading frames (ORFs) similar to the exfoliative toxin (ET) gene, glutamyl endopeptidase gene, and edin-B gene in tandem and the phage resistance gene, flanked by hsdM, hsdS (restriction and modification system), and IS256. The protein encoded by the ET-like gene showed 40, 59, and 68% amino acid sequence identities with exfoliative toxin A (ETA), exfoliative toxin B (ETB), and Staphylococcus hyicus ETB (ShETB), respectively. When injected into neonatal mice, the recombinant protein derived from the ET-like gene induced exfoliation of the skin with loss of cell-to-cell adhesion in the upper part of the epidermis as observed in histological examinations, just as was found in neonatal mice injected with ETA or ETB. Western blot analysis indicated that the recombinant protein is serologically distinct from ETA and ETB. Therefore, the product encoded by this new ORF is a new ET member produced by S. aureus and is termed ETD. ETD did not induce blisters in 1-day-old chickens. In the skins of mice injected with ETD, cell surface staining of desmoglein 1 (Dsg1), a cadherin type cell-to-cell adhesion molecule in desmosomes, was abolished without affecting that of desmoglein 3 (Dsg3). Furthermore, in vitro incubation of the recombinant extracellular domains of Dsg1 and Dsg3 with the recombinant protein demonstrated that both mouse and human Dsg1, but not Dsg3, were directly cleaved in a dose-dependent manner. These results demonstrate that ETD and ETA induce blister formation by identical pathophysiological mechanisms. Clinical strains positive for edin-B were suggested to be clonally associated, and all edin-B-positive strains tested were positive for etd. Among 18 etd-positive strains, 12 produced ETD extracellularly. Interestingly, these strains are mainly isolated from other sources of infections and not from patients with bullous impetigo or staphylococcal scalded-skin syndrome. This strongly suggests that ETD might play a pathogenic role in a broader spectrum of bacterial infections than previously considered.

Exudative epidermitis-inducing exotoxins, originally described by Amtsberg (1979), have been identified and purified from *S. hyicus* strains in Japan and Denmark and have been designated as SHETA and SHETB and ExhA, ExhB, ExhC, and ExhD, respectively. The prevalence of the exfoliative toxin genes *exh*A, *exh*B, *exh*C, and *exh*D has been described for *S. hyicus* strains isolated from various countries. However, little is known about the distribution of SHETA- and SHETB-encoding genes in *S. hyicus* or the combined occurrence of SHETA and SHETB and the exfoliative toxin-encoding genes described in Denmark.Staphylococcus (S.) hyicus strains isolated in Russia (n = 23) and Germany (n = 17) were investigated for the prevalence of the previously described genes sheta and shetb (Kanbar *et al.* 2008). Sheta was detected in 16 S. hyicus strains. Sheta-positive strains were mainly found among strains isolated from exudative epidermitis, and frequently together with the exfoliative toxin-encoding genes exhD and exhC. Partial sequencing of sheta in a single

S. hyicus strain revealed an almost complete match with the sheta sequence obtained from GenBank. None of the S. hyicus strains displayed a positive reaction with the shetb-specific oligonucleotide primer used in the present study. According to the present results, the exotoxin encoding gene sheta seems to be distributed among S. hyicus strains in Russia and Germany. The toxigenic potential of this exotoxin, which does not have the classical structure of a staphylococcal exfoliative toxin, remains to be elucidated. Genes coding for four different exfoliative toxins from S. hyicus (ExhA, ExhB, ExhC, and ExhD) were cloned and sequenced (Ahrens and Andresen,2004).. The coding sequence of the four toxin genes ranged from 816 to 834 bp. The amino acid sequences of these four toxins were homologous to the earlier described exfoliative toxins SHETB from S. hyicus and ETA, ETB, and ETD from Staphylococcus aureus. The homology between the S. hyicus toxins was at the same level as the homology to the exfoliative toxins from S. aureus. The toxins showed similarity to serine proteases, including preservation of the catalytic tract in ExhA, ExhB, and ExhC. However, in ExhD, Asp in the putative catalytic tract was replaced with Glu.

Exfoliative toxins produced by S. aureus have been shown to selectively cleave human or mouse desmoglein 1, a desmosomal adhesion molecule, that when inactivated results in blisters. Amagai *et al.*(2002) demonstrated that exfoliative toxin A specifically cleaves desmoglein 1, a desmosomal adhesion molecule, that when inactivated results in blisters. The authors determined the target molecule for exfoliative toxin B. Exfoliative toxin B injected in neonatal mice caused superficial epidermal blisters, abolished cell surface staining of desmoglein 1, and degraded desmoglein 1 without affecting desmoglein 3 or E-cadherin. When adenovirus-transduced cultured keratinocytes expressing exogenous mouse desmoglein 1 or desmoglein 3 were incubated with exfoliative toxin B, desmoglein 1, but not desmoglein 3, was cleaved. Furthermore, cell surface staining of desmoglein 1, but not that of desmoglein 3, was abolished when cryosections of normal human skin were incubated with exfoliative toxin B, suggesting that living cells were not necessary for exfoliative toxin B cleavage of desmoglein 1. Finally, in vitro incubation of the recombinant extracellular domains of desmoglein 1 and desmoglein 3 with exfoliative toxin B demonstrated that both mouse and human desmoglein 1, but not desmoglein 3, were directly cleaved by exfoliative toxin B in a dose-dependent fashion. These findings demonstrate that exfoliative toxin A and exfoliative toxin B cause blister formation in staphylococcal scalded skin syndrome and bullous impetigo by identical molecular pathophysiologic mechanisms.Fudaba *el ul.*(2005) attempted to identify the molecular target of Exhs in porcine skin. Each of recombinant Exhs injected in the skin of pigs caused superficial epidermal blisters or crust formation. Cell surface staining of desmoglein 1, but not that of desmoglein 3, was abolished when cryosections of normal porcine skin were incubated with one of Exhs suggesting that Exh selectively degrade porcine desmoglein 1. In vitro incubation of the recombinant extracellular domains of desmoglein 1 and desmoglein 3 of human, mouse or canine origin demonstrated that only mouse desmogleins 1alpha and 1beta were cleaved by ExhA and ExhC at high concentration. Furthermore, injection of ExhA and ExhC at high concentration caused superficial blisters in neonatal mice. These findings strongly suggest that Exhs cause blister formation of porcine skin by digesting porcine desmoglein 1 in a similar fashion to exfoliative toxins from S. aureus.

Diagnosis

An indirect ELISA was developed for the detection of toxigenic strains as an alternative method to the use of phage typing for selection of S. hyicus isolates to be used in autogenous vaccine against exudative epidermitis in pigs(Andresen 1999). The indirect ELISA was evaluated by investigating the presence of toxin among a total of 655 S. hyicus isolates from 69 pig skin samples, one from each of the 69 pig herds with outbreak of exudative epidermitis. Toxigenic S. hyicus were detected in 74% of the cases by ELISA. From each of the five cases, in which initially no toxigenic S. hyicus were found, a further 40 S. hyicus-like colonies were tested in ELISA. Testing of this number of colonies has a >99% probability of disclosing toxigenic S. hyicus. Toxin-producing isolates were found in only two of the five cases investigated. This may indicate the existence of one or more variants of the exfoliative toxin of S. hyicus that are not detected in the indirect ELISA or that S. hyicus may be displaced from lesions of exudative epidermitis. Andresen and Ahrens (2004) developed a multiplex PCR for detection of genes encoding the exfoliative toxins ExhA, ExhB, ExhC and ExhD from Staphylococcus hyicus and to estimate the prevalence of exfoliative toxins among Staph. hyicus isolates from Danish pig herds with exudative epidermitis (EE).A multiplex PCR employing specific primers for each of the genes encoding four different exfoliative toxins was developed and evaluated using a collection of Staph. hyicus with known toxin type and a number of other staphylococcal species. A total of 314 Staph. hyicus isolates from pigs with EE were screened by multiplex PCR and the combined results of the present and previous investigations showed that ExhA, ExhB, ExhC and ExhD was found in 20, 33, 18 and 22%, respectively, of 60 cases of EE investigated.This study has provided a new tool for detection of toxigenic Staph. hyicus and a more comprehensive picture of the prevalence of the Staph. hyicus exfoliative toxins in Danish pig herds.The multiplex PCR can be used in studies on the prevalence of toxigenic Staph. hyicus elucidating the epidemiology of EE in pigs. The multiplex PCR is currently being used for selection of Staph. hyicus isolates for production of autogenous vaccine.

Various pyogenic infections

Coagulase positive *S.aureus* normally causes pyoderma in dogs and rarely in cats. The organism is now called as *S.intermedius* (Phillips and Kloos 1981). Both virulent and nonvirulent strains of this species occur.*Staphylococcus pseudintermedius* is a member of the coagulase-positive staphylococci, and is the commonest cause of canine pyoderma.(Tse *et al.*2011). Futagawa *et al.* (2009) identified the exfoliative toxin in strains of S.pseudointermedius. Recently, an exfoliative toxin gene (exi) was identified in *Staphylococcus pseudintermedius* isolated from canine pyoderma. This novel exfoliative toxin, which targets a cell-cell adhesion molecule in canine epidermis and might be involved in a broad spectrum of canine pyoderma (Iyori *et al.*2010). Animals are predisposed to the disease by various factors such as immunodeficiency, parasitic infestation, skin damage and allergy. Recurrent infectionds do occur and repeated exposure to staphylococci leads to delayed hypersensitivity to the peptidoglycan. The cell mediated response intensifies inflammatory responses while spatially confining them. Antibody induced hypersensitivity is also thought to be generated in pyoderma.

In typical staphylococcal infection, pus filled abscess are formed in which participating cells have been found to be destroyed by the various toxins produced by staphylococci and inflammatory cell activity. This interaction between leukocytes and bacterial cells produces pus. Abscess is surrounded by the fibrin strands. In chronic infection fibrous material predominates with areas of suppuration.

Phosphate urolithiasis of dogs and mink is commonly associated with *S.intermedius* infections. This pathogen also occur in respiratory, genital lymphatic, bone and joint infections, wounds and infection of eye lids and conjunctiva.

Bumble foot of birds is a chronic pyogranulomatous process in the subcutaneous tissues of foot resulting in thick walled swelling on one or more joints. In turkeys it causes bacteremia localizing in joints and tendon sheaths.

Cutaneous and pyemic staphylococcosis are problems in wild and domestic rabbits.

Diagnosis

Various samples which need to be collected for examination comprise of aspirates from unopened lesions, swabs, preferably in transport media and milk (from cases of mastitis). For septicaemic cases blood and urine are appropriate.

On gram stained films, staphylococci appear as gram-positive cocci in clusters, twos or short chains. Isolation can be attempted on blood agar. Colonies are smooth small to big and showing multiple haemolysis.. *Staphylococcus aureus* forms a fairly large yellow colony on rich medium; *S. epidermidis* has a relatively small white colony. *S. aureus* is often hemolytic on blood agar; *S. epidermidis* is non hemolytic. Staphylococci are facultative anaerobes that grow by aerobic respiration or by fermentation that yields principally lactic acid. Bovine blood is best for the detection of beta toxins. Typing of isolates can be attempted using bacteria phage lysis. Phage typing set have been developed for human, bovine and avian *S.aureus.*

Treatment and Control

Treatment varies according to the clinical disease observed. Abscess and empyemas are drained of pus surgically. For pyoderma topical application of antiseptics may be adequate.

For systemic treatment antibiotic are given. Methicillin resistance has emerged as an important problem in these organisms, with significant concerns about animal and public health (Weese and Duijkeren, 2010). Staphylococci are also commonly resistant to penicillin, streptomycin and tetracyclines. Effective antimicrobials include derivates of penicillin, chloramphenicol, erythromycin, cephalosporins, vancomycin and lincomycin. Antibiogram of the isolate need to be known if antibiotic treatment does not work satisfactorily. Clavulanic acid/amoxicillin combination is very effective. *S. aureus* exhibits resistance to antiseptics and disinfectants, such as quaternary ammonium compounds, which may aid its survival in the hospital environment. For staphylococcal cystitis, penicillin is considered effective provided the causative agent is susceptible. For treatment of greasy pig disease, cloxacillin is used topically and systemically. Low concentrations of menthol can markedly inhibit the expression of α-hemolysin, enterotoxins A and B, and toxic shock syndrome toxin 1 in *S. aureus*. It has been demonstrated that menthol may be useful in managing *S. aureus* infections when used in combination with β-lactam antibiotics, which can often increase *S. aureus* toxin secretion when used at subinhibitory concentrations. In addition, the menthol basic structure has potential applications in the development of new anti-virulence drugs (Qiu *et al.* 2011).

S. aureus strains from cases of mastitis are sensitive to penicillin, however, the treatment with this antibiotic has provided disappointing results due to inaccessibility of bacteria in the interacinar tissues or obstructed ducts and alveoli. For treatment of resistant strains ampicillin and amoxicillin are effective. Cloxacillin and nefacillin are less effective against non-lactamase staphylococci. Clavulonic acid added to amoxicillin overcomes this problem of B-lactamase producing staphylococci. Cephalosporins and erythromycin are effective against beta lactamase producing staphylococci. Third generation cephalosporins are effective against gram-negative bacteria (Radostitis etal. 1994).

Coagulase-negative Staphylococcus (CNS) isolates (n=168) obtained from milk from heifers and dairy cows were screened for minimum inhibitory concentration (MIC) to antimicrobials used commonly for mastitis therapy (Sawant *et al.*2009). Of the 10 CNS species included in the study, the predominant species were Staphylococcus chromogenes (n=61), Staphylococcus epidermidis (n=37), Staphylococcus hyicus (n=37), and Staphylococcus simulans (n=16). The majority of CNS was susceptible to ampicillin, oxacillin, cephalothin, and ceftiofur. Erythromycin and pirlimycin were also very effective in vitro inhibitors of CNS. The only exception was observed with S. epidermidis. Of 37 S. epidermidis evaluated, 13 (35%) exhibited efflux-based resistance to erythromycin (> or =16 microg/ml) encoded by msrA and one isolate carried ermC encoding ribosomal methylase-based resistance to both erythromycin (> or =64 microg/ml) and pirlimycin (> or =64 microg/ml). A total of 17 S. epidermidis, 11 S. chromogenes, and one S. hyicus exhibited phenotypic resistance to ampicillin (> or =0.5 microg/ml). Constitutive beta-lactamase production was observed in all ampicillin resistant isolates except 4 S. epidermidis that exhibited inducible beta-lactamase production. Induced beta-lactamase production was also observed in 13 S. epidermidis that were phenotypically susceptible to the entire MIC panel. All isolates that produced beta-lactamase either constitutively or by induction carried blaZ. S. epidermidis (n=12, 32%) that were resistant to methicillin (oxacillin > or =0.5 microg/ml) carried low affinity penicillin-binding protein encoded by mecA. Most multi-drug resistant (MDR) S. epidermidis (> or =2 resistance genes) were resistant to ampicillin, erythromycin and methicillin. All except one MDR S. epidermidis had icaAB, which encodes for polysaccharide intercellular adhesion. Based on pulsed field gel electrophoresis, MDR S. epidermidis were closely related genotypically, and were isolated from different cows on the same farm suggesting clonal dissemination. Bovine S. epidermidis share antimicrobial resistance patterns and virulence determinants of strains observed in human infections. Studying CNS at the species level can provide valuable information about species-specific differences that can be vital data for effective mastitis therapy and management..Kumar *et al.*(2010) detected the distribution of antibiotic-resistant genes of S. aureus isolates. Isolates (128) of S. aureus from mastitic milk were collected, tested for antibiotics with disc-diffusion method, and resistant genes mecA, linA, msrA msrB, vatA, vatB, vatC ermA, ermC tetK, tetM and aacA-D were detected by PCR. The phenotypic antibiotics resistance percent in S. aureus isolates was classified as tetracycline (36.7), gentamycin (30.5), streptomycin (26.6), kanamycin (25.8) and penicillin G (22.7). All the isolates were susceptible to vancomycin. Among isolates, 10.2% were observed as methicillin-resistant. The distribution of antibiotic-resistant genes was linA (51.6) followed by msrB (46.1), tetK + M (34.4), msrA and aacA-D (26.6%). Different antibiotic-resistant genes combinations (mecA/linA-2; mecA/aacA-D/tetK/linA/msrB-3; mecA/linA/msrA/msrB-3; aacA-D/linA/msrA/msrB-4; aacA-D/linA/msrB-7; linA/msrA/msrB-10; tetK/linA/msrA/msrB-11; aacA/tetK/linA/msrB-12 isolates) were observed. All the isolates lacked amplification of vatA, vatB, ermA and ermC genes. Molecular typing resulted genetic variation in protein A (6-12 repeats) and coagulase genes (A-E patterns) were observed. Coagulase A and D genotypes were more prevalent in antibiotic-resistant isolates, while E, B and C in susceptible ones. The significant observation was the prevalence of methicillin-resistant S. aureus, which were resistant to multiple antibiotics. Findings revealed the status of resistant isolates in herd that might be helpful in treatment, controlling of resistant strains and culling of cows for mastitis reduction. Further Kumar *et al.*(2011) carried out characterizations of pathogenic factors (adhesin and toxin genes) and antibiotic susceptibility of isolates using gene amplification and disc diffusion assays, respectively. A high prevalence of MRSA was observed in the tested isolates (13.1%). The isolates were also highly resistant to antibiotics, i.e. 36.4% were resistant to streptomycin, 33.6% to oxytetracycline, 29.9% to gentamicin and 26.2% each to chloramphenicol, pristinomycin and ciprofloxacin. A significant variation in the expression of pathogenic factors (Ig, coa and clf) was observed in these isolates. The overall distribution of adhesin genes ebp, fib, bbp, fnbB, cap5, cap8, map and cna in the isolates was found to be 69.1, 67.2, 6.5, 20.5, 60.7, 26.1, 81.3 and 8.4%, respectively. The presence of fib, fnbB, bbp and map genes was considerably greater in MRSA than in methicillin-susceptible S. aureus (MSSA) isolates. The proportions of toxin genes, namely, hlb, seb, sec, sed, seg and sei, in the isolates were found to be 94.3, 0.9, 8.4, 0.9, 10.2 and 49.5%, respectively. The proportions of agr genes I, II, III and IV were found to be 39.2, 27.1, 21.5 and 12.1%, respectively. A few isolates showed similar antibiotic-resistance patterns, which could be due to identical strains or the dissemination of the same strains among animals. These findings can be utilized in mastitis treatment programmes and antimicrobials strategies in organized herd.

Control measures adopted besides the treatment are effective in spread of the infection. Hygiene in the milking shed attains greatest importance. Dry period therapy and post-milking teat dipping in 1% iodine is essential. Teat dipping in 0.5% chlorhexidine in 5-10% glycerine is completely effective against staphylococcal mastitis. Of special importance is the premilking teat washing and drying. There is no effective vaccine against mastitis which could be advocated for use although experimentally many have been tested. A vaccine based on fibronectin binding protein induces protective immunity against mastitis in cattle and might also be used as a vaccine in humans.

Hyperimmune serum or monoclonal antibodies directed towards surface components (e.g., capsular polysaccharide or surface protein adhesions) could theoretically prevent bacterial adherence and promote phagocytosis by opsonization of bacterial cells. Also, human hyperimmune serum could be given to hospital patients before surgery as a form of passive immunization.

In general, bacterin-toxoid vaccines, vaccines of DNA-recombinant protein and recombinant protein alone have been investigated. It is suggested that vaccines that employ new technologies (DNA and/or recombinant protein vaccines) and some long-standing bacterins have achieved good results, which supports their use in the prevention and control of bovine mastitis caused by S. aureus. An experimental bivalent vaccine against *Staphylococcus aureus* is reported to be safe and immunogenic for approximately 40 weeks in humans with end-stage renal disease undergoing hemodialysis. The vaccine called StaphVAX is composed of *S. aureus* type 5 and 8 capsular polysaccharides conjugated to nontoxic recombinant *Pseudomonas aeruginosa* A trivalent staphylococcal polysaccharide conjugate vaccine called TriStap has been developed. It contains the two main capsular types, 5 and 8, found in the outer coating of more than 80% of *S. aureus* strains, and conjugated to nontoxic recombinant *Pseudomonas* exotoxin A. To enhance the efficacy of this vaccine, a surface polysaccharide, 336, is added. *S. aureus* Type 336 accounts for the approximately 20% of *S. aureus* infections that do not form a polysaccharide capsule in the human bloodstream.

A double-blind, placebo-controlled study was conducted to compare two vaccines using different adjuvants with regard to their ability to stimulate antibody production against the alpha- and beta-toxins and the exopolysaccharide of Staphylococcus aureus (Tollersrud *et al.*2002). The vaccines contained identical antigens, consisting of inactivated whole bacteria of two strains of S. aureus in addition to alpha- and beta-toxoid. One vaccine contained mineral oil, while the other used a water-soluble acrylic acid polymer resin (Carbopol) as adjuvant. Saline served as the placebo. One hundred and forty ewes were vaccinated twice before lambing, by subcutaneous injection with vaccine or placebo in the region of the supramammary lymph node, and were observed and sampled over a period of 6 months. The vaccine containing mineral oil as adjuvant induced significantly greater immune responses to the α and β toxins than did the vaccine containing Carbopol. The latter vaccine induced higher levels of antibodies to exopolysaccharide. The degree of local adverse reactions did not differ between the two groups.

Third generation vaccines have been tested for control of mastitis. Gong *et al.* (2010) evaluated the potential of recombinant binding region A of clumping factor A (rClfA-A) to be an effective component of a vaccine against mastitis induced by Staphylococcus aureus in the mouse. rClfA-A and inactivated S. aureus were each emulsified in Freund's adjuvant, mineral oil adjuvant, and Seppic adjuvant; phosphate-buffered saline was used as a control. Seven groups of 12 mice each were immunized intraperitoneally three times at 2-week intervals. The titers of IgG and subtypes thereof (IgG1 and IgG2a) in the rClfA-A-immunized group were more than 1,000-fold higher than those in the killed-bacteria-immunized group ($P < 0.01$). Of the three adjuvants used, mineral oil adjuvant induced the highest antibody levels for both antigens ($P < 0.001$). Furthermore, the anti-rClfA-A antibody capacities for bacterial adhesion and opsonizing phagocytosis were significantly greater in the rClfA-A-immunized group than in the killed-bacteria-immunized group ($P < 0.05$). Lactating mice immunized with either rClfA-A or inactivated vaccine were challenged with *S. aureus* via the intramammary route. The numbers of bacteria recovered from the murine mammary glands 24 h after inoculation were significantly lower in the rClfA-A group than in the killed-bacteria-immunized group ($P < 0.001$). Histologic examination of the mammary glands showed that rClfA-A immunization effectively preserved tissue integrity. Thus, rClfA-A emulsified in an oil adjuvant provides strong immune protection against S. aureus-induced mastitis in the mouse. To construct a universal vaccine against mastitis induced by either Streptococcus agalactiae (*S. agalactiae*) or *Staphylococcus aureus* (*S. aureus*), the B-cell epitopes of surface immunogenic protein (Sip) from S. agalactiae and clumping factor A (ClfA) from *S. aureus* were analyzed and predicted. Sip-ClfA, a novel chimeric B cell epitope-based gene was obtained by overlapping PCR, and then the recombinant Sip-ClfA (rSip-ClfA) was expressed and purified. rSip-ClfA and inactivated *S. agalactiae* and *S. aureus* were formulated into different vaccines with mineral oil as the adjuvant and evaluated in mouse models. The rSip-ClfA vaccination induced higher Immunoglobulin G (IgG) titers compared with inactivated bacteria groups (Xu *et al.* 2011). Furthermore, rSip-ClfA immunization was characterized as the dominant IgG1 subtype, whereas both bacterial immunizations produced similar levels of IgG1 and IgG2a. The antiserum capacities to opsonize adhesion and phagocytosis were significantly greater in the rSip-ClfA immunization group than in the killed bacterial immunization groups ($P < 0.05$). The immunized lactating mice were challenged with either *S. agalactiae* or *S. aureus* via the intramammary route. At 24h postinfection, the numbers of bacteria recovered from the mammary glands were over 5-fold lower in the rSip-ClfA group than those in both inactivated bacterial groups ($P < 0.01$). Histopathological examination of the mammary glands showed that rSip-ClfA immunization provided better protection of mammary gland tissue integrity against both *S. agalactiae* and S. aureus challenge. Thus, the recombinant protein rSip-ClfA would be a promising vaccine candidate against mastitis induced by either S. agalactiae or S. aureus.

References

Ahrens P. and Andresen L.O. 2004.Cloning and sequence analysis of genes encoding Staphylococcus hyicus exfoliative toxin types A, B, C, and D. J. Bacteriol. **186:** 1833-1837.

Amagai M., Yamaguchi T., Hanakawa Y., Nishifuji K., Sugai M. and Stanley J.R..2002.Staphylococcal exfoliative toxin B specifically cleaves desmoglein 1. J. Invest. Dermatol. **118:** 845-850.

Amtsberg G.1979. Nachweis von Exofoliation auslösenden Substanzen in Kulturen von *Staphylococcus hyicus* des Schweines und *Staphylococcus epidermidis* Biotyp 2 des Rindes. *Zentralbl. Veterinarmed. B.* **26:** 257-272.

Andresen L.O.1999.Development and evaluation of an indirect ELISA for detection of exfoliative toxin ExhA, ExhB or ExhC produced by Staphylococcus hyicus. Vet. Microbiol. **68**(3-4): 285-92.

Andresen L.O. and Ahrens P.2004. A multiplex PCR for detection of genes encoding exfoliative toxins from Staphylococcus hyicus. J. Appl. Microbiol. **96:** 1265-70.

Birgersson, A., Johnsson, P. and Holberg, O. 1992. Species identification and some characteristics of coagulase negative staphylococci isolated from bovine udders. Vet. Microbiol. **31:** 181-89.

Devriese, L.A. and Olding, P. 1976. Characteristics of Staphylococcus strains isolated from different animal species. Res. Vet. Sci. **21:** 284-91.

du Preez, J.H. 1985. Teat canal infections. Kieler Milchwirtsch for schungsber **37:** 267-273.

Foster, T.J. 1992. The use of mutant for defining the role of virulence factor in vivo. In Molecular Biology of Bacterial Infections: current status and future perspectives. Ed. C.E. Hormaeche, C.W. Penu and C.J. Smyth. Pp173-91. Cambridge University Press, Cambridge, U.K.

Fudaba Y., Nishifuji K., Andresen L.O., Yamaguchi T., Komatsuzawa H., Amagai M. and Sugai M.2005.Staphylococcus hyicus exfoliative toxins selectively digest porcine desmoglein 1. Microb. Pathog. **39:** 171-6. Epub 2005 Oct 28.

Futagawa-Saito K, Makino S, Sunaga F, Kato Y, Sakurai-Komada N, Ba-Thein W, Fukuyasu T.2009.Identification of first exfoliative toxin in Staphylococcus pseudintermedius. FEMS Microbiol Lett. **301:** 176-180.

Gong R., Hu C., Xu H., Guo A., Chen H., Zhang G. Shi L.2010.Evaluation of clumping factor A binding region A in a subunit vaccine against Staphylococcus aureus-induced mastitis in mice. Clin Vaccine Immunol. **17:** 1746-52. Epub 2010 Sep 8.

Gudding R, McDonald JS, Cheville NF.1984.Pathogenesis of Staphylococcus aureus mastitis: bacteriologic, histologic, and ultrastructural pathologic findings.Am J Vet Res. **45:** 2525-2531

Hajek, V. 1971. The differentiation of pathogenic staphylococci and a suggestion for their taxonomic classification Zentralbe Bacteriol. Parasitekde (Abt 1 orig) **217a:** 176-182.

Hogen, J.S., White, D.G. and Pankey, J.W. 1987. Effect of teat dipping on intramammory infections by staphylococci other than *S.aureus*. J. Dairy Sci.**70:** 873-879.

Iyori K, Hisatsune J, Kawakami T, Shibata S, Murayama N, Ide K, Nagata M, Fukata T, Iwasaki T, Oshima K, Hattori M, Sugai M, Nishifuji K.2010.Identification of a novel Staphylococcus pseudintermedius exfoliative toxin gene and its prevalence in isolates from canines with pyoderma and healthy dogs. FEMS Microbiol Lett. **12:** 169-175

Jonsson, P. and Wadstrom, T. 1993. Staphylococcus. In Pathogenesis of Bacterial Infections in animals Ed. C.L. Gyles and C.O. Thoen pp21-35. Iowa State University Press, Ames, U.S.A.

Jarp, J. 1991. Classification of coagulase negative staphylococci isolated from bovine clinical and sub-clinical mastitis. Vet. Microbiol. **27:** 151-158.

Kanbar T., Voytenko A.V., Alber J., Lämmler C., Weiss R. and Skvortzov V.N.2008.Distribution of the putative virulence factor encoding gene sheta in Staphylococcus hyicus strains of various origins. J. Vet. Sci. **9:** 327-329.

Kato F, Kadomoto N, Iwamoto Y, Bunai K, Komatsuzawa H, Sugai M..2011.The Regulatory Mechanism for Exfoliative Toxin Production in Staphylococcus aureus. Infect Immun. Jan 31 [http://www.ncbi.nlm.nih.gov/pubmed/21282415].

Kumar R., Yadav BR., Anand S.K. and Singh R.S.2011.Molecular surveillance of putative virulence factors and antibiotic resistance in Staphylococcus aureus isolates recovered from intra-mammary infections of river buffaloes. Microb. Pathog.. 2011 Apr 1. [http://www.ncbi.nlm.nih.gov/pubmed/21440053].

Kumar R., Yadav B.R. and Singh R.S.2010.Genetic determinants of antibiotic resistance in Staphylococcus aureus isolates from milk of mastitic crossbred cattle. Curr. Microbiol. **60:** 379-386. Epub 2009 Dec 3.

Kumar R., Yadav B.R. and Singh RS.2011.Antibiotic resistance and pathogenicity factors in Staphylococcus aureus isolated from mastitic Sahiwal cattle. J. Biosci. 2011 **36:** 175-188.

Kuroda M, Yamashita A, Hirakawa H, Kumano M, Morikawa K, Higashide M, Maruyama A, Inose Y, Matoba K, Toh H, Kuhara S, Hattori M, Ohta T.2005.Whole genome sequence of Staphylococcus saprophyticus reveals the pathogenesis of uncomplicated urinary tract infection. Proc Natl Acad Sci U.S.A. **102:** 13272-13277.

Matsuoka E, Tanaka Y, Kuroda M, Shouji Y, Ohta T, Tanaka I, Yao M.2011.Crystal structure of the functional region of Uro-adherence factor A from Staphylococcus saprophyticus reveals participation of the B domain in ligand binding. Protein Sci. **20:** 406-416.

Nagahata H., Kawai H., Yuki W., Higuchi H., Kawai K., Yayou K. and Chang C.J.2011.Altered Leukocyte Responsiveness in Dairy Cows with Naturally Occurring Chronic Staphylococcus aureus Mastitis. J. Vet. Med. Sci. Mar 11. [http://www.ncbi.nlm.nih.gov/pubmed/21415573].

Nawrotek P, Borkowski J, Boroñ-Kaczmarska A, Furowicz AJ.2005. [The characteristics of staphylococcal enterotoxins produced by strains isolated from mastitic cows, including epidemiological aspects]. Przegl Epidemiol. **9:** 891-902.

Nofrarías M., Pujols J., Segalés J., Gibert X. and Majó N.2006.Changes in peripheral blood leukocyte populations in pigs with naturally occurring exudative epidermitis. Res. Vet. Sci. **81:** 211-214. Epub 2006 Feb 20.

Oliveira M., Bexiga R., Nunes S.F., Carneiro C., Cavaco L.M., Bernardo F. and Vilela C.L.2006.Biofilm-forming ability profiling of Staphylococcus aureus and Staphylococcus epidermidis mastitis isolates. Vet. Microbiol. **118:** 133-140. Epub 2006 Aug 21.

Oliveira M., Bexiga R., Nunes S.F. and Vilela C.L.2011.Invasive potential of biofilm-forming Staphylococci bovine subclinical mastitis isolates. J .Vet. Sci. **12:** 95-97.

Phillips, W.E. Jr. and Kloos, W.E. Identification of coagulase positive *staphylococcus intermedius* and *Staphylococcus hyicus* subsp. *hyicus* isolated from veterinary clinical specimens. J. Clin. Microbiol. **14:** 671-673.

Pyörälä S, Taponen S.2009.Coagulase-negative staphylococci-emerging mastitis pathogens. Vet Microbiol. **134:** 3-8.

.Qiu J, Luo M, Dong J, Wang J, Li H, Wang X, Deng Y, Feng H, Deng X.2011.Menthol diminishes *Staphylococcus aureus* virulence-associated extracellular proteins expression. Appl Microbiol Biotechnol. 2011 Feb 2[http://www.ncbi.nlm.nih.gov/pubmed/21287163].

Radostitis, O.M., Blood, D.C. and Gay, C.C. 1994. Mastitis caused by miscellaneous staphylococci: In veterinary medicine. A text book of the diseases of cattle, sheep, pigs, goats and horses. Pp. 577-582. ECBS with Bailliere Tindall. The Bath Press, Avon, Great Britain.

Sawant A.A., Gillespie B.E. and Oliver S.P.2009.Antimicrobial susceptibility of coagulase-negative Staphylococcus species isolated from bovine milk. Vet. Microbiol. **134:** 73-81. Epub 2008 Sep 11.

Stevens DL, Ma Y, Salmi DB, McIndoo E, Wallace RJ, Bryant AE. 2007.Impact of antibiotics on expression of virulence-associated exotoxin genes in methicillin-sensitive and methicillin-resistant Staphylococcus aureus. J Infect Dis. **195**(2): 202-211.

Taponen S, Björkroth J, Pyörälä S. 2008.Coagulase-negative staphylococci isolated from bovine extramammary sites and intramammary infections in a single dairy herd. J Dairy Res. **75:** 422-429.

Taponen S, Pyörälä S. 2009.Coagulase-negative staphylococci as cause of bovine mastitis-not so different from Staphylococcus aureus? Vet. Microbiol. **134:** 29-36.

Tse H, Tsoi HW, Leung SP, Urquhart IJ, Lau SK, Woo PC, Yuen KY.2011.Complete genome sequence of the veterinary pathogen Staphylococcus pseudintermedius strain HKU10-03 isolated from a case of canine pyoderma. J Bacteriol. 2011 Jan 28. [http://www.ncbi.nlm.nih.gov/pubmed/21278300].

Tollersrud T., Nørstebø P.E., Engvik J.P., Andersen S.R., Reitan L.J. and Lund A. 2002. Antibody responses in sheep vaccinated against Staphylococcus aureus mastitis: a comparison of two experimental vaccines containing different adjuvants. Vet Res Commun. **26:** 587-600.

Vasudevan P., Nair M.K., Annamalai T. and Venkitanarayanan K.S.2003.Phenotypic and genotypic characterization of bovine mastitis isolates of Staphylococcus aureus for biofilm formation. Vet Microbiol. **92:** 179-185.

Weese JS, van Duijkeren E. 2010.Methicillin-resistant Staphylococcus aureus and *Staphylococcus pseudintermedius* in veterinary medicine. Vet Microbiol., **140:** 418-429.

Xu H., Hu C., Gong R., Chen Y., Ren N., Xiao G., Xie Q., Zhang M., Liu Q., Guo A. and Chen H.2011.Evaluation of a novel chimeric B cell epitope-based vaccine (rSip-ClfA) in mice against mastitis induced by either Streptococcus agalactiae or Staphylococcus aureus. Clin. Vaccine Immunol. Apr 20. [http://www.ncbi.nlm.nih.gov/pubmed/21508165].

Yamaguchi T., Nishifuji K., Sasaki M., Fudaba Y., Aepfelbacher M., Takata T., Ohara M., Komatsuzawa H., Amagai M. and Sugai M.2002.Identification of the Staphylococcus aureus etd pathogenicity island which encodes a novel exfoliative toxin, ETD, and EDIN-B. Infect. Immun. **70:** 5835-5845.

□□□

Chapter 2

Listeriosis

Dr. S.K. SRIVASTAVA
Former, Division of Bacteriology & Mycology
Indian Veterinary Research Institute, Izatnagar-243122
Bareilly (U.P.)

Listeriosis is a acute disease of animals caused by the genus Listeria. Clinical symptom commonly associated with listeriosis are fever, encephalitis, abortion, stillbirth and septicaemia, mastitis, spinal myelitis or keratoconjuctivitis. Encephalitis is most frequently encountered in ruminants. It was first reported by Mahajan in 1936 under the circling disease amongst the sheep. However, the first documented case of listeriosis due to *L.monocytogenes* was reported in 1950 from sheep in Madras (Vishwanathan and Ayyer 1950). It has also been isolated from pigs (Rahman *et al.* 1985), goats (Katiyar 1960, Dutta & Malik 1978), buffaloes (Namboothiripad etal. 1978) and infertile cows (Srivastava etal 1985). *Listeria ivanovii* has been reported from cases of abortion in sheep in Himanchal Pradesh (Sharma etal 1996), endometritis cases in sheep and goats (Mahajan & Katoch 1997) and also from an outbreak of abortion in a flock of 254 crossbred sheep in Hisar, India (Chand and Sadana 1999). It has been reported by Dhanda *et al.* 1959 & Sharma *et al.* 1996. Aghi *et al.* (2004) showed the presence of several Listeria spp. in samples of faces and manure from cattle, sheep & poultry and sewage in India. These studies have shown a low prevalence of the disease. The high prevalence of *Listeria* spp., including *L. monocytogenes,* in the farm environments may favor emergence and evolution of novel, and possibly more virulent, *L. monocytogenes* strains. Continued monitoring of animal listeriosis cases and outbreaks may not only improve animal health but also aid in the early discovery of newly emerging *L. monocytogenes* strains.

Etiology

Listeria genus includes 6 species. *L.monocytogenes* and *L.ivanovi* are pathogenic, whereas *L. innocua, L.grayi, L.welshimeri* and *L.seeligeri* are regarded as non-pathogenic species. *L.monocytogenes* has 13 serovars of which serovar 4b is most commonly associated with major outbreaks (Yadav & Rao 2009). Initial EcoRI ribotyping and serotyping indicated that an outbreak was caused by an unusual L. monocytogenes serotype 4b strain, which was classified into lineage III. Further characterization of this isolate by DNA sequencing-based subtyping methods indicated that the strain responsible for this outbreak represented a unique genotype as supported by its classification into a new sigB allelic type, which has not been identified previously among >290 isolates, and by compelling phylogenetic evidence. While lineage III isolates are generally rare, they seem to be more common among L. monocytogenes isolates from animals with clinical signs of listeriosis (Bundrant *et al.* 2011).4b is also a major serovar associated with ruminant listeriosis (Farber and Peterkin 1991). Listeria is a gram positive, non-sporulating rods arranged in palisades in smears from young culture. The organisms are motile due to peritrichous flagella. Optimal growth temperature is between 30 to 37°C but the organism can grow and reproduce at temperature between -0.4°C and 45°C. It can grow between pH 4.5 and 9.6 although growth at low pH is minimal at low temperatures. The organisms grow well under aerobic conditions but growth is better in an atmosphere containing 10% CO_2.

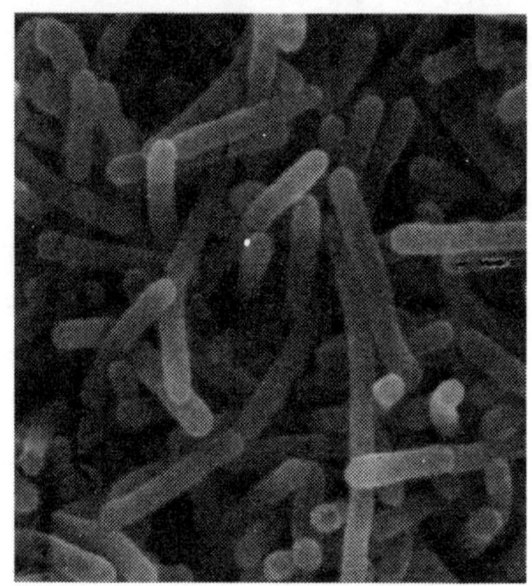
Listeria monocytogenes

Growth is rich in the presence of blood, serum or glucose. On blood agar, *L. monocytogenes* produces a narrow zone of beta haemolysis. The organism also produce a CAMP reaction with *Staphylococcus aureus* and *Rhodococcus equi*. Virulence cluster of *Listeria* spp. comprise of 6 coherent chromosomal genes encoding 2 phospholipases cytolysin, a metalloprotein and a surface protein Act A. Beta haemolysis (Cytolysin) seems to be the property of virulent strains only. This haemolysin is termed as listeriolysin O which is believed to be a major virulence factor. It is a 58 kDa protein. Virulent strains can also be identified on their basis to multiply in macrophages and monocytes.

Listeriosis is primarily a disease of ruminants particularly sheep although other livestock animals such as horses and pigs may also be affected.

Encephalitis (Circling disease) is the most common manifestation in sheep. Abortion storms may also be caused in animals.

The disease is common and assumes epidemic proportion in many countries of North America, Europe and Austria. In India it is a common problem of sheep.

The disease has been reported either as a single case or outbreaks which occurs sporadically. Abortions are more common in cattle with an attack rate which frequently reaches 10% (Radostits *et al.* 1994). Braun *et al.* (2002) reported listeriosis in sheep and goats showing typical clinical symptoms viz. Vestibular ataxia, circling, head tilt and unilateral cranial nerve deficits. Evans *et al.* (2004) reported eye infection in 3 cattle and a horse due to *L.monocytogenes*. Septicaemia is usually rare in animals except in non-ruminants. Spinal myelitis is recorded as occurring in 0.8-2.5% of sheep in affected flock and in all ages of sheep (Seaman *et al.* 1990). Other manifestations of the disease are conjunctivitis, pneumonia, mycocarditis, endocarditis and still birth. It is also reported in human beings. In poultry the disease usually causes sudden death particularly among young birds. Healthy carriers are frequently seen. A common finding at necropsy is the presence of multiple areas of degeneration in the heart muscle, focal necrosis in the liver and kidneys and generalized oedema. Occasionally CNS is involved. It swine it usually takes form of acute disease characterized by meningoencephalitis. The symptoms are fever, trembling and a stilled gait affecting particularly the forelegs. Some animals suffer from dyspnoea and cough and abortion may occur during pregnancy. Septicaemia is most frequently.

Epidemiology

Listeria organisms are ubiquitous in environment and can be commonly isolated from feces, sewerage, sludge, soil, silage, surface water, plants, animal feed and other farm environments. In a study carried out in Gujrat state, Listeria was reported to be isolated from 16 samples out of 1002 studied. *L.monocytogenes* from 7 & *L. innocua* was isolated for 9 samples comprised of blood, fecal swabs, vaginal swabs (Yadav and Roy, 2009). In temperate climates the prevalence of *L.monocytogenes* in the feces of ruminants appear to vary with the season. It also increases during period of environmental stress and due to stress of lambing. The number of organisms in the feces is influenced by the number present in the feed. Sheep experimentally fed *Listeria* organisms were found to have the organisms in the fore stomach within 4 hours of feeding and whole GI tract with in 24 hours. Fecal shedding lasted for 10 days. The organism persisted in retro-pharyngeal lymph nodes for 14 days. The organisms were present in all the organs of stomach but not gall bladder (Zundel & Bernard, 2006). Gastrointestinal listeriosis is common in sheep (Otter *et al.* 2004). In the septicaemic form and abortion, ingestion of pathogens appears to be the way the organisms are transmitted to the animals. The encephalitic form of the disease results from the infection of the terminals of the trigeminal nerves due to abrasions of the buccal mucosa from course feed or from the infected food cavities. The number of microorganisms in feed and their massive multiplication appears to a factor that increases risk factor, although the feeding of contaminated grass or silage is the major risk factor. Silage seems to provide a suitable environment for growth and maintenance of L.monocytogenes. Low quality silage having a pH of more than 4.0 is more likely to harbour *L. monocytogenes* than good quality silage with pH of less than 4.0. An association between silage consumption and listeriosis in ruminants was first recognized in 1922, when investigators warned of a disease resembling listeriosis known in Iceland as "votheysveiki," or silage sickness

Risk factors involve those factors which lower the immune status of animals such as poor nutritional status, sudden changes of weather, stress of late pregnancy and parturition. Over crowding and unsanitary conditions also predisposes the animals to listeriosis.

Most of the animals may carry the organism in the feces; however, the number may vary based on several factors. It is difficult to enumerate the number of bacteria in faces. The main potential hazard to humans and animals is due to shedding of bacteria that can then persist in the environment and be aerosolized. A non-negligible proportion of seronegative animals that delivered normally could excrete *C. burnetii*. The organisms may also be present in milk of the animals and may serve as carriers and infect their offspring soon after the birth. Rodolakis *et al.*(2007) studied the shedding of Coxiella burnetii in bovine, caprine, and ovine milk using PCR, in 3 herds for each species, the bulk tank milk samples of which were positive at the time of their selection. Milk samples of 95 cows, 120 goats, and 90 ewes were sampled over 16 wk, as was the bulk tank milk. The shedding of *C. burnetii* in vaginal mucus and feces was checked at the beginning of the experiment and 2 months later. The clinical signs in the selected herds as well as the duration and the shedding routes differed among the 3 species. The cows were asymptomatic and shed *C. burnetii* almost exclusively in milk. In one of the caprine herds, abortions due to *C. burnetii* were reported. The goats excreted the bacteria mainly in milk. In contrast, the ewes, which came from flocks with abortions due to Q fever (*C. burnetii* infection), shed the bacteria mostly in feces and in vaginal mucus. This could explain why human outbreaks of Q fever are more often related to ovine flocks than to bovine herds. These excretions did not seem more frequent when the samples were taken close to parturition. The samples were taken from 0 to 421 d after parturition in bovine herds and from 5 to 119 d and 11 to 238 d after parturition in the caprine and ovine herds, respectively. The shedding in milk was sometimes intermittent, and several animals shed the bacteria but were negative by ELISA: 80% of the ewes were seronegative, underscoring the lack of sensitivity of the ELISA tests available for veterinary diagnosis. The detection of antibodies in milk seems more sensitive than it is in serum. Pease (1967) reported that the bacteria are carried as L form unable to be detected by common bacteriological methods. However, in case the immunological status is lowered due to above listed causes the disease may occur.

The high number of healthy carriers are also implicated from meat hygiene point of view. Meat may act as source of infection to human. Meat and vegetables fertilized with animal manure are important source of contamination for humans. Carrier animals are source of infection for human beings (Borucki *et al.* 2004).

Pathogenesis

Ingestion of the causative agent is the main route of infection for animals. It is usually through the silage or other contaminated food may be involved. The infection has a "epithelial phase" in which they penetrates the epithelial cells and readily multiply, thus being protected from phagocytosis by leukocytes and antibodies (Racz etal 1972). Excessive multiplication damages the epithelial cells, releasing the bacteria which are later phagocytozed by the polymorphonuclear cells and macrophages. Listeria being a facultative intracellular pathogen stay in the phagosomes for a while. Bacterial superoxide dismutase protects against the bactericidal activity of the respiratory burst of phagocytes and listerolysin O disrupts lysosomal membrane allowing organisms to grow in the cytoplasm. This causes severe degeneration and destruction of the epithelial cells because of the release of toxic phagosome contents (Lysosomal enzymes). The *Listeria* cell wall, a 80kDa surface protein internalin, interacts with a epithelial cell receptor protein, E-cadherin which facilitates phagocytosis into phagocytic cells and endocytosis in non-phagocytic cells. Subsequently, the haemolytic enzyme, listeriolysin O, is produced in phagosomes that lyse the cholesterol containing membranes of the cells thus allowing bacteria to escape into the cytoplasm of host cells. There are evidence that gamma interferon treated activated cells restricts the ability of *L.monocytogenes* to escape from phagolysosome (Portnoy etal 1989). This is followed by the polymerization of host cell action which moves them to the cell membrane where they push against the cell and produces protrusions. This is followed by ingestion of cells protrusions by adjacent macrophages and other cells. The *Listeria* are subsequently released and multiply to repeat the cycle. Lecithinase produced by *L.monocytogenes* may play a role in cell to cell spread by lysing the cell membrane of the host and temperature regulated positive regulatory factor which coordinates the expression of several virulence associated genes. The macrophage activation might prevent the intracellular multiplication of listriae as well increase the ability of macrophages to investigate ingested organisms. In additions to the cells described above, various soluble mediators play a role in anti-listeria resistance. Experimental studies have shown that gamma-IFN, IL-1, 1L-2, TNF-α, GM-CSF enhance experimental resistance in mice.

L. monocytogenes is able to survive inside macrophages by escaping into the cytoplasm from the phagosome by virtue of a 58-kDa listeriolysin O (LLO) and several enzymes encoded by genes located adjacent to the *hly* gene coding for LLO.

LLO, the major virulence factor of *L. monocytogenes*, shows a pH-dependent hemolytic activity , and this activity is blocked by oxidation or small amounts of cholesterol. The ability to produce LLO is unique to virulent strains of *L. monocytogenes*), and the LLO-producing, virulent strain has been shown to induce the expression of various cytokines in the infected host, such as tumor necrosis factor alpha (TNF-α), interleukin-1α (IL-1α), IL-6, and gamma interferon (IFN-γ). These inflammatory cytokines produced during the early stage of infection with *L. monocytogenes* are believed to be necessary for the nonspecific protection of mice. Though inflammatory cytokines may contribute to the protection to some extent, nonspecific protection never results in the complete clearance of replicating bacteria, and the generation of antigen-specific, T-cell-mediated immunity is required for the complete resolution and establishment of long-lived acquired protection. Using various *Listeria* strains with different LLO production abilities, it has been shown that the generation of cell-mediated acquired immunity in mice is achieved after infection with LLO-producing, virulent strains but not with the LLO-nonproducing [LLO (-)] strain or killed bacteria.

Barlow and McGoran (1985) reported that sheep under high risk environmental conditions, a breach in the integrity of the buccal dental terminals of trigeminal nerves is caused or by shedding of permanent or desiduous teeth or periodontitis. *Listeria* thus penetrates alveoli and reach the fine dental terminals of the trigeminal nerves thereafter moving centripetally towards the brain via an intracellular route being shielded from the host immune system. Bacteria move within individual nerve fasciculi while traveling towards the brain stem (Charlton & Garcia 1977). The cells then move along nerve fiber tracts in axoplasm. Damaged neurons are also visible. At this stage induction of type IV reaction results in pathologic lesions in the brain of calves (Kuchembuck 1978).

Iron seems to play an important role in *Listeria* pathogenesis. In hosts treated with iron supports *Listeria* multiply rapidly and to greater extent than non-treated animals (Sword 1966). Feeding of silage also probably increases the serum iron which seems to decrease the immunity. Serum proteins also seems to be effected by the feeding of silage. The encephalitis in sheep is usually unilateral. Spread of infection along the optic nerve may result in endophthalmitis in sheep and cattle.

Abortion in sheep due to *L.ivanovii* has only been recorded as a sporadic disease in cattle similar to *L.monocytogenes*. Out breaks are recorded in sheep and are manifested with abortions, still birth but particularly with the birth of live infected lambs which soon die. The uterus of probably all the animals is susceptible to the infection at all stages of pregnancy which can result in placentitis, metritis, fetal infection & neonatal death. The metritis has little or no effect on subsequent reproduction, however, *Listeria* may be shed for one month or more via vagina and milk. Abortion usually occurs during the last trimester of pregnancy. Listeriosis is also responsible for subclinical mastitis in cattle. In a study cases suffered from a subclinical mastitis characterized by an elevated somatic cell count, a persistent shedding of *Listeria* and by a normal appearance of the milk. The animals did not show any systemic reaction, but all animals developed an atrophy of the infected mammary gland. Histological examinations revealed a chronic interstitial mastitis with diffuse infiltration of lymphocytes, plasma cells and macrophages. All internal organs showed no abnormalities, no *Listeria* could be isolated. *Listeria* could however be isolated from the affected mammary parenchyma and from the mammary lymph node. The results of the bacteriological examination could be confirmed by means of PCR. Using PFGE, all the isolates from the same animal were identical. Immunohistochemical examination of the ovine mammary glands achieved a very strong immunoreactivity for CD5 cells (Winters *et al.* (2004).

Diagnosis

Often the clinical symptoms and signs are characteristic of listeriosis in animals. Meningo-encephalitis can be difficult to diagnose, but occurring of circling disease in sheep is quite characteristic. It is accompanied with blinking of eye lids appearing intermittently and flaccid lips. The most important changes are an increase in leukocytes with dominance of macrophages and lymphocytes and an increase in glucose and total protein (Gronstol 1986) *L.monocytogenes* is rarely isolated from the cerebrospinal fluid. This is often marked with ketonuria. The CSF has an increased protein concentration and a mild pleocytosis composed of macrophages. *L.monocytogenes* can be isolated from medulla and brain stem of dead animals. A cold enrichment of brain samples for 1 month may help in isolation of organism particularly when the concentration of organism is low due to antibiotic treatment.

Isolations of organisms from cases of abortions are often successful. Organisms are isolated from internal organs of aborted foetus. The organisms can be isolated from vaginal secretions for up to 2 weeks. Cases of mastitis may be acute, chronic or symptomless. One or more teat or sometime the entire udder may be affected. Isolation of *L.monocytogenes* from mastitic udder is easy. In cases of septicaemia attempts may be made to isolate the organisms from feces, urine and milk of the infected animals.

Cultural examination of *Listeria* is not difficult. Special media are not required. Use of blood agar or tryptose agar is preferred. However, for processing of samples such as feces, vaginal secretions, food and environmental samples the use of selective media is necessary. Media, requiring cold enrichment before isolation should be preferably Brain heart infusion, Tryptose Phosphate broth or Thioglycollate medium supplemented with selective substances such as nalidixic acid, polymyxin or cycloheximide are used. Where injured organisms are likely to be present, a pre-enrichment step is required (Curtis and Lee 1995). Listeria colonies are small, smooth and beta haemolytic and the organisms show tumbling motility when observed following growth on nutrient broth. The pathogen can be isolated from blood, cerebrospinal fluid, aborted fetus, feces, vomitus & vaginal secretions of infected individuals. Identification of organism is based on biochemical methods and serotyping. The detection of antibodies to listeriolysin O has been suggested to be a useful test for serodiagnosis in cattle (Barbuddhe 1996) and buffaloes (Shakuntala *et al.* 2007). The immunopotential for serodiagnosis of phosphatidylinositol - specific phospholipase C was found to be weaker than listeriolysin O (Chaudhuri *et al.* 2001).

Immunofluorescence is effective for rapid identification of *L.monocytogenes* in smears from animals died or aborted of listeriosis and from milk, meat and other sources. Serological tests viz; agglutination and complement fixation tests have been used. Usually a titer of 1:200 is observed in normal animals. Therefore, titers higher than this are suggestive of clinical disease. In sheep, the titers way persist for years which may return to normal after abortion with in a month's period. ELISA may prove more reliable for diagnostic and investigative purpose. Bourry *et al.* (1997) Carried out serological diagnosis of bovine, caprine, and ovine mastitis caused by *Listeria monocytogenes* by using an enzyme-linked immunosorbent assay. Using goat and ewe milk samples, the sensitivity and specificity of the test were 100 and 88%, respectively. Barbuddhe *et al.* (2002) successfully studied the occurrence of Listeria monocytogenes in meat and milk samples, and antilisteriolysin O (ALLO) antibodies in sera of buffaloes.Recently, a immunohistochemistry technique has been reported to be an improved diagnostic tool than cultural examination in ruminants affected with encephalitis (Loeb 2004). Several polymerase chain reactions have also been standardized for the diagnosis (Norton 2002). A combined serological and PCR method for the detection of Listeria monocytogenes infection in symptomatic and asymptomatic ovine flocks was evaluated (Amagliani *et al.* 2006). Seventy-eight milk samples and 157 serum samples were analysed using a *L. monocytogenes* PCR detection kit and an anti-listeriolysin O IgG immunoassay kit. The combined use of these commercial kits allowed a rapid and effective detection of *L. monocytogenes* infection in both the early stage, before seroconversion, and in a later phase, even after antibiotic therapy.

Treatment and Control

L.monocytogenes is susceptible to penicillin, erythromycin and trimethoprim/sulfonamide. High doses are required to be given because the organisms reside in brain and it is not possible to achieve higher minimum concentration in brain if high doses are not given. Antibiotics should be started as soon as the disease is suspected. However, considering the cost involved it may not be advisable. Mastitis has proven refractory to treatment in several instances. Other antibiotics such as oxytetracyclin, gentamycin are also effective. Cephalosporins are not recommended. If latent udder infection occur, significant number of listeriae might be shed in the milk following parturition. In case of abortions the cow may clear the infection without treatment. For control use of silage should be restricted or at least well fermented silage should be given for consumption. The animals should be tested for fecal shedding and the shedders should be segregated and periodically tested. Low levels of tetracyclines are recommended as a control measure.

Since silage feeding is a major risk factor preparation of good quality silage itself reduces the cases of listeriosis. While making the silage soil contamination should be avoided when filling the clamp. Use of additives to improve fermentation is useful. Decayed silage, silage with pH above than 5.0 or an ash content of more than 70mg/kg of dry matter should be avoided.

There is no satisfactory vaccine for listeriosis. In India no vaccine is used although in Norway a live attenuated vaccine has been in use in sheep since last many years. The use of this vaccine has reduced the incidence in sheep from 4% to 1.5%. Commercial killed vaccines are available in some countries. At farms where feeding of silage is essential use of an autogenous killed vaccine may be given to control the cases of listeriosis. Dong *et al.*(2009) compared, in a mouse model, the immunogenicity of *Listeria monocytogenes* that were lethally inactivated by gamma-irradiation, traditional heat or formalin treatment.

BALB/c mice were inoculated intraperitoneally with these killed vaccine The serum antibody level of mice inoculated with gamma-irradiated LM was the highest, up to 1:1280 as determined by ELISA, while the level of mice immunized with heat-killed or formalin-killed LM was 1:640 or 1:160, respectively. The protective efficacy of gamma-irradiated,heat-killed or formalin-killed vaccines candidates were 100%, 35% or 30%. As judged by the bacterial elimination in the organs, mice inoculated with gamma-irradiated LM were the most efficiently protected group. Adoptive T cell transfer assay showed that gamma-irradiated LM can trigger T cell protective immune response. The results indicated the superiority of gamma-irradiation over traditional heat or formalin treatment in generating LM killed vaccine candidate. gamma-irradiation may be applied to numerous bacterial vaccine candidates, and could have important potential in development of killed vaccines. Datta *et al.* (2006) evaluated gamma-irradiated Listeria monocytogenes as a killed bacterial vaccine, testing the hypothesis that irradiation preserves antigenic and adjuvant structures destroyed by traditional heat or chemical inactivation. Irradiated Listeria monocytogenes (LM), unlike heat-killed LM, efficiently activated dendritic cells via Toll-like receptors and induced protective T cell responses in mice. Like live LM, irradiated LM induced Toll-like-receptor-independent T cell priming. Cross-presentation of irradiated listerial antigens to CD8(+) T cells involved TAP- and proteasome-dependent cytosolic antigen processing. These results establish that killed LM can induce protective T cell responses, previously thought to require live infection. Gamma-irradiation may be potentially applied to numerous bacterial vaccine candidates, and irradiated bacteria could serve as a vaccine platform for recombinant antigens derived from other pathogens, allergens, or tumors.

However, since *Listeria* is an intracellular pathogen use of live attenuated vaccines is most effective than killed vaccines. *Listeria monocytogenes* virulence and the capacity for inducing specific protection is ensured by the protein listeriolysin O. The importance of gamma-interferon, tumor necrosis factor alpha, interleukin 12 and other mediators in ensuring the differentiation of (CD4(+) T-cells into Th1-helpers and cytotoxic *T-lymphocytes* in animals infected with L. monocytogenes is described in detail. Hopeful results have been obtained in experiments on the immunization of mice with killed bacteria with listeriolysin O or interleukin 12. Works describing the use of modified *L. monocytogenes* strains as vectors for the creation of vaccines against different infections seem to show good prospects. It is known that only listeriolysin O (LLO)-producing Listeria monocytogenes strains are able to induce protective immunity, but the underlining relationship between LLO produced by virulent strains and generation of protective immunity in the infected host remains poorly understood. In the present study, it was found that LLO gene expression was only detected in the mice infected with virulent strain which was able to induce protective immunity, while non-virulent strains or killed bacteria were not able to generate protective immunity. When mice were immunized with LLO plus killed bacteria in the presence of incomplete Freund's adjuvant, the protective immunity was partially generated, and adoptive transfer experiment confirmed that this protection was antigen specific (Xiong *et al.*,1998). Reverse-transcription polymerase chain reaction revealed that LLO plus killed bacteria induced the expression of interferon-gamma (IFN-gamma) and interleukin-12 (IL-12). These results also showed CD4+ T cells were the principal cells constituting protective immunity. Taken together, it may be concluded that LLO produced from virulent strains of *L. monocytogenes* was essential for the generation of protective immunity, and that LLO plus killed bacteria induced IFN-gamma and IL-12 expression which resulted in the generation of protective immunity.

Miller *et al.* (1996) demonstrated the striking potentiating effects of IL-12 when it is combined with listerial immunogens. Although LM alone does not elicit strong T-cell responses, the results presented here demonstrate that the combination of LM and IL-12 elicited vigorous Listeria-specific Th1-type T-cell responses when administered intraperitoneally. The intensity of these responses, as well as the cytokine profiles of the Listeria-specific peritoneal T cells and macrophages, was remarkably similar to that of Listeria-infected/ immune mice. These studies also revealed that typically nonimmunogenic forms of soluble listerial antigen preparations (cLLO, SLP) and LLO peptide homologs elicited intense Listeria-specific T-cell responses when administered with IL-12. In conjunction with the generation of specific T-cell responses following injection of IL-12 in combination with either killed Listeria or soluble listerial antigen preparations, macrophages from these mice expressed upregulated quantities of class II MHC and produced increased amounts of IL-12 following restimulation in vitro. Protection studies established that the Listeria-specific T-cell responses elicited by the HKLM + IL-12 mixture conferred protective immunity of mice to a lethal dose of viable L. monocytogenes. Studies designed to investigate the regulation of IL-12 production by peritoneal macrophages revealed that activated macrophages are particularly sensitive to bacterial products. However, nonviable or replication-incompetent bacteria or bacterial products injected alone were unable to influence the ability of macrophages to produce IL-12. The ability of activated macrophages to respond to HKLM was dramatically upregulated upon addition of IFN-gamma and markedly downregulated in the presence of the Th2 cytokines, IL-4 and IL-10. In light of what is known about the ability of IL-12 to induce IFN-gamma production by NK cells and gamma delta T cells, these results suggest that the exogenous addition of IL-12 may help initiate a cytokine cascade which enables the immune system to interact productively with an antigen that is typically nonimmunogenic when administered alone. These findings demonstrate that IL-12 may prove to be a powerful and broadly useful adjuvant component of particulate and soluble antigen-based vaccines directed towards many types of intracellular pathogenic microorganisms. Subsequently, Miller *et al.*(1998) demonstrated that multiple injections of heat-killed L. monocytogenes and IL-12 elicit memory responses that confer long-lived (> or = 3 months) protective immunity and that immunity can be transferred adoptively with cells from immunized mice injected into naive mice. These studies have also demonstrated that the powerful adjuvanticity of IL-12 is observed with soluble as well as particulate immunogens and is operative in mouse strains that have different MHC haplotypes. These findings suggest that IL-12 may be a useful adjuvant component of vaccines for a wide variety of pathogens in animal and human systems.

Significant research has been done in the area of vaccination in man using mice model. In a study mice were immunized with L. monocytogenes , an LLO-nonproducing avirulent strain, along with LLO encapsulated in liposome (LLO-liposome). LLO-liposome was highly potent in the induction of various cytokines, including IFN-gamma. Immunization of mice with either LLO-liposome or the viable strain ATCC 15313 alone did not induce protection against challenge infection (Tanabe *et al.*1999). In contrast, the combination of LLO-nonproducing bacteria plus LLO-liposome induced a significant level of protective immunity mediated mainly by Th1-type cells capable of producing a large amount of IFN-gamma in an antigen-specific manner. The protection afforded by the combination was not dependent on LLO-specific cytotoxic T cells. These results support the idea that the inability of an LLO-nonproducing avirulent strain or killed bacteria to induce the generation of protective T cells is due not to the lack of a central T-cell epitope(s) but to the lack of ability to induce the production of endogenous cytokine during the early stage of immunization; the results also suggest that an appropriate use of LLO at least in an animal model may be effective in the induction of antigen-specific Th1-dependent protective immunity to various kinds of intracellular parasitic bacteria.

Whether IFN-gamma contributes to the per-cell protective capacity of memory CD8(+) T cells againstLM has not been formally tested. Messingham *et al.* (2007) generated LM Ag-specific memory CD8(+) T cells via immunization of wild-type (WT) and IFN-gamma-deficient (gamma knockout (GKO)) mice with LM peptide-coated dendritic cells and compared them phenotypically and functionally. Immunization of WT and GKO mice resulted in memory CD8(+) T cells that were similar in number, functional avidity, TCR repertoire use, and memory phenotype. The protective capacity of memory CD8(+) T cells from immunized WT and GKO mice was evaluated after adoptive transfer of equal numbers of WT or GKO cells into naive BALB/c mice followed by LM challenge. The adoptively transferred CD8(+) T cells from GKO donors exhibited a decreased ability to reduce bacterial numbers in the organs of recipient mice when compared with an equivalent number of Ag-matched WT CD8(+) T cells. This deficiency was most evident early (day 3) after infection if a relatively low infectious dose was used; however, transferring fewer memory CD8(+) T cells or increasing the LM challenge dose revealed a more pronounced defect in protective immunity mediated by the CD8(+) T cells from GKO mice. These studies identified a decrease in Ag-specific target cell lysis in vivo by CD8(+) T cells from GKO mice as the mechanism for the decreased protective immunity after LM challenge. Further studies suggest that the lack of IFN-gamma production by the Ag-specific CD8 T cells themselves diminishes target cell sensitivity to cytolysis, thereby reducing the lytic potency of IFN-gamma-deficient LM-specific memory CD8(+) T cells.

Bahey *et al.*(2008) utilized L. lactis as a live vector for expression of listeriolysin O (LLO), a major Listeria monocytogenes antigen and virulence factor. A variety of plasmid constructs were designed to permit either constitutive or nisin-inducible expression of secreted or non-secreted LLO in L. lactis. Recombinant strains were subsequently tested in a murine model for vaccination efficacy against L. monocytogenes infection. CD8(+) T lymphocytes specific for the LLO(91-99) epitope were detected when strains were administered via the intraperitoneal (IP) but not the oral route. Challenge with live L. monocytogenes revealed different levels of protection among the three vaccine strains tested with the nisin-inducible LLO-secreting L. lactis strain providing the greatest protection against secondary infection. This work highlights the usefulness of the GRAS (Generally Regarded As Safe) organism L. lactis as the basis of a live vaccine vector against L. monocytogenes. The work suggests that LLO-expressing L. lactis strains may also have the potential to act as a platform for directing other co-expressed antigens towards the cytosolic MHC class I pathway for enhanced stimulation of the CD8(+) T-cell response.The pore-forming haemolysin listeriolysin O (LLO), the main virulence factor of Listeria monocytogenes, allows bacteria to escape from the harsh environment of the phagosome to the cytoplasm of the infected cell. This leads to processing of bacterial antigens predominantly through the cytosolic MHC class I presentation pathway. Bahey -El-Din *et al.*(2010) examined the immune response and protective efficacy of an L. lactis strain co-expressing LLO and a truncated form of the listerial P60 antigen (tP60). Oral immunization revealed no significant protection against listeriosis with L. lactis expressing LLO, tP60 or the combined LLO/tP60. In contrast, intraperitoneal vaccination induced an LLO-specific CD8(+) immune response with LLO-expressing L. lactis but no significant improvement in protection was observed following vaccination with the combined LLO/tP60 expressing L. lactis strain. This may be due to the low level of tP60 expression in the LLO/tP60 strain.

References

Aghi, H.M., Garg, S.R. and Usha, Mandokhot 2004. Occurrence of Listeria in animal fecal matter, farm yard manure and sewage. Indian J. Anim. Sci. **74:** 737-738.

Amagliani G, Giammarini C, Omiccioli E, Merati EG, Pezzotti G, Filippini G, Brandi G, Magnani M.2006. A combination of diagnostic tools for rapid screening of ovine listeriosis. Res Vet Sci. **81:** 185-189.

Bahey-El-Din M, Casey PG, Griffin BT, Gahan CG.2008.Lactococcus lactis-expressing listeriolysin O (LLO) provides protection and specific CD8(+) T cells against Listeria monocytogenes in the murine infection model. Vaccine. **26:** 5304-14. Epub 2008 Aug 6.

Bahey-El-Din M., Casey P.G., Griffin B.T. and Gahan C.G.2010.Expression of two Listeria monocytogenes antigens (P60 and LLO) in Lactococcus lactis and examination for use as live vaccine vectors. J Med Microbiol. **59**(Pt 8): 904-12. Epub 2010 May 20.

Barbuddhe, S.B. 1996. Studies on the kinetics and efficacy of listeriolyin D for the serodiagnosis of *Listeria monocytogenes* infection. Ph.D. thesis submitted to Deemed University, Indian Veterinary Research Institute, Izatnagar, India.

Barbuddhe SB, Chaudhari SP, Malik SV. 2002.The occurrence of pathogenic Listeria monocytogenes and antibodies against listeriolysin-O in buffaloes. J Vet Med B Infect Dis Vet Public Health. **49:** 181-184.

Bourry A, Cochard T, Poutrel B. 1997.Serological diagnosis of bovine, caprine, and ovine mastitis caused by Listeria monocytogenes by using an enzyme-linked immunosorbent assay. Clin Microbiol. 1997 **35:** 1606-1608.

Borucki, M.K., Reynolds, J., Gay C.C. Mc, Elwain, K.L, Kim, S.H., Knowles, D.P. and Hu, J.X. 2004. Dairy farm reservoir of *L.monocytogenes* sporadic and epidemic strains. Jour. Food Protec. **67:** 2496-2499.

Braun, U., Stehle, C. and Ehrensperger, F. 2002. Clinical findings and treatment of listeriosis in 67 sheep & goats. Vet. Rec. **150:** 38-42.

Bundrant BN, Hutchins T, den Bakker HC, Fortes E, Wiedmann M. 2011.Listeriosis outbreak in dairy cattle caused by an unusual Listeria monocytogenes serotype 4b strain. J Vet Diagn Invest. **23:** 155-158.

Chand, P. and Sadana, J.R. 1999. Outbreaks of *Listeria ivanovii* abortion in sheep in India. Vet. Rec. **145:** 83-84.

Charlton, K.M. and Garcia, M.M. 1977. Spontaneous listeric encephalitis and neuritis in sheep. Light microscopic studies. Vet. Pathol. **14:** 297-313.

Chaudhuri, S.P., Malik, S.V.S., Banu Rekha, G. and Barbuddhe, S.B. 2001. Detection of anti-listeriolycin O and *Listeria monocytogenes* in experimentally infected buffaloes. Trop. Anim. Health Prod. **33:** 285-293.

Curtis, G.B.W. and Lee. W.H. 1995. Culture media and methods for isolation of *Listeria monocytogenes*. Int. J. Food Microbiol. **26:** 1-13.

Datta S.K., Okamoto S., Hayashi T., Shin S.S., Mihajlov I., Fermin A., Guiney D.G., Fierer J. and Raz E.2006.Vaccination with irradiated Listeria induces protective T cell immunity. Immunity. **25:** 143-152.

Dhanda, M.R., Lall, S.M., Seth, R.N. and Chandrasekhriah, H. 1959. A case of listeric abortion in an ewe. Indian Vet. J. **36:** 113-123.

Dong H. Jiao X., Pan Z., Yin Y., Sun L. and Liu S.2009. [Immunogenicity comparision of Listeria monocytogenes inactivated by gamma-irradiation or traditional treatments]. Wei Sheng Wu Xue Bao. **49:** 269-73.[Article in Chinese]

Dutt, P.K. and Malik, B.S. 1978. Some epidemiological studies on listeriosis in man and animals in India. Ind. J. Public Health. **22:** 321-322.

Evans, K., Smith, M., McDonough, P., Wiedmann, M. 2004. Eye infections due to *Listeria monocytogenes* in three cows and one horse. Jour. Vet. Diag. Invest. **16:** 464-469.

Farber, J.M. and Peterkin, P.I. 1991. *Listeria monocytogenes*, a food borne pathogen. Microbiol. Rev. **55:** 476-511.

Gronstol, H. 1986. Listeria: In pathogenesis of Bacterial infections of animals. Ed. Gyles C. & C.O. Thoen pp. 48-55. Iowa State University Press, USA.

Katiyar, R.D. 1960. Listeriosis amongst sheep and goats in U.P. Indian Vet. J. **37:** 620-623.

Kuchembuck, M.R. 1978. Immunological, clinical and pathological studies in bovine experimental listeriosis. Ph.D. diss. Univ. of Minnesota, Minneapolis, USA.

Loeb, E. 2004. Encephalitic listeriosis in ruminants: immunohistochemistry as a diagnostic tool. Jour. Vet. Med. **51:** 453-455.

Mahajan, M.R. 1936. Animal Administration Report. V.I.O. Hyderabad (1936-485 37).

Mahajan, M.R. and Katoch, R.C. 1997. Aerobic microbial flora associated with endometritis in sheep and goats. Indian J. Anim. Sci. **67:** 290-291.

Messingham K.A., Badovinac V.P., Jabbari A. and Harty J.T.2007.A role for IFN-gamma from antigen-specific CD8+ T cells in protective immunity to Listeria monocytogenes. J. Immunol. **179:** 2457-2466.

Miller M.A., Skeen M.J. and Ziegler H.K..1996.Protective immunity to Listeria monocytogenes elicited by immunization with heat-killed Listeria and IL-12. Potential mechanism of IL-12 adjuvanticity. Ann. N. Y. Acad. Sci. **797:** 207-227.

Miller M.A., Skeen M.J. and Ziegler H.K.1998.Long-lived protective immunity to Listeria is conferred by immunization with particulate or soluble listerial antigen preparations coadministered with IL-12. Cell. Immunol. **184:** 92-104.

Norton, D.M. 2002. Polymerase chain reaction based methods for detection of *L.monocytogenes*: towards real time screening for food and environmental samples. J. Assoc. Office Anal. Chem. **85:** 505-515.

Otter A, Houlihan MG, Daniel RG, Kirby FD, Schock A, Higgins RJ.2004. Ovine gastrointestinal listeriosis. Vet Rec. **154:** 479.

Pease, P.E. 1967. Tolerated infection with the sub-bacterial phase of Listeria. Nature (London). **215:** 936-938.

Portnoy, D.A., Sehreiber, R.D., Conndly, P. and Titney, L.G. 1989. Gamma-Interferon limits access of *L.monocytogenes* to the macrophage cytoplasm. J. Exp. Med. **170:** 2141-2146.

Racz, P., Tennor, K. and Mero, E. 1972. Experimental Listeria enteritis. An electron microscopic study of the epithelial phase in experimental Listeria infection. Lab Invest. **26:** 694-700.

Radostits, O.M., Blood, D.C. and Gay, C.C. 1994. Listeriosis. In Veterinary Medicine. A text book of the diseases of cattle, sheep, pigs, goats and horses. 660-666; ELBS. Bailliere Tindall, UK.

Rahman, T., Sharma, D.K., Goswami, B.K., Upadhyay, T.N. and Chowdhury, B. 1985. Occurrence of listerial meningoencephalitis in pigs. Indian Vet. J. **62:** 7-9.

Rodolakis A, Berri M, Héchard C, Caudron C, Souriau A, Bodier CC, Blanchard B, Camuset P, Devillechaise P, Natorp JC, Vadet JP, Arricau-Bouvery N.2007.Comparison of Coxiella burnetii shedding in milk of dairy bovine, caprine, and ovine herds. J Dairy Sci. **90:** 5352-5360.

Seaman JT, Carter GI, Carrigan MJ, Cockram FA.1990. An outbreak of listerial myelitis in sheep.Aust Vet J. **67:** 142-143.

Shakuntala, I., Malik. S.V.S., Barbuddhe, S.B. and Rawool 2006. Isolation of *Listeria monocytogenes* from buffaloes with reproductive disorders and its confirmation by polymerase chain reaction. Vet. Microbiol. **117:** 229-234.

Sharma, M., Batta, M.K., Katoch, R.C., Asrani, R.K., Nagal, R.C. and Joshi, V.B. 1996. *Listeria monocytogenes* abortions among migratory sheep and goats in Himanchal Pradesh. Indian J. Anim. Sci. **66:** 1117-1119.

Srivastava, N.C., Gupta, S.K. and Uppal, P.K. 1985. *Listeria monocytogenes* infection in infertile cows. Indian Vet. J. **62:** 545-547.

Sword, C.P. 1966. Mechanism of pathogenesis in *Listeria monocytogenes* infection. Influence of Iron. J.Bacteriol. **92:** 536-542.

Tanabe Y., Xiong H., Nomura T., Arakawa M. and Mitsuyama M.1999.Induction of protective T cells against Listeria monocytogenes in mice by immunization with a listeriolysin O-negative avirulent strain of bacteria and liposome-encapsulated listeriolysin O. Infect Immun. **67:** 568-575.

Vishwanathan, G.R. and Ayyar, V.V. (1950). Indian Vet. J. **26:** 362.

Winter P, Schilcher F, Bagò Z, Schoder D, Egerbacher M, Baumgartner W, Wagner M.2004. Clinical and histopathological aspects of naturally occurring mastitis caused by Listeria monocytogenes in cattle and ewes. J Vet Med B Infect Dis Vet Public Health. **51:** 176-179.

Xiong H., Tanabe Y., Ohya S. and Mitsuyama M.1998.Administration of killed bacteria together with listeriolysin O induces protective immunity against Listeria monocytogenes in mice. Immunology. **94:** 14-21.

Yadav, M.M. and Roy, A. 2009. Prevalence of Listeria spp. including *Listeria monocytogenes* from apparently healthy sheep of Gujarat State, India. Zoonoses Public Health. **56:** 515-524.

Zundel, E. and Bernard, S. 2006. *Listeria monocytogenes* translocates throughout the digestive tract in asymptomatic sheep. J.Med. Microbiol. **55:** 1717-1723.

□□□

Winter P, Schleicher L, Bago Z, Schoder D, [illegible] M (2004) Clinical and histopathological [illegible]
SE 126–129

[illegible]

[illegible]

[illegible]

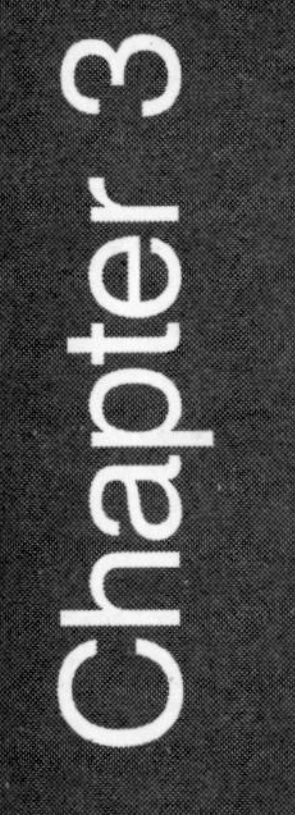

Diseases Caused by Clostridium spp.

Dr. S.K. SRIVASTAVA
Former, Division of Bacteriology & Mycology
Indian Veterinary Research Institute, Izatnagar-243122
Bareilly (U.P.)

Diseases caused by Clostridium spp.

Clostridia are gram positive non-encapsulated rods, anaerobic or aerotolerant. The genus contains more than 100 species and only a few are important from animal diseases point of view. The disease producing clostridia are motile except *Clostridium perfringens*. All species form endospores and have a strictly fermentative type of metabolism. Most clostridia will not grow under aerobic conditions and vegetative cells are killed by exposure to O_2, but their spores are able to survive long periods of exposure to air.

The clostridia are ancient organisms that live in virtually all of the anaerobic habitats of nature where organic compounds are present, including soils, aquatic sediments and the intestinal tracts of animals.

Clostridia are able to ferment a wide variety of organic compounds. They produce end products such as butyric acid, acetic acid, butanol and acetone, and large amounts of gas (CO_2 and H_2) during fermentation of sugars. A variety of foul smelling compounds are formed during the fermentation of amino acids and fatty acids.

They can be divided into 4 major groups according to the type of the disease produced in animals.

1. The histotoxic clostridia cause a variety of tissue and muscle infections following wounds or other trauma. Examples are blackleg and malignant oedema.

2. The hepatotoxic clostridia produce toxins in liver and cause the disease. Examples are bacillary hemoglobinuria and black disease.
3. The enterotoxigenic clostridia produce enterotoxaemia and food poisoning. They are also occasionally histotoxic. For example enterotoxaemia caused by *C.perfringens* type D.
4. The neurotoxic clostridia caused disease by the production of potent neurotoxins. Botulism and tetanus are 2 examples.

Although most important clostridial infections are acquired by ingestion or via wounds, some arise endogenously, for example enterotoxaemia in sheep.

Histotoxic clostridia are *Clostridium perfringens, C.chauvoei, C.septicum, C.novyi, C.haemolyticum* and *C.sordellii*. Typically all these clostridia are involved in infections of muscles, tissues and liver or intestines.

Three types of wound infections may be caused, wound contamination alone, anaerobic cellulitis and gas gangrene (Smith 1975). Of these three types gas gangrene is often severe. Gas gangrene is initiated by deep wound to large muscle masses. Presence of low redox potential provides a favourable milieu for the growth of the anaerobic clostridia. The presence of other bacteria in the wound may also support the growth.

Clostridium perfringens

C. perfringens is part of the normal intestinal flora of humans and animals and is widespread in soil. Hence it is difficult to incriminate this organism in case of the disease. Type A usually causes gas gangrene (Smith 1975). Toxins of the organism are responsible for the destruction of tissues and phagocytes. The toxin involved in gas gangrene is known as á-toxin, which inserts into the plasma membrane of cells, producing gaps in the membrane that disrupt normal cellular function.*C. perfringens* can participate in polymicrobial anaerobic infections. After ingestion, bacteria multiply and lead to colic, diarrhea, and sometimes nausea. In horses it causes equine clostridiosis which is characterized by an acute profuse watery diarrhoea and high mortality in adult horses. Colic and gastroenteritis has been produced by intravenous injection of ponies with enterotoxin of *C.perfringens*. Cellulitis due to *C.perfringens* and accompanied by immune-mediated haemolytic anemia has been described in horses (Reef 1983). Isolation of large numbers of *C. perfringens* type A from intestinal contents, in the absence of other enteric pathogens, is the most reliable criterion on which to base a diagnosis. Recently, beta2 (CPB2) toxin-producing *C. perfringens* type A has been linked to disease in piglets and other animals. However, implication of CPB2 in pathogenesis of porcine infections is based principally on isolation of *C. perfringens* carrying cpb2, the gene encoding CPB2, and the specific role of CPB2 in enteric disease of pigs remains to be fully defined. Clostridium difficile can also be a normal inhabitant of the intestine of healthy pigs, and diagnosis of enteric infection with this microorganism is based on detection of its toxins in feces or intestinal contents (Songer and Uzal 2005).*C.perfringens* is also associated with diarrhoea in pigs. These lesions and symptoms are due to a 54 kDa alpha-toxin which possess phospholipase C and sphingomyelinase activity and consequent haemolytic action. Alpha toxin is the most important virulence factor of *C. perfringens*. It is also protective in animals. Damage to tissues is mediated by hydrolysis of lecithin and sphingomyelin in membranes of various cells (Smith 1979). Experimentally, the alpha toxin can produce gas gangrene in guinea pigs. The toxin damages phospholipids of microsomes and mitochondria (Demello *et al.*, 1974). Additionally, Kappa toxin, a collegenase produced by *C.perfringens* destroys collagen in blood vessels. Amino acids that are released by the action of collegenase facilitate the growth of *C.perfringens* in the damaged tissues. *C.perfringens* takes up large amount of oxygen from its surroundings and this is probably responsible for vascular damage, resulting in hemo-concentration and shock (Smith 1979). Amino acid degradation leads to massive amount of gas production in muscles which forms pockets which leads to tissue necrosis.

Clostridium chauvoei

C. chauvoei is responsible for causing blackleg. It is an acute infection characterized by inflammation of skeletal and cardiac muscles, severe toxemia and high mortality. *C.chauvoei* are gram positive highly motile, sporulating bacteria. Spores are highly resistant to environmental changes and disinfectants and remain in soil for many years. Mixed infections with *C. chauvoei* and *C. septium* are often observed but *C.septicum* has not been incriminated as the cause of the diseases. There is no consensus on the pathogenesis of blackleg infection that occurs in ruminants, but toxins and neuraminidase produced by Clostridium chauvoei are believed to play a significant role in the pathogenesis of the disease. Several toxic compounds are produced by *C.chauvoei*. Alpha toxin, a lethal necrotizing protein that causes haemolysis of sheep red blood cells; beta toxin is responsible for marked destruction of nuclei in muscle cells observed in local lesions (Dixit and Khera 1968). It also produces gamma toxin, a hyaluronidase and a delta toxin, an oxygen labile haemolysin. A 65 kDa neuraminidase toxin has been reported. It cleaves sialic acid from RBC ghosts of sheep, horse, goats, cattle, pig and mice. The enzyme is activated by Ca^{++} and Mg^{++} (Useh *et al.* 2006). Sialidases, or neuraminidases (EC 3.2.1.18), are enzymes that cleave N-acetylneuraminic acid from carbohydrate polymers, such as mucin, glycoproteins, gangliosides and other sialoglycoconjugates, located on many mammalian cell membranes.

The mature sialidase is generally composed of three main domains. At its N-terminal end, it contains the F5/8 type C domain, alternatively designated CBM32 (carbohydrate binding module 32) or discoidin domain, that appears to be primarily involved in binding of terminal galacto-configured sugar residues and is also found in the *C. perfringens* sialidase NanJ. The central domain contains a CBM40 module (or lectin-like sialic acid binding domain) that was shown to be specific for binding sialic acid residues in NanJ of *C. perfringens*. The enzymatically active site of sialidases is in the C-terminal end that contains the usual catalytic residues that are common to all sialidases, including a catalytic nucleophile tyrosine, an arginine triad that interacts with the carboxylate group of sialic acid, a tryptophan residue that forms a weak H-bond with the glycerol side chain of sialic acid, and an aspartic acid that forms H-bonds with the four OH-groups of sialic acid. Furthermore, the enzymatically active domain contains four "Asp-boxes" characterized by the motif Ser-X-Asp-X-Gly-X-Thr-Trp, and the first arginine of the catalytic triad of sialidases generally belongs to a RIP (Arg-Ile-Pro) motif. Sialidase may have an important role in blackleg by degrading tight junctions upon cleavage of sialic acids at a high rate, thus allowing the bacterium to spread through host tissue. A sialidase activity has been reported in *C. chauvoei*, but the sialidase enzyme has not yet been characterized in detail. Furthermore, the molecular and genetic basis of sialidase in *C. chauvoei* is still unclear. A sialidase from Clostridium chauvoei (Jakari strain), an indigenous bacterial strain that causes blackleg in Nigerian cattle and other ruminants was isolated and partially purified by chromatography on DEAE cellulose, hydroxyapatite and phenyl agarose columns Useh *et al.*2006). The enzyme migrated as a 65-kDa protein after electrophoresis on sodium dodecyl sulphate polyacrylamide gels. It was optimally active at pH 4.5 and 40 degrees C with an activation energy (Ea) of 13.40 kJ mol(-1). It had Km and Vmax values of 170 microM and 200 micromole h(-1) mg(-1) respectively with fetuin as substrate. When sialyllactose (Neu5Ac2,3 lactose) was used as substrate the Km and Vmax values were 8 microM and 5 micromoles min (-1) mg(-1) respectively. The Clostridium chauvoei sialidase cleaved sialic acids from RBC ghosts of sheep, horse, goat, cattle, pig and mice as well as mouse brain cells, albeit at different rates. The enzyme was activated by Ca2+ and Mg2+ and inhibited by the group-specific reagents diethylpyrocarbonate (DEP) and N-ethylmalemide (NEM). The sialidase inhibitors, 2,3 didehydroneuraminic acid (Neu5Ac2,3en) and paranitrophenyl oxamic acid (pNPO) inhibited the enzyme competitively with Ki values of 40 and 30 microM respectively.

Vilei *et al.* (2011) have analyzed the sialidase activity of the NanA protein of C. chauvoei and cloned the sialidase gene nanA. Sialidase is encoded as a precursor protein of 722 amino acids with a 26 amino acid signal peptide. The mature sialidase has a calculated molecular mass of 81 kDa and contains the carbohydrate binding module 32 (CBM32, or F5/8 type C domain), the sialic acid binding module CBM40 and the enzymatically active sialidase domain found in all pro- and eukaryotic sialidases. Sialidase activity does not require the CBM32 domain. The NanA protein is secreted by *C. chauvoei* as a dimer. The NanA gene was found to be conserved and sialidase activity was found in *C. chauvoei* strains isolated over a period of 50 years from various geographical locations. Antiserum directed against a recombinant 40 kDa peptide containing CBM40 and part of the enzymatically active domain of NanA neutralized the secreted sialidase activity of all *C. chauvoei* strains tested.

Using ammonium sulphate fractionation, the Clostridium chauvoei hemolysin was purified by cation exchange chromatography and sephacryl S-100 gel filtration by Mudenda *et al.*(2006). The molecular mass of the hemolysin, determined by SDS-PAGE was found to be approximately 27kDa. The activity of the hemolysin was determined in erythrocytes of various animals, with sensitivities observed in the order of cow, sheep, chicken, rabbit, rat, mouse, dog and horse. Temperature affected the sensitivity of erythrocytes to *C. chauvoei* hemolysin. These results may reflect distinct characteristics of the hemolytic activity of *C. chauvoei* hemolysin and that the hemolysin may be pore-forming.

Flagellar proteins play an important role in the pathogenesis. Differential centrifugation and cesium chloride-equilibrium centrifugation were used to purify the flagella from the strain Okinawa of the formalin-fixed Clostridium chauvoei. SDS-PAGE profile of purified flagella showed that a major protein band with a molecular mass of 46 kDa, corresponding to the flagellin monomer, and at least two minor protein bands with molecular masses of approximately 73 and 100 kDa were found(Kojima *et al.*1999). The amino acid composition of *C. chauvoei* flagellin was similar to the flagellin of Salmonella typhimurium and Bacillus subtilis. In addition, *C. chauvoei* flagellin monomer shared limited sequence homology with the N-terminal amino acid sequence reported for other bacterial flagellins. N-terminal sequences of two minor bands corresponded to the flagellin monomer, indicating that higher molecular mass bands were polymeric forms of the flagellin monomer.

Blackleg is a soil borne disease however portal of entry is supposed to be the alimentary mucosa after ingestion of contaminated feed. The bacteria are present in various organs of the animals including feces which contaminate the soil. Dead decomposed animals also contaminate the soil. Blacklegs develop when spores lodged in normal tissues proliferate following trauma or anoxia. Activation of spores requires some predisposing factors. Access of spores in the blood requires the help of macrophages which are later lodged in liver and intestines. Young cattle on a high plane of nutrition are highly susceptible. Excessive exercise also appears to provide an environment in muscles that permit germination of *C.chauvoei* spores. Stress factors which lead to the activation of spores are unknown.

In sheep when blackleg lesions occur in the limb there is stiff gait and disliking moving due to severe lameness in one or more limbs. Subcutaneous oedema are also observed with gaseous crepitation. Animals show fever and skin discolouration is evident. Muscles are dark, with a rancid odour and gas bubbles due to staining of muscles with hemoglobin and butyric acid.

In cattle, rapid depression, high fever and anorexia are seen. Edema and emphysema of affected muscles is pronounced. Skin is discoloured and dry with scaly appearance, Generalized lesions may also be observed involving heart muscles, the diaphragm, brisket and udder. Animals may die without showing any lesions.

Diagnosis

The standard method for C. chauvoei diagnosis is the detection of culture and biochemical identification, which requires a pure culture. In most muscle samples from cattle dead from blackleg the amount of C. chauvoei in samples is high and the bacterium can easily be cultured, although some samples may be contaminated. Conventional microbiological methods are hampered by the slow growth of *C. chauvoei*, which is often overgrown by other anaerobes or swarming *C. septicum* colonies, as both might be present in a sample. Immunological detection methods are reported to be prone to cross-reactions between the two species. In addition, production of antisera for their detection is complex because it involves the use of laboratory animals.

Detection by PCR would be faster and independent of contaminating flora. Digested residues from biogas plants provide an excellent fertilizer, but it is known that spore-forming bacteria such as *Clostridium* spp. are not reduced by pasteurization. The use of digested residues as fertilizer may contribute to the spread of *C. chauvoei*. Soil, manure and substrate from biogas plants are contaminated with other anaerobic bacteria which outgrow *C. chauvoei*. Therefore, detection by PCR is would be useful. The study by agge *et al.* (2009) applied a PCR-based method to detect of *C. chauvoei* in 25 muscle and blood samples, 114 manure samples, 84 soil samples and 33 samples from the biogas process. Muscle tissues from suspected cases of blackleg were analysed both by the standard culture method followed by biochemical identification and by PCR, with and without preculture. To investigate whether muscle tissue samples are necessary, samples taken by swabs were also investigated. Samples from a biogas plant and manure and soil from farms were analyzed by culture followed by PCR. The farms had proven cases of blackleg. For detection of *C. chauvoei* in the samples, a specific PCR primer pair complementary to the spacer region of the 16S-23S rRNA gene was used. *Clostridium chauvoei* was detected in 32% of muscle samples analyzed by culture with identification by biochemical methods and in 56% of cases by culture in combination with PCR. *Clostridium chauvoei* was detected in 3 (out of 11) samples from the biogas plants collected before pasteurisation, but samples taken after pasteurization and after digestion all tested negative. Clostridium chauvoei was not detected in any soil or silage samples and only one manure samples tested positive. The diagnostic method used for *C. chauvoei* was not applicable in estimating the risk of blackleg on particular pastures from manure or soil samples, but found to be highly useful for clinical samples.

Amplification of the 16S-23S rDNA spacer region by polymerase chain reaction (PCR) was used for the rapid detection of Clostridium chauvoei and C septicum. To assess its specificity, PCR was performed with total DNA from 42 strains of clostridia and three strains of other genera (Sasaki *et al.* 2001). PCR products specific to C *chauvoei* or to C *septicum* were generated from homologous cultures only. Clostridium chauvoer-specific or C *septicum-specific* amplicons were also generated from tissues of cows experimentally infected with C *chauvoei* or C *septicum* and in DNA samples from cows clinically diagnosed as having blackleg or malignant oedema. These results suggest that a species-specific PCR may be useful for the rapid and direct detection of C *chauvoei* and C *septicum* in clinical specimens. C. *chauvoei* and C. *septicum* are closely related taxa and share many phenotypic properties hampering diagnosis by using traditional microbiological methods. Thus, there is a need for a fast and reliable identification method for specific detection of both species in clinical samples. The multiplex real-time PCR assay reported by Lange *et al.* (2010) is based on the detection of the spo0A gene and enables the simultaneous identification of C. *chauvoei* and C. *septicum*. The assay design includes an amplification control DNA template for the recognition of PCR-inhibitors. Assay validation was performed using a collection of 29 C. *chauvoei*, 38 C. septicum strains and 26 strains of other Clostridium species. Furthermore, the real-time PCR assay was successfully tested on tissue samples from 19 clinical blackleg cases. The assay allowed the reliable detection of one picogram DNA which represents approximate 239 genome equivalents.

Vaccines

Immunity to C. chauvoei is considered to be mainly anticellular, and for this reason there is scarce information about the immunogenicity of extracellular proteins. In the work by Mattar *et al.* (2007) variations in protein profiles, immune response by ELISA and protective capacity of culture supernatants of three *C. chauvoei* strains, collected at different growth phases, are reported. Sera raised against extracellular antigens also recognised cellular antigens of the same molecular masses. Partially purified cell-free supernatants and those concentrated 10 times by ultrafiltration (C-CFS), obtained at the early stationary phase of growth, induced a strong immunoprotective response, even at low doses, that was more marked for *C. chauvoei* strain ATCC 10092 ($p \leq 0.05$). With C-CFS formulations, a clear relationship was observed between IgG titres, protective capacity and concentration of the antigen doses, indicating a specific immune response. One of the major protective antigen of the organism is the flagellar protein. Using an Escherichia coli expression library of the *C. chauvoei* Okinawa strain, Kojima *et al.* (2000) isolated the fliC gene encoding the flagellin protein. DNA sequence analysis revealed an open reading frame of 413 amino acid residues with a calculated molecular mass of 43819Da. Comparison of the sequence with those of flagellins from other bacteria showed considerable homology in the N-terminal and C-terminal domains. The glutathione-S-transferase (GST)-flagellin fusion protein and the purified FliC protein after removing the GST part with thrombin reacted with both polyclonal antisera and the non-protective monoclonal antibody (Mab), Mo-114. However, the protective Mab, Mo-41, which may recognize its conformational epitope, failed to react with both the GST-flagellin fusion protein and the purified FliC. Furthermore, the GST-flagellin fusion protein and the purified FliC induced very little protective immunity in mice. These results suggested that a conformation-dependent epitope play an important role in the development of immunity against blackleg.

Clostridium septicum

This is an important cause of wound infections in animals. Several clostridial species are involved alongwith *Clostridium septicum*. These are *C. chauvoei, C. perfringens, C. sordelli* and *C. novyi*. The disease caused is called malignant oedema or gas gangrene. These species may cause the disease alone or in combination. In this condition cellulitis occur with minor muscle involvement associated with foul odour. The condition caused is emphysema with necrotic myositis or gas gangrene. In sheep braxy is caused by *C.septicum* associated with eating frozen food. Clinical signs include high fever, anorexia, necrotic lesions and haemorrhagic oedema of the abomasal and duodenal walls. The disease is rare in India in which the abomasum is invaded by the organism. *Clostridium septicum* belongs to the pathogens involved in the gas edema complex and is very similar to *C. chauvoei*.

All ages and species of animals are infected and the infection occurs sporadically. The organisms are present in the environment and intestinal tract. Source of infection is soil where the resistant spores live for a long period. Soil contamination is the common predisposing factor. Deep wound leading to the trauma provides a suitable environment for the growth of the microorganism. Any wound may lead to the infection, such as during surgical intervention or vaccination. Outbreaks have been reported in cattle and sheep following parturition. Contaminated sheep dips may result in outbreaks of the disease. Castration wounds in pigs and cattle may also lead to gas gangrene. Unless treatment is initiated in the early stages the mortality is high.

Spontaneously occurring clostridial myonecrosis involving *C. septicum* has recently reemerged as a concern for many poultry producers. However, despite its increasing prevalence, the epidemiology of infection and population structure of *C. septicum* remains largely unknown. Clostridial dermatitis of turkeys (CDT) has emerged as a major issue across most geographic regions of the World. The prevalence and severity of dermatitis has increased over the last several years, since the time it was first reported in 1993. Cellulitis in poultry can be associated with *Staphylococcus aureus* or *Escherichia coli*, but the more recent field situation in turkeys is specifically associated with *Clostridium* spp. The prevalence of cellulitis is relatively low; however, the disease can be devastating in the individual flocks affected. *Clostridium septicum, Clostridium perfringens, Clostridium sordelli,* and *S. aureus* can cause cellulitis. Escherichia coli, Streptococcus spp., and other bacteria have occasionally been isolated from birds diagnosed with cellulitis. CDT appears as excessive mortality in older birds around 16-18 weeks of age. It has been reported from field experience as early as 7 wk of age. Clinical signs of CDT can range from sudden death to inappetence, depression, leg weakness, recumbency, and ataxia. The disease is characterized by reddish to dark or greenish discoloration of the skin around the thighs, abdomen, keel, tail region, back, and wings. The lesions can extend into the underlying muscles, and there can be gas bubbles under the skin which result in crepitation. Some cases present with dead birds having "bubbly tail," fluid-filled blisters associated with broken feather follicles around the base of the tail. Bubbly tail in breeder toms might not cause excessive mortality, but the lesions are so severe that the birds cannot be used for semen collection. Incidence of mortality from this condition can be severe and acute (i.e., rapid onset of high mortality). The dead birds decompose very quickly. Microscopically, there is necrosis, with or without inflammation of the skin, especially in the dermis and occasionally in the skeletal muscles, associated with large numbers of rod-shaped bacteria. Overcrowding, aggressive birds, poor-wet litter, decreased down time, a contaminated environment including feed and water, poor hygienic conditions, and contaminated vaccines and vaccine equipment, etc., can predispose birds for CDT. Intravenous administration (approximately 10(8) cells/ml) of 1 of 4 isolates of *Clostridium septicum* from cellulitis lesions rapidly caused the classic lesions of cellulitis followed by death within 36 hr at high doses (Tellez *et al* 2009). When the supernatant alone was injected into turkey poults, signs of depression and ataxia were temporarily observed for up to 20 hr after injection, but no cellulitis lesions were detected. An enzyme-linked immunosorbent assay was developed to measure antibody levels against the isolated *C. septicum*. a multilocus sequence typing (MLST) approach was utilized to examine evolutionary relationships within a diverse collection of *C. septicum* isolates recovered from poultry flocks experiencing episodes of gangrenous dermatitis. The 109 isolates examined represented 42 turkey flocks and 24 different flocks of broiler chickens as well as *C. septicum* type strain, ATCC 12464. Isolates were recovered predominantly from gangrenous lesions although isolates from livers, gastrointestinal tracts, spleens and blood were included. The loci analyzed were csa, the major lethal toxin produced by C. septicum, and the housekeeping genes gyrA, groEL, dnaK, recA, tpi, ddl, colA and glpK. These loci were included in part because of their previous use in MLST analysis of *Clostridium perfringens* and Clostridium difficile. Results indicated a high level of conservation present within these housekeeping gene fragments when compared to what has been previously reported for the aforementioned clostridia. Of the 5352 bp of sequence data examined for each isolate, 99.7% (5335/5352) was absolutely conserved among the 109 isolates. Only one of the ten unique sequence types, or allelic profiles, identified among the isolates was recovered from both turkeys and broiler chickens suggesting some host species preference. Phylogenetic analyses identified two unique clusters, or clonal complexes, among these poultry isolates which may have important epidemiological implications for poultry producers in the United States. This work by Neumann and Rehberger (2009) indicates a predominantly clonal population structure for *C. septicum* although some evidence of recombination was also observed.

Gangrenous dermatitis (GD) is an emerging disease of increasing economic importance in poultry resulting from combined infection by Clostridium septicum and Clostridium perfringens type A. Lack of a reproducible disease model has been a major obstacle in understanding the immunopathology of GD. To gain better understanding of host-pathogen interactions in GD infection, Li *et al.* (2010) evaluated various immune parameters in two groups of birds from a recent commercial outbreak of GD, the first showing typical disease signs and pathological lesions (GD-like birds) and the second lacking clinical signs (GD-free birds). The results revealed that GD-like birds showed: reduced T-cell and B-cell mitogen-stimulated lymphoproliferation; higher levels of serum nitric oxide and alpha-1-acid glycoprotein; greater numbers of K55(+), K1(+), CD8(+), and MHC class II(+) intradermal lymphocytes, and increased K55(+), K1(+), CD8(+), TCR1(+), TCR2(+), Bu1(+), and MHC class II(+) intestinal intraepithelial lymphocytes; and increased levels of mRNAs encoding proinflammatory cytokines and chemokines in skin compared with GD-free chickens. These results provide the first evidence of altered systemic and local (skin and intestine) immune responses in GD pathogenesis in chickens.

The toxins produced by *C.septicum* are similar to that produced by *C.chauvoei* (Aikat and Dible 1960). Alpha toxin, a 48 kDa protein, is capable of causing capillary damage. It causes haemolysis and is lethal and necrotizing to tissues. Production of the alpha toxins by various strains varies. Immunologically all strains produce a similar protein. Results in mice have demonstrated it to be a partially protective factor. Alpha-toxin is an important agent of the virulence of *Clostridium septicum*. Hang'ombe *et al.*(2004) examined cytotoxicity for alpha-toxin to various mammalian cells with recombinant toxin fused with a histidine-tag at the amino-terminal. The recombinant toxin retained the activity indistinguishable from the native form. Mammalian nucleated cells examined in this study are more sensitive to the protoxin than to the trypsinized toxin, except RAW 264.7 and P3U1 cells of myeloid lineage. Cellular proteins of various molecular sizes interacted with the toxin. The size and SDS-PAGE pattern of the proteins were different among cell lines but they were liberated from the cells by the treatment with phosphatidylinositol-specific phospholipase C. The toxin appeared to target and utilizes detergent resistant membranes (DRMs) for binding and subsequent oligomerization. In discontinuous sucrose density gradient, we demonstrated by immunoblotting that the toxin bound to DRMs contained in L929 cells and caused the oligomer formation. Furthermore, cholesterol depletion with cholesterol-interacting agents reduced toxin oligomerization and lowered cytotoxicity of the toxin towards cells. These results suggest that alpha-toxin preferentially exploits DRMs for oligomerization.

The activity of *Clostridium septicum* alpha-toxin was determined in erythrocytes of various animals, with sensitivities observed in the order of mouse, rat, canine, equine, rabbit, chicken, bovine, swine and ovine (Hang'Ombe *et al.*, 2005). Temperature and protease treatment affected the sensitivity of erythrocytes to alpha-toxin. Proteinase K treatment decreased the sensitivity of murine, canine, equine and bovine erythrocytes, but ovine erythrocytes did not change the sensitivity to alpha-toxin activity. On the other hand, the activity of alpha-toxin on swine erythrocytes increased after treatment with proteinase K, trypsin, chymotrypsin or lysyl endopeptidase. Toxin overlay assay showed that alpha-toxin bound to erythrocyte membrane proteins with a molecular mass of 30 to 45-kDa in mouse, equine, bovine, swine and chicken, whereas in rat erythrocyte membranes the toxin reacted with 100-kDa protein. The treatment of murine and swine erythrocyte membranes with phosphatidylinositol-specific phospholipase C resulted in liberation of the toxin-binding protein from the individual membranes in a native state. These results show that alpha-toxin associates with specific erythrocyte membrane proteins in any animal species, and are subsets of glycosylphosphatidylinositol-anchored proteins in various animal species. These results may reflect distinct characteristics of the hemolytic activity of alpha-toxin in response to various erythrocytes.Knapp *et al.*(2010) analyzed channel formation of the recombinant septicum alpha-toxin and characterized its activity on living cells. Recombinant septicum alpha-toxin induces the formation of ion-permeable channels with a single-channel conductance of about 175pS in 0.1M KCl in lipid bilayer membranes, which is typical for a large diffusion pore. Septicum alpha-toxin channels remained mostly in the open configuration, displayed no lipid specificity, and exhibited slight anion selectivity. Septicum alpha-toxin caused a rapid decrease in the transepithelial electrical resistance of MDCK cell monolayers grown on filters, and induced a rapid cell necrosis in a variety of cell lines, characterized by cell permeabilization to propidium iodide without DNA fragmentation and activation of caspase-3. Septicum alpha-toxin also induced a rapid K(+) efflux and ATP depletion. Incubation of the cells in K(+)-enriched medium delayed cell death caused by septicum alpha-toxin or epsilon-toxin, another potent pore-forming toxin, suggesting that the rapid loss of intracellular K(+) represents an early signal of pore-forming toxins-mediated cell necrosis.

The other toxins identified are Beta toxin, a deoxyribonuclease and leukocidal; a gamma toxin, which is hyaluronidase; a delta toxin, which is a haemolyzing and necrotizing factor. Neuraminidase produced by *C.septicum* (Gadalla and Collee 1968) is produced in vivo and may contribute to pathogenicity.

Diagnosis

Although *C. septicum* is readily cultured from diseased tissues it can be difficult to enumerate due to its tendency to swarm over the surface of agar plates. In one study a quantitative real-time PCR assay was developed in order to more accurately measure the levels of *C. septicum* in healthy as well as GD associated poultry samples. The assay was specifically designed to target the *C. septicum* alpha toxin gene, csa, which is, to our knowledge, carried by all strains of *C. septicum* and has been shown to be essential for virulence. Genomic DNAs from a diverse collection of bacterial species, including closely related Clostridium chauvoei, *Clostridium carnis, Clostridium tertium* as well as several strains of *Clostridium perfringens*, all failed to produce a positive reaction. An approximate reproducible limit of detection in spiked extracts of at least 10(3) cfu/g of *C. septicum* was observed for a variety of different sample types. *C. septicum* levels in broiler chicken field samples estimated from the results of qPCR were statistically correlated to culture based enumerations obtained from those same tissues (Neumann *et al.* 2010). A real-time PCR assay based on the 16S rRNA gene sequence was designed for differentiation of blackleg-causing *Clostridium chauvoei* and *Clostridium septicum*, a phylogenetically closely related bacterium responsible for malignant edema (Halm *et al.* 2010). In order to exclude false-negative results, an internal amplification control was included in the assay. A set of three probes, one specific for *C. chauvoei*, one specific for *C. septicum*, and one specific for both species, permitted unequivocal detection of *C. chauvoei* in tests of 32 Clostridium sp. strains and 10 non-Clostridium strains. The assay proved to be sensitive, detecting one genome of *C. chauvoei* or *C. septicum* per PCR and 1.79 x 10(3) C. chauvoei cells/g artificially contaminated muscle tissue. In tests of 11 clinical specimens, the real-time PCR assay yielded the same results as an established conventional PCR method.

Clostridium novyi

The species is also known as *C. oedematiens*. There are four types which are distinguished on the basis of toxins produced. These are discussed below;

Type A : Causes gas gangrene and is widespread in human, cattle and sheep. It causes big head in rams.

Type B : Causes Black Disease and has been reported from various countries. It is associated with liver fluke infection in sheep.

Type C : It causes osteomyelitis and has been reported in buffaloes in some Asian countries.

Type D : This is also known as *C.haemolyticum*. It causes bacillary haemoglobinuria in cattle.

C.novyi cells synthesize 5 toxins, alpha, beta, gamma, delta and epsilon. Strains of type A produce all but beta toxin. Strains of type B produce alpha and beta-toxins only. Strains of type C are non-toxigenic and not associated with any diseases.

The disease is caused in cattle, sheep and several other animal species. Extensive oedema is characteristic. Only a small number of clostridia are often detected in cases of the disease. It is due to high activity of the toxins which is responsible for the disease symptoms.

Black disease (Infectious necrotic hepatitis) is an acute disease of animals caused by the toxins of the organisms produced in damaged liver tissues. Field outbreaks of the disease are usually precipitated by invasion of liver by immature liver fluke which damage the tissues and facilitates spore germination and bacterial multiplication leading to tissue necrosis. Fatal infection with *C.novyi* can also occur through the navel in lambs and the uterus in ewes.

Alpha toxin, a 200 kDa protein, is produced in the local areas of necrosis in the liver and is absorbed into the circulation and results in systemic infection besides causing local reactions such as necrosis and increased vascular permeability. Experimentally, intravenous injections of alpha toxin in mice causes oedema and hypovolemic shock which is considered to be the cause of death (Bette *et al.* 1989). The toxin probably alters the microfilament system of the cell (Oksche *et al.* 1992). There are alternations in cell shape along with partial loss of F actin and redistribution of vinculin which are the sites of attachment of microfilaments on membranes. As regards the chemical nature of other toxins, the beta-toxin is a lecithinase, gamma toxin is a necrotizing phospholipase D, delta toxin is an oxygen labile haemolysin and epsilon toxin is a lipolytic enzyme. Zeta toxin is a poorly characterized haemolysin and theta toxin is a lipase produced in trace amounts by type B strains of *C.novyi*. Eta toxin is a tropomyosinase which breakdown tropomycin and destroys infected animals (Gyles 1993).

C.novyi type D (*C.haemolyticum*) causes the disease due to the production of large amount of lethal, necrotizing and haemolytic beta toxin. The organism is soil borne similar to other clostridia species and types. The cultures of the organism produce severe muscle necrosis and haemoglobinuria when injected intra-muscularly in cattle. In infected areas the organisms usually resides in the healthy livers of the animals. In the liver the organisms can be identified using immunoperoxidase technique (Uzal *et al.*, 2010). An injury caused due to the liver fluke or *Cysticercus tennuicollis* results in anaerobic conditions. The hypoxia generated may trigger the infection by production of large amount of beta toxin (Phospholipase C) by the organism. The development of an organized thrombus in a subterminal branch of the portal vein produces the anemic infarct in which bacteria are found which produce large amount of toxin causing toxaemia. In the later stage bacteremia develops which causes severe haemolysis. Van Kempen and Kenndey (1969) have suggested that following damage of liver tissues by the liver fluke, necrosis of cells takes place which favours induction of spore germination by *C.haemolyticum* present in kupffer cells. Toxins are produced which lyse the kupffer cells to release the bacteria and further production of phospholipase C toxin occurs.

The disease is not produced in areas where conditions are not favourable for the flukes or snails. Death in animals is brought about by lysis of enthrocytes by the toxin and the animal dies of anoxia.

Clostridium sordellii

C.sordelli is associated with acute myositis and abomasitis in animals. It has been isolated from cases of fatal metritis in ewes. It has been also isolated from lesions typical of malignant oedema of cattle and sheep. The organism can be recovered from lesions in muscle and liver. There are considerable oedema of subcutaneous tissues and facial planes surrounding the muscle. Subendocardial haemorrhages in the left ventricle and a terminal septicaemia have been observed in experimentally infected cattle (Gyles, 1993). Similar to other clostridia, toxic substances are produced that account for sign of the disease. An edema-producing factor is most important (Arsecularatne *et al.*, 1969). Other toxin enzymes such as phospholipase C, a lysolecitinase, a oxyen sensitive haemolysin, a neuraminidase and DNAse. DNAse may cause destruction of cells (Smith 1975 b). Its lethal toxin kills mice by inducing major increase in lung vascular permeability (Blandine Geny *et al.*, 2007).

Diagnosis of histotoxic clostridia

Cases of blackleg can occur year after year on contaminated pastures. A method to determine the prevalence of *C. chauvoei* spores on pasture would be useful.The standard method for *C. chauvoei* detection is culture and biochemical identification, which requires a pure culture. In most muscle samples from cattle dead from blackleg the amount of *C. chauvoei* in samples is high and the bacterium can easily be cultured, although some samples may be contaminated. Detection by PCR would be faster and independent of contaminating flora.Isolation and identification of *C.chauvoei* and *C.septicum* is laborious. Initially the organism can be grown in Robertson cooked meat medium and later plated on any anaerobic media. A reliable fluorescent antibody (FA) technique is carried out for identification of organisms in tissues or cultures. For laboratory animal pathgenicity testing, guinea pig inoculation is carried out with *C.chauvoei*. The animal dies with in 48 hours and tissues yield large amount of organisms. For *C.septicum*, guinea pigs and rabbits may be used. Long chains of filaments are seen in impression smears from the tissues of the infected animals. *C.novyii* type A and *C.haemolyticum* is also identified by FA technique. *C. sordelli* and *C.perfringens* type A are isolated and identified by conventional procedures. On blood agar plates, *C. perfringens* grown anaerobically produces â-haemolytic, flat, spreading, rough, translucent colonies with irregular margins. A Nagler agar plate, containing 5-10% egg yolk, is used to identify strains that produce á-toxin, a diffusible lecithinase that interacts with the lipids in egg yolk to produce a characteristic precipitate around the colonies. One-half of the plate is inoculated with antitoxin to act as a control in the identification.PCR detection of *Clostridium chauvoei* in pure cultures and formalin fixed, paraffin embedded tissues was carried out by Uzal *et al.*, (2003). A polymerase chain reaction (PCR) system using common primers designed from multiple alignment of the 16S rRNA and 23S rRNA genes of Clostridium species was developed by Sasaki *et al* (2000) to identify pathogenic clostridia. The PCR was performed with total DNA from 26 strains which included seven different Clostridia species. These bacteria were differentiated at species level by the different PCR product patterns. To characterise the 16S-23S rDNA spacer regions of these clostridia further, most PCR products of these bacteria were sequenced. The smallest PCR products of each bacterium represented the fundamental 16S-23S rDNA spacer region; larger PCR products of each bacterium were caused by insertion sequences, i.e. tRNA gene sequences. The authors' observations indicate that the PCR patterns of the 16S-23S rDNA spacer regions have the potential to be used as an identification marker of pathogenic clostridia in gas gangrene. Amplification of the 16S-23S rDNA spacer region by polymerase chain reaction (PCR) was used for the rapid detection of Clostridium chauvoei and C septicum (Sasaki *et al.* 2001). To assess its specificity, PCR was performed with total DNA from 42 strains of clostridia and three strains of other genera. PCR products specific to *C chauvoei* or to *C septicum* were generated from homologous cultures only. Clostridium chauvoer-specific or *C septicum*-specific amplicons were also generated from tissues of cows experimentally infected with *C chauvoei* or *C septicum* and in DNA samples from cows clinically diagnosed as having blackleg or malignant oedema. These results suggest that a species-specific PCR may be useful for the rapid and direct detection of *C chauvoei* and *C septicum* in clinical specimens.

A PCR has been described for detection and identification of *Clostridium* chauvoei from clinical sample, bovine feces and biogas plants, (Bagge *et al.*, 2009) for diagnosis of the disease.

Treatment and Control

When an outbreak of blackleg occurs all animals in the susceptible age range should be vaccinated and treated prophylactically. Treatment of clinical cases is usually unsuccessful. Formalinized whole broth cultures, alum precipitated, is used to confer long lasting immunity in animals. Protection is both antibacterial and antitoxic. A soluble heat labile protective antigen is associated with the alpha-toxin. A double bacterin containing *C.chauvoei* & *C.septicum* is very effective against blackleg and malignant oedema.Ontiveros *et al* (2008) studied immunogenic capacity of a 156-kDa recombinant protein of *Clostridium chauvoei* that showed 80% protection against this disease in guinea pigs. This immunogenic protein was cloned in the expression vector pBluescript and was used to immunize *C. chauvoei*-free bovine animals that were kept in an endemic area.

Penicillin is also effective against *C.septicum.* Other broad spectrum antibiotics are also used. Local application of penicillin into affected muscle may limit spread of the lesion and contain the disease.

For control of black disease elimination of liver flukes by destruction of snails is effective. Formalinized bacterins and toxoids are of value. *C.novyi* type A is included in some vaccines for the prevention of gas gangrene.

Treatment of bacillary haemoglobinuria requires use of broad spectrium antibiotics. Early treatment should be followed. Supportive treatment such as blood transfusion, parenteral fluid and electrolyte solution is of considerable importance. Bulls should not be used for service for at least 3 weeks because of the danger of sudden death due to liver rupture. The disease is controlled by elimination of liver flukes through destruction of snails. Formalinized alum precipitated whole broth cultures are used to confer an active immunity. The vaccination is done 4-6 weeks before the expected occurrence of the disease. To overcome the problem of local reaction, vaccination at several sites is recommended or it should be distributed by massage after the administration. The carcass of animal dying off the disease must be either buried deep in the ground or burnt. Revaccination is advocated at every 6 months. Vaccinations against all the diseases caused by clostridia should be given subcutaneously.

Vaccines prepared from *C.septicum, C.chauvoei, C.novyi, C.hemolyticum* and *C.sordellii* are available commercially. *C.perfringens* is only infrequently associated with the wound infections in animals. The choice of the vaccine is based on the organism causing the disease in a given area. The immunity developed in the animals following the vaccination is against bacterial structures (flagellin and toxins).

Enterotoxaemic *Clostridium perfringens*

Clostridium perfringens is an anaerobic bacilli but strict anaerobic conditions are not required. Various toxins produced by different types of *C. perfringens* are listed in the table below;

Type	Major Toxins	Disease
A Classical	Alpha (phospholipase C) + several minor toxins	Gas gangrene in animals, colitis in horses, necrotic enteritis in fowl.
Food Poisonıng	Enterotoxin	Human Food poisoning
B 2 varieties	Beta (+epsilon and minor toxins)	Lamb dysentery, haemorrhagic enterotoxaemia in adult sheep and goats in Iran.
C	Beta (Several minor toxins)	Enteritis in Lambs, calves, foals, piglets; struck in sheep; necrotic enteritis in man & fowl.
D	Epsilon	Enterotoxaemia in sheep, goats and possibly cattle.
E	Iota	Pathogenicity in sheep & cattle not confirmed.

[Source: Nilo, L. (1993)]

Besides the toxins listed above 8 other toxins or antigenic substances may be produced. The important among is enterotoxin followed by Kappa (collagenase); mu (hyaluronidase) and two hemolysins, delta and theta. All the *C.perfringens* types are present in environment and the animal and human intestinal tract. Some may not survive in soil for a long time, but survive in intestinal tract. Survival in the environment is aided by the formation of spores which are resistant to the environmental changes.

Type A strains of *C perfringens* are commonly found as part of the normal intestinal microflora of animals and lack some of the powerful toxins produced by strains of other types. Nonetheless, they produce the lethal and necrotizing á toxin and are incriminated in necrotic enteritis in poultry and dogs, in colitis in horses, and in diarrhea in pigs. *C perfringens* type A is clearly implicated in a rarely occurring hemorrhagic diarrhea in dogs. The disease is characterized by a necrotic enteritis in which there is massive destruction of the villi and coagulation necrosis of the small intestine. These organisms are also associated with chronic intermittent diarrhea in dogs but have not been confirmed as the causal agent. Typically, large numbers of large, gram-positive rods are visible in fecal smears, and large numbers of *C.perfringens* type A are recovered on anaerobic culture of feces. Other known enteric pathogens are usually absent. Untyped *C.perfringens* has also been shown to proliferate in the intestines of dogs with parvoviral enteritis, but its contribution to disease is not clear. Production of enterotoxin by type A strains of *C.perfringens* can induce diarrhea in humans, but this has not been demonstrated in dogs. Type A strains from pigs with diarrhea have produced enterotoxin in vitro, and anti-enterotoxin antibodies in sows indicate that enterotoxin is produced in vivo in pigs. Enterotoxin has also been demonstrated in the feces of pigs with diarrhea but not in feces of healthy pigs. However, recent studies have shown that *C.perfringens* isolated from pigs with diarrhea are typically nonenterotoxigenic but produce the cytotoxic β2 toxin, which has been suggested to play a role in disease. Experimental disease has been produced in pigs challenged orally with *C.perfringens* type A.

Among all the enterotoxaemias, type D is most important; caused by epsilon toxin. It affects sheep of all ages. Clinically the disease is characterized by diarrhea, convulsion, paralysis and rapid death. It is world wide in nature. The presence of *C. perfringens* type D in the intestine does not in itself result in disease unless other factors intercede which promote proliferation and production of toxin. The disease is world wide in distribution. The mode of entry of toxigenic *C..perfringens* is by ingestion or presence of the causative agent in the intestine. In most of the cases the affected sheep are on highly nutritious diet and are generally healthy. Lambs on well fed heavy milking ewes are particularly susceptible. In such animals the organisms proliferate rapidly in intestine and produce lethal quantities of 32 kDa plasmid coded epsilon toxin. One of the circumstances of production of disease is the passage of large quantities of starch granules into the duodenum when animals over eat. Heavy milk feeding may also have the same affect. It is not known why *C.perfringens* type D strain can overgrow type A strain since the latter is in high number initially. The epsilon toxin is released as prototoxin of low toxicity is initially released which is later activated by digestive enzymes such as trypsin and chymotrypsin, increasing the activity 1000 fold. The conversion of prototoxin to fully active toxin occurs by the cleavage of the N-terminal peptide. A large plasmid etx, encodes epsilon toxin. A single type D isolate can carry multiple virulence plasmids (Sayeed *et al.*, 2007). Large amount of epsilon cause increase in the permeability of the intestine leading to the absorption of large amount of its own toxin and other toxins into the systemic circulation (Bullen 1970). The first effect of the toxin is to cause profuse diarrhoea and secondarily to produce stimulation and then depression of central nervous system including that of brain capillaries. This results in rapid extravasation of fluid into the brain and increased intracerebral pressure. This is revealed by incoordination and convulsions (Griner 1961). Serous cavities such as lungs, pericardium are also affected. The damage to the vascular endothelium leads to the accumulation of protein rich fluid effusions in heart, brain and lung.

The epsilon toxin binds to receptors through sialoglycoprotein to the luminal surface of the vascular endothelium of brain and cells lining the loops of Henle, distal convulated tubules of the kidney and to hepatic sinusoids (Nagahama and Sakurai 1992; Nilo 1993) and causes degeneration of cells. This allows alteration of fluid dynamics and leakage of plasma proteins resulting in perivascular and intercellular edema followed by focal to diffuse areas of degeneration and necrosis (Buxton and Morgan 1976). Treatment of brain membrane fraction with lipase resulted in complete loss of binding suggesting that interaction may require an appropriate lipid environment (Nagahama & Sakurai 1992).

The hyperglycemia and glycosuria seen in cases of enterotoxaemia is due to glycogenolysis of liver glycogen reserves. There is severe hemo-concentrations of pyruvate, lactate and α-ketoglutarate. This glycogenolysis is due to the increased production of cyclic adenosine 3′, 5′ monophosphate (CAMP) which in turn causes breakdown of glycogen to glucose. It could also be due to the brain edema that stimulates a release of catecholamines (epinephrine, norepinephrine, dopamine) via the adrenal medulla. These activate adenyl cyclase, boosting the production of CAMP which in turn causes glycogenolysis and hyperglycemia leading to glycosuria. In kidneys there are rapid autolytic post-mortem changes in the damaged tissues.

In goats, the clinical disease varies from peracute to chronic form which show bloody diarrhoea, associated with haemorrhagic or necrotic enterocolitis (Blackwell *et al.,* 1991). Predisposing factors contributing to the disease enterotoxaemia include a gut environment suitable for bacterial growth in the intestine and a slowing in the movement of material through the intestinal tract. This can be caused by increased feed intake, new or better pasture, dramatic change in diet, or grain based diets. Enterotoxaemia is most likely to occur during periods of greatest pasture growth and feed availability. The disease in goats is mostly caused by *Clostridium perfringens* type D, although the role of the toxins of this microorganism in the pathogenesis of the disease is not fully understood. The disease occurs in three forms, peracute, acute and chronic, the cardinal clinical sign of the acute and chronic forms being diarrhoea. The main biochemical alterations are hyperglycaemia and glycosuria, while at necropsy the disease is often characterized by haemorrhagic colitis. The typical histological changes observed in the brain of sheep with enterotoxaemia are not considered to be a common feature of enterotoxaemia in goats. Although the pathogenesis of caprine enterotoxaemia has not yet been properly defined, it is usually accepted that the presence of *C. perfringens* type D in the small bowel, together with a sudden change to a diet rich in carbohydrates, is the main predisposing factor for the disease.The symptoms are produced both in natural and experimental infection. One such difference between sheep and goat may be because in ovine the epsilon toxin is more promptly absorbed by ovine than caprine intestine. Work has suggested that epsilon toxin modifies ion and water transport in the small and large intestine of goats and sheep through different mechanisms (Miyakawa and Uzal 2003).

Next most important disease is caused by *C.perfringens* type C. Different varieties of this type have been found in different geographical locations throughout the world (Niilo 1980). Infection with *C. perfringens* type C results in severe enteritis with diarrhoea and dysentery in young lambs, calves, pigs and foals. In Great Britain, it is responsible for causing struck especially when fed in abundance. In calves & goats it causes enterotoxaemia. Pig enterotoxaemia caused by this organism is recorded in pigs during the first week of life. Similarly foal enterotoxaemia is also caused by *C.perfringens* type C.

Both, the bacterial cells and their toxins are needed to initiate disease. *C.perfringens* produce a potent beta-toxin which has activity different from the activity of enterotoxin of type A and epsilon-toxin of type D. The toxin has a molecular weight of approximately 30 kDa and is sensitive to proteolytic enzymes, thus, the full effect of the toxin can be observed under diminished proteolytic enzyme activity (Niilo 1988). Experimentally administered soybean flour used as a protease inhibitor converts the experimentally induced enteritis from non fatal to fatal one. Beta toxin causes increased capillary permeability resulting in increased absorption in blood circulation. This causes increased blood pressures and reduced heart rate leading to atrioventricular block (Sakurai *et al.*, 1981). Recombinant purified beta toxin is glutathione S-transferase (Steinpors dotti *et al.*, 1995). The organisms are ingested by animals, thereafter they proliferate and attaches to the damaged jejunal villi. The toxin is produced and degeneration of mitochondria and damage to terminal capillaries should also be there to facilitate bacterial adherence (Johanssen *et al.*, 1986). The destruction and desquamation of epithelium further facilitates the invasion by bacteria leading to more toxin production which causes more structural tissue damage and haemorrhages. Beta toxin causes cell necrosis and the necrotic tissues are infiltrated and densely covered with *C.perfringens* cells. The intestinal lesions vary from necrotic to haemorrhagic, due to ulceration of the intestinal mucosa.

Clostridium perfringens type B causes lamb dysentery in young animals. Lamb up to 3 weeks and calves up to 10 days of age are most susceptible. In foals it causes the disease with in first few days of life. The course is rapid and mortality is nearly 100%. It is haemorrhagic and causes fatal enterotoxaemia. The disease is prevalent in most of the countries of Asia, Europe and Middle

East. The causative organism occurs in soil and alimentary tract of young animals. The disease is precipitated by some unknown factors. In general rapidly growing well nourished animals are most susceptible. Lamb dysentery is most prevalent in cold weather and on farms where ewes are kept closely confined in small fields for lambing.

Toxigenic strains of *C.perfringens* type B produces beta toxin which is responsible for the disease syndrome. The beta toxin is highly sensitive to trypsin which is a component of normal pancreatic proteases. The trypsin susceptibility of beta-toxin explains in part the predilection of the disease for new born since colostrum on which they survive contains anti-trypsin substances. Beta-toxin is a necrotizing toxin and initially produces damage to the microvilli with degeneration of mitochondria and destruction of epithelial cells similar to type C beta toxin. Extra intestinal lesions include congestion, edema, serosal effusions and haemorrhages in various organs.

C.perfringens type A also causes enterotoxaemia in animals, however, its significance as a disease entity has not been proven. There is acute profuse diarrhea and high mortality. In haemolytic disease, there is an acute onset of severe depression, jaundice, hemoglobinuria, dyspnea & severe abdominal pain. Food is the source of organism which later multiplies and sporulates in intestine which is necessary for the production of enterotoxin. The digestive enzymes do not have any effect on the enterotoxin. The toxin is not released by intact cells. The enterotoxin is a 35 kDa polypeptide having activity on small intestinal mucosa causing profuse fluid loss and diarrhea. Bacterial cells do not invade the intestinal cells. Suitable conditions are required for the enterotoxin to act upon the cells. The toxin binds to the protinacious receptors on the cell membrane followed by the insertion in the plasma membrane of the host cells. Following this, a complex comprising of one toxin molecule and 2 membrane proteins (70 & 50 kDa) with a final size of 160 kDa is formed (Wnek and Mclane 1989). This initial receptor binding is located with in a 30 amino acid sequence at the C-terminal region of the toxin. The region between amino acid sequences 26 and 171 is involved with insertion and cytotoxicity of the toxin. The cytotoxicity can be enhanced by removal of the first 25 sequences of N-terminal region. This binding of toxin to membrane proteins causes alterations in cell membrane permeability leading to rapid changes in intracellular levels of ions and other small molecules.

Subsequently, there is transport reversal manifested by out pouring of water, sodium and chloride ions and inhibition of glucose uptake (McDonel 1979). There may be a change in intestinal motility. All this result in clinical diarrhoea.

The hemolytic disease caused in sheep & cattle in various countries lay some credibility due to the activity of the primary toxin of *C.perfringens* type A, alphatoxin, which possess phospholipase C and sphingomyelinase activity and consequent hemolytic action.

Diagnosis

In cases of enterotoxaemia, numerous Gram positive large organisms are seen in smears from the small intestine. History, clinical signs, and gross postmortem findings are useful tools for establishing a presumptive diagnosis of clostridial enterotoxemia in sheep and goats. Definitive diagnosis requires laboratory confirmation. Isolation of some types of *C. perfringens* (e.g., B and C) can be of diagnostic value, but other types (e.g., A) are so commonly found in the intestine of normal animals that isolation is meaningless from a diagnostic point of view. The most accepted criterion in establishing a definitive diagnosis of enterotoxemia is detection of *C. perfringens* toxins in intestinal contents. Also, histopathological examination of brain is very useful for diagnosis of type D disease, as lesions produced by epsilon toxin in the brains of sheep and goats are pathognomonic for type D enterotoxemia. Ancillary tests, such as measuring urine glucose or observing Gram-stained smears of intestinal mucosa, can be used. However, although such tests have a presumptive diagnostic value when positive, they cannot be used to rule out a diagnosis of enterotoxemia when negative.

Toxin-antitoxin assay is carried out by inoculating in mice to detect toxins in the intestinal content. Injection of mixture of 3 parts of test fluid to one part of known antitoxin to various *C.perfringens* types is given. An intradermal test may also be carried out in the skin of guinea pigs. The type of *C.perfringens* involved is determined by the protection or neutralization pattern observed (Table). The test is performed on both trypsinized and untrypsinized toxin.

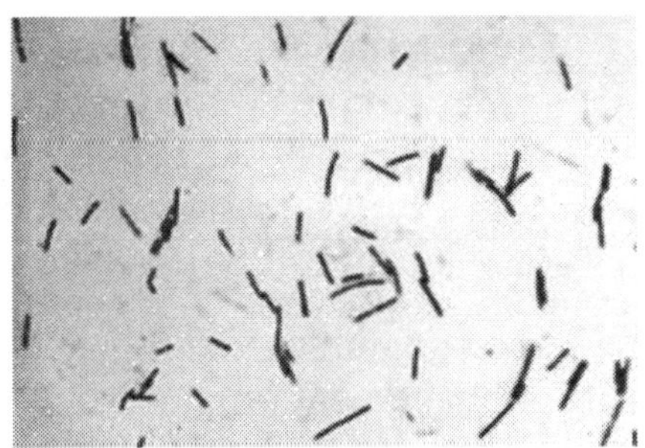

Clostridium perfringens

An enzyme linked Immunosorbent Assay can be performed in place of the neutralization test in order to diagnose serologically. Lee *et al* (2011) reported that two antigenic *C. perfringens* proteins, EF-Tu and PFO can be useful ELISA antigens for *C. perfringens*-afflicted infections in commercial poultry. Recombinant proteins were better than the native proteins.

Intestinal content type	Major lethal toxins	Antitoxins				
		A	B	C	D	E
A	Alpha	+	+	+	+	+
B	Alpha, beta, epsilon	-	+	-	-	-
C	Alpha, beta	-	+	+	-	-
D	Alpha, epsilon	-	+	-	+	-
E	Alpha, iota	-	-	-	-	+

Isolation and Identification of the causative organism can also be carried out using suitable bacteriological media. All strains of *C.perfringens* give a positive Nagler reaction due to the presence of alpha toxin.

C.perfringens produces few spores, unless grown on special media and is non-motile. It produces a characteristics double zone of hemolysis due to the production of 2 toxins. The narrow clear zone next to the colony is produced by theta toxin and the alpha-toxin causes the partial, larger outer zone. Deoxyribonucleic acid probes specific for genes that are responsible for the toxins are being evaluated. A latex test for detecting enterotoxin of type A is available commercially. DNA primers specific for the various genes encoding the toxins have been developed for detection in feces or cultures by using the polymerase chain reaction (Pen Jian Guo *et al.* 2009).

Treatment and Control

Considering the acuteness of the disease, the antimicrobial treatment is not usually useful. Antitoxin of appropriate type may be given to sick animals and to those at risk. Antitoxins prepared in horses against types B, C & D are available. Protection is effective for 2-3 weeks only. Prophylactic dosages given subcutaneously can be doubled and given intravenously for therapy.

Young animals should be weaned slowly in addition to other changes in diet. Management practices aimed at reducing digestive upsets will also help control the disease. Restricting access to grain, concentrates, lush feed, molasses and food scraps will all reduce the disease level. Sudden changes to diet should be avoided. Diets high in grain should be supplemented with adequate roughage. Ensuring against overeating is an effective preventive measure. Feeding of broad spectrum antibiotics decreases the prevalence in lambs.

Bacterins are available for protection in sheep. Alum precipitated formalinized whole broth cultures prepared from strains of type C and D are used to produce an active immunity. The vaccine is effective for one year only and revaccination is required. During outbreaks antitoxin and toxoid are often given and a second dose of toxoid is administered some weeks later. Protection of lambs against type D enterotoxaemia requires 2 vaccinations at monthly intervals. An investigation was undertaken to evaluate the immune response of sheep to 2 types of enterotoxaemia vaccines prepared by incorporating bentonite clay and alum separately as adjuvants. *Clostridium perfringens* type D was used for preparation of vaccines. Two groups of sheep were immunized separately with both vaccine formulations, and the immune response of sheep against all the formulations was assayed by mouse neutralization test (MNT). It was evident from the result that both types of vaccines protected sheep against enterotoxaemia up to 120th day post vaccination (MNT titre of 2 IU/ ml) without booster dose of vaccination. Bentonite clay adjuvanted enterotoxaemia vaccine was found superior to alum precipitated vaccine in terms of cost, availability and production of higher immune response at 30th day of post vaccination (Basavalingappa *et al.* 2008).

Bernath *et al.* (2009) demonstrated that a booster at 8 weeks of an aluminum hydroxide adjuvanted vaccine provide protective immunity in sheep. In another study, the immunity was found to last for 3-4 months and then revaccination is required to prolong the immune status (Pavan Kumar *et al.*, 2008). Ewes are given 2 doses of toxoid 6 weeks before lambing. Lambs are immunized with bacterin or toxoid during the first week of life.

Clostridium tetani

C.tetani is the causative agent of tetanus in animals and man and disease manifestations are basically due to the release of a toxin. *C.tetani* is a strict anaerobe that grows like rods in young cultures but grows as long filaments in older cultures. The organism is motile owing to the presence of numerous peritrichous flagella on vegetative cells. The organisms form spores under strict anaerobic conditions. The organism is gram positive and form terminal spores within a swollen sporangium giving it a distinctive drumstick appearance. Although the bacterium has a typical Gram-positive cell wall, it may stain Gram-negative or Gram-variable, especially in older cells.. The spores are resistant to several disinfectants including heating at 100°C for 30-60 minutes but can be destroyed by autoclaving. The disease is world wide in distribution. Most cases of the disease occur in Asia & Africa due to poor hygienic conditions. Satish & Swaminathan (2009) isolated several clostridial species including *C.tetani* from various sources in South India and reported a great genetic diversity in respect of excretory proteins patterns.

C.tetani are normally present in the feces of animals, especially horses and in soil contaminated by the feces. The bacterium is not ubiquitous and is confined to certain regions only. Probably the nature of soil is the determining factor. An alkaline calcareous clay constitution of soil contains tetanus spores whereas these are not found in acidic soil as well as house dust. The spores of *C.tetani* germinate both aerobically and anaerobically when put in a favourable environment (Shoesmith and Holland 1972).

The portal of entry of the cells is usually through deep puncture wounds. When outbreaks of the so called "idiopathic tetanus" occurs in young cattle without a wound being seen. .It is believed that the toxin is produced in the intestine or is ingested preformed in the feed. The entry of the infection is such cases may be through wounds in the mouth following feeding on rough fibrous feed. It has been suggested that tetanus may be present in the rumen and produce neurotoxin which may cause the disease. The incubation period varies from 1 to 3 weeks with occasional cases occurring as long as several months after the infection is introduced. In sheep and lambs, The disease appears 3-10 days after shearing or docking. The clinical picture is more or less same in all the animals. Animals first develop muscle stiffness accompanied by muscle tremor and later on spasm develops. There is an alert or anxious expression contributed by erect carriage of the ears, retraction of eyelids, dilation of nostrils and exaggerated response to the external stimuli. There is drooling of saliva and animal may stop eating. Constipation is observed and retention of urine is normally seen. There may be rigidity in muscles of the back and tail, extension of the body or protrusion of the nictating membrane. As the disease progresses respiration becomes impared and respiration failure may lead to death. The severity of the disease depends on the quantity of toxins that reaches the central nervous systems.

Pathogenesis

The infective organisms remain deposited at the site of entry and proliferate. The bacterium is non-invasive. The duration of this may vary according to the local conditions. The characteristic symptom of "lockjaw" involves spasms of the masseter muscle. It is an early symptom which is followed by progressive rigidity and violent spasms of the trunk and limb muscles. Spasms of the pharyngeal muscles cause difficulty in swallowing. Death usually results from interference with the mechanics of respiration. Following proliferation the neurotoxin is produced. The length of the incubation period and severity of the disease is determined on the basis of the amount of toxin formed in the primary lesion; toxigenecity of the infecting strain; the amount of toxin reaching the neural pathways; the toxin transferring capacity of the neural pathways and susceptibility of the receptors of the central nervous system which is animal species dependent. The toxins produced are of 2 types, tetanospasmin and tetanolysin. The former is a neurotoxin and the later, a haemolysin. Tetanolysin is produced in low concentration and does not play any significant role in pathogenesis. The toxigenicity is due to the presence of a 75 kb plasmid which carries tox gene. Tetanus neurotoxin is approximately 150 kDa protein that has A-B structure formation properties; the A domain is a zinc metalloprotease and the B encodes a translocation domain and C- *terminal* receptor binding domain (Chen *et al.,* 2009). The toxin is synthesized as a single polypeptide chain with a molecular mass of 150,700 Da. The toxin is intracellular in nature; cleavage of it causes three-fold increase in the activity. In old cultures the toxin is released following lysis of bacterial cells; the toxin is nicked by endogenous proteases. This toxin, termed as extracellular toxin consists of a light chain of 52,288 Da held by a disulfide and non-covalent bonds to a heavy chain with a molecular mass of 98,300 Da. Either constituent toxin itself is non-toxic.

The toxin binds to the nervous tissues through ganglioside via a disialyl group attached to the inner galactose residue of the toxin, however, the ganglioside site is debatable; rather a trypsin sensitive receptor component has been reported (Yavin and Nathan 1986). Montecucco (1986) suggested both, the ganglioside and a protein receptor may be involved in the binding. Recently Chen *et al.* (2009) showed that gangliosides are functional dual receptors for neurotoxin.

At the site of the wound, the toxin reaches the adjoining muscles where it is bound to the presynaptic terminals of the motor axons followed by distribution to all the muscles through lymphatics and blood vascular systems. Transport of the toxin to the central nervous system (CNS) depends on binding to presynaptic membrane receptors and internalization into the membrane and retroaxonal transport within the smooth endoplasmic recticulum carrier system. The toxin reaches the neuronal body and persists there for a long period (Bezzini 1993). Pathogenic action of the toxin is due to its unique ability to pass transsynaptically from the nerve body to the axon terminals and its ability to selectively bind to the pre-synaptic membranes and to interfere with the release of afferent neurotransmitters, glycine and gamma-aminobutyric acid causing the innervated muscle to remain in sustained clonic or tonic spasms. At later stages, excitory neurotransmission is also affected (Bizzini 1993). When small amount of toxin is given in the muscle local tetanus usually occurs characterized by the occurrence of spasm at the local site. The toxin then travels along the tissue spaces of the peripheral nerves to the anterior horns of the spinal cord and may spread anteriorly in the spinal cord (Kryzhanovsky 1981).

Toxin produced in wound by the bacteria reaches primarily the motor nerve endings and is transported intraaxonally retrograte to the some of the neurons in CNS followed by binding presynaptic oxonal terminals of neurons.

Initially it blocks the release of glycine and gamma-amino butyric acid. This results in hyperactivity of motor neurons and leads to muscle spasticity. There is also flaccid paralysis of the diaphragm occasionally observed in affected individuals leading to asphyxia.

No structural lesions are produced as a result of affect of tetanus toxin but it is accompanied by various changes in metabolism. Major changes occur in fluid, acid-base and electrolyte balance and general metabolism. Variations in the level of enzymes are also recorded (Kryzhanovsky 1981). The clinical picture is same is all animals.

Diagnosis

A gram-stained smear from a suspect wound may reveal the typical "drumstick" type of bacteria. It is only suggestive of the presence of tetanus organism because the morphology is not unique to *C.tetani.*

Bacteriologically the wound exudate is plated on blood agar for anaerobic culture. Increased agar concentration (4%) inhibits swarming and a drop of antitoxin inhibits hemolysin on that portion of the plate. Replicated cooked meat broth cultures are incubated and some are heated at 80°C for up to 20 minutes. All are incubated at 37°C for 4-5 days and subcultured periodically on blood agar. Suspect isolates are identified by differential tests and toxin production is confirmed in 2 mice by intramuscular inoculation one of which has received specific antitoxin.

Treatment and Control

Treatment aims at

1. Neutralization of circulating toxin.
2. Suppression of toxin production.
3. Life support and symptomatic relief to the patient.

For achieving first objective injection of adequate doses of antitoxin is given, usually 10,000 to 300,000 units for horses. In animals vaccination can be performed at all ages by injecting 2 doses of tetanus toxoid at 1 month intervals and a third dose 1 year later. Booster injection are repeated every 5th year. Intrathecal administration is also suggested. Toxoid may be administered at different site. Wound care and large doses of parenteral penicillin or metronidazole is given to stop toxin production. Other alternatives are erythromycin, tetracycline, Chloramphenicol and Clindamycin.

Nursing care with appropriate tranquilizors and sedation to prevent titanic seizures is important. Recovery from tetanus does not usually confer permanent immunity because of the production of a very small amount of toxin. Another reason is that the toxin as it is produced in situ by *C. tetani* is readily bound by its receptors on the terminals of the nerves innervating the infected area. Development of natural antitetanus immunity is likely to be related to prolonged ingestion of tetanus spores which are present in highly contaminated areas.

Clostridium botulinum

Botulism is a neuro paralytic intoxication that is caused by a heterogenous groups of bacteria called *C.botulinum;* A to G. *C.botulinum* type G has been renamed as *C.argentinense*. The organism has an unremarkable morphologically. At a pH near or above neutrality it produces subterminal oval spores. *C.botulinum* is a strict anaerobe that can survive extreme environmental conditions by producing spores. Spores are unevenly distributed in food items, animal tissues and feces of some animals. Factors that affect the distribution of various types of *C.botulinum* include temperature, water activity, soil pH and organic matter (Smith and Sugiyama 1988). At the whole organism level, substantial differences between the six botulinum neurotoxin-forming clostridia have been reported (Peck 2009). For example, the genomes of proteolytic *C. botulinum* (*C. botulinum* Group I) and non-proteolytic *C. botulinum* (C. botulinum Group II) are highly diverged and show neither synteny nor homology. It has also emerged that the botulinum neurotoxin-forming clostridia are not overtly pathogenic (unlike *C. difficile*), but saprophytic bacteria that use the neurotoxin to kill a host and create a source of nutrients. One important feature that has contributed to the success of botulinum neurotoxin-forming clostridia is their ability to form highly resistant endospores. The spores, however, also present an opportunity to control these bacteria if escape from lag phase (and hence growth) can be prevented. This is dependent on extending understanding of the biology of these processes. Differences in the genetics and physiology of spore germination in proteolytic *C. botulinum* and non-proteolytic *C. botulinum* have been identified. The biological variability in lag phase and its stages has been described for individual spores, and it has been shown that various adverse treatments extend different stages of lag phase. For example, heat treatment primarily extended germination, while incubation at a chilled temperature primarily extended outgrowth. The neurotoxin gene is present within a cluster of associated genes, and can be located on the chromosome, a plasmid or a bacteriophage. Two basic types of neurotoxin cluster have been identified. Evolution of the neurotoxin gene and cluster has occurred independently of the organism, and involved a series of recombination events but is still poorly understood. Factors affecting the regulation of neurotoxin formation also remain poorly understood, and will be the focus of much future research.

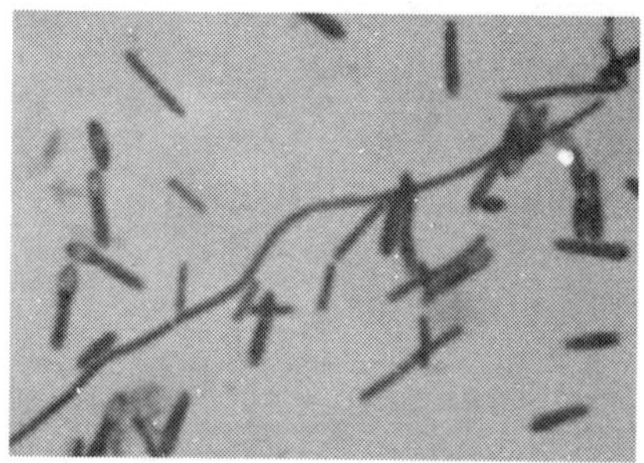

Clostridium botulinum

The disease affects sheep and cattle in areas where they suffer from phosphorous or protein deficiency. The disease occurs in number of animals at a time and is usually fatal. Botulism is generally caused as a food born intoxication caused by consumption of preformed toxins. However, the disease can also be caused as a result of homing of bacteria in intestine followed by the production of the neurotoxins. Silage feeding in animals has led to an increase in cases of *C.botulinum* Group I-III in dairy cattle. The organisms multiply in silage and gastrointestinal tract. Milk also contains spores and toxin and outbreaks in humans due to consumption of contaminated milk has been reported (Lindstrom *et al.,* 2010).

At least 7 different neurotoxins are produced by *C.botulinum* designated as A, B, C, D, E, F and G (Smith and Sugiyama 1988). These toxins are pharmacologically same but serologically distinct with a few exceptions. Common antigens are present in some C and D toxins and E and F toxins.

Strains of *C.botulinum* are denoted by the type of toxin produced but some strains produce more than one toxin. Type C strains produce C_2 or both (Eklund *et al.*, 1987). Some type D strains also produce low titers of C_2 toxin. Some *C. botulinum* strain that produce more than one toxin comprise of A_B, B_A and B_F. The subscript indicating minor neurotoxin being produced. Basic requirements for toxin production are an anaerobic environment, a suitable energy source and a pH above 4.8. Other physiological and cultural characteristics vary between serotypes (Smith and Sugiyama 1988). The toxins are produced intracellularly and released on autolysis. In vitro the production is maximum at the stationary phase. The toxin production and bacterial growth have different nutritional requirements.

The production of neurotoxin C and D is specific phage dependent (Eklund *et al.,* 1987). UV exposed bacteria lose their ability to produce toxin C & D but not C_2. The TOXt phage isolated from type D strains can lysogenize type C strain and induce them to produce type D toxin and vice-versa. The relationship with type C and D host strains is unstable; therefore, the TOXt phages have been described as pseudolysogenic (Eklund *et al.,* 1987). The DNA of the phage is not integrated with the bacterial genome, however, like lysogenic phages they can suppress the lysis of cells through several generations. The stability of the host-phage relationship depends on the bacterial strains, environmental conditions such as temperature and the growth phase of the bacteria (Eklund *et al.*, 1987).

The neurotoxin is produced as an inactive, single chain protein with a molecular weight of 140-170 kDa, that on nicking by protease (trypsin) is nicked into 2 chains, as a dichain molecule, composed of a heavy chain (85-100 kDa) and a light chain (50-59 kDa) held together by a non-covalent bonds and one or more disulfide bonds. The dichain molecule is more toxic than the single chain molecule. Krysinski and Sugiyama (1981) have suggested that nicking and activation are not related and may be a separate phenomenon. An alkaline pre-induced conformational change in the dichain molecule may be necessary for the activation (Das Gupta 1988).

Cattle acquire the infection (toxin) from diverse source such as animal carcasses, hay or silage, poultry litter and brewers grain. The disease is known by various names, such as lamsiekte in South Africa, bulbar paralysis in Australia, and loin disease in USA. The cattle in these areas often become phosphorous deficient and develop pica, forcing them to eat unusual food such as bones and flesh. The consumption of bones & flesh may be lethal if the carcass is toxic. The lamsiekte form of botulism also occurs in protein deficient sheep in South Africa and Australia. Similarly forage poisoning occurs due to consumption of hay or silage contaminated with the toxin laden carcass. Neurotoxin type C is usually involved. Horse botulism outbreak may also follow due to type C & D neurotoxin after consumption of contaminated forage. Poultry waste used as manure may be the source of neurotoxin for cattle and horses. In foals the disease is known as shaker foal syndrome. It occurs in foals of mares that are fed an excessive nutritious diet supplemented with protein, vitamins and minerals or those exposed to stress such as inclement weather. Botulism in poultry is associated with neurotoxin type C, occasionally type A is involved. Cannibalism of decaying carcasses was the cause of outbreaks in broiler chickens, but it is difficult to trace back the cause in most of the cases (Dohmes 1987). Recently, it has been investigated that *C.botulinum* in the intestine may contribute as an important source of intoxication in broiler chicken. Caecum is probably the site of production of the toxin. Chicken fed type C spores produces toxin in fecal dropping which on coprophagy develop botulism and die (Huyn and Sakaguchi 1989).

Pathogenesis

The toxins of *C.botulinum* are neurotoxins and produce functional paralysis without the development of histological lesions. When toxin is injected much smaller doses are required to cause death than when it is ingested, probably due to digestion of some of the toxin by the proteolytic enzymes in the gut.

After the experimental administration of botulinum toxins in goats clinical signs appear on the second or 3rd day. If small doses of toxins are administered over a number of days cumulative effect are produced.

In toxicoinfectious botulism, the spores are germinated in tissues followed by toxin production. Shaker foal syndrome is caused by this mechanism. Clinically, the foal shows sudden onset of the weakness and prostration, with the foal going down and unable to rise. It shows muscle tremor, recumbancy and complete prostration. Death is due to the respiratory failure.

Neurotoxin released after the lysis of bacterial cells is produced as pro-toxin activated by proteases (Bacterial or tissue). At peripheral cholinergic nerve junction it inhibits acetylcholine release, thereby blocking transmission of neural impulses. The toxin is acid and pepsin resistant but inactivated by protein denaturing agents. The toxin produced by the bacterial cells has at least 3 steps to exert their action. Ist critical step is the binding of the toxin to the cell membrane and further accumulation at the neuromuscular junction. The binding sites are confined to presynaptic nerve cell membranes (Dolly *et al.*, 1984; Black and Dolly 1986). Although, the receptors for neurotoxins have not been defined, however, it is believed that not all the toxin types have same receptors (Kozaki 1979). This explains the different susceptibility of the various animal species to the different types of botulinum toxin. Probably the binding domain resides on the heavy chain. Both H & L chains are required for paralytic activity indicating that the H chain helps in the binding and the L chain causes paralysis, following endocytosis through the receptors. Endocytosis is a two step process in which the receptor bound toxin is first encapsulated into an endosome and then penetrates the endosomal membrane by a pre-dependent mechanism to enter the cytoplasm (Rocke 1993). This mechanism appears to be mediated by the aminoterminus of H chain.

The light chain of type B neurotoxin is a zinc endopeptidase that cleaves synaptobrevin, a protein located in the membrane of the synaptic vesicle (Schiavo *et al.*, 1992). Hydrolysis of this protein leads to degeneration of synapse. Degeneration takes several months. Synaptobrevin is critical for the release of acetylcholine from synaptic vesicles. The osmolyte bimethyl amine N-oxide increases the proteolytic activity of L chain (Nuss *et al.*, 2010). Type A & E neurotoxin have no effect on this protein. The neurotoxin inhibit the release of neurotransmitter (Simpson 1981).

Closridium botulinum type C_2 toxin is an NDP-ribosyl transferase, causing depolymerization of the actin cytoskeleton in eukaryotic cells. The C_2 toxin is a binary toxin consisting of the enzymatic subunit C_2I and the binding submit C2 II. Proteolytical activation of the binding unit triggers the formation of heptameric structures (C_2IIa) which blind to cellular receptors. C_2I is able to bind to C_2 II oligomers and the whole complex is internalized by a raft dependent mechanism (Pust *et al.,* 2010). This endocytosin involve clathrin and Rho.

Each molecule the toxins that cause botulism is specifically neutralized by its **antitoxin**. Botulinum toxins can be toxoided and make good antigens for inducing protective antibody. As with tetanus, immunity to botulism does not develop, even with severe disease, because the amount of toxin necessary to induce an immune response is lethal. Repeated occurrences of botulism has been reported. Once the botulinum toxin has bound to nerve endings, its activity is unaffected by antitoxin. Any circulating (unfixed) toxin can be neutralized by intravenous injection of antitoxin. Therefore, individuals known to have ingested food with botulism should be treated immediately with antiserum.

Diagnosis

Diagnosis of botulism depends on the demonstration of toxins in blood or tissue before death or from a fresh carcass. Isolation of the bacterial cells from intestinal contents is not definitive. Demonstration of toxins in feed stuffs, fresh stomach contents or vomitus supports a diagnosis of botulism.

If the level of toxin is high in an animal at sometimes it can be demonstrated in urine and serum by mouse inoculation. For extracting toxins, the suspected material is treated with saline overnight and the mixture is centrifuged. The clear supernatant is filter sterilized and trypsinized for 45 minutes. Guinea pigs or mice are injected intraperitoneally with the clear fluid (extract), mixture of extract and antitoxin and extract heated at 100^{0}C for 10 minutes. Death due to botulism will occur with in 10 hours to 3 weeks preceded by muscular weakness, limb paralysis and respiratory difficulties. No signs are visible in animals given mixture of extract and antitoxin.

For isolation of bacteria the suspected material (feed, tissue etc.) are heated for 30-40 minutes at 65^{0}C to 80^{0}C to induce germination. Type E spores require in addition, treatment with lysozyme (5mg/ml of medium). Blood agar plates are inoculated with the material and cultured anaerobically. Colonies appear on plates after 48-72 hours. Grams staining reveals gram-positive sporulating bacilli. Identification is possible by carrying out biochemical reactions and testing for toxin production. Molecular techniques targeted to the neurotoxin genes are ideal for the detection and identification of C. *botulinum,* but they do not detect biologically active neurotoxin and should not be used alone.Lindstrom *et al.* (2001) described a multiplex PCR assay for the detection of Clostridium botulinum types A, B, E, and F in food and fecal material was developed. The method employs four new primer pairs with equal melting temperatures, each being specific to botulinum neurotoxin gene type A, B, E, or F, and enables a simultaneous detection of the four serotypes. A total of 43 *C. botulinum* strains and 18 strains of other bacterial species were tested. DNA amplification fragments of 782 bp for C. botulinum type A alone, 205 bp for type B alone, 389 bp for type E alone, and 543 bp for type F alone were obtained. Other bacterial species, including *C. sporogenes* and the nontoxigenic nonproteolytic *C. botulinum*-like organisms, did not yield a PCR product. Sensitivity of the PCR for types A, E, and F was 10(2) cells and for type B was 10 cells per reaction mixture. With a two-step enrichment, the detection limit in food and fecal samples varied from 10(-2) spore/g for types A, B, and F to 10(-1) spore/g of sample material for type E. Of 72 natural food samples investigated, two were shown to contain *C. botulinum* type A, two contained type B, and one contained type E. The assay is sensitive and specific and provides a marked improvement in the PCR diagnostics of C. botulinum. A focused oligonucleotide microarray featuring 62 probes targeting strain variable regions of the *Clostridium botulinum* strain ATCC 3502 genome sequence was developed to differentiate *C. botulinum* type A strains (Raphael *et al.* 2010). The strain variable regions were selected from deletions identified among a panel of 10 type A strains compared to the strain ATCC 3502 genome sequence using high density comparative genomic hybridization microarrays. The focused microarray also featured specific probes for the detection of the neurotoxin genes of various serotypes (A-G), toxin gene cluster components (ha70 and orfX1), and fldB as a marker for proteolytic clostridia (Group I). Eight pairs of strains selected from separate type A botulism outbreaks were included in the 27 subtype A1-A4 strains examined in this study. Each outbreak related strain pair consisted of strains isolated from different sources (stool and food). Of the eight outbreak related strain pairs, six groups of strains with indistinguishable hybridization patterns were identified. Outbreak related strains were shown to have identical hybridization patterns. Strain pairs from three separate outbreaks involving strains harboring both the type A neurotoxin gene (bont/A) and an unexpressed type B neurotoxin gene (bont/B) shared the same probe hybridization profile. The focused microarray format provides a rapid approach for neurotoxin gene detection and preliminary determination of the relatedness of strains isolated from different sources.

Treatment and Control

Inoculation of antimicrobials is of no use. Intravenous administration of antitoxin in laboratory animals is useful if given during the early stage of infection, especially into mink and duck. In large animals, it is difficult to prevent the infection by antitoxin treatment. Guanidine and aminopyridine stimulates acetyl choline release and germine intensifies neural impulses. Clinical reports on their use are few and mixed.

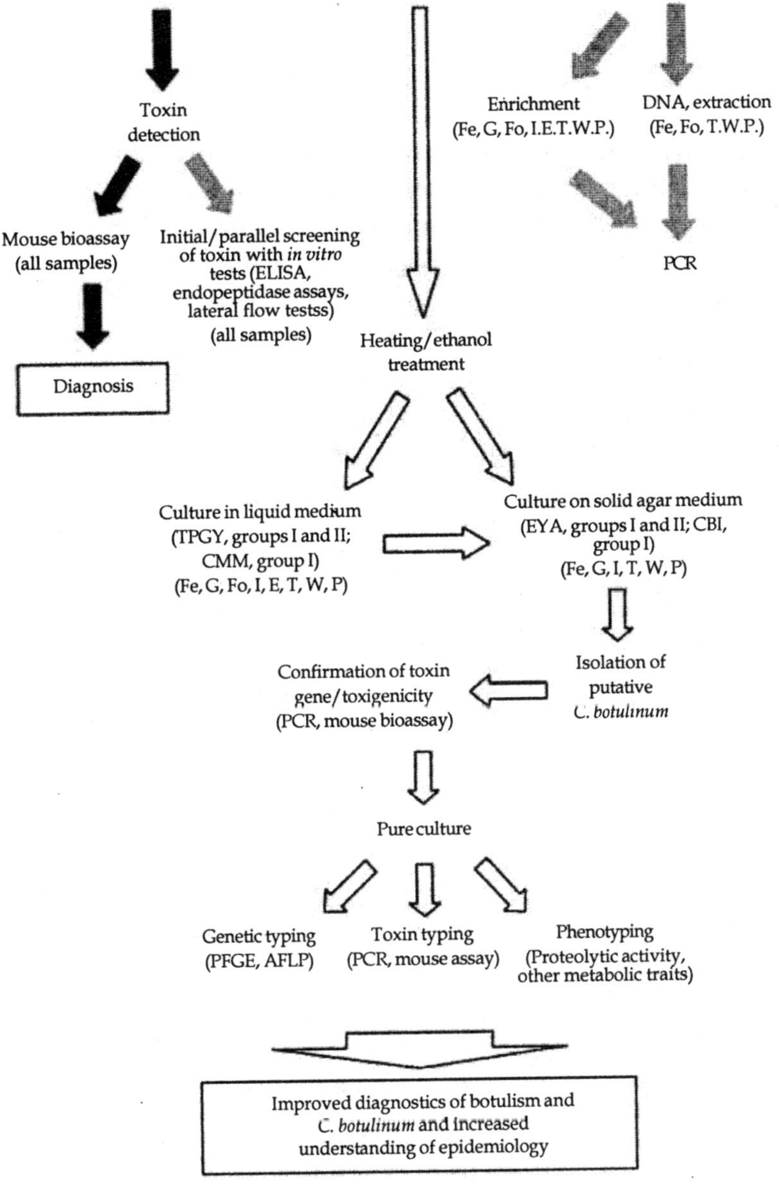

Diagnosis of *C. botulinum*

Botulinum toxin can be inactivated with formaldehyde to produce a toxoid that is immunogenic. Toxoids have been used successfully as vaccines to prevent botulism in domestic and captive reared animals. Vaccination of cattle with C_1 and D has been effective in preventing lamsiekte in South Africa and Australia. In young horses, Shaker foal syndrome has been prevented by vaccinating pregnant mares with type B toxoid a few weeks prior to parturition (Johnston and Whitlock 1987).

Toxoids are used for preventing the disease in cattle and mink with success. Bivalent or trivalent antitoxins are available for prophylactic use. They are of questionable value after clinical signs have developed.

Recombinant neurotoxin vaccines with adjuvants developed as multivalent vaccine have been tested for stability (Vessely *et al.,* 2009), and could be used for the vaccination in animals and man. In order to reduce the degeneration of the toxin using formaline, a novel non toxic method of alkylation with iodoacetamide in the presence of reversibly denaturing condition has been described. This way the potency of the antitoxin increased many fold (Jones *et al.,* 2008).

Control requires avoidance of spoiled or otherwise suspicious foals. Cooking at 100ºC for 10 minutes destroys the toxin.

References

Aikat, B.K. and Dible, J.H. 1960. The local and general effects of cultures and culture filtrate of *Clostridium oedematiens, Cl. septium, Cl. sporogenes* and *Cl. histolyticum*. J. pathol. Bacteriol. **79:** 227-241.

Arsecularatue, S.N., Panabokke, R.G. and Wijesundra, S. 1969. The toxins responsible for the lesions of *Clostridium sordelli* gas gangrene. J. Med. Microbiol. **2:** 37-53.

Bagge, E., Sternberg Lewerin, S. and Johansson K.K. 2009. Detection and identification by PCR of *Clostridium chouvoei* in clinical isolates, bovine feces and substrates from biogas plants. Acta. Vet. Scand. **51:** 8.

Basavalingappa ., B. , Rishnamurthy, S. K., Suryanarayana ,G. V., Byregowda V. V. S., Shrikrishna Isloor, Mayannaasha,. S. M. and Krishnappa G.2008.Immune response of sheep to bentonite clay and alum-adjuvanted enterotoxaemia vaccines. Ind.Jour.Anim. Sci. **78:** 201-203.

Bernath, S., Fabian, K., Kadar, I, Szita, G. and Barna, T. 2004. Optimum time interval between the first vaccination and the booster of sheep for *Clostridium perfringens* type D. Acta. Veterinaria Brno. **73:** 473-475.

Bette, P., Frevert, J., Mauler, F., Suttrop, N. and Habermann, E. 1989. Pharmacological and biochemical studies of cytotoxicity of *Clostridium novyei* type A alpha toxin. Infect. Immun. **57:** 2507-2513.

Bizzini, B. 1993. *Clostridium titani*: In pathogenesis of bacterial diseases in animals. pp. 97-105. Ed. C.L. Gyles & C.O. Thoen. Iowa State University Press, Ames, Iowa, USA.

Black, J.D. and Dolly, J.O. 1986. Interaction of 125 I-labelled nurotoxins with nerve terminals. I. ultrastructural autoradiographic localization and quantitation of distinct membrane acceptors for types A & B on motor nerves. J. Cell. Biol. **103:** 521-534.

Blackwell, T.E., Butler, D.G., Prescott, J.F. and Wilcock, B.P. 1991. Differences in signs and lesions in sheep and goats with enterotoxaemia induced by intraduodenal infusion of *Clostridium perfringens* type D. Am. J. Vet. Res. **52:** 1147-1152.

Blandine, Geny, Hout, K., Catherine, K., LetriciaZ., Christelle, M., Nedege, C., Marek, S., *et al.*, 2007. *Clostridium sordelli* lethal toxin kills mice by inducing a major increase in lung vascular permeability. Am. J. pathol. **170:** 1003-1017.

Bullen, J.J. 1970. Role of toxins in host-parasite relationships. In Microbial Toxins, Vol. I. Ed. S.J. Ajl, S. Kadis & T.C. Montie, pp. 233-76. New York, Academic Press.

Buxton, D. and Morgan, K.T. 1976. Studies of lesions produced in the brain of colostrum deprived lambs by *Clostridium welchii (Cl. perfringens)* type D toxin. J. Comp. Pathol. **86:** 435-447.

Chen, C., Fu Z.., Kim, J.J., Barbieri, J.T. and Baldwin, M.R. 2009. Glycosides as high affinity receptors for tetanus neurotoxin. J. Biol. Chem. **284:** 26569-26577.

Das Gupta, B.R. 1988. The structure of botulinum neurotoxins: In botulinum neurotoxin and tetanus toxin Ed. L.L. Simpson pp. 296-314. New York, Academic Press, New York.

Demelo, F.J., Anderson, R., Hitchcock, C.R. and Hagein, J.J. 1974. Ultrastructure study of clostridial myositis. Arch Pathol. **97:** 118-125.

Dixit, S.N. and Khera, S.S. 1968. Pathogenesis of *Clostridium chauvoei* infection in guinea pigs. Indian J. Exp. Biol. **6:** 80-83.

Dohms, J.E. 1987. Laboratory investigations of botulism in poultry. In Avian Botulism. An international perspective, Ed. M.W. Eklund and V.R. Dowell. Jr. pp. 296-314. Springfield Ill. Charles C. Thomas.

Dolly, J.O., Black, J., Williams, R.S. and Melling, J. 1984. Acceptors for botulinum neurotoxin reside on motor nerve terminals and mediate its internalization. Nature **307:** 457-460.

Eklund, M.W., Poysky, F.T., Oguma, K., Lida, H. and Inoue, K. 1987. Relationship of bacteriophage to toxins and haemagglutinin production by *Clostridium botulinum* types C and D and its significance in avian botulism outbreaks. In Avian Botulism. An international perspective, ed. M. W. Eklund and V.R. Dowell. Jr. pp. 191-222, Springfield, Ill. Charles C. Thomas.

Gadalla, M.S.A. and Collee, J.G. 1968. The relationship of neuraminidase of *Clostridium septicum* to the hemagglutinin and other soluble products of the organism. J. Pathol. Bacteriol. **96:** 169-185.

Griner, L.A. 1961. Enterotoxaemia of sheep. I. Effect of *Clostridium perfringens* type D toxins on the brain of sheep and mice. Am. J. Vet. Res. **22:** 129-142.

Gyles, C. L. 1993. Histotoxic Clostridia: In pathogenesis of Bacterial Infections in Animals. Ed. C.L. Gyles and C.O. Thoen. pp 106-113. Iowa State University Press. Ames, Iowa.

Halm A., Wagner M., Köfer J. and Hein I.2010.Novel real-time PCR assay for simultaneous detection and differentiation of Clostridium chauvoei and Clostridium septicum in clostridial myonecrosis. J. Clin. Microbiol. **48:** 1093-8. Epub 2010 Feb 3.

Hang'ombe M.B., Kohda T., Mukamoto M. and Kozaki S. 2005.Relationship between Clostridium septicum alpha-toxin activity and binding to erythrocyte membranes. J. Vet. Med. Sci. **67:** 69-74.

Hang'ombe M.B., Mukamoto M., Kohda T., Sugimoto N. and Kozaki S.2004.Cytotoxicity of Clostridium septicum alpha-toxin: its oligomerization in detergent resistant membranes of mammalian cells. Microb. Pathog. **37:** 279-86. Epub 2004 Nov 13.

Huyn, S. and Sakaguchi, G. 1989. Implications of coprophagy in pathogenesis of chicken botulism. Jpn. J. Vet. Sci. **51:** 582-586.

Johannsen, U., Menger, S., Erwerth, W. And Koehler, B. 1986. Untersuchngen zur *Clostridium perfringens* type C Enterotoxaemia der Sangferkel. 3 Arch. Exp. Veterinaermed **40:** 895-909.

Johnston, J. and Whitlock, R.H. 1987. Botulism. In current therapy in Equine Medicine-Two. Ed. N.E. Robinson pp. 367-70. Philedelphia: W.B. Saunders Co.

Jones, R.G., Liu Y., Ringsby, P. and Sesardic, D. 2008. An improved method for development of toxoid vaccine and antitoxins. J. Immunol. Method. **337:** 42-48.

Knapp O., Maier E., Mkaddem S.B., Benz R., Bens M., Chenal A., Geny B., Vandewalle A. and Popoff M.R.2010.Clostridium septicum alpha-toxin forms pores and induces rapid cell necrosis. Toxicon. **55:** 61-72. Epub 2009 Jul 24.

Kojima A., Amimoto K., Ohgitani T. and Tamura Y. 1999.Characterization of flagellin from Clostridium chauvoei. Vet. Microbiol. **67:** 231-237.

Kojima A., Uchida I., Sekizaki T., Sasaki Y., Ogikubo Y., Kijima M. and Tamura Y.2000.Cloning and expression of a gene encoding the flagellin of Clostridium chauvoei. Vet Microbiol. **76:** 359-372.

Kozaki, S. 1979. Interaction of botulinum types A, B and E derivative toxins with synaptosomes of rat brain. Naunyn Schmiedebergs Arch. Pharmacol. **308:** 67-70.

Krysinski, E.P. and Sugiyama, H. 1981. Nature of intracellular type A botulinum neurotoxin. Appl. Environ. Microbiol. **41:** 675-678.

Kryzhanovsky, G.N. 1981. Pathophysiology In tetanus- Important new concepts. Vol. 1. pp. 109-82. Amsterdam, Oxford, Princeton: Excerpta medica.

Lange M., Neubauer H. and Seyboldt C.2010.Development and validation of a multiplex real-time PCR for detection of Clostridium chauvoei and Clostridium septicum. Mol. Cell Probes. **24:** 204-10. Epub 2010 Mar 31.

Lee K, Lillehoj HS, Li G, Park MS, Jang SI, Jeong W, and Jeoung HY, An DJ, Lillehoj EP.2011.Identification and cloning of two immunogenic Clostridium perfringens proteins, elongation factor Tu (EF-Tu) and pyruvate:ferredoxin oxidoreductase (PFO) of C. perfringens. Res Vet Sci. 2011 Feb 21[http://www.ncbi.nlm.nih.gov/pubmed/21345474].

Li G., Lillehoj H.S., Lee K.W., Lee S.H., Park M.S., Jang S.I., Bauchan G.R., Gay C.G., Ritter G.D., Bautista D.A. and Siragusa G.R.2010.Immunopathology and cytokine responses in commercial broiler chickens with gangrenous dermatitis. Avian Pathol. **39:** 255-264.

Lindstrom, M.,Keto R., Makkula A.,Navas M., Hielm S.and Korkeala H.2001.Multiplex PCR assay for detection and identification of Clostridium botilinum types A,B,E,and F in food and fecal material. Appl. Environ.Microbiol. **67:** 5694-5699.

Lindstrom, M., Myllykoski, J., Sivela, S., Korkeala, H. 2010. Clostridium botulinum in cattle and dairy products. Crit. Rev. Food Sci. Nutr. **50:** 281-304.

Mattar M.A., Cortiñas T.I. and Stefanini A.M.2007.Extracellular proteins of Clostridium chauvoei are protective in a mouse model. Acta. Vet. Hung. **55:** 159-170.

McDonel, J.L. 1979. The molecular mode of action of *Clostridium perfringens* enterotoxin. Am. J. Clin. Nutr. **32:** 210-218.

Miyakawa, F. and Uzal, F.A. 2003. The early effects of *Clostridium perfringens* type D Epsilon toxin in ligated intestinal loops of goats and sheep. Vet. Res. Commun. **27:** 231-241.

Montecucco, C. 1986. How do tetanus and botulinum toxins bind to neuronal membranes? Trends Biochem. Sci. **11:** 314-317.

Mudenda Hang'ombe B., Kohda T., Mukamoto M. and Kozaki S.2006.Purification and sensitivity of Clostridium chauvoei hemolysin to various erythrocytes. Comp. Immunol. Microbiol. Infect. Dis. **29:** 263-268. Epub 2006 Aug 17.

Nagahama, M. and Sakurai, J. 1992. High affinity binding of *Clostridium perfringens* epsilon toxin to rat brain. Infect. Immun. **60:** 1237-1240.

Neumann A.P. and Rehberger T.G.2009. MLST analysis reveals a highly conserved core genome among poultry isolates of Clostridium septicum. Anaerobe. **15:** 99-106.

Neumann A.P., Dunham S.M., Rehberger T.G. and Siragusa G.R. 2010.Quantitative real-time PCR assay for Clostridium septicum in poultry gangrenous dermatitis associated samples. Mol Cell Probes. **24:** 211-218. Epub 2010 Apr 23.

Niilo, L. 1980. *Clostridium perfringens* in animal disease: A review of current knowledge. Can. Vet. J. **21:** 141-148.

Niilo, L. 1988. *Clostridium perfringens* type C enterotoxaemia. Can. Vet. J. **29:** 658-664.

Niilo, L. 1993. Enterotoxaemic *Clostridium perfringens*. In pathogenesis of Bacterial diseases in animals. Pp. 114-123. Ed. C.L. Gyles and C.O. Thoen. Iowa State University Press, Ames, USA.

Nuss, J.E. Wanner, L.M., Tressler, L.E. and Bavari, S. 2010. The osmolyte trimethylamine N-oxide (TMAO) increases the proteolytic activity of botulinum neurotoxin light chain A, B & C: implications for enhancing analytic assay sensitivity. J. Biomol. Screen. **15:** 928-936.

Oksche, A., Nakov, R. and Habermann, E. 1992. Morphological and biochemical study of cytoskeletal changes in cultured cells after extracellular application of *Clostridium novyii* alpha toxin. Infect. Immun. **60:** 3002-3006.

Ontiveros Corpus Mde L., Hernández Andrade L., López Mendez J., Tenorio Gutierrez V.2008.Prevention of Blackleg by an immunogen of Clostridium chauvoei. Ann. N. Y. Acad. Sci. **1149:** 303-305.

Pang, Jian Guo, Quang Jing Ning and Fang, J. [Isolation and development of a PCR method for the detection of *Clostridium perfringens* in dogs]. Chinese J. Vet. Sci. Technol. **34:** 45-50.

Pavan Kumar, T., Sunitha, G., Krishnamohan, A.V. and Hanumanth Reddy, G. 2008. Seromonitoring by indirect ELISA of sheep vaccinated against enterotoxaemia. Ind. Vet. J. **85:** 1253-1255.

Peck M.W.2009.Biology and genomic analysis of Clostridium botulinum. Adv Microb Physiol. **55:** 183-265.

Pust, S., Barth, H. and Sanding, K. 2010. *Clostridium botulinum* C_2 toxin is internalized by Clathrin and Rho-dependent mechanisms. Cell Microbiol. Aug, 2, [http://www.nebi.nlm.nih.gov/pubmed/20690924].

Raphael B.H., Joseph L.A., McCroskey L.M., Lúquez C., Maslanka S.E.2010.Detection and differentiation of Clostridium botulinum type A strains using a focused DNA microarray. Mol Cell Probes. **24**(3): 146-153.

Reef, V.B. 1983. *Clostridium perfringens* cellulitis and immune mediated hemolytic anaemia in a horse. J. Am. Vet. Med. Assoc. **182:** 251-254.

Rocke, T.E. 1993. *Clostridium botulinum*. In pathogenesis of bacterial infections in animals. Ed. C.L. Gyles and C.O. Thoen, pp. 86-96, Iowa; Iowa State University Press.

Sakurai, J., Fujii, Y., Matsura, M. and Endo, K. 1981. Pharmacological effect of beta toxin of *Clostridium perfringens* type C on rats. Microbiol. Immunol. **25:** 423-432.

Sasaki Y, Yamamoto K, Kojima A, Norimatsu M, Tamura Y.2000. Rapid identification and differentiation of pathogenic clostridia in gas gangrene by polymerase chain reaction based on the 16S-23S rDNA spacer region. Res Vet Sci. **69:** 289-294.

Sasaki Y., Yamamoto K., Amimoto K., Kojima A., Ogikubo Y., Norimatsu M.,Ogata H.and Tamura Y.2001.Amplification of the 16S-23S rDNA spacer region for rapid detection of Clostridium chauvoei and Clostridium septicum. Res Vet Sci. **71**(3): 227-229.

Satish, S., and Swaminathan, K. 2009. Genetic diversity among toxigenic clostridia from soil, water, meat and associated polluted sites in South India. Ind. J. Med. Microbiol. **27:** 311-320.

Sayeed, S., Jihong, Li and Meclane, B.A. 2007. Virulence plasmid diversity in *Clostridium perfringens* type D isolates. Infect. Immun. **75:** 2391-2398.

Schiavo, G. Benfenati, F., Poulain, B., Rosetto, O., Polverino de Laurets, P., Das Gupta, B.R. and Montecucco, C. 1992. Tetanus and botulism B neurotoxins block neurotransmitter release by proteolytic cleavage of synaptobrevin. Nature **359:** 832-835.

Shoesmith, J.G. and Holland, K.T. 1972. The germination of spores of *Clostridium tetani*. J. Gen. Microbiol. **70:** 253-261.

Simpson, L.L. 1981. The origin, structure and pharmacological activity of botulinum toxin. Pharmacol. Rev. **33:** 155-188.

Smith L. D.S. 1975a. Clostridial wound infections. In the pathogenic Anaerobic Bacteria 2nd ED. Pp. 321-24, Springfield Ill. Charles C. Thomas.

Smith L. D.S. 1979. Virulence factors of *Clostridium perfringens*. Rev. Infect. Dis. **1:** 254-260.

Smith, L. D.S. 1975b. *Clostridium sordelli*: In the Pathogenic Anaerobic Bacteria. 2nd Ed. pp. 291-98 spring field Ill., Charles C. Thomas.

Smith, L.D.S. and Sugiyama, H. 1988. Botulism, the organism, its toxins, the disease. Springfield Ill. Charles C. Thomas.

Steinporsdotti, V., Fridriksdoftir, V., Gunnarson, E. and Andersson, O.S. 1995. Expression and purification of *Clostridium perfringens* beta toxin glutathione S-transferase fusion protein. FEMS Microbiology letters. **130:** 273-278.

Songer J.G. and Uzal F.A. 2005.Clostridial enteric infections in pígs. J Vet Diagn Invest. **17:** 528-536.

Tellez G., Pumford N.R., Morgan M.J., Wolfenden A.D. and Hargis B.M.2009.Evidence for Clostridium septicum as a primary cause of cellulitis in commercial turkeys. J. Vet. Diagn. Invest. **21:** 374-377.

Useh, N.M., Ajanusi, J.O., Esievo, K.A.N. and Nok, A.J. 2006. Characterization of a sialidase (neuraminidase) isolated from *Clostridium chauvoei* (Jakari strain) Cell Biochem. Function **24:** 347-352.

Uzal, F.A., Belak, K., Rivera, E., Robles, C.A. and Feinstein, R.E. 2010. Bacillary haemoglobinuria diagnosis by the peroxidase- antiperoxidase (PAP) technique. Jr. Vet. Med. **39:** 595-598.

Uzal, F.A., Hugenholtz, P., Blackall, L.L., Petray, S., Moss, S., Assis, R.A., Fernandez Miakawa, M. and Carloni, G. 2003. PCR detection of *Clostridium chauvoei* in pure cultures and in formalin fixed paraffin embedded tissues. Vet. Microbiol. **91:** 239-248.

Vankempen, K.R. and Kennedy, P.C. 1969. Experimental bacillary hemoglobinuria II. Pathogenesis of the hepatic lesions in rabbits. Pathol. Vet. **6:** 59-67.

Vesseley, C., Estey, T., Randolph, T.W., Henderson, I., Cooper, J., Nayar, R., Braun, L.J. and Carpenter, J.F. 2009. Stability of a trivalent recombinant protein vaccine formulation against botulism neurotoxin during storage in aqueous solution. J. Pharm. Sci. **98:** 2970-2993.

Vilei E.M., Johansson A., Schlatter Y., Redhead K. and Frey J.2011.Genetic and functional characterization of the NanA sialidase from Clostridium chauvoei. Vet. Res. **42:** 2.

Wnek, A.P. and Mclane, A.B. 1989. Preliminary evidence that *Clostridium perfringens* type A enterotoxin is present in a 160,000 M complex in mammalian membranes. Infect. Immun. **57:** 574-581.

Yavin, E. and Nathan, A. 1986. Tetanus toxin receptors of nerve cells contain a trypsin-sensitive components. Eur. J. Biochem. **154:** 403-407.

□□□

Chapter 4

Diseases Caused by *Corynebacterium* spp.

Dr. S.K. SRIVASTAVA
Former, Division of Bacteriology & Mycology
Indian Veterinary Research Institute, Izatnagar-243122
Bareilly (U.P.)

Corynebacterium spp. are responsible for causing a wide variety of pyogenic infections in animals, namely cattle, buffalo, sheep, goats & swine. Occasionally disease is caused in horses. The organism enters the body through abrasion, wounds and insect bites & may cause localized or systemic infection. There are several species of *Corynebacterium* responsible for causing the disease. The following list provides name of various species of *Corynebacterium*. There are more than 30 species of *Corynebacterium* but only a few are regularly responsible for disease in animals.

S.N.	Corynebacterium spp.	Disease produced	Chief Host
1	*Corynebacterium (Actinomyces, Arcanobacterium) pyogenes*	Purulent disease, Mastitis, metritis	Cattle, Sheep & Swine
2	*C. bovis*	Commensal, mild mastitis	Cattle, Goats
3	*C. diphtheriae*	Diphtheria, pharyngitis	Man
4	*C. (Rhodococcus) equi*	Granulomatons pneumonia	Horse
5	*C. (Arcanobacterium) haemolyticum*	Pharyngitis, skin infection	Human
6	*C. pseudotuberculosis (C.ovis)*	Abscesses, lymphadenitis	Sheep & Goat
7	*C. (Eubacterium, Actinobaculum) suis*	Cystitis, pyelonephritis	Swine
8	*C. ulcerans*	Pharyngitis	Human
9	*C. renael* *C. pilosum* *C. cystitidis*	Cystitis, pyelonephritis -do-	Cattle, Sheep Cattle, Sheep Cattle, Sheep

The role of some of the important species as a causative agent in various diseases has been described in the following sections. The organisms are aerobic, gram-positive, club shaped rods (Coryneform bacteria) arranged in Chinese letter style.

Corynebacterium renale group

C.renale in association with *C.pilosum* and *C.cystitidis* are considered to be the apportunist pathogens responsible for causing sporadic cases of cystitis and ascending pyelonephritis (Yanagawa 1986). The disease is named as contagious bovine pyelonephritis. Three immunologic types of *C.renale* I, II & III are now recognized. Due to the lack of genetic and chemotaxonomic identification methods, distinguishing the different species from the group remained impossible. Rather phenotypic identification of the organisms was the normal identification process used before. Only in the late 1970s, due to new methods such as genetic analyses (16S rRNA & rDNA sequencing, nucleic acid hybridization, etc), chemotaxonomic methods (detection of mycolic acids, peptidoglycan analyis, cellular fatty acid studies, menaquinone characterization, etc.) and phenotypic techniques (identification systems, organic compound assimilation tests, etc) was the group distinguished as three different species On the basis of taxonomic studies, each type has been given a species name; type I, *C. renale*, type II, *C. pilosum*, type III, *C. cystitidis*. They can be distinguished by biochemical reactions. Type I appears to be most pathogenic type capable of producing complement fixing antibodies which cross react with *Mycobacterium johnii*. *C. renale* is a facultatively anaerobic Gram positive organism, characterized by non-encapsulated, non-sporulated, immobile, straight or curved rods with a length of 1 to 8 µm and width of 0.3 to 0.8 µm, which form ramified aggregations in culture (looking like "Chinese characters"). The bacterium is sensitive to the majority of antibiotics, such as the penicillins, ampicillin, cephalosporins, quinolones, chloramphenicol, tetracyclines, cefuroxime and trimethoprim. Arai *et al.* (1997) showed the relationship between infection stone and Corynebacterium species in vitro and in vivo. Urease activity of urease-splitting Corynebacterium species was evaluated by 2 methods; an increase in pH of urine after inoculation of Corynebacterium species and direct measurement of urease activity of 10(7) CFU organisms from amounts of ammonia by indophenol method. Formation of infection bladder stone was induced in male Wistar rats by implanting a zinc disc and inoculating 10(6) CFU organisms surgically into the bladder. Urine was alkalinized by the inoculation of Corynebacterium renale, *C. pilosum* and group D2 Corynebacterium. *C. renale* and *C. pilosum* had strong urease activity, and group D2 Corynebacterium had moderate activity. C. pseudodiphtheriticum did not produce the elevation of urinary pH and had little urease activity. Infection stones were formed in 100% of rats by inoculation of C. renale and C. pilosum and 88% of rats by group D2. Urinary pH was elevated in all inoculated rats. In conclusion, C. renale, C. pilosum and group D2 Corynebacterium may play a role in formation of infection stones.

Corynebacterium renale

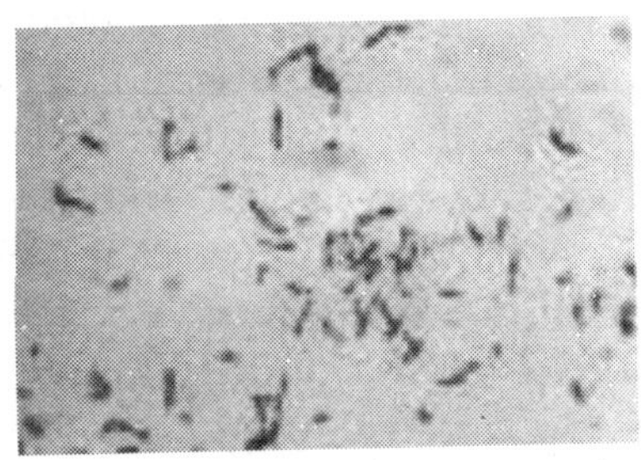

C. renale

The peptidoglycan of *C. renale* contains meso-diaminopimelic acid (m-DAP) as the constituent of amino acid (Mahon *et al.*, 2007). This species also contains mycolic acids, arabinose and galactose in their cell walls, as well as, distinctive cellular fatty acids and menaquiniones (Winn *et al.*, 2006). In addition, there are proteins anchored to this organism's cell wall in three ways: 1) by their C-terminal ends, 2) by way of charge or hydrophobic interactions, and 3) by their N-terminal region (lipoproteins) (2). Thus, the cell wall of *C. renale* can be considered highly complex, because it is made up of proteins with specific binding functions and enzymatic activity that have the ability to generate energy. The complete genome of *C. renale* has yet to be sequenced. But due to new DNA technological advances, the 16S rRNA's genes of *C. renale* have been sequenced. The 16S rRNA contains approximately 1400 nucleotide bases. Moreover, through the sequencing of 16S rRNA of multiple organisms, it has led to the discovery of many new species of *Corynebacterium*; as well as, separated *Corynebacterium species* thought to be one. In addition, *C. renale* contains plasmids (Srivastava *et al.* 2006). This organism contains a small, cryptic plasmid called pCR1. It is the smallest corynebacterial plasmid known to date. This plasmid has been sequenced and contains 1441 nucleotide bases. Another plasmid *C. renale* has is known as pCR2. This plasmid, as well, has been sequenced and contains 3181 nucleotide bases. In a later study, Srivastava *et al.* (2011) reported that Corynebacterium renale harbors four small cryptic plasmids, pCR1, pCR2, pCR3 and pCR4, and can be a good system for understanding host-plasmid interactions. In this study, effect of plasmid loss and their subsequent introduction on various properties of the host was evaluated. Loss of plasmids caused a reduction in bacterial size and also slowed down their growth rate, ì, and respiratory rate, r. Both ì and r values were partially recovered in C. renale R, obtained by retransformation of the cured strain with all the four cryptic plasmids. Further delineation revealed that a 3153bp plasmid pCR2 alone is sufficient for the observed increase in ì in C. renale R. The advantages conferred by the remaining three plasmids may be are two subtle to be seen under laboratory conditions. Overall, the observations point to the gross metabolic crisis in the host partly as a result of loss of plasmids.

The disease most commonly occurs in mature cows. *Corynebacterium pilosum* and *C.renale* are member of the normal flora of lower urogenital tract and causes cystitis and pyelonephritis. *C.cystitidis* causes most severe form of cystitis (Hiramune *et al.,* 1971). Cases of cystitis are commonly caused by *C.renale*. Twenty-one rejected kidneys from 2426 slaughtered dairy cows (0.87 per cent) had gross signs of pyelonephritis that were confirmed by histopathology (Rosenbaum *et al.,* 2005). Altmaier *et al.* (1994) reported a case of Osteomyelitis and disseminated infection caused by Corynebacterium renale in a goat. Elias *et al.* (1993) infected with Corynebacterium renale type II by either the intravenous or intraurethral routes using infection rates of 1.75 x 10(10), 7.08 x 10(19) or 5 x 10(23) organisms. All inoculated goats were anorexic, lost weight and became dull or depressed. Albuminuria, pyuria and epithelial casts were noted in the urine. Following intravenous challenge the animals showed a dose-related elevation of serum ammonia, urea, and creatinine with significant changes in haemoglobin concentration, packed cell volume and leucocyte counts. A mild to severe (sometimes haemorrhagic) cystitis and urethritis and a mild nephrosis were noted post mortem and mucoserous or mucogelatinous non-purulent discharges were present in the renal pelvis. The findings are compared to the naturally occurring *C. renale* pyelonephritis in cattle and the suitability of the goat as a model for that disease is suggested.With all species infection is transmitted venereally and indirectly by contaminated urine. Infection may also be endogenous. All 3 species have the ability to adhere to the uro-genital tract mediated by pili. Minor antigenic cross reaction have been observed between pili of *C.pilosum* and *C.renale* (Kudo *et al.,* 1987). Piliated organisms are more resistant to phagocytosis by mouse neutrophils in vitro than non-piliated cells but opsonized cells do not show this difference (Kubota and Yanagawa 1988). Cystitis may occur without pyelonephritis. Ureteritis is also seen. Cystitis may develop after parturition and is more common in individuals on a high protein diet. Bovine pyelonephritis is sporadic and global in distribution. Because of the ease at which pyelonephritis can be produced by causing stagnation of urine, it is a possibility that some obstruction in the urinary tract is the primary cause of the disease.

An extra cellular protein, Renalin with a strong non-enzymatic affinity for ceramide (a product of phospholipase action on sphingomyelin) may play a role in lysis of cell membrane (Bernheimer and Angad 1982). Iron seems to play a role in regulation of virulence of *C.renale* (Henderson *et al.,* 1978). Loss of pili upon repeated in vitro passage in the presence of anti-pilus antibodies has been demonstrated (Koga *et al.,* 1988). There is no difference between the piliated and non-piliated cells as regards their virulence for mice suggesting that probably pili are not the obligate factor in virulence of *C.renale*. Probably studies carried out in natural host might reveal some intricate mechanisms involved in the action of pili in causation of the disease. Vulva supports the firm adhesion of the organisms suggesting that the portal of entry may be through this organ.

Epidemiology

Sporadic cases have been reported from Europe, North America, Australia, Japan, Iraq and countries of Asia. Outbreaks have been seldom reported even in those herds where carriers occur. Management plays some role in occurrence of the disease in animals. Pyelonephritis is basically a disease of cattle whereas sheep and goats are seldom affected. All ages of mature cows are affected. In cows clinical cases are more frequent during early lactation. A significant lower risk of pyelonephritis has been recorded in cows that have post-parturient uterine disease occurring more commonly during winter, however, in India, it has been recorded more in summer. Similarly disease is more in highly fed high producing dairy herd. Clinically sick or normal carrier cows are probably the principal source of infection. The incidence of cows excreting *C.renale* in their urine is higher in herds than in clinically free herds. The disease may also spread venereally; bulls normally carrying the organisms in prepuce and urethra. Unless treatment is introduced in the herd the disease may turn fatal in animals.

Takahashi *et al.*(1995) used comparative 16S rRNA gene sequencing to assign four isolates of spontaneous urinary calculus in young laboratory rats. The phylogenetic relationships among the rat isolates and selected species of corynebacteria were also inferred. Based on the homology and evolutionary distance analysis, the 16S rRNA genes of the rat isolates were almost identical with that of Corynebacterium renale ATCC 19412. Also the results of the phylogenetic analysis showed a close relationship among the isolates and *C. renale*, but they were clearly different from *C. pilosum, C. cystitidis, C. kutscheri and Rhodococcus equi*. The results of the present study and previously published biochemical data demonstrate that the organism involving urinary infections in young rats is identified to be *C. renale*.

Pathogenesis

Transmission between animals occurs when contaminated droplets of urine are splashed on the vulvar area of a susceptible animal from an infected carrier. However, research has also shown that *C. renale* can be found in healthy animals of diseased herds without affecting them. Depression, muscle wasting, weakness and frequent urine dribbling are the main characteristics of UTI in calves. Affected cows show weight loss and an abrupt reduction in feed intake and milk production.Ascending infection is caused in animals which involves bladder, ureter and one or both kidneys. The bladder wall, ureter and kidneys are greatly thickened and enlarged. Haemorrhages, necrosis and ulceration are extensive and abscesses may be found throughout the kidney. The urine is purulent and blood stained, particularly the last portion voided.

During the infection the corynebacteria associate with urethral epithelium through pili and ascend to the bladder more frequently during pregnancy or injury caused during parturition. The various parts of the bovine urinary tract, the renal pelvis, the ureter, the urinary bladder, the urethra, the vaginal vestibule and the vulva, were examined for the capacity of the epithelial cells to bind Corynebacterium renale and *C. pilosum* (Hayashi *et al.*, 1985). *C. renale* adhered best to the epithelial cells of the vulva, and then to those of the ureter and renal pelvis. *C. pilosum* also adhered best to the epithelial cells of the vulva, followed by those of the vaginal vestibule. The results indicate that the most important target tissue for these bacteria may be the vulva, and the results correlate with the fact that *C. renale* frequently causes pyelonephritis and ureteritis, while *C. pilosum* causes the same diseases less frequently and behaves like normal flora of the vaginal vestibule.

The adhesion of *C. renale* bacteria to bovine epithelial cells was studied with two clones of the bacteria piliated (P+) and non-piliated (P-) (Takai *et al.*1980). The percentage of cells with the attached P+ bacteria was much greater than the number of cells with attached P- bacteria. The adhesion of P+ bacteria was found to be pH dependent and is supported by the following facts. One that the number of attached bacteria was high at a pH above 7.6 and low at a pH below 6.8. And two, the adhering P+ bacteria were eluted immediately after the pH was decreased from 7.4 to 6.4. In addition, the P+ bacteria adhered to the cells immediately after the pH was increased back to 7.4. This study also found that the adhesion of P+ bacteria was inhibited by anti-plus antiserum, but that it was not inhibited by amino acids, sugars, and not influenced by calcium and magnesium. The P- bacteria hardly attached to the epithelial cells, irrespective of the pH and other factors. This adherence is not due to the difference in the hydrophobicity of the piliated and non-piliated strains (Ito *et al.*1987). Piliated (P+) and non-piliated (P-) clones of Corynebacterium renale and *C. pilosum* were similar in hydrophobicity as measured by hydrophobic interaction chromatography, bacterial adherence to hydrocarbons and the salt aggregation test. Hydrophobicity of P+ and P- clones was found to be high when measured by hydrophobic interaction chromatography and bacterial adherence to hydrocarbons, but low when measured by the salt aggregation test.

A plasmid gene library of Corynebacterium renale piliated strain No. 109P+ was prepared in Escherichia coli in order to study the chemical structure of the pili of *C. renale* (Abe *et al.*, 1990). Of 3,000 recombinant clones tested, 5 reacted with anti-pili anti-serum. The gene products of these clones reacted with anti-pili monoclonal antibodies 8/4, 5/2 and B20/3 but lacked the reactivity with 13/4. SDS-PAGE analysis revealed that the expressed protein had a molecular mass of 48 kilodalton and deletion analysis showed that the encoding region for this protein was localized within a 1.4 kilobase gene including a promoter sequence. Immunoelectron microscopy showed that mouse antibodies raised to the expressed protein bound to the entire surface of the pili of C. renale. Nath and Deb(1995) reported that *Corynebacterium renale,* harbors multiple small plasmids designated pCR1, pCR2, pCR3, and pCR4 with sizes of 1.4, 3.2, 4.4, and 5.7 kb, respectively. Plasmid pCR1 of 1.4 kb is the smallest plasmid reported in this group of bacteria and is present in high copy number. Attempts to clone whole pCR1 in Escherichia coli were unsuccessful but two of its fragments (750 and 650 bp) could be separately cloned in it. The 4.4-kb plasmid, pCR3, bears considerable restriction pattern similarity to a 4.4-kb plasmid belonging to the pBL1 group of cryptic plasmid of corynebacteria but has no sequence homology, suggesting that pCR3 represents a new member of the 4.4-kb group of *corynebacterial plasmids.*

Because, this organism multiples in sterile bovine urine, it becomes strongly alkaline. This is because of *C. renale* contains the enzyme urease (Timoney *et al.,* 1988). In particular, urease catalyzes the hydrolysis of urea into carbon dioxide and ammonia. Organisms that tend to produce urease tend to be gastrointestinal or urinary tract pathogens, since urease enables them to neutralize the acid present in their acidic environments. In addition, *C. renale* can also perform catalase production. Catalase is a common enzyme that catalyzes the decomposition of hydrogen peroxide to water and oxygen. Hydrogen peroxide is a harmful by-product of many normal metabolic processes and so to prevent damage it is converted into less dangerous compounds. Bacteria utilize urea present in the urine and multiply rapidly producing cystitis and further ascend to the kidney where in most cases infection spread. Urea breakdown with production of ammonia initiates an inflammatory process, high alkalinity in urine (pH 9.0) and suppression of antibacterial defense possible through complement inactivation by ammonia. A study was initiated to see if the iron content of the *C. renale* cultivation's medium had any effect on the growth of the bacteria or their ability to produce pyelonephritis in model rats. It had previously been reported that poor or no growth of several different strains of *C. renale* was observed in minimal medium with added iron (Henderson *et al.,* 1978). Through the study it was observed that the iron content of the media had a definite effect on the *C. renale* recovered from the renal tissue of the rats. It was shown that *C. renale* was unable to produce pyelonephritis when grown in medium where the iron content was below an undetermined critical level. When grown in a low-iron defined medium, *C. renale* proved to be avirulent for rats, but when cultivated in a high iron defined medium, the organism, was extremely virulent. Since the iron concentration was the only factor which varied in each group, it seems reasonable to assume that iron serves a role as a "virulence factor" in producing pyelonephritis.

The gram-positive cell wall contains polysaccharides and lipids. These with lipoteichoic acids interacting with macrophages cells resulting in the release of proinflammatory cytokines. More often the onset is gradual with a fluctuating temperature, capricious appetite, loss of condition and fall in milk yield over a period of weeks. There may be hypoalbuminemia and hyper gammaglobulinemia. Neutrophilia may be present but is not constant to all cases. There is an elevated serum creatinine and urea (Markusfeld *et al.,* 1989). Characteristic necropsy findings are limited to kidneys, ureter and bladder. Enlargement of kidneys occur with light coloured necrotic areas appearing on the surface and the pelvis. Ureter is grossly enlarged containing blood and pus. Cows with pyelonephritis and urethritis have a serum antibody response to these bacteria. Organisms with urinary sediments from animals with upper urinary tract involvement were coated with the antibody IgG (Timoney *et al.*1988). This antibody is probably derived from the plasma that the inflammatory tissue exudates. The host's protective response, however, is infective and untreated animals seldom recover. The local appearance of various immunoglobulin (Ig) isotypes in the urinary tract during ascending pyelonephritis was studied in rats experimentally infected with Corynebacterium renale(De Buysscher *et al.*1985). The indirect fluorescent antibody assay was used to detect IgG, IgM, IgA, IgE, and C3 on *C renale* present in the urine of the experimental animals. Corynebacterium renale coated with IgM and IgG antibodies was found beginning on the 4th day after induced infection, with IgG being the more abundant isotype. Coating with IgA occurred as early as the 4th day, but was less dense than coating with IgG. The presence of C3 on C renale was concurrent with IgM and IgG coating. A significant quantity of IgE could not be identified on antibody-coated *C renale.* Thus, IgG is the major component of the humoral immune response in this model of ascending pyelonephritis. The IgM early during infection and IgA later during infection seem not to be a major component of the immune response in this model.

Diagnosis

High alkalinity (pH 9.0) of urine accompanied by red blood cells in the urine are positive signs of the disease. Microscopically, packets of pleomorphc gram-positive diphtheroids are seen. Culturing of the etiological agent on a suitable culture medium is easy. The organisms produce positive urease test.

Glucose is fermented by *C.renale* group. Amplified rDNA restriction analysis(ARDRA) may represent a possible alternative for identification of coryneforms, since this technique enabled the identification of most coryneforms tested and since DNA extraction (i.e. cell lysis by boiling), amplification, restriction and electrophoresis can be carried out within 8 hours. This might allow quick identification of C. *diphtheriae* and other possible pathogens of the genus Corynebacterium (Vaneechoutte *et al.*1995)).

Young colonies are initially small and the colony characteristics of each of the 3 species are somewhat different. Those of *C.renale* become opaque and ivory whereas those of *C.pilosum* are cream coloured to yellow. The colonies of *C.cystitidis* are semitransparent. Sonography can be applied for the diagnosis of pyelonephritis (Floeck 2007). Ultrasonographic changes include enlarged kidneys, echogenic material, and flocculent fluid within a dilated and deformed renal sinus and a poor cortical medullary differentiation. Azotemia was detected in 10 and hematuria and proteinuria in all animals. Sonography supplements the clinical examination and clinicopathological analysis by providing additional information on renal disease (Floeck, 2007).

Treatment and Control

Early treatment with antibiotics is useful. Penicillin at 15,000 units/kg body weight is effective if administered daily for 3-5 weeks. Administration of mono basic sodium phosphate (100 g daily for several days) causes improvement. The relapse is common and the relief through antibiotic treatment is temporary.Trimethoprim-sulfadoxine (16 mg combined/kg, IM, BID) for = 3 wk is also effective. The dosage, frequency, and length of administration for both of these drugs is extra-label, and adequate precautions must be taken to prevent antibiotic residues from entering the human food chain. The organisms form biofilm consisting of micro-colonies encased in extracellular polysaccharide material. Biofilms composed of Arcanobacterium (Actinomyces) pyogenes, *Staphylococcus aureus, Staphylococcus hyicus,* Streptococcus agalactiae, *Corynebacterium renale,* or Corynebacterium pseudotuberculosis are not killed by the antibiotics but as planktonic bacteria they were sensitive at low concentrations (Olson et al 2002).No specific control measures are usually effective but segregation of affected animals and disinfection of infected surroundings, bedding etc. is helpful in reducing the bacterial population. Where natural service is practiced, it should be discontinued and replaced with artificial insemination. Although this too is not always safe as *C.renale* has been formed to be present in semen of bulls (Kapoor, 2003). Treatment of ulcerative posthitis in sheep is effective by clipping and cleaning of hair around the prepuce followed by application of antiseptics and change in diet. Administration of testosterone every 3 months are useful.

Corynebacterium pseudotuberculosis infection

Caseous hymphadenitis is the disease primarily caused by *C.pseudotuberculosis*. It is characterized by the formation of abscesses in lymph nodes. It is usually a local problem but often becomes generalized. It also causes ulcerative lymphangitis in cattle and horses and contagious and suppurative arthritis of lambs. There are a few reports of the organism causing mastitis (Peng Xiam Feng *et al.*, 2003). Caseous lymphadenitis (CLA) of sheep, has been a significant disease in the majority of sheep-rearing regions for over a century. Because of the chronic and often sub-clinical nature of the infection, it has proved difficult to control and prevalence is high in many parts of the world, which in turn leads to significant economic losses for farmers.

Etiology

C.pseudotuberculosis, a facultative intracellular parasite, has 2 biotypes based on their ability to reduce nitrate; a nitrate positive, and a nitrate negative. Both biotypes produce an exotoxin, phospholipase D which is a sphingomyleinase and is a pathogenicity factor. Isolates from cattle are heterogenous in nature. It is leucotoxic that damages endothelial cells and promotes spread from initial site of infection to regional lymph nodes. It is lethal to several species of laboratory animals. In vitro it is haemolytic to sheep and bovine red blood cells. Another exotoxin released by *C.pseudotuberculosis* is a serine protease which is a protective factor. *C.pseudotuberculosis* posses a cluster of 4 genes, fag A-D encoding protein that are involved with iron uptake. Deletion of this genes results in a decrease in virulence. In addition it also contains a cord factor like material on the surface but its role in virulence is not known (Carne *et al.*, 1956). The organism can survive in pus infected soil for up to 8 months, in infected shearing sheds for approximately 4 months and on straw, hay and other fomites for approximately 2 months (Augustine and Renshaw 1987). *Corynebacterium pseudotuberculosis* is gram-positive, catalase positive, non-spore forming, non-motile rod shaped bacteria. Metachromatic granules are found in the cells. The bacteria are grouped together in a characteristic way which has been described as "palisades" or "Chinese letters". arrangement. They may also appear elliptical. They are aerobic or facultatively anaerobic, chemoorganotrophs, with a 51-65% genomic G:C content. They are pleomorphic through their life cycle: they come in various lengths and frequently have thickenings at either end, depending on the surrounding conditions.

D'Afonseca *et al.* (2010) used a genomic library of *C. pseudotuberculosis* to generate 1440 genomic survey sequences (GSSs); these were analyzed in silico with bioinformatics tools, using public databases for comparative analyses employing non-redundant unique sequences as a query for BLAST searches against the genome, the translated genome and the proteome of four other Corynebacterium species that have been completely sequenced. The authors were able to characterize approximately 8% of the genome of *C. pseudotuberculosis*, including previously undescribed functional group genes, based on the COG database; the GSSs classification into categories gave 13% information storage and processing, 14% cellular processes and 23% metabolism. A close relation between *C. pseudotuberculosis* and *C. diphtheriae* conserved-gene synteny in Corynebacteria species.

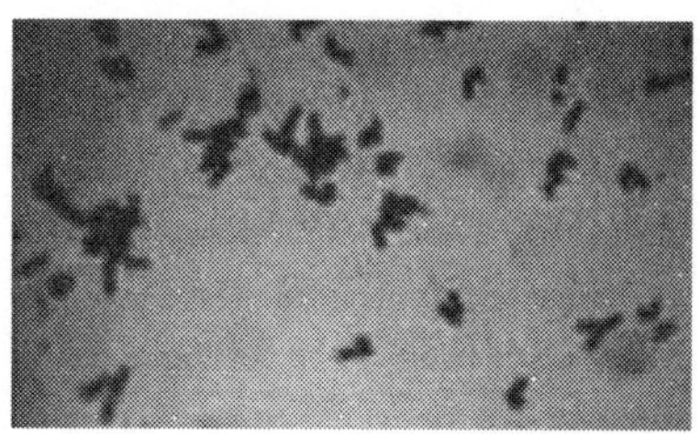

C. pseudotuberculosis

In horses, *C pseudotuberculosis* causes ulcerative lymphangitis (an infection of the lower limbs), chronic abscesses in the pectoral region, and contagious acne. It is one of the most common and economically important infectious diseases of horses in through out the world.

Epidemiology

High prevalence of the disease has been reported from most countries of the world. The disease is prevalent in all those countries where sheep & goat husbandry is practiced at a large scale. Cases are more in adult animals which increase with age. Studies in USA have shown that sheep appears to have a higher prevalence, than goats.

Economic losses occur due to condemnation of infected carcasses and devaluation of hides.

The sources of infection are discharges from the ruptured abscessed superficial lymph nodes and nasal and oral secretions from the diseased animals. The organism enters the healthy susceptible animals through the ruptured skin or skin wounds and cuts caused by shearing. Infection can also be transmitted through the contaminated shearing apparatus. Infection can acquired through nasal or oral secretion of sheep with pulmonary infection. The sheep dip is another way for transmitting the disease. The bacterium can survive in commercial sheep dip for 24 hours and may be transmitted through the intact skin. In goats shearing is not a risk factor, however, in Angora goats this could be so. Pulmonary abscesses are not so prevalent in goats than sheep and therefore might not play an important role in transmitting the disease.

The disease is most often introduced to a flock by entry of an apparently healthy carrier from an infected flock, by contact on shared pastures, or via contaminated fomites such as shearing equipments.

Pathogenesis

Virulence is attributed to phospholipase D leukotoxin and cell wall lipids both of which initiate inflammatory response. PLD damages neutrophils, macrophages and endothelial cells. The PLD deficient mutants do not produce caseous lymphadenitis (Hodgson *et al.*, 1992). The chromosomal gene encoding the phospholipase D from *Corynebacterium pseudotuberculosis* (biovar ovis) isolate Whetten 1 was replaced with an allele containing a nonsense mutation. The virulence of the mutant strain (W1.31r1) and the isogenic parental strain were then compared by inoculation of goats. The wild-type strain caused abscessation at the site of infection, which then spread to the regional lymph node, while W1.31r1 had a reduced ability to establish a primary infection and was incapable of dissemination (McNamara *et al.*, 1994). These results confirm that phospholipase D is a virulence determinant of *C. pseudotuberculosis* that increases the persistence and spread of the bacteria within the host.

Phospholipase D (Pld), a major virulence determinant of C. pseudotuberculosis, is believed to play a critical role in dissemination of bacteria from the site of infection to the lymph nodes. Although the pld gene has been studied for some time, it is only recently that it has been identified as being down-regulated following heat shock from 37 to 43 degrees C. To gain insights into the mechanisms of Pld action, Mckean *et al.* (2007) investigated how it was regulated under varying environmental conditions. Studies measuring pld mRNA levels or utilizing a reporter construct containing the pld promoter upstream of a gfp gene were performed. These showed that pld was upregulated in a cell-density-dependent manner, was regulated by heat shock at all cell-culture densities, and was highly expressed in a tissue-culture macrophage-infection model. Finally, the expression of Pld by intracellular C. *pseudotuberculosis* was shown to play a small but significant role in the reduction of macrophage viability following infection. This study demonstrates that the regulation of C. *pseudotuberculosis* pld is complex. This regulatory complexity may play an important role in allowing the pathogen to successfully adapt to the changing host environment during infection, migration, establishment and disease progression.

Caseous lymphadenitis is a chronic recurring disease. A slowly enlarging localized and non-painful abscess may develop either at the point of entry into the skin or in the regional lymph nodes from which it may spread via the blood or lymphatic system and cause abscessation of internal lymph nodes or organs (Pepin *et al.*, 1991[a]). The pathogenesis of Caseous Lymphadenitis is a slow process, and produces a chronic rather than an acute disease state. Acute phase proteins (APP) such as haptoglobin (Hp) serum amyloid A (SAA) and alpha1 acid glycoprotein (AGP) are produced by the liver and released into the circulation in response to pro-inflammatory cytokines. The concentration of Hp in serum increases in experimental CLA but it is not known if SAA and AGP respond in parallel or have differing response profiles. In one study (Eckersall *et al.*, 2007) the concentration in serum of Hp, SAA and AGP in 6 sheep challenged with 2 x 105 cells of *C. pseudotuberculosis* showed significant increases (P < 0.05) compared to 3 unchallenged control sheep. By day 7 post infection. (p.i.) the Hp and SAA concentrations reached mean (+/- SEM) values of 1.65 +/- 0.21 g/L and 18.1 +/- 5.2 mg/L respectively. Thereafter, their concentrations fell with no significant difference to those of the control sheep by day 18 p.i.. In contrast, the serum AGP concentration in infected sheep continued to rise to a peak of 0.38 +/- 0.05 g/L on day 13 p.i., after which a slow decline occurred, although the mean concentration remained significantly higher (P < 0.05) than the control group up to 29 days p.i. Specific IgG to phospholidase D of *C. pseudotuberculosis* became detectable at 11 days p.i. and continued to rise throughout the experiment. In conclusion,the serum concentrations of Hp, SAA and AGP were raised in sheep in an experimental model of CLA. An extended response was found for AGP which occurred at a point when the infection was likely to have been transforming from an acute to a chronic phase. The results suggest that AGP could have a role as a marker for chronic conditions in sheep. Four genes, fagA, B, C and D, encoding products with 32-47% identity to proteins involved in bacterial iron uptake systems, were identified immediately downstream of the Corynebacterium pseudotuberculosis phospholipase D gene (Billington *et al.*, 2002). beta-Galactosidase assays on a *C. pseudotuberculosis* strain carrying a fagA-lacZ fusion indicated that the putative fagABC operon was poorly expressed in iron-rich media. However, similar experiments in iron-limited media resulted in an approximately three-fold increase in beta-galactosidase activity, suggesting that this operon is regulated by iron in vitro. Although no defect in iron utilization could be determined for a *C. pseudotuberculosis* fagB(C) mutant in vitro, this mutant showed reduced virulence compared to wild-type in a goat model of caseous lymphadenitis. Thus, expression of the fag genes in the host appears to contribute to virulence.

The toxins are absent from abscesses or neutralized. Initial infection may not cause any clinical sign or may be accompanied by high fever, anorexia, anemia and cellulites at the infection sites. The bacterial cells are capable of multiplying in the phagolysosomes. *Corynebacterium pseudotuberculosis* strains survive within macrophages more than 48 hours. During that time bacteria were released as a result of the process that lead to death of phagocytes. This property varied among strains. There is no increase of microtubule-associated protein I light chain 3 (MAP I LC3) activity in macrophages infected with examined strains comparing with uninfected cultures and cultures treated with autophagy inducer (rapamycin) that served as negative and positive controls, respectively. The study with confocal microscopy did not show the increasing of caspase-3 activity in the infected macrophages and their nucleus did not reveal the fragmentation (stefanska *et al.* 2010). The permeability of local vessels increases. Superficial abscess may enlarge and rapture and discharge infectious pus. The pus is creamy to dry and crumbly (cheesy). Old abscesses consist of dead macrophages with peripheral neutrophils, giant cells and fibrous tissues. Lesions almost always contain *C.pseudotuberculosis*. Mostly prescapular and prefemoral lymph nodes are involved, and transmission usually occurring when the flock is gathered for group treatment such as shearing. In housed sheep and goats superficial abscesses develop mainly in the head and neck region. Abscessation may recur at the same sites. Cell mediated and humoral immunity develop and immune macrophages engulf the bacteria & kill resulting in spread of the pathogen to other locations. Internal abscesses should be considered as a potential diagnosis for "thin ewe syndrome", in which an adult ruminant losses condition in want of adequate nutrition. The visceral form is more extensive in sheep than goats, mostly involving abscess of pulmonary parenchyma and mediastinal lymph nodes. Abscessation of other organs such as brain, scrotums, vertebral body etc. may occur giving rise to related complications. Clinical disease is more prevalent in adults and up to 40% animals in a flock may be infected. Ulcerative lymphangitis in horses and mules and sometime in cattle appears as nodule most often involving the superficial lymphatics around the fetlock. The organisms enter via the injuries.

Diagnosis

The diagnosis is usually based on clinical signs and flock history. For confirming the diagnosis an aspirate of an intact abscess should be submitted for bacteriological examination. *C.pseudotuberculosis* can easily be isolated on any suitable medium alongwith other pyogenic microorganisms such as *Staphylococcus aureus*, *Streptococcus* spp., *Arcanobacterium pyogenes*, *Pasteurella multocida* and occasionally anaerobes such as *Fusobacterium necrophorum*. On blood agar *C.pseudotuberculosis* produces small off white haemolytic colonies that can be pushed intact on the agar surface. Inhibition of Staphylococcal beta toxin and synergistic haemolysis with *Rhodococcus equi* confirm the identification. A differential diagnosis for emaciated animals also should include ovine progressive pneumonia, caprine arthritis and encephalitis.

Serology is also useful in diagnosis of the disease. Tests include agglutination, complement fixation, haemolysis inhibition, gel diffusion and toxin-neutralization. Organism can be identified on the basis of cell fatty acids. Most tests detect antibodies to phospholipase D exotoxin. Infected animals may have false negative results likely because the infection is well walled off in the abscesses or if they are severely debilitated. Antibody titers also appear in colostrums which disappear by 3-6 months of age. Goats tend to have higher titer than sheep. The applicability of the quantification of gamma interferon (IFN-γ) levels for the detection of animals infected with Corynebacterium pseudotuberculosis and for determining caseous lymphadenitis (CLA) clinical status was evaluated (REbaucas *et al.,* 2011). Peripheral blood leukocytes were collected from CLA nonendemic areas animals, from CLA seropositive animals without clinical signs of the disease, and from seropositive animals presenting CLA clinical signs. The leukocytes were stimulated with *C. pseudotuberculosis*-secreted antigens that were concentrated by the three-phase partitioning technique. An ovine IFN-γ enzyme-linked immunosorbent assay was used to quantify IFN-γ production. Goats and sheep with CLA had higher IFN-γ levels than uninfected seronegative animals. Leukocytes from sheep with CLA chronic abscesses produced higher IFN-γ levels when compared with seropositive sheep without CLA clinical signs, but this difference was not significant in goats. The sensitivity of the assay was 55.8% and 56%, whereas the specificity was 100% and 93%, for goats and sheep, respectively. In conclusion, IFN-γ is a potential marker for the determination of CLA infection status in small ruminants. The IFN-γ response of sheep whole blood to *C. pseudotuberculosis* antigens offers promise for use in a test-and-removal approach to eradication of CLA in sheep (Prescott *et al.,* 2002). A surface plasmon resonance-based biosensor assay for the detection of antibodies to the phospholipase D (PLD) exotoxin of *C. pseudotuberculosis* in sheep serum was generated by Stapleton *et al.* (2009). It employed a recombinant form of PLD, which was immobilized, and all aspects of the assay including minimization of non-specific binding, and the regeneration of the chip, were optimised. The applicability of the assay was initially demonstrated using sera collected from experimentally infected sheep and from sheep with no prior history of infection. The assay was then evaluated on a panel of clinical samples and the results obtained compared very favourably to those obtained by a double sandwich ELISA (over 90% similarity) and clearly verified its analytical value.

Genus and species specific primers have been developed to conduct PCR for amplifying DNA. Setinkaya *et al.* (2002) carried out A PCR using specific primers and found that it can be used for specific diagnosis of caseous lymphadenitis in sheep and goats. Although cross-reaction with *C. ulcerans*, a human/bovine species, was observed, the PCR assay used in this study may successfully be applied for the diagnosis of CL in goats and sheep as an alternative to conventional methods, owing to its advantages of specificity and speed.

Treatment & Control

Penicillin is effective but usually not administered because it can't penetrate the abscesses. Surgical excision too is not very effective as the abscesses reappear. Administration of a combination of rifamycin SV, intramuscularly 10mg/kg body weight twice a day for 10 days and oxytetracycline (20mg/kg body weight) is effective in the treatment of the disease (Senturk and Tamizel, 2006).

Following approaches are useful in prevention of the infection.

Reducing transmission of the organism from infected to susceptible animals in useful. Emaciated animals and those having recurring abscesses should be culled. Valuable animals may be segregated and abscesses opened and flushed with an iodine solution. Any lancing of abscesses should be done such that the purulent material can be collected and environmental contamination prevented. Young animals should be reared in isolation from older infected animals. Shearing equipment should be decontaminated. Skin wounds from shearing or fighting should be treated topically with iodine and sutured, if necessary.

Commercial vaccines are available which reduce the incidence and prevalence of the disease but do not prevent all new infections nor cure the disease. Currently all the vaccines contain phospholipase D toxoid and some also contain killed *C.pseudotuberculosis* cells. Vaccination should be initiated after the colostral immunity has waned. Colostral immunity can be improved by administering a booster to pregnant ewes one month prior to the lambing/ kidding. A primary series (2 injections 4 weeks apart) is required in young stock or previously unvaccinated adults. Repeat vaccination is advocated annually that will help reducing the prevalence of the disease. The vaccines in potentially infected goats should be used cautiously as adverse effects may be caused. In a study sheep were immunised with *Corynebacterium pseudotuberculosis* vaccines prepared from cell-free toxoid or from toxoid with formalin-killed cells of *C pseudotuberculosis* added. Resistance of sheep to infection was tested 6 months after immunisation by inoculation with caseous lymphadenitis pus. The outcome was assessed 3 months later by slaughter and inspection of the sheep for lesions of caseous lymphadenitis. immunised sheep were adequately protected against infection as shown by a significant reduction in the number of sheep exhibiting lesions compared with control sheep, and by fewer abscesses in affected vaccinated sheep than in affected control sheep. The protective potency of the vaccines was not improved by the inclusion of cells of *C pseudotuberculosis* (Eggleton *et al.*, 1991). Using a virulent United Kingdom Corynebacterium pseudotuberculosis isolate, an ovine experimental model of caseous lymphadenitis was developed, in which the manifestation of disease was equivalent to the naturally observed infection in this country (Fontaine et al. 2006). Subsequently, the capacity of several experimental vaccines to protect against experimental challenge was determined. Sheep were immunised with a recombinant derivative of phospholipase D, deriving from the virulent UK isolate, a formalin-killed bacterin of the same strain, or a bacterin supplemented with recombinant phospholipase D. Following homologous experimental challenge, the phospholipase D and bacterin vaccines were observed to confer statistically significant protection against infection, and appeared to restrict dissemination of challenge bacteria beyond the inoculation site in the majority of animals. More importantly, the combined vaccine succeeded in providing absolute protection against infection, whereby challenge bacteria were eradicated from all vaccinates. In addition to the experimental vaccines, a commercially available CLA vaccine, unlicensed for use in the European Union, was assessed for its capacity to protect against heterologous challenge. The vaccine conferred significant protection, although the dissemination of infection beyond the inoculation site was not restricted as it had been with the previous vaccines. However, no animals immunised with this vaccine manifested infection within the lungs; thus, a potentially important route of disease transmission was eliminated.

Rose *et al.* (2002) reported a DNA vaccine when given to sheep that gave rise to protective immunity. The plasmid DNA encoding inactivated phospholipase D when given intramuscularly elicited a strong immunity than given by gene gun or sub-cutaneous routes. The protected sheep had high level of IgG_2 response compared with the unprotected animals.

Side by side culling and hygienic precautions should be taken. Eradication is difficult to achieve, however, it could be controlled by eradication of infected carriers. One study aimed at validation of a whole blood interferon-gamma (IFN-gamma) enzyme immunoassay (EIA) (Bovigam, Pfizer) in naturally infected sheep for use in eradication of infection from a flock (Sunil et al 2008). This assay used formalin-inactivated whole bacterial cells as antigen. The sensitivity of the whole cell assay was improved by increasing both the volume of blood and the number of bacterial cells. The assay was validated in experimentally infected sheep and in a flock of known-negative sheep, as well as in a naturally infected flock, a proportion of which was vaccinated with a commercial CLA vaccine. The test had a sensitivity of 91% and a specificity of 98%. Postmortem data supported the results in test-negative animals. Visit-to-visit variation in IFN-γ EIA OD in the naturally infected flock as well as CLA disease status was used to develop an algorithm for the eradication of CLA from a known infected flock. The whole blood IFN-γ assay show a promose for eradication of CL in animals.

Once the disease is at a low prevalence, vaccination should be stopped and all seropositive animals and non vaccinated animals culled. Prevention of disease entry into a clean flock is based on serologic screening and isolation of incoming animals. Seropositive unvaccinated animals should not be allowed to enter the flock. If management allows removal of young stock at birth and rearing separately from the infected flock has been shown to be an effective means of eradication. The infected flock is then culled as quickly as economics allow. Preventive measures at uninfected farm require shearing hygiene and purchase only of uninfected stock.

Corynebacterium bovis

C.bovis is a commensal bacteria found in the reproductive tract of some cows and bulls and on the ductular epithelium. Corynebacterium bovis often colonizes the teat canal, without causing true intramammary infection. Brooks et al.(1983) concluded that the rate of infection with mastitis pathogens was not significantly different in quarters previously colonized with only *C. bovis* compared to previously uninfected quarters. *C.bovis* is an aerobic, gram-positive bacteria with a tendency to increase the population during lactating period. A typing method for *Corynebacterium bovis* based on pulsed-field gel electrophoresis (PFGE) is described and applied to type 162 strains isolated from mastitic milk from 57 Friesian dairy herds in northern Spain (Garcia-Crespo *et al.*, 2005). Isolates were identified to the species level using the API-Coryne system and a polymerase chain reaction-restriction fragment length polymorphism of the 16S rDNA amplicon. Seven different pulsotypes were identified; none of them were similar to that of the reference strain (ATCC 7715). The most frequent pulsotype was pattern I (51.9%) followed by pattern II (29.6%). The majority of the herds showed infection with one single pulsotype, but 12 herds yielded 2 pulsotypes, and one herd had 3 pulsotypes. No relationship was found between the geographical location of the herd and the pulsotype. It is a lipid-requiring Corynebacterium spp. Data indicate that the coryneform bacteria isolated from bovine mammary glands are a heterogeneous group of organisms. Routine identification of *C. bovis* should include Gram-stain, cell morphology, catalase production, nitrate reduction, stimulated growth on 1% Tween 80 supplemented media, and beta-galactosidase production as the minimum requirements(Watts *et al.*, 2000). Watts *et al.*, (2001) examined the phylogeny of *C. bovis* using 47 strains isolated from bovine mammary glands. Phylogenetic studies were performed by direct sequencing of the 16S ribosomal RNA and comparison to sequences of reference strains. All strains identified as C. bovis demonstrated similarity of 98% or higher to the ribosomal RNA gene sequences of the type strain of *C. bovis*. Phylogenetic analyses indicated that all strains tested clustered with members of the Corynebacterium urealyticum group confirming that *C. bovis* is a legitmate member of the genus Corynebacterium. Further investigation into the diversity within the species using repetitive element palindrome PCR indicated only minor differences between the strains tested. It was predicted that endonuclease restriction with HindIII and SmaI could be used to differentiate *C. bovis* from all other known lipophilic Corynebacterium species (Huxley *et al.*, 2004). The method was successfully employed to identify 741 of 762 (97.2%) lipophilic Corynebacterium species as *C. bovis*. Twenty one (2.8%) were identified as species other than *C. bovis*. Using this technique, it was demonstrated that it is not safe to assume that all lipophilic coryneform organisms isolated from bovine milk samples are *C. bovis*. This method is an alternative to more traditional methods of identification in large scale studies until methods such as 16S rRNA gene sequencing become more widely available.

C.bovis is not regarded as a significant pathogen in causing mastitis because of its low pathogenicity. It provokes a mild neutrophil response that may protect the udder against more pathogenic bacteria. Of 272 bovine udder quarters studied for mastitis, 19 of them naturally infected with *Corynebacterium bovis* alone, were compared with 16 others infected by *C. bovis* together with other bacteria and another 36 non-infected quarters(Ngatia et al 1991). While there was no significant difference in milk somatic cell counts between the quarters infected by C. bovis alone and those affected by C. bovis together with other bacteria (33.37 +/- 20.28 X 10(3) and 33.86 +/- 23.18 X 10(3)/ml of milk, respeetively), there was a significant difference between these and the non-infected quarters (5.60 +/- 3.23 X 10(3)/ml of milk). Microscopically, quarters infected by either *C. bovis* alone or *C. bovis* in combination with other bacteria had inflammatory changes in the teat cisterns, Furstenberg's rosettes and/or mammary parenchyma. The non-infected quarters had no changes. In all 82 quarters no pathological changes could be seen in the teat canals.

Interestingly infection with Corynebacterium bovis was associated with increased milk yield in goats (Koop et al. 2010). A real-time PCR-based test was performed on milk samples with an individual quarter somatic cell count above 500,000 cells/ml that were either negative (n=51 samples) or that led to the isolation of minor pathogens in culturing: *Corynebacterium bovis* (n=79 samples) or *non-aureus staphylococci* (NAS, n=32) (Bexiga et al.2011). A mastitis pathogen, beyond the result obtained with standard bacteriology, was detected on 47% of the no-growth samples, on 35% of the samples from which C. bovis had been isolated and on 25% of the samples from which NAS had been isolated. Interestingly in one study it has been found that infection by *S.aureus* was inhibited but animals showed increased susceptibility to streptococcal infection (Pankey *et al.* 1985). Lam *et al.* (1997) demonstrated that minor pathogens have a protective effect against infection with major pathogens in bovine mastitis. The protective effect of *C. bovis* against subsequent infection with major pathogens appears to be greater than the effect of coagulase-negative Micrococcaceae. *C. bovis* has been found to cause mild mastitis during the middle of lactation probably due to the quality of milk whereas during the dry period its growth is inhibited. It rarely causes udder disease but is randomly found in milk samples. Taponen et al (2009) demonstrated that in nearly half of the clinical mastitis cases in which conventional culture failed to detect bacteria, mastitis pathogens including *C. bovis*, were still present, often in substantial quantities. The clearly elevated N-acetyl-beta-d-glucosaminidase activity values of the milk samples, together with clinical signs of the infected cows and quarters, confirmed the diagnosis of clinical mastitis and indicated that real-time, PCR-based bacterial findings are able to reveal bacteriological etiology. It was concluded that all common mastitis bacteria can occur in large quantities in clinical mastitis samples that exhibit no growth in conventional culture, and that the real-time PCR assay is a useful tool for bacteriological diagnosis of such milk samples. Low bacterial concentration is commonly speculated to explain the no-growth milk samples. Because it is highly susceptible to teat disinfection it has been suggested that its presence on teat could be used to assess the teat-dipping efficacy.Foret et al.(2005) concluded that teat dips containing 0.25 % iodine significantly reduces the *C. bovis* count in teat canal. *C.bovis* is a lipophilic organism that grows best in the presence of long chain fatty acids. On media containing milk, colonies appear in abundance. Data suggest that mammary secretions support growth of *Corynebacterium bovis* during lactation but inhibit growth during the nonlactating period. Inhibition of growth in secretions collected during the nonlactating period may be associated with the high rate of spontaneous elimination of *Corynebacterium bovis* intramammary infection from cessation of milking to parturition. Conversely, enhanced growth in milk may be related to persistent *Corynebacterium bovis* intramammary infections during lactation (Oliver and Juneja 1990).

References

Abe S., Saito T., Koga T., Ono E., Yanagawa R., Ito T., Kida H. and Shimizu Y. 1990. Cloning and expression of a pili gene of Corynebacterium renale in Escherichia coli. Nippon Juigaku Zasshi. **52:** 11-18.

Altmaier K.R., Sherman D.M., Schelling S.H., Fister R.D. and Lamb C.R.1994.Osteomyelitis and disseminated infection caused by Corynebacterium renale in a goat. J. Am. Vet. Med. Assoc. **204:** 934-937.

Arai Y., Tomoyoshi T. and Takeuchi H.1997. [An experimental study of infection stone formation by Corynebacterium species]. Hinyokika. Kiyo. 43:115-21.[Article in Japanese].

Bernheimer, A.W. and Angad, L.S. 1982. Mechanism of haemolysis by renalin: a CAMP like protein from *C.renale*. Infect. Immun. **36:** 1253-1256.

Bexiga R., Koskinen M.T., Holopainen J., Carneiro C., Pereira H., Ellis K.A. and Vilela C.L.2011.Diagnosis of intramammary infection in samples yielding negative results or minor pathogens in conventional bacterial culturing. J.Dairy Res. **78:** 49-55.

Billington S.J., Esmay P.A., Songer J.G.and Jost B.H 2002.Identification and role in virulence of putative iron acquisition genes from Corynebacterium pseudotuberculosis. FEMS Microbiol. Lett. **208:** 41-45.

Brooks B.W., Barnum D.A. and Meek A.H.1983.An observational study of Corynebacterium bovis in selected Ontario dairy herds. Can. J. Comp. Med. 1983 **47:** 73-78.

Carne, H.R., Wickham, N. and Kater, J.C. 1956. A toxic lipid from the surface of Corynebacterium ovis. Nature UK **178:** 701-702.

Cetinkaya B., Karahan M., Atil E., Kalin R., De Baere T.and Vaneechoutte M.2002.Identification of Corynebacterium pseudotuberculosis isolates from sheep and goats by PCR. Vet Microbiol. **88:** 75-83.

D'Afonseca V., Prosdocimi F., Dorella F.A., Pacheco L.G., Moraes P.M., Pena I., Ortega J.M., Teixeira S., Oliveira S.C., Coser E.M., Oliveira L.M., Corrêa de Oliveira G., Meyer R., Miyoshi A.and Azevedo V..2010.Survey of genome organization and gene content of Corynebacterium pseudotuberculosis. Microbiol. Res. **165:** 312-20.

De Buysscher E.V., Appleton J.A. and Kadis S.1985.Appearance of immunoglobulin classes and complement (C3) during Corynebacterium renale-induced experimental pyelonephritis in the rat. Am J Vet Res. **46:** 401-403.

Eckersall P.D., Lawson F.P., Bence L., Waterston M.M., Lang T.L., Donachie W.and Fontaine M.C.2007.Acute phase protein response in an experimental model of ovine caseous lymphadenitis. BMC Vet. Res. **3:** 35.

Eggleton D.G., Middleton H.D., Doidge C.V.and Minty DW.1991.Immunisation against ovine caseous lymphadenitis: comparison of Corynebacterium pseudotuberculosis vaccines with and without bacterial cells. Aust. Vet. J. **68:** 317-319.

Elias S., Abbas B.and el San-Ousi S.M.1993.The goat as a model for Corynebacterium renale pyelonephritis. Br. Vet. J. **149:** 485-493.

Floeck M.2007.Sonographic application in the diagnosis of pyelonephritis in cattle. Vet Radiol. Ultrasound. **48:** 74-77.

Fontaine M.C., Baird G., Connor K.M., Rudge K., Sales J. and Donachie W.2006.Vaccination confers significant protection of sheep against infection with a virulent United Kingdom strain of Corynebacterium pseudotuberculosis. Vaccine. **24:** 5986-5996.

Foret C.J., Corbellini C., Young S.and Janowicz P.2005.Efficacy of two iodine teat dips based on reduction of naturally occurring new intramammary infections. J. Dairy Sci. **88:** 426-432.

García-Crespo D., Navas J., Gradillas G. and Juste RA.2005.Technical note: molecular typing of Corynebacterium bovis isolates by pulsed-field gel electrophoresis. J. Dairy Sci. **885:** 1705-1707.

Hayashi A., Yanagawa R. and Kida H.1985.Adhesion of Corynebacterium renale and Corynebacterium pilosum to the epithelial cells of various parts of the bovine urinary tract from the renal pelvis to vulva. Vet. Microbiol., **10:** 287-292.

Henderson, L.C., Kadis, S. and Chapman, W.L. 1978. Influence of iron on *C.renale* induced pyelonephritis in a rat experimental model. Infect. Immun. **21:** 540-545.

Hiramune, T., Inui, S., Murase, N. and Yanagawa, R. 1971. Virulence of 3 types of *Corynebacterium renale* in cows. Am. J. Vet. Res. **32:** 235-242.

Hodgson A.L.M., Krymult J., Corner, LA., Rothel, J.S. and Rodford, A.J. 1992. Rational attenuation of *Corynebacterium pseudotuberculosis*: Potential cheesy gland vaccine and live delivery vehicle. Infect. Immun. **60:** 2900-2905.

Huxley J.N., Helps C.R. and Bradley A.J. 2004.Identification of Corynebacterium bovis by endonuclease restriction analysis of the 16S rRNA gene sequence. J. Dairy Sci. **87:** 38-45.

Ito H., Ono E. and Yanagawa R.1987.Comparison of surface hydrophobicity of piliated and non-piliated clones of Corynebacterium renale and Corynebacterium pilosum. Vet. Microbiol. **14:** 165-171.

Kapoor, S. 2003. Isolation of aerobic bacteria in frozen semen of cattle and buffaloes. Ind. J. Comp. Microbiol. Immunol. Infect. Dis. **24:** 207-208.

Kapoor, S. 2003. Isolation of aerobic bacteria in frozen semen of cattle and buffaloes. Ind. J. Comp. Microbiol. Immunol. Infect. Dis. **24:** 207-208.

Koop G., van Werven T., Schuiling H.J. and Nielen M.2010.The effect of subclinical mastitis on milk yield in dairy goats. J. Dairy Sci. **93:** 5809-5817.

Kubota, T. and Yanagawa, R. 1987. Comparison of susceptibility to phagocytosis by mouse peritoneal macrophages between *C.renale* piliated and non-piliated clones. Jpn. J. Vet. Sci. **49:** 663-672.

Kudo, Y., Yanagawa, R. and Hiramune, T. 1987. Isolation and characterization of monoclonal antibodies against pili of *C.renale* and *C.pilosum*. Vet. Microbiol. **13:** 75-5.

Lam T.J., Schukken Y.H., van Vliet J.H., Grommers F.J., Tielen M.J. and Brand A.1997. Effect of natural infection with minor pathogens on susceptibility to natural infection with major pathogens in the bovine mammary gland.Am. J. Vet. Res. **58:** 17-22.

Mahon, Connie R, Donald C. Lehman, & George Manuselis. 2007. Diagnostic Microbiology. 3rd ed. St. Louis: Saunders Elsevier.

Mariasfeld, O. *et al.*, 1989. Br. Vet. J. **31:** 515.

McKean S.C., Davies J.K.,and Moore R.J.2007.Expression of phospholipase D, the major virulence factor of *Corynebacterium pseudotuberculosis,* is regulated by multiple environmental factors and plays a role in macrophage death. Microbiology. **153:** 2203-2211.

McNamara P.J., Bradley G.A.and Songer J.G.1994.Targeted mutagenesis of the phospholipase D gene results in decreased virulence of *Corynebacterium pseudotuberculosis*. Mol. Microbiol. **12:** 921-930.

Menzies, P.I., Muckle, C.A., Brogden, K.A. and Robinson, L. 1991. A field trial to evaluate a whole cell vaccine for the prevention of caseous lymphadenitis in sheep and goat flocks. Can. J.Vet. Res. **55:** 362-366.

Nath N. and Deb J.K.1995Partial characterization of small plasmids from Corynebacterium renale. Plasmid. **34:** 229-233.

Ngatia T.A., Jensen N.E.and Berg B.B.1991.Changes in the bovine udder quarters naturally infected by Corynebacterium bovis. Br. Vet. J. **147:** 463-468.

Oliver S.P.and Juneja V.K.. 1990.Growth of Corynebacterium bovis in mammary secretions during physiological transitions of the bovine mammary gland. J. Dairy Sci. **73:** 351-356.

Olson M.E., Ceri H., Morck D.W., Buret A.G. and Read R.R.2002.Biofilm bacteria: formation and comparative susceptibility to antibiotics. Can. J. Vet. Res. 2002 **66:** 86-92.

Pankey, J.W., Nickerson, S.C., Boddie, R.L. and Hogan, J.S. 1985. Effect of Corynebacterium infection on susceptibility to major mastitis pathogens. J. Dairy Sci. **68:** 2684-2693.

Peng, Xian Feng, Zeng Zhen Ling, Chen Zhang Lin.2003. [Screening of therapeutic drugs for clinical mastitis in dairy cattle and their efficacy] Chinese Journal Vet. Sci. **23:** 193-195.

Pepin, M., Fontaine, J.J., Pardon, P., Marley, J. And Parodi, A.L. 1991a. Histopathology of the early phase during experimental pseudotuberculosis infection in lambs. Vet. Microbiol. **29:** 123-134.

Pepin, M., Pardon, P., Lantier, F., Marley, J., Levieux, D. and Lamand, M. 1991b. Experimental *C.pseudotuberculosis* infection in lambs: Kinetic of bacterial dissemination and inflammation. Vet. Microbiol. **26:** 381-392.

Prescott J.F., Menzies P.I.and Hwang Y.T.2002.An interferon-gamma assay for diagnosis of Corynebacterium pseudotuberculosis infection in adult sheep from a research flock. Vet. Microbiol. **88:** 287-297.

Rebouças M.F., Portela R.W., Lima D.D., Loureiro D., Bastos B.L., Moura-Costa L.F., Vale V.L., Miyoshi A., Azevedo V. and Meyer R.2011.*Corynebacterium pseudotuberculosis* secreted antigen-induced specific gamma-interferon production by peripheral blood leukocytes: potential diagnostic marker for caseous lymphadenitis in sheep and goats. J. Vet. Diagn. Invest. **23:** 213-220.

Rose, R. D.E., Tennet, J., Mc Waters, P., Chaplin, P.J., Wood, P.R., Kimpton, W., Chavill, R. and Scheerlinck, J.P.Y. 2002. Efficacy of DNA vaccination by different routes of immunization in sheep. Vet. Immunol. Immunopathol. **90:** 55-63.

Rosenbaum A., Guard C.L., Njaa B.L., McDonagh P.L., Schultz C.A,and Warnick LD, White ME.2005.Slaughterhouse survey of pyelonephritis in dairy cows. Vet. Rec. **157:** 652-655.

Senturk, S. and Temizel, M. 2006. Clinical efficacy of rifamycin SV combined with oxytetracycline in the treatment of caseous lymphadenitis in sheep. Vet. Rec. **159:** 216-217.

Srivastava P., Singh P., Nath N.and Deb J.K.2011.Physiological and biochemical consequences of host-plasmid interaction—a case study with Corynebacterium renale, a multiple cryptic plasmid containing strain. Plasmid. **65:** 110-117.

Srivastava, P, Nath N, and Deb JK. 2006.Characterization of Broad Host Range Cryptic Plasmid pCR1 from Cornyebacterium renale. Plasmid 56. **1:** 24-34. [http://www.ncbi.nlm.nih.gov/sites/entrez].

Stapleton S., Bradshaw B. and O'Kennedy R.2009.Development of a surface plasmon resonance-based assay for the detection of Corynebacterium pseudotuberculosis infection in sheep. Anal.Chim. Acta. **651:** 98-104.

Stefañska I., Gieryñska M., Rzewuska M. and Binek M. 2010. Survival of Corynebacterium pseudotuberculosis within macrophages and induction of phagocytes death. Pol J Vet Sci. **13:** 143-149.

Sunil V., Menzies P.I., Shewen P.E.and Prescott J.F.2008.Performance of a whole blood interferon-gamma assay for detection and eradication of caseous lymphadenitis in sheep. Vet. Microbiol. **128**(3-4): 288-297.

Takahashi T., Tsuji M., Kikuchi N., Ishihara C., Osanai T., Kasai N., Yanagawa R. and Hiramune T. 1995.Assignment of the bacterial agent of urinary calculus in young rats by the comparative sequence analysis of the 16S rRNA genes of corynebacteria. J. Vet. Med. Sci. **57:** 515-517.

Takai, S, Ryo Yanagawa and Yukitoshi Kitamura. 1980.pH-dependent Adhesion of Piliated Corynebacterium renale to Bovine Bladder Epithelial Cells." Infection and Immunity **28:** 669-674.

Taponen S., Salmikivi L., Simojoki H., Koskinen M.T.and Pyörälä S.2009.Real-time polymerase chain reaction-based identification of bacteria in milk samples from bovine clinical mastitis with no growth in conventional culturing. J. Dairy Sci. **92:** 2610-2617.

Timoney, John F, James H. Gillespe, Frederic W. Scott and Jeffrey E. Barlough. 1988. Hagan and Bruner's Microbiology and Infectious Diseases of Domestic Animals. Ithaca: Cornell University Publishing.

Vaneechoutte M., Riegel P., de Briel D., Monteil H., Verschraegen G., De Rouck A.and Claeys G.E.1995.Valuation of the applicability of amplified rDNA-restriction analysis (ARDRA) to identification of species of the genus Corynebacterium. Res. Microbiol. **146**(8): 633-641.

Watts J.L., Lowery D.E., Teel J.F., Ditto C., Horng J.S. and Rossbach S.2001.Phylogenetic studies on Corynebacterium bovis isolated from bovine mammary glands. Dairy Sci. 2001 **84:** 2419-2423.

Watts J.L., Lowery D.E., Teel J.F.and Rossbach S.2000.Identification of corynebacterium bovis and other coryneforms isolated from bovine mammary glands. J. Dairy Sci. **83:** 2373-2379.

Winn Jr, Washington, Stephen Allen, William Janda, Elmer Koneman, Gary Procop, Paul Schreckenberger, and Gail Woods.2006. Koneman's Color Atlas & Textbook of Diagnostic Microbiology. 6th ed. Philadelphia: Lippincott Williams & Wilkins.

Yanagawa, R. 1986. Causative agent of bovine pyelonephritis: *Corynebacterium renale, C.pilosum* & *C.cystitidis*. In progress in Veterinary Microbiology & Immunology Vol:2 Ed. R. Pandey pp. 158-174 Basel: S. Kanger.

□□□

Chapter 5

Arcanobacterium Pyogenes (Actinomyces Pyogenes) Infection

Dr. S.K. SRIVASTAVA
Former, Division of Bacteriology & Mycology
Indian Veterinary Research Institute, Izatnagar-243122
Bareilly (U.P.)

Arcanobacterium pyogenes is involved in causation of mastitis and metritis in animals. Uterine bacterial infection after parturition causes endometritis, perturbs ovarian function and leads to infertility in cattle. Although endometritis is caused by mixed infections, endometrial pathology is associated with the presence of *A. pyogenes. A. pyogenes* is an opportunistic pathogen of a number of important livestock species, and usually infects from an endogenous, commensal source. Thus, as with other normal flora opportunistic pathogens, the regulation of *A. pyogenes* virulence factors is likely important during both commensal and pathogenic interactions with the host. *A. pyogenes* is a small, gram positive rod that lack a capsule and meta- chromatic granules. The cell wall lack coryneform constituents but contains lysine, rhamnose and glucose. In cattle, sheep, swine infertility has also been observed with abortion (Bonnett 1991, Hinton 1972). This genus is closely related to Corynebacterium and Actinomyces. Like Corynebacteria the cells are pleomorphic. There is some controversy that this organism alone is not responsible for the disease as concurrent infection with gram-negative anaerobes, *Fusobacterium necrophorum* and *Bacteriodes melaninogenicus* has been often seen. *Peptostreptococcus indolicus* has also been incriminated in causation of disease. However, inoculation of pure cultures of *A. pyogenes* into non-pregnant uterus leads to the endometritis with a persistent corpus luteum. Moreover, isolation of *A. pyogenes* has been frequently achieved from cases of endometritis, pyometritis and purulent discharges. It is found on mucous membranes and the skin of susceptible species. Silva *et al.* (2008) carried out characterization of *A. pyogenes* based on BOX-PCR typing and on screening of eight virulence factor genes (plo, nanP, nanH, cbpA, fimA, fimC, fimE, fimG) by conventional PCR. *A. pyogenes* clonal types identified from isolates recovered from the uterus of postpartum dairy cows differed among herds. Although some clonal types were strictly associated with the development of clinical metritis, others were identified from isolates recovered from normal puerperium and clinical metritis cows. Moreover, the presence of the eight virulence factor genes was not related with the ability to induce clinical metritis, suggesting that the type of *A. pyogenes* may not be a determinant factor in the development of the disease. It was suggested that host intrinsic factors, the synergism between *A. pyogenes* and other bacteria and the differential gene expression of virulence factor genes may play a more relevant role in the establishment of puerperal uterine infections. Barbour *et al.* (2010) studied Koch's postulate of *Arcanobacterium pyogenes* recovered from the necrotic lung of a kid and compared the immunogenicity of this isolate in local and imported Saanen goats. The disease was successfully reproduced in intrathoracically challenged hamsters which showed lung congestion and liver abscesses, while hamsters that were intraperitoneally challenged showed only the formation of intestinal abscesses. The percentage of histopathologic legions in 12 observed microscopic fields per lung of three groups of hamsters (unchallenged controls, challenged intrathoracically and challenged intraperitoneally) showed a significant increase in lung necrosis of the intrathoracically challenged group, followed by intraperitoneally challenged hamsters, in comparison to unchallenged controls ($p<0.\ 05$). In addition, the frequency of mucus accumulation in alveolar ducts followed the same respective pattern ($p>0.\ 05$), while there was no significant difference in the frequency of neutrophil infiltration ($p>0.\ 05$). The isolate was successfully recovered from the lungs and livers of hamsters challenged by both routes. Saanen does showed significant seroconversion using the indirect haemagglutination (HA) test and slide agglutination test (SAT) and at three weeks following priming and boosting with *A. pyogenes* antigens ($p<0.\ 05$); however, only SAT showed significant seroconversion in local does at three weeks post booster ($p<0.\ 05$).

Frequently chronic mastitis, chronic suppurative pneumonia, with mycoplasmas and species of *Pasteurella* and *Mannheimia*, septic arthritis, vegetative endocarditis (cattle), endometritis and pyometra; umbilical infections; infections of the wounds and surgical incisions; and seminal vesiculitis (bulls and boars) are observed. It may be shed from apparently normal udders and is frequently recovered from tonsils and retropharyngeal lymph nodes. Infections occur subsequent to the entrance of the organisms to the tissues as a result of injuries. Dissemination to other organs may be hematogenous.

The cases of abortion are associated with autolysis of fetus and the organisms are isolated from all internal organs. Abortion can occur at any stage of pregnancy. This organism has the tendency to spread from its normal habitat on mucosal surfaces commonly causing abscess at any site.

The organism has been frequently associated with mastitis in many countries. A. (*Corynebacterium*) *pyogenes* has been associated with mastitis in India (Tuteja *et al.*, 2001). It is an opportunistic pathogen causing many types of purulent affections in young and immunocompromized hosts. It causes "summer mastitis" in cold countries and is communicable among dairy cattle during dry period. It often takes a destructive course causing abscess formation and sloughing. Summer mastitis spread by flies attracted to traumatized teats. Fly borne *A. pyogenes* can survive for over two weeks.

Arcanobacterium pyogenes is an established but often unrecognized human pathogen. A. pyogenes may also be misidentified as Arcanobacterium haemolyticum, which gives remarkably similar results in conventional biochemical tests. In a study, Kavitha *et al.* (2010) reported three cases of wound infections associated with *A. pyogenes* and also on the bacteriological characteristics which are relevant for identification of these isolates. The negative reverse CAMP test, the ability to produce acid from xylose and to hydrolyse gelatin and the positive beta-glucuronidase test clearly differentiated A. pyogenes from other closely related species. Only a few confirmed cases have been reported throughout the world and therefore the diagnostic evaluation of this organism is emphasized.

Pathogenesis

A. pyogenes produces a haemolysin which is lethal to several laboratory animals on intravenous inoculation. This also causes skin necrosis. Pure preparations of the haemolysin have revealed that it is 36000 to 90,000 daltons in Mol. Wt. (Takeuchi *et al.*, 1979). Infection of animals produces antitoxin in the infected animals. Antibodies also develop in animals against another *C. pyogenes* protein, a gelatinase activity containing protease. Santos *et al* (2010) reported antimicrobial resistance in *A. pyogenes* isolated from the uteruses of postpartum Holstein dairy cows and identified virulence factors. Seventy-two *A. pyogenes* isolates were phenotypically characterized for antimicrobial resistance to amoxicillin, ampicillin, ceftiofur, chloramphenicol, florfenicol, oxytetracycline, penicillin, spectinomycin, streptomycin and tetracycline by the broth microdilution method. Presence of virulence factor genes of *A. pyogenes* was investigated. Isolates exhibited resistance to all antimicrobial agents tested; high levels of resistance were found to amoxicillin (56.9%); ampicillin (86.1%), chloramphenicol (100%), florfenicol (59.7%), oxytetracycline (54.2%), penicillin (86.1%) and tetracycline (50%). Of all isolates, 69 (95.8%) were resistant to at least 2 of the antimicrobial agents tested and multidrug resistance (resistant to at least 3 antimicrobials) was observed in 64 (88.9%) of the A. pyogenes isolates. The major multidrug resistance profile was found for chloramphenicol-ampicillin-penicillin-florfenicol-amoxicillin-tetracycline, which was observed in 21 (29.2%) multidrug resistant isolates. No isolate was resistant to all nine antimicrobial agents tested but four isolates (5.6%) were resistant to eight antimicrobials. The information highlights the need for prudent use of specific antimicrobial agents. All four virulence factor genes occurred in isolates from normal puerperium and clinical metritis; however, the fimA gene was present in significantly higher frequency in isolates from metritis cows.

The pathogenesis of these bacteria requires further investigations. This organism possesses a number of virulence factors that contribute to its pathogenic potential Pyolysin (a58 kDa haemolytic exotoxin) is thought to be a major virulence determinant and a protective factor. It resembles the thio-activated cytolysins produced by *Listeria* and clostridia. Antitoxin can be demonstrated in naturally infected animals. Pyolysin leads to abscess formation, empyemia and pyogranulomas. Abscesses are often heavily encapsulated and variable in size. The pyolysin is cytolytic for immune cells, including macrophages. Expression of pyolysin (PLO) is required for virulence and this molecule is the most promising vaccine candidate identified to date. Four monoclonal antibodies (mAbs) to PLO were prepared for the analysis of functional domains of this toxin (Imaizumi *et al.* 2001). Two (mAbs S and H) of these markedly inhibited the hemolytic activity of PLO, but the inhibiting activity of the other two antibodies (mAbs C and G) was weaker. Subsequently, nine truncated PLOs were derived from recombinant Escherichia coli by various deletions from the N-terminus. Strong hemolytic activity was recognized in truncates of PLO following the deletion of 30 or 55 amino acids, but not in the truncate with deletion of 74 residues. Truncated PLOs were used in immunoblotting experiments to locate the epitopes for the mAbs. The epitope for mAbs C and G lies within the undecapeptide region (amino acids 487-505) of the C-terminus of PLO, which seems to be the binding site to erythrocytes. In contrast, the epitopes for mAbs S and H, which showed strong neutralizing activity, were found to lie in the N-terminal regions of the PLO ranging from 55 to 73 and 123 to 166 amino acids, respectively. From these results, it seems that the N-terminal region of PLO, in particular, the region of amino acids 55-74 is important for hemolytic activity.

The plo gene, encoding the *A. pyogenes* pyolysin is localized to a 2. 7-kb genomic islet of reduced %G+C content and alternate codon usage frequency. This islet, conserved among isolates from diverse hosts and geographical locations, separated the housekeeping genes smc and ftsY, which are found adjacent in many prokaryotes. The ftsY and ffh genes, located downstream of the plo islet, encode components of the signal recognition particle (Rudineck *et al.*, 2003). Mutational analysis suggest that these genes were essential for viability in *A. pyogenes*. The *A. pyogenes* ffh gene was unable to complement a conditional ffh mutant of Escherichia coli and its overexpression was toxic in E. coli. Mutagenesis of the islet-encoded orf121 did not affect plo expression, indicating that it may not be involved directly in the regulation of plo expression (Rudineck *et al.*, 2003). Regardless, the presence of the plo gene as part of a genomic islet inserted between genes essential for normal growth may provide selective pressure for the retention of this important virulence factor.

Insertional inactivation of the plo gene results in loss of expression of PLO with a concomitant loss in hemolytic activity (Jost *et al.* 1999). The plo mutant, PLO-1, has an approximately 1.8-log10 reduction in the 50% infectious dose compared to that for wild-type A. pyogenes in a mouse intraperitoneal infection model. Studies involving cochallenge of wild-type and PLO-1 bacteria resulted in recovery of similar numbers of both strains, suggesting that PLO production is required for survival in vivo. Recombinant, His-tagged PLO (His-PLO) is cytotoxic for mouse peritoneal macrophages and J774 cells in a dose-dependent manner. Protection against challenge with A. pyogenes could be afforded by vaccination with formalin-inactivated His-PLO, suggesting that PLO is a host-protective antigen, as well as a virulence determinant. PLO is the most divergent member of the cholesterol-binding pore-forming family of toxins. PLO is also divergent in a C-terminal undecapeptide motif which is almost invariant among other members of the family. This divergent undecapeptide motif is required for the full cytolytic activity of PLO and is also responsible for its oxygen-resistant nature. Insertional inactivation of the plo gene results in a significant reduction in virulence in an intraperitoneal mouse model of infection. The virulence of the plo mutant can be restored by providing PLO in trans, suggesting that PLO is a major virulence factor in A. pyogenes pathogenesis in mice. Results of vaccination trials with crude antigens against A. pyogenes infection in domestic animals and mice have been equivocal at best (Billington *et al.*, 2001). However, a recombinant PLO-based subunit vaccine protected mice from experimental A. pyogenes infection, indicating that PLO is also an important host protective antigen. Analysis of PLO production in broth culture indicated that expression of PLO was induced during early stationary phase, and that this correlated with an increase in plo-specific mRNA (Rudnick *et al.*, 2008). Analysis of a plo-cat transcriptional fusion indicated that transcription of plo was also induced during early stationary phase. Primer extension analysis and 5' RACE suggested that two putative promoter sequences, P1 and P2 were active. Analysis of site-directed mutants of these promoters in the plo-cat fusion indicated that P2 was the major-stationary phase promoter. Deletions of the plo promoter region from the plo-cat fusion implicated three direct repeat (DR) sequences as important for plo transcription. Mutagenesis of both DR1 and DR2 resulted in reduction in plo transcription, while the presence of only DR3 in deletions of the plo promoter region repressed transcription from P2. Gel shift experiments indicated that a soluble factor from A. pyogenes binds to the plo promoter region and that the DRs may act as binding sites for a transcriptional regulator.

A. pyogenes also possesses a number of adherence mechanisms, including two neuraminidases, the action of which are required for full adhesion to epithelial cells, and several extracellular matrix-binding proteins, including a collagen-binding protein, which may be required for adhesion to collagen-rich tissue However, a neuraminidase-deficient mutant of *A. pyogenes* only had a reduced ability to adhere to host epithelial cells, indicating that other factors are involved in adhesion. Studies have identified the first *A. pyogenes* adhesin, CbpA, a protein located on the bacterial surface which has the ability to bind collagen and promotes adhesion to the host cells (Pietrocola *et al.*, 2007). The protein has an N-terminal ligand-binding region (region A) and a C-terminal repetitive domain (region B). In this study we found that CbpA bound to almost all the collagen types tested but not to other proteins, and it displayed a propensity to interact with several collagenous peptides derived by CNBr cleavage of type I and II collagens. The K(D) values of CbpA for type I and II collagens and collagen peptides determined by solid-phase binding assay and intrinsic tryptophan fluorescence were in the range of 1-15 nM. It was also found that CbpA and its A region bound fibronectin, and that collagen and fibronectin interacted with distinct subsites. Anti-CbpA antibodies were effective at inhibiting both binding of isolated CbpA and bacterial adhesion to immobilized collagen, suggesting that CbpA is a functional collagen-binding adhesin. Analysis of the immunological cross-reactivity of CbpA with antibodies against other bacterial collagen-binding proteins indicated that CbpA is immunologically related to ACE from Enterococcus faecalis but not to CNA from Staphylococcus aureus or Acm from Enterococcus faecium. Far-UV and near-UV circular dichroism spectra showed that full-length CbpA and its region A are mainly composed of beta-sheet with only a minor alpha-helical component and that both the proteins have a well-defined tertiary structure. Far Western blotting revealed the presence of an approximately 120-kDa *A. pyogenes* cell wall protein that binds collagen type I. The 3. 5-kb gene that encodes the 124. 7-kDa CbpA protein was cloned, and sequence analysis indicated that CbpA contains a typical MSCRAMM protein domain structure. Recombinant, six-His-tagged CbpA (HIS-CbpA) was capable of binding collagen types I, II, and IV but not fibronectin. In addition, CbpA was involved in the ability of A. pyogenes to adhere to HeLa and 3T6 cells, as a cbpA knockout strain had 38.2 and 57.0% of wild-type adhesion, respectively (Esmay *et al.*, 2003). This defect could be complemented by providing cbpA on a multicopy plasmid. Furthermore, HIS-CbpA blocked A. pyogenes adhesion to HeLa or 3T6 cells in a dose-dependent manner. cbpA was only present in 48% of the *A. pyogenes* strains tested (n = 75), and introduction of plasmid-encoded cbpA into a naturally cbpA-deficient strain increased the ability of this strain to bind to HeLa and 3T6 cells 2.9- and 5.7-fold, respectively. These data indicate that CbpA, a collagen-binding protein of *A. pyogenes*, plays a role in the adhesion of this organism to host cells. *A. pyogenes* also expresses fimbriae, which are similar to the type 2 fimbriae of Actinomyces naeslundii, and forms biofilms (Jost and Billington 2005). However, the role of these factors in the pathogenesis of *A. pyogenes* infections remains to be elucidated. *A. pyogenes* also invades and survives within epithelial cells and can survive within J774A. 1 macrophages for up to 72 h, suggesting an important role for *A. pyogenes* interaction with host cells during pathogenesis. The two component regulatory system, PloSR, up-regulates pyolysin expression and biofilm formation but down-regulates expression of proteases, suggesting that it may act as a global regulator of A. pyogenes virulence. A protease, which may be identical to the gelatinase produced by the organism, has been suggested as a virulence factor. Any offensive odours are contributions of anaerobic pathogens such as *S. necrophoxin, Bacteroides* spp. Since *A. pyogenes* is a permanent resident of susceptible species, the occurrence of the disease is governed by some precipitating factors. The cholesterol-dependent cytolysins (CDCs) are part of a large family of pore-forming proteins that include the human proteins perforin and the complement membrane attack complex. The activity of all family members is focused on membranes, but the proteins are themselves involved in a diverse range of phenomena (Gilbert 2010). The way in which pore formation depends on specific characteristics of the membrane under attack as well as of the protein doing the attacking is emphasised. The cholesterol-dependent cytolysins (CDCs) have been the focus of a renewed keen research interest for over ten years now. Their importance has been even further enhanced by the homology now identified between them and the membrane attack complex/perforin (MACPF) family of proteins, which includes several components of the complement cascade as well as perforin itself. Well-known examples include listeriolysin, perfringolysin, streptolysin and pneumoysin. Listeriolysin from *L. monocytogenes* is responsible for the escape of bacteria from the phagosome to colonise the cytoplasm and has been applied as a protein adjuvant in the development of vaccines against cancer and tuberculosis, for example. Perfringolysin from *C. perfringens* has become perhaps the most studied CDC4 and has an important role in pathology associated with infection (gangrene).

Streptolysin from *S. pyogenes* is another intensely studied CDC and has been applied widely in experimental permeabilisation of biological membranes. Pneumolysin is a major virulence determinant for *S. pneumoniae*, allowing bacterial invasion of tissues and mediating inflammation and the activation of the complement cascade. However, CDCs have now, for example, been identified in the bacteria Arcanobacterium pyogenes and Gardnerella vaginalis and there also appear to be homologues outside prokaryotes such as the sea anemone Metridium senile pore-forming toxin metridiolysin. The homology with the MACPF family was unknown until the first structures of the canonical fold of that family were solved, revealing the now characteristic MACPF/CDC fold of a twisted 3-sheet around which helices are clustered. Without any significant other sequence homology, the fold of this superfamily of pore-forming and membrane-binding proteins has been conserved by compensatory mutation around a handful of key conserved glycines. The glycines presumably act as critical hinges during the dramatic refolding that CDCs are known to undergo and which is presumably the selective advantage of this specific structure that has caused it to be conserved over such a vast evolutionary timescale. While not all MACPF domains are involved in pore formation-for example, C6 and C8beta—they are all apparently involved in action on membranes. The dramatic refolding undergone by CDCs is tightly coupled to their oligomerisation and results in the conversion of the helices hemming the core 3-sheet of the MACPF/CDC domain into a pair of beta-hairpins which in tandem and alongside those from other subunits within the oligomer insert into the membrane to create a pore. It is obviously the basic assumption that where nonCDC members of the superfamily-such as complement proteins and perforin-act on membranes they do so by a mechanism involving similar refolding. Even where a member of the MACPF/CDC superfamily is not known to form a pore, or has been shown. not to-at least alone-the same conformational change could have other adaptive functions during activity on or at membranes. However, the bicomponent nature of some pore-forming toxins alerts us that showing an absence of activity for one pure protein does not mean that they do not contribute to pore formation quite directly, since that may require the presence of another MACPF/CDC family member or members from the same specific system. Complement acts by a combination of the C5b-8 complex of proteins preassembled on a target membrane recruiting C9 to form a lesion, which may be a complete ring of C9 associated with the C5b-8 or an arc-electron microscopy images show both possibilities. Perforin acts in concert with granzymes, to trigger apoptosis when delivered by cytotoxic cells at their targets (damaged, transformed and infected host cells). Incomplete rings are visible for perforin also and there are many unresolved issues concerning its mechanism and the dependence ofgranzymes on it for their delivery.

When cows develop endometritis after birth, *Escherichia coli* and *Arcanobacterium pyogenes* are usually the most prominent bacteria present in bovine uterine lochial secretions. *A. pyogenes* alone is rarely found in the course of a disturbed puerperium. This was confirmed in one study, since average and high-grade uterine contaminations were always associated with the presence of both bacteria (Zarbe *et al.*, 2001). The contamination grade was positively correlated with uterine polymorphonuclear granulocyte (PMN) numbers and negatively correlated with blood PMN numbers. Whether E. coli and *A. pyogenes* affect the phenotype and function of bovine PMN in a similar or differential way was subject to in vitro studies. PMN were tested in the presence of washed bacterial fragments or culture supernatants taken as a source for soluble and/or secreted bacterial products. Fragments and soluble products differed only quantitatively in their effects on PMN. Usually, long-time exposure (24h) of PMN to fragments induced the strongest effects. Accelerated death of granulocytes was only moderately induced by both E. coli and A. pyogenes products. Both *E. coli* and *A. pyogenes* products induced the enhanced expression of a membrane molecule detected by mAb IL-A110 and of CD11b. Expression of other surface structures remained largely unchanged (MHC class I, CD11c). Functional parameters of PMN (phagocytosis; generation of reactive oxygen species, ROS; antibody-independent cellular cytotoxicity, AICC) generally declined after pre-incubation for 24h with products of E. coli or A. pyogenes. Interestingly, soluble products of A. pyogenes stimulated the phagocytosis of PMN. However, co-incubation with E. coli products abrogated this stimulatory effect. The results supply evidence for similar modes of action of the gram-negative E. coli and the gram-positive A. pyogenes on bovine PMN. Alterations in PMN function and phenotype are mainly triggered by direct contact between bacterial fragments and PMN. Inhibition experiments with polymyxin B demonstrated that *E. coli*-mediated effects were not solely due to the action of lipopolysaccharide. The dominant functional depression of neutrophils by *E. coli* products strengthens the suggestion that the earlier appearance of E. coli in the uterus may support the co-infection of this organ by *A. pyogenes* at later times.

Diagnosis

Diagnosis is best achieved by culturing the suspected clinical material on a suitable agar, preferably blood agar. It is a facultative, anaerobe requiring 3-4 days to produce discernible colonies which are translucent, hemolytic up to 1mm in diameter. With age colonies become opaque and dry. *A. pyogenes* is catalase negative, lactose fermenting bacteria which digests proteins (gelatin, casein, coagulated serum). Most strains peptonize litmus milk and are CAMP positive. It is often difficult to grow bacteria in many milk samples showing subclinical mastitis. A study was made of 79 mastitic milk samples with no-growth bacteria in conventional culture, originating from cows with clinical mastitis (Taponen *et al* 2009). Of the 79 samples, 34 (43%) were positive for 1 (32 samples) or 2 (2 samples) of the target bacteria. The positive findings included 11 Staphylococcus spp. (staphylococci other than Staphylococcus aureus), 10 Streptococcus uberis, 2 Streptococcus dysgalactiae, 6 Corynebacterium bovis, 3 Staph. aureus, 1 Escherichia coli, 1 Enterococcus, and 1 Arcanobacterium pyogenes. The positive samples contained as many as 10(3) to 10(7) bacterial genome copies per milliliter of milk. This study demonstrates that in nearly half of the clinical mastitis cases in which conventional culture failed to detect bacteria, mastitis pathogens were still present, often in substantial quantities.

A study was designed to identify phenotypically and genotypically 61 *Arcanobacterium pyogenes* isolated from bovine mastitis and from various other origins(Hijazin *et al.*, 2011). The *A. pyogenes* isolates showed the typical cultural and biochemical properties of this species and displayed CAMP-like synergistic hemolytic activities with various indicator strains. The species identity could be confirmed genotypically by amplification and sequencing of the superoxide dismutase A encoding gene sodA of reference strains representing 8 species of genus Arcanobacterium and subsequent design of *A. pyogenes* sodA gene-specific oligonucleotide primer. The A. pyogenes sodA gene-specific oligonucleotide primer allowed, together with previously described *A. pyogenes* 16S-23S rDNA intergenic spacer region-specific oligonucleotide primer, a reliable molecular identification of all 61 A. pyogenes of various origins. The additionally performed PCR-mediated amplification of 5 known and putative virulence factor encoding genes revealed that 100, 20, 87, 75, and 98% of the A. pyogenes carried the genes plo, cbpA, nanH, nanP, and fimA, which allowed an individual strain characterization. This might help also to elucidate the role the putative virulence factors which play in bovine mastitis and in various other infections caused by this bacterial pathogen. Silva *et al.* (2008) characterized A. pyogenes field isolates recovered from the uterus of cows with either normal puerperium or clinical metritis, in an attempt to identify factors that might be associated with the establishment and persistence of the disease. This characterization was based on BOX-PCR typing and on screening of eight virulence factor genes (plo, nanP, nanH, cbpA, fimA, fimC, fimE, fimG) by conventional PCR. Finally, a relationship between clonal types, virulence factors and presence of disease was investigated. *A. pyogenes* clonal types identified from isolates recovered from the uterus of postpartum dairy cows differed among herds. Although some clonal types were strictly associated with the development of clinical metritis, others were identified from isolates recovered from normal puerperium and clinical metritis cows.

Moreover, the presence of the eight virulence factor genes was not related with the ability to induce clinical metritis, suggesting that the type of *A. pyogenes* may not be a determinant factor in the development of the disease. We suggest that host intrinsic factors, the synergism between A. pyogenes and other bacteria and the differential gene expression of virulence factor genes may play a more relevant role in the establishment of puerperal uterine infections.

Treatment and Control

For treatment of the infection penicillin, ampicillin, tetracyclines, trimethoprim-sulfonamides and other antimicrobial drugs are used. Resistant strains have been reported because of the nature of infections ;abscess with thick fibrous capsules. In such cases the response to antimicrobial drugs is poor. Billington and Jost (2006) studied tetracycline resistant genes in strains of *A. pyogenes.* The tet(W) gene is associated with tetracycline resistance in a wide range of bacterial species, including obligately anaerobic rumen bacteria and isolates from the human gut and oral mucosa. However, little is known about how this gene is disseminated and the types of genetic elements it is carried on. The authors examined tetracycline-resistant isolates of *A. pyogenes,* all of which carried tet(W), and identified three genetic elements designated ATE-1, ATE-2, and ATE-3. These elements were found in 25%, 35%, and 60% of tetracycline-resistant isolates, respectively, with some strains carrying both ATE-2 and ATE-3. ATE-1 shows characteristics of a mobilizable transposon, and the tet(W) genes from strains carrying this element can be transferred at low frequencies between *A. pyogenes* strains. ATE-2 has characteristics of a simple transposon, carrying only the resistance gene and a transposase, while in ATE-3, the tet(W) gene is associated with a streptomycin resistance gene that is 100% identical at the DNA level with the aadE gene from the Campylobacter jejuni plasmid pCG8245. Both ATE-2 and ATE-3 show evidence of being carried on larger genetic elements, but conjugation to other strains was not observed under the conditions tested. ATE-1 was preferentially associated with *A. pyogenes* strains of bovine origin, while ATE-2 and ATE-3 elements were primarily found in porcine isolates, suggesting that these elements may circulate in different environments. In addition, four alleles of the tet(W) gene, primarily associated with different elements, were detected among *A. pyogenes* isolates. Malinowski *et al.* (2011) carried out bacteriological examination of uterine swabs collected from cattle with metritis, according to commonly accepted procedures with the additional use of API tests. Sensitivity to antibiotics was tested by the disk diffusion method and performed in Mueller-Hinton agar. *A. pyogenes* strains were the most sensitive to amoxicillin/clavulanic acid (Amc) (97.3%), bacitracin (96.7%), ceftiofur (95.8%) and cephapirin (77.5%). Liu *et al.* (2009) aimed to identify, determine the susceptibility, and detect gene cassettes of Arcanobacterium (Actinomyces) pyogenes isolates from cows with endometritis. Arcanobacterium pyogenes isolates were identified first by using the API Coryne Vit system test, and further through PCR. Minimum inhibitory concentrations of 23 antimicrobial agents against A. pyogenes were tested using standard broth microdilution assays according to the protocols of the Clinical and Laboratory Standards Institute. The genes of integrons I and II were amplified by PCR using specific primers. Thirty-two *A. pyogenes* isolates were isolated from 136 endometritic cows in the Hohhot region. Antibiotic susceptibility tests revealed that all isolates were highly sensitive to fluoroquinolones (100%), macrolides (approximately 81.2 to 100%) and florfenicol (90.6%), aminoglycosides (approximately 15.6 to 81.2%), and tetracyclines (approximately 43.7 to 68.7%). However, 53.1% were resistant to clindamycin, approximately 50 to 65. 6% were resistant to penicillins, and approximately 37.5 to 71.9% were resistant to cephalosporins. One hundred percent were resistant to sulfonamides and bacitracin zinc. The integrons were further confirmed by sequencing. No class II integrons were detected, whereas 50% (n = 16) of the *A. pyogenes* isolates were positive for the presence of the intI I gene, but only 13 contained gene cassettes. Sequence analysis of gene cassettes revealed 6 gene cassettes, 4 of which encode resistant determinants of aminoglycosides (aadA1, aadA5, aadA24, and aadB) and 1 of which encodes the resistance gene of chloramphenicol (cmlA6). The function of the sixth identified cassette, designated ORF1, is unknown. The gene cassette arrays aadA24-ORF1, aadA5, and aadA1-addB-cmlA6 were found in 46. 13% (6/13), 38. 46% (5/13), and 38. 46% (5/13) of the isolates, respectively. These cassettes segregated according to a consistent pattern, with aadA5 always alone, ORF1 always with aadA24, and aadA1-aadB and cmlA6 always together. Most of the positive integrons existed in the multiresistant isolates (n = approximately 3 to 7), indicating that the integrons played an important role in the dissemination and spread of antimicrobial resistance.

Prophylactic treatment of heifers and dry cows with long acting penicillin is effective in preventing mastitis. Several vaccines consisting of A. pyogenes alone or mixed with several vaccine candidates of bacteria have been tested. A vaccine composed of two immunogens and five bacterins comprising of leukotoxoid and bacterin of Mannheimia haemolytica type A, outer membrane protein and bacterin of Pasteurella multocida type A, and bacterins of Haemophilus somnus, *Mycoplasma bovis,* and *Arcanobacterium pyogenes* was develod(Cho *et al.* ,2008). ELISA antibody titers to five bacterial antigens in vaccinated guinea pigs increased, compared with those in unvaccinated ones. BRV was safe for calves and pregnant cattle in this study. In calves challenged with *M. haemolytica* and *P. multocida,* the average daily weight gain and antibody titers of vaccinated calves increased, and respiratory symptoms (P<0. 05) and treatment frequency (P<0. 01) of vaccinated calves significantly decreased, compared with those of unvaccinated calves. Interestingly, the antibody titers of M. haemolytica leukotoxoid and Mycoplasma bovis were closely related with the reduction of respiratory symptoms. Genetic vaccines have also been tested. Three genetically toxoided, nonhemolytic PLO molecules, HIS-PLO. F(497), HIS-PLO. Delta P(499), and HIS-PLO. A(522), were found to be nontoxic, and vaccinated mice were protected from infection, indicating the potential of these toxoids as vaccines9Jost *et al.* 2003).

Immune response to *A. pyogenes* are not well understood. Infection or vaccination confers no useful resistance. The usefulness of pyolysin as a vaccine remains to be demonstrated.

Rhodococcus equi pneumonia

R equi is a facultative, intracellular, nonmotile, non–spore-forming, gram-positive coccobacillus (an organism that has the ability to exist as a coccus or bacillus or intermediate form). It is called *Rhodococcus* because of its ability to form a red (salmon-colored) pigment, *R equi* can be weakly acid-fast and bears a similarity to diphtheroids. The organism is commonly found in dry and dusty soil and can be important for diseases of domesticated animals (horses and goats). The frequency of infection can reach nearly 60 percent. *R. equi* is an important pathogen causing pneumonia in foals. Since 2008, it is known that *R. equi* can infect wild boar as well as domestic pigs. *Corynebacterium equi* was assigned to a new genus *Rhodococcus* long time ago but has come in use recently. Goodfellow *et al.*, (1981) reported that *R. equi* strains differ in their pathogenicity to the natural host. The organism causes chronic granulomatous pneumonia but acute cases have also been reported. It is a soil bacteria and multiplies in soil contaminated with feces particularly horse manure. It is enzootic at several horse farms and becomes the cause of foal pneumonia. The disease has a world wide distribution; prevalence at farms can be as high as 50%. At horse farms population of *R. equi* is high and it builds up thousand times. It is known to survive in moist soils for more than 15 months.

Rhodococcus equi infection primarily causes chronic pyogranulomatous pneumonia in 1 to 4 month old foals. Disease does not occur in adult horses unless there is a severe immunodeficiency. *R. equi* has also rarely caused infections in immunodeficient humans (such as those people with *HIV*. It is often confused with *Rotavirus*, a highly contagious virus that causes diarrhoea in foals. *R. equi* may occasionally also cause disease in other body systems.

Inflammation of the eye (uveitis), bone infection, inflammation of the joints, diarrhoea and abdominal abscess formation are noted infections outside of the lungs.

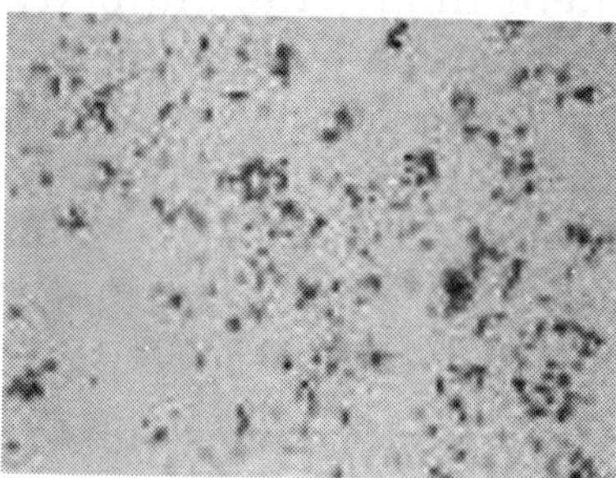

Rhodococcus equi, stained film

There occur several serotypes based on their capsular antigen which is polysaccharide in nature. No apparent relationship between the serotypes and virulence and species of the animal infected has been observed. The organism produces exoenzymes, a cholesterol oxidase and phospholipase C which may be the virulence factors of the organisms. Presence of a 20 kb plasmid may be associated with the virulence of the organisms (Prescott 1991). Cell wall corynemycolic acid and cell wall lipids such as phosphotidyl inositol & phosphotidyl ethanolamine are other virulence factors and may have implications in pathogenesis. A virulence plasmid (85-90 kb) has been associated with virulence. It is correlated with a cell surface protein, Vap, the role of which is not known. It is a 15-17 kDa protein.

The modes of transmission of the infection include ingestion, inhalation and infection through umbilicus. The organism colonizes the horse intestinal canal during the first 2 months of age and shed organisms in the feces. Inhalation of the organisms in the dust is the important route of infection. However, ingestion of soil containing metal is also responsible for occurrence of the disease Swallowing of infected pulmonary fluid in foals less than 5 weeks of age is also associated with the intestinal form of the disease resulting in enteritis or immunity against the disease. Intestinal lesions form due to massive exposure to infection over a sustained period. There are ulcerative lesions on the intestinal mucosa. Rarely bacteremia develops resulting in development of suppurative foci in many organs. Occasionally there may be infection of skin, joints & spleen. In non-pneumonic foals it may cause an ulcerative colitis.

Pneumonic foals often develop enteric disease after swallowing infected sputum. The prognosis varies with the age of the foals. In animals less than 2 months of age it is poorest. Aside from the respiratory form, abortions, uterine infections, have been observed. It is a common cause of submandibular and cervical lymphadenitis of swine. Lesions resemble those of tuberculosis.

Mode of transmission

The lifecycle of the organism is quite simple. *R. equi* inhabits the soil and obtains entry into the foal's respiratory tract primarily by inhalation of airborne bacteria. Entry may also occur through ingestion of soil where the bacteria gains entry to the blood stream and it seeds the lungs. The disease progresses very slowly as large abscesses begin to grow throughout the lung. As the infection matures the foals begin to show signs of pneumonia: fever, cough, depression. However, many of the symptoms are quite insidious until the disease has progressed to a life threatening state.

- The organism replicates within the respiratory tract and then is coughed up and swallowed by the foal. Replication continues as the bacteria travel though the intestinal tract after which time large amounts of *R. equi* are defecated and subsequently regain entry into the soil. Although adults are only very rarely infected, it is known that mares will also contaminate the soil by ingesting bacteria and passing larger numbers in their faeces. Studies have not shown there to be a relationship between which mares are shedding the bacteria in their faeces and which foals become infected with *R. equi* pneumonia.

Although *Rhodocococcus equi* is found in the soil of most farms, pneumonia caused by this organism can be endemic, sporadic or unrecognized depending upon the farm studied. Several factors may influence the incidence of the disease including the degree of contamination on the farm, density of horses, climatic conditions and virulence of the isolate. The infection is acquired through inhalation.

Virulence factors

The most common route of infection in horses is likely via inhalation of contaminated dust particles. Inhaled virulent strains of *R. equi* are phagocytosed by alveolar macrophages. During normal phagocytosis, bacteria are enclosed by the phagosome, which fuses with the lysosome to become a phagolysosome. The internal environment of the phagolysosome contains nucleases and proteases, which are activated by the low pH of the compartment. The macrophage produces bacteriocidal compounds (e. g. , oxygen radicals) following the respiratory burst. However, like its close relative *Mycobacterium tuberculosis*, *R. equi* prevents the fusion of the phagosome with the lysosome and acidification of the phagosome. Additionally, the respiratory burst is inhibited. This allows *R. equi* to multiply within the phagosome where it is shielded from the immune system by the very cell that was supposed to kill it (Hondalus and Mosser, 1994). After about 48 hours, the macrophage is killed by necrosis, not apoptosis. Necrosis is pro-inflammatory attracting additional phagocytic cells to the site of infection, eventually resulting in massive tissue damage.

All strains isolated from foals and the majority of human, cattle and pig isolates contain a large plasmid. This plasmid has been shown to be essential for infection of foals, and presumably plays a similar role for infection of other hosts, although this has not been established yet. Strains that lack the virulence plasmid are unable to proliferate in macrophages. This virulence plasmid has been characterized in detail from equine (horse) and porcine (pig) strains, although only the former has been functionally characterized (Letek *et al* 2008). These circular plasmids consist of a conserved backbone that is responsible for replication and bacterial conjugation of the plasmid. This portion of the plasmid is highly conserved and found in non-pathogenic *Rhodococci* plasmids. In addition to the conserved region, the virulence plasmids contain a highly variable region that has undergone substantial genetic rearrangements, including inversion and deletions. This region has a different GC-content from the rest of the plasmid, and is flanked by genes associated with mobile genetic elements. It is therefore assumed to be derived from a different bacterial species than the backbone of the plasmid via lateral gene transfer. Nearly all isolates from pigs are of 20-kd virulence-associated protein antigen (VapB) origin, which is of intermediate virulence. In human beings, only about 20-25% of isolates have been reported to express VapA.

The variable region of the virulence plasmid contain genes that are highly expressed following phagocytosis of *R. equi* by macrophages. It is believed that this variable region is a pathogenicity island that contains genes that are essential for virulence.

A hallmark of the pathogenicity island (PAI) is that many genes within it do not have homologues in other species. The most notable of these are the virulence associated protein (*vap*) genes. All foals infected with *R. equi* produce high levels of antibodies specific for *vapA*, the first *vap* gene to be characterised. Deletion of *vapA* renders the resulting strain avirulent (Jain *et al.* 2003). In addition to *vapA*, the pathogenicity island encodes a further five full length *vap* homologues, one truncated *vap* gene and two pseudo *vap* genes. The porcine pathogenicity island contains five full length *vap* genes, including the *vapA* homologue, *vapB*. In addition to these unique genes, the pathogencity island contains genes that have a known function, in particular two regulatory genes encoding the LysR-type regulator VirR and the response regulator Orf8. These two proteins have been shown to control expression of a number of pathogenicity island genes including *vapA*. Other genes have homology to transport proteins and enzymes. However, the functionality of these genes has not yet been established, nor how the proteins encoded within pathogenicity island subvert the macrophage.

Pathogenesis

Age related occurrence of the infection is very characteristic. This is either due to waning maternal immunity in association with immature immunity.

Failure of passive transfer of colostrum derived antibodies may be the predisposing factor of the development of the infection.

R. equi is a facultative intracellular pathogen and cells such as neutrophils and pulmonary macrophages play an important role in providing primary defenses to the foal. It survives inside the macrophages to cause granulomatous inflammation and eventually destroys them. Opsonic antibodies are important for providing defenses against the disease. However, the capacity of pulmonary macrophages of foals to kill *R. equi* is impaired and the bacteria persist in the macrophages for some time possibly due to failure of phagosomes to fuse with lysosomes. There is also a lack of superoxide anion response (Brumbaugh *et al.* , 1990). Continued persistence of *R. equi* in macrophages leads to chronic bronchopneumonia with extensive abscessation and an associated suppurative lymphadenitis. The organisms also cause non-specific degranulation of lysosomes *invitro,* which if *invivo,* would contribute to neutrophils influx and tissue destruction characteristics of advanced lung lesions (Hietala and Ardans 1987).

Both virulent and avirulent strains are encountered. Virulent strains posses 15-17 vap protein antigens.

The infection is marked by the development of ELISA antibodies, which opsonize the organisms for killing by phagocytes. These antibodies confer immunity in animals. It is also opsonized by complement component C_3b generated by alternate pathway Opsonized *R. equi* then associate with macrophages by way of the Mac-1 complement receptor. Once inside the macrophage it survives there. As regards the cellular immunity the importance of CD4+ and cD8+ lymphocytes in clearing infection as well as the dominant role of CD8+T cells has been established in nude mice (Nordmann *et al.* , 1992).

Diagnosis

Developments of suppurative bronchopneumonia with a history of the occurrence of the infection in foals at certain farms are suggestive of *R. equi* infection. Clinical signs can be characteristic of the disease and include fever, cough, depression, labored breathing and tracheal rattle (noise in the windpipe due to mucus accumulation). Unfortunately, many of these foals do not begin to show symptoms of the infection until the disease has progressed to a severe state. Confirmation of the disease is dependant on accumulating information regarding previous disease on the farm (how likely is this case also to be caused by *R. equi*).

The other diseases such as strangles, equine herpes virus 1 and equine viral arteritis have somewhat shorter course of infection. In strangles and equine viral arteritis lungs are not involved, however, *Streptococcus zooepi demicus* and *S. equi* infection may sometime involve lungs and therefore cultural examination is required. Routine laboratory evaluation of CBC and serum chemistry reveals nonspecific abnormalities consistent with infection and inflammation. Neutrophilic leukocytosis and hyperfibrinogenemia are common, and the severity of these findings relates to prognosis. Thoracic radiographic evaluation may reveal a pattern of perihilar alveolization, consolidation, and abscessation. The presence of nodular lung lesions and mediastinal lymphadenopathy in foals 1-5 months of age is highly suggestive of *R equi*. Bacterial culture of transtracheal wash samples is required for definitive diagnosis. Cytologic evaluation of transtracheal wash samples reveals intracellular coccobacilli, identification of which indicates initiation of appropriate antimicrobial therapy pending culture results.

The organism can be culturally diagnosed. It grows well on blood agar aerobically at 37^{0}C. In 48 hours, the colonies are smooth, mucoid, translucent & 3-5 mm in diameter. On some media a pink pigment is produced. The organisms are gram-positive rods which are catalase & urease positive. CAMP test can be employed to identify *R. equi*. Partial haemolysin of *R. equi* enhance the haemolysin of phospholipase D of *Corynebacterium pseudotuberculosis* or B-haemolysis of *Staphylococcus aureus.* There are 12 species of *Rhodococcus* that differ considerably in morphology, growth characteristic, biochemical activity and capacity to produce disease. Only *R. equi* is an important animal pathogen.

Sonmez *et al.* (2011) developed an immunocytochemical procedure for the early detection and demonstration of Rhodococcus equi in smears of tracheal aspirates taken from live foals in field conditions. Tracheal wash samples were collected from thoroughbred foals, aged 1-5 months and studied. Some foals were suspected of having R. equi infection on the basis of clinical examination (n=56) and others were unaffected control animals (n=54). Serum samples were also collected from each foal for testing for the presence of R. equi-specific antibody by enzyme linked immunosorbent assay (ELISA). Thirty-six of the control foals (66.7%) and 37 of the affected foals (66.1%) were seropositive for R. equi. Immunocytochemical labelling was detected in the smears from 73.2% of the affected foals and 70.4% of the control foals. For both ELISA and immunocytochemistry (ICC), there was no significant difference between the affected and control foals (P>0. 05) and there was no significant difference between the two test modalities (P>0. 05). ICC may therefore have similar diagnostic utility when compared with ELISA.

An enzyme-linked immunosorbent assay (ELISA) was developed against Rhodococcus equi using Triton X-114 detergent extracted whole cell material, in which the virulence associated protein (VapA) predominated

(Prescott *et al.*, 1996). Enzyme linked immunosorbent assay titres corresponded to antibody reacting with VapA on Western blots. There was considerable variation in antibody titres of nonimmunised mares and in the time when the colostrally derived antibody of their foals had declined to low or undetectable titres. In general, antibodies in foals declined to their lowest levels at age 4-8 weeks. Seroconversion occurred in foals of 8-10 weeks age, but the precise time depended on maternal titre and the month in which the foal was born. Foals reaching age 8 weeks in late summer showed more marked seroconversion than foals born earlier. The ELISA was used to follow the response to immunisation with the same Triton X-114 extracted material. Six mares immunised before parturition with the antigen in aluminium hydroxide adjuvant developed high titres, up to > 102,400 and transferred them to their foals through colostrum. Their foals responded to immunisation with 0.5-1.0 mg antigen 3, 5, 7 and 9 weeks after birth. Antibody titres following immunisation with similar dosage reached up to > 102,400 in a separate group of foals of nonimmunised mares. Nonvaccinated control foals seroconverted at age 6-8 weeks. The VapA based ELISA is useful to follow the course of natural infection with R. equi or immunisation with VapA based antigen.

A specific PCR assay for the rapid and reliable identification of *R. equi* is based on the amplification of a fragment of the *ChoE* gene encoding cholesterol oxidase, an enzyme believed to be a major virulence factor of *R. equi*. Mutational analysis indicated that *Cho*E is the membrane-damaging factor responsible for the typically shovel-shaped synergistic hemolysis (CAMP-like) reaction elicited by *R. equi* in the presence of sphingomyelinase C-producing bacteria, such as *Listeria ivanovii, Bacillus cereus*, and *Staphylococcus aureus*. This CAMP-like reaction can be used as a phenotypic marker for the rapid presumptive identification of *R. equi*.

Indirect fluorescent antibody technique (IFA)using a monoclonal antibody against the 15- to 17-kDa virulence-associated antigens (VapA) of *R. equi* and PCR targeting the structural gene of VapA detected bacteria in tracheal aspirates less sensitively than the isolation technique although they were more rapid. Therefore a combination of tracheal aspiration and bacterial isolation is the most valuable method for routine diagnosis of *R. equi* pneumonia in foals.

Treatment and Control

Treatment with erythromycin combined with rifampicin is effective. Animals with diffuse alveolar or intestinal lesions respond favourably than animals with cavitary lung lesions. The intracellular presence of R. equi and the formation of granulomatous and suppurative inflammatory tissue mean that prolonged treatment is needed. The pharmacological properties of the combination of erythromycin and rifampicin have improved the survival of foals infected with R. equi; however, erythromycin can cause adverse reactions in foals and mares, which has prompted the search for alternative therapies(Boswinkel *et al.*, 2006). The combination of azithromycin or clarithromycin with rifampicin seems to be a promising alternative. However these combinations are expensive and adverse effects remain to be determined, especially in the dams of treated foals. Thus correct diagnosis and appropriate use of drugs are essential for the treatment of R. equi infection in foals. During prolonged treatment plasma fibrinogen concentration can be used to monitor efficacy. Antibiotics given orally are more effective than given parenterally. Trimethoprim-sulfadizine combination may also be effective. Idiosyncratic hyperthermia and tachypnea can occur with erythromycin administration during periods of warm environmental conditions, and anorexia, bruxism, and salivation may be observed. Life-threatening, antibiotic-induced enterocolitis, due to *Clostridium difficile*, has been observed in the dams of nursing foals treated with erythromycin. Azithromycin is a newer generation macrolide with greater bioavailability than erythromycin. Azithromycin is administered orally (10 mg/kg, SID) with rifampin until clinical signs stabilize, then every other day until resolution of disease. The duration of antimicrobial therapy typically ranges from 4-9 wk.

Occurrence of antibiotic resistant strains are common. Giguere *et al.* (2010) found that 24 of 38 (63.2%) isolates were resistant to >or= 1 antimicrobial. Two isolates were resistant only to rifampin, whereas 22 isolates were resistant to azithromycin, erythromycin, clarithromycin, and rifampin. The overall prevalence of antimicrobial-resistant isolates in submissions received from Florida and Texas was 3.7% (12/328). The survival proportion of foals infected with resistant R equi isolates (2/8 [25.0%]) was significantly less, compared with the survival proportion in foals that received the same antimicrobial treatment from which antimicrobial-susceptible isolates were cultured (55/79 [69.6%]). Odds of nonsurvival for foals infected with resistant R equi isolates were 6.9 (95% confidence interval, 1.3 to 37) times the odds for foals infected with susceptible isolates. Interpretation of the results emphasized the importance of microbiological culture and antimicrobial susceptibility testing in foals with pneumonia caused by R equi.

Supportive therapy includes provision of a clean, comfortable environment and highly palatable, dust-free feeds. Judicial IV fluid therapy and saline nebulization facilitates expectoration of pulmonary exudates. NSAID should be administered as needed to maintain rectal temperature <103.5°F (39.7°C). Nasal insufflation with oxygen is necessary in foals with severe respiratory compromise. Bronchodilator therapy may or may not improve arterial oxygenation. Prophylactic antiulcer medication is indicated in foals that are stressed by respiratory difficulty, pain, frequent handling, hospitalization, and transportation.

The survival rate of *R equi* pneumonia is approximately 70-90% with appropriate therapy. The case fatality rate without therapy (or with inappropriate antimicrobial therapy) is ~80%. Parameters for discontinuation of medical therapy include clinical signs, serum fibrinogen concentration, and radiographic resolution of pulmonary consolidation and abscessation.

Prescott *et al.* (1997) evaluated the efficacy of virulence-associated protein of Rhodococcus equi in immunizing foals against R equi pneumonia. Virulence-associated protein extracted from R equi was used to prepare an acetone-precipitated. Triton X-extracted (APTX) antigen. After determination of the efficacy of passive immunization, in untreated foals or in foals given plasma from a horse vaccinated with APTX antigen or from a nonvaccinated horse, a field trial was done to evaluate the efficacy of vaccination of 8 mares, twice with APTX before parturition, and of their foals at ages 3 and 5 weeks; 6 mares and their foals served as unvaccinated controls. All 2-day-old foals were given plasma from local donor horses inoculated with a locally produced bacterin. Serum opsonizing activity produced by vaccination with APTX was determined. Passively immunized foals were challenge exposed with an aerosol of virulent R equi. Foals of the field trial were exposed to enzootic R equi infection. Results indicated that inoculation with APTX resulted in high IgG antibody liters with opsonizing activity. Passive immunization of foals with plasma from an immunized horse enhanced bacterial clearance from the lungs, compared with that in foals not given plasma or given plasma without APTX antibodies. Vaccination of mares and foals exposed to natural infection resulted in development of R equi pneumonia in 4 of 8 vaccinated foals, but in only 1 of 6 unvaccinated foals. In conclusion vaccination with APTX antigen led to high-titer, opsonizing antibody. Plasma from a vaccinated horse appeared to enhance clearance of *R. equi* from the lungs of foals. Paradoxically, vaccination of mares and their foals with APTX antigen did not protect foals and may have enhanced *R. equi* pneumonia in the foals. immunization with either proteins from an *R. equi* strain containing virulence-associated protein A (VapA), an immunodominant surface-expressed lipoprotein encoded by a virulence plasmid crucial for virulence in foals, or a whole killed virulent *R. equi* preparation was carried out (Cauchard *et al.*, 2004). Forty-eight pregnant mares were distributed into three groups, i.e. 24 immunized with *R. equi* VapA protein antigen associated with a water-based nanoparticle adjuvant (Montanide IMS 3012), 8 immunized with whole killed *R. equi*, and 16 non-immunized as control. Serum IgG and opsonizing capacity were evaluated during pregnancy in mares, and up to day 45 post-delivery in foals in which *R. equi* infections were recorded in the first 6 months of life.

Pregnant mares immunized with virulent R. equi proteins developed higher serum IgG and opsonic activity which were transferred to the foals than either in the whole *R. equi* immunized or the control group. Four foals developed pneumonia in the control group while none in immunized groups. Results support evaluation of VapA protein antigen associated with a water-based nanoparticle adjuvant as a candidate vaccine for immunization of pregnant mares resulting in passive antibody-mediated protection of foals. Lopez *et al.* (2003) developed a DNA vaccine expressing the vapA gene (pVR1055vapA) that induced an anamnestic response characterized by virulence associated protein A (VapA)-specific IgG antibodies in sera and bronchoalveolar lavage fluid (BALF) as well as VapA-specific proliferation of pulmonary lymphocytes when tested in adult ponies. In contrast, none of the adults receiving the control plasmid responded. To determine if pVR1055vapA induced VapA-specific responses in the foal, the targeted age group for vaccination against R. equi, 10 naïve foals were randomly assigned at birth to two groups of five. At 8-15 days of age (day 1), foals were vaccinated by intranasal and intradermal (i.d.) routes with either pVR1055vapA or the negative control pVR1055vapA_rev. All foals were DNA boosted at day 14 and protein boosted at day 30 with either recombinant VapA or recombinant CAT (control group). Prior to the protein boost, neither group developed VapA-specific immune responses. However, at day 45, two of the VR1055vapA-vaccinated foals had increased titers of VapA-specific IgGb, IgM and IgGa in the sera, and IgG in the BALF. The induction of the opsonizing isotypes IgGa and IgGb has been previously shown to be associated with protection against R. equi. No VapA-specific immune responses were detected in the control group. This study indicates that the DNA vaccine effectively stimulates anamnestic systemic and pulmonary immune responses in adult horses. The results in foals suggest that the DNA vaccine also primed a subset of immunized neonates.

There are 3 basic strategies to decrease the incidence of *R equi* pneumonia on endemic farms: decreased exposure to the organism, early detection of clinical cases, and enhanced passive immunity for neonatal foals. Foals should be maintained in well-ventilated, dust-free areas, avoiding dirt paddocks and overcrowding. Pneumonic foals should be isolated and their manure composted. Herd surveillance programs for early detection of pneumonic foals on endemic farms include twice weekly physical examination and auscultation, and monthly CBC and fibrinogen concentration. Foals with WBC count >14,000 cells/μL should be further evaluated for *R equi*. Administration of hyperimmune plasma might reduce the incidence and severity of *R equi* within the herd, but it is not completely effective in preventing disease. Hyperimmune plasma (1 L) is administered IV within the first week of life, followed by a second liter at approximately 25 days of age.

For prevention of the disease, contributory factors should be avoided such as exposure to dust, contaminated soil etc. Whenever there are epidemics of the disease preventive antibiotic treatment may be initiated. Routine clinical and physical examination of animals at risk is useful in detecting the cases at an early stage, thereby leading to the initiation of therapy. *R. equi* has proven itself quite resistant to various approaches of preventing the disease. Most likely time of infection to be during the first 2 weeks of life. Foals are administered the antibiotics during the first 2 weeks of life. Initial research conclusions indicate this may reduce, but not completely eliminate, infection in foals.

Another approach is the administration of hyperimmune plasma to foals during the first few days of life and then again at 3 weeks of age. Studies show that it may reduce incidence of the disease by up to one third and that it may also lead to a reduction in severity of the pneumonia if the foals are infected. The other method in preventing the disease is early detection.

References

Barbour E. K., Itani H. H., Shaib H. A., Saade M. F., Sleiman F. T., Nour A. A. and Harakeh S. 2010. Koch's postulate of Arcanobacterium pyogenes and its immunogenicity in local and imported Saanen goats. Vet. Ital. **46:** 319-327.

Billington S. J. , Jost B. H. 2006. Multiple genetic elements carry the tetracycline resistance gene tet(W) in the animal pathogen Arcanobacterium pyogenes. Antimicrob, Agents Chemother. 2006 **50:** 3580-3587.

Billington S. J. , Songer J. G. and Jost B. H. 2001. Molecular characterization of the pore-forming toxin, pyolysin, a major virulence determinant of Arcanobacterium pyogenes. Vet. Microbiol. **82:** 261-274.

Bonnett B. N., Martin S. W., Gannon V. P., Miller R. B. and Etherington W. G. 1991. Endometrial biopsy in Holstein-Friesian dairy cows. III. Bacteriological analysis and correlations with histological findings. Can J Vet Res. **55:** 168-173.

Boswinkel M., Sloet van Oldruitenborgh-Oosterbaan M. M. 2006. [Diagnosis and therapy of Rhodococcus equi infection in the horse]. Tijdschr. Diergeneeskd. **131:** 602-611.

Brumbaugh G. W., Davis L. E., Thurmon J. C. and Savage D. C. 1990. Influence of Rhodococcus equi on the respiratory burst of resident alveolar macrophages from adult horses. Am. J. Vet. Res. **51:** 766-771.

Cauchard J., Sevin C., Ballet J. J,. and Taouji S. 2004. Foal IgG and opsonizing anti-Rhodococcus equi antibodies after immunization of pregnant mares with a protective VapA candidate vaccine. Vet. Microbiol. **104:** 73-81.

Cho Y. S. , Lee H. S. , Lim S. K. , Joo Y. S. , Kim J. M. and Kim J. H. 2008. Safety and efficacy testing of a novel multivalent bovine bacterial respiratory vaccine composed of five bacterins and two immunogens. J. Vet. Med. Sci. **70:** 959-964.

Esmay P. A., Billington S. J., Link M. A., Songer J. G. and Jost B. H. 2003. The Arcanobacterium pyogenes collagen-binding protein, CbpA, promotes adhesion to host cells. Infect Immun. 4368-4374.

Giguère S., Lee E., Williams E., Cohen N. D., Chaffin M. K., Halbert N., Martens R. J., Franklin R. P., Clark C. C. and Slovis N. M. 2010. Determination of the prevalence of antimicrobial resistance to macrolide antimicrobials or rifampin in Rhodococcus equi isolates and treatment outcome in foals infected with antimicrobial-resistant isolates of R equi. J. Am. Vet. Med. Assoc.; **237:** 74-81.

Gilbert R. J. 2010. Cholesterol-dependent cytolysins. Adv. Exp. Med. Biol. **677:** 56-66.

Goodfellow, M. , Weaver, C. R. , and Minniken, D. E. 1981. Numerical classification of some rhodococci, corynebacteria and related organisms. J. Gen. Microbiol. **128:** 731-745.

Hietala, S. K. and Ardans, A. A. 1987. Interactions of *Rhodococcus equi* with phagocytic cells from *R. equi* exposed and non-exposed foals. Vet. Microbiol. **14:** 279-294.

Hijazin M., Ulbegi-Mohyla H., Alber J., Lämmler C., Hassan A. A., Abdulmawjood A., Prenger-Berninghoff E., Weiß R. and Zschöck M. 2011. Molecular identification and further characterization of Arcanobacterium pyogenes isolated from bovine mastitis and from various other origins. J Dairy Sci. **94:** 1813-1819.

Hinton, M. 1972. Vet. Bull. **42:** 1753.

Hondalus M. K. and. Mosser. D. M 1994. Survival and replication of Rhodococcus equi in macrophages. Infect. Immun. **62:** 4167-4175.

Imaizumi K., Serizawa A., Hashimoto N., Kaidoh T. and Takeuchi S. 2001. Analysis of the functional domains of Arcanobacterium pyogenes pyolysin using monoclonal antibodies. Vet. Microbiol. **81:** 235-242.

Jain, S. , Bloom, B. R. and. Hondalus. M. K. 2003. Deletion of *vapA* encoding Virulence Associated Protein A attenuates the intracellular actinomycete Rhodococcus equi. Mol. Microbiol **50:** 115-128.

Jost B. H. and Billington S. J. 2005. . Arcanobacterium pyogenes: molecular pathogenesis of an animal opportunist. Antonie Van Leeuwenhoek. **88:** 87-102.

Jost B. H., Songer J. G. and Billington S. J. 1999. An Arcanobacterium (Actinomyces) pyogenes mutant deficient in production of the pore-forming cytolysin pyolysin has reduced virulence. Infect. Immun. **67:** 1723-1728.

Jost B. H., Trinh H. T., Songer J. G. and. Billington S. J. 2003. Immunization with genetic toxoids of the Arcanobacterium pyogenes cholesterol-dependent cytolysin, pyolysin, protects mice against infection. Infect. Immun. **71:** 2966-2969.

Kavitha K. , Latha R. , Udayashankar C. , Jayanthi K. and Oudeacoumar P. 2010. Three cases of Arcanobacterium pyogenes-associated soft tissue infection. J. Med. Microbiol. **59:** 736-739. Epub 2010 Mar 18.

Letek, M., Ocampo-Sosa, M. A. A, Sanders, U. Fogarty, T. Buckley, D. P. Leadon, P. Gonzalez, M. Scortti, W. G. Meijer, J. Parkhill, S. Bentley, and. Vázquez-Boland. J. A. 2008. Evolution of the Rhodococcus equi vap pathogenicity island seen through comparison of host-associated vapA and vapB virulence plasmids. J. Bacteriol. **190:** 5797-5805.

Liu M. C., Wu C. M., Liu Y. C., Zhao J. C., Yang Y. L. and Shen J. Z. 2009. Identification, susceptibility, and detection of integron-gene cassettes of Arcanobacterium pyogenes in bovine endometritis. J Dairy Sci. **92:** 3659-66.

Lopez A. M., Hines M. T., Palmer G. H., Knowles D. P., Alperin D. C. and Hines S. A. 2003. Analysis of anamnestic immune responses in adult horses and priming in neonates induced by a DNA vaccine expressing the vapA gene of Rhodococcus equi. Vaccine. **21:** 3815-3825.

Malinowski E., Lassa H., Markiewicz H., Kaptur M., Nadolny M., Niewitecki W. and Ziêtara J. 2011. Sensitivity to antibiotics of Arcanobacterium pyogenes and Escherichia coli from the uteri of cows with metritis/endometritis. Vet. J. **187:** 234-238. Epub 2010 Feb 2.

Nordmann, P., Ronco, E. and Nauciel, C. 1992. Role of T. lymphocytes subsets in *Rhodococcus equi* pneumonia. Infect. Immun. **60:** 2748-2752.

Pietrocola G., Valtulina V., Rindi S., Jost B. H. and Speziale P. 2007. Functional and structural properties of CbpA, a collagen-binding protein from Arcanobacterium pyogenes. Microbiology. 2007 **153:** 3380-3389.

Prescott J. F., Fernandez A. S., Nicholson V. M., Patterson M. C., Yager J. A., Viel L. and Perkins G. 1996. Use of a virulence-associated protein based enzyme-linked immunosorbent assay for Rhodococcus equi serology in horses. Equine Vet. J. **28:** 344-349.

Prescott J. F., Nicholson V. M., Patterson M. C., Zandona Meleiro M. C., Caterino de Araujo A., Yager J. A. and Holmes MA. 1997. Use of Rhodococcus equi virulence-associated protein for immunization of foals against R equi pneumonia. Am. J. Vet. Res. **58:** 356-359.

Prescott, J. F. 1991. Rhodococcus equi – an animal and human pathogen. Clin. Microbiol. Rev. **40:** 20-34.

Rudnick S. T., Jost B. H. and Billington S. J. 2008. Transcriptional regulation of pyolysin production in the animal pathogen, Arcanobacterium pyogenes. Vet Microbiol. **25:** 96-104.

Rudnick S. T., Jost B. H., Songer J. G. and Billington S. J. 2003. The gene encoding pyolysin, the pore-forming toxin of Arcanobacterium pyogenes, resides within a genomic islet flanked by essential genes. FEMS Microbiol. Lett. **225:** 241-247.

Santos T. M., Caixeta L. S., Machado V. S., Rauf A. K., Gilbert R. O. and Bicalho RC. 2010. Antimicrobial resistance and presence of virulence factor genes in Arcanobacterium pyogenes isolated from the uterus of postpartum dairy cows. Vet. Microbiol. **145** (1-2): 84-89.

Silva E., Gaivão M., Leitão S., Jost B. H., Carneiro C., Vilela C. L., Lopes da Costa L. and Mateus L. 2008. Genomic characterization of Arcanobacterium pyogenes isolates recovered from the uterus of dairy cows with normal puerperium or clinical metritis. Vet. Microbiol. **132:** 111-118.

Sonmez K. , Gurel A. and Takai S. 2011. Immunocytochemical Detection of Rhodococcus equi in Tracheal Washes of Foals. J. Comp. Pathol. [http://www. ncbi. nlm. nih. gov/pubmed/21238974].

Takeuchi, S. , Azuma, R. and Suto, T. 1979. Purification and some properties of haemolysin produed by *Corynebacterium pyogenes*. Jpn. J. Vet. Sci. **41:** 511-516.

Taponen S., Salmikivi L., Simojoki H., Koskinen M. T. and Pyörälä S. 2009. Real-time polymerase chain reaction-based identification of bacteria in milk samples from bovine clinical mastitis with no growth in conventional culturing. J. Dairy Sci. **92:** 2610-2617.

Tuteja, F. C. , Kapur, M. P. , Sharma, A. and Manuja, B. 2001. Mastitis pathogens from apparently healthy buffaloes and their relation to somatic cell count of milk. Ind. J. Comp. Microbiol. Immunol. Infect. Dis. **22:** 162-163.

Zerbe H. , Ossadnik C. , Leibold W. and Schuberth H. J. 2001. Influence of Escherichia coli and Arcanobacterium pyogenes isolated from bovine puerperal uteri on phenotypic and functional properties of neutrophils. Vet Microbiol. **79:** 351-365.

□□□

Chapter 6

Diseases Caused by *Streptococcus* spp.

Dr. S.K. SRIVASTAVA
Former, Division of Bacteriology & Mycology
Indian Veterinary Research Institute, Izatnagar-243122
Bareilly (U.P.)

The *Streptococcus* constitute of gram-positive spherical bacteria occurring in short or long chains. These are facultatively anaerobic in their gaseous requirement but grow best under aerobic environment. They show considerable ecological, nutritional and serological diversity. Warm blooded animals carry a resident flora of streptococci on the mucous membrane of the upper respiratory, lower genital and most of the alimentary tract. Classification is based on a combination of various characteristics; prominent among these are carbohydrate and protein antigen composition, fermentation of sugars, biochemical reaction, growth characteristics and DNA homology. "Lancefield" serological grouping is most useful in classifying the streptococci in various groups based on carbohydrate antigen possessed on the surface. Lancefield groups have been designated as A – H and K – V. Streptococci are responsible for causing pyogenic infection in cattle, buffalo, horses, swine, dogs and cats. It is also a common cause of mastitis in cattle and buffaloes. Both, potentially pathogenic and non-pathogenic species occur in nature.

Freshly isolated group A and C *Streptococci* have a hyaluronic acid capsule that is non-antigenic and is antiphagocytic. Under the capsule is the cell wall consisting of mosaic of proteins (M, T, R proteins), peptidoglycan and group specific carbohydrate. Peptidoglycan can trigger inflammation, fever and lymphocyte proliferation. It is dermonecrotic and cytotoxic in vitro.

Exotoxins of *Streptococci pyogenes* include haemolysins (Streptolysin O and S) DNAse, NADase, protease, streptokinase (a fibrinolysin) and a phage coded pyogenic toxin responsible for rash of scarlet fever. Most evoke immune response in course of infection.

Effects on sheep or bovine blood are used to divide streptococci into 3 groups;

1. Alpha haemolytic streptococci produce a zone of green discolouration around colonies. It does not cause lysis of cells. Most Commensal streptococci are of this type.
2. Beta haemolytic streptococci destroy erythrocytes and produce a clear zone around colonies. Most pathogenic types are Beta - haemolytic eg. *S.pyogenes.*
3. Gamma - haemolytic are non-haemolytic.

Streptococci of veterinary interest are tabulated below;

Species	Lancefield group	Main host species affected	Chief Disease
Caused			
S.pyogenes	A	Human, Cattle	Pharyngitis, tonsillitis, pyoderma, erysipelas puerpural fever, rheumatic fever, glomerulonephritis, mastitis
S. agalactiae	B	Dairy cattle, Human	Mastitis, neonatal infections
S.equi subsp. *equi*	C	Horses	Strangles
S.dysgalactiae subsp..equisimilis	G	Swine, Horses	Miscellaneous suppurative conditions, lymphadenitis, metritis, porcine arthritis
S.equi subsp. *zooepidemicus*	C	Horses	Secondary pneumonias, miscellaneous suppurative conditions, genital and neonatal conditions
S.dysgalactiae subsp. dysgalactiae	G	Dairy cattle	Mastitis
Group E	E	Swine	Jowl Abscesses
S.canis	G	Carnivores, laboratory animals	Feline lymphadenitis, miscellaneous pyogenic conditions

S.suis	R (=type 2) S (=type 1)	Swine, Horses	Neonatal infections, septicaemias, pneumonia
S.uberis	-	Cattle	Mastitis
S.pneumoniae	-	Primates, lab animals, horses	Pneumonia, Septicaemia

Streptococci contain a variety of virulence factors. These are tabulated below;

Bacterial species	**Virulence factors**
S.pyogenes	Capsular polysaccharide, M protein, haemolysin, CAMP factor, Streptokinase
S.agalactiae	Capsular polysaccharide, R protein, CAMP factor
S.dysagalatiae	Hyaluronidase, streptokinase, fibronectin binding protein
S.equi subsp. *equi*	Hyaluronic acid capsule, M protein, haemolysin, streptokinase, plasmin receptors, Leukocidal toxin
S.equi subsp. *zooepidemicus*	Capsule, M protein, haemolysin, streptokinase
S.equisimilis	M protein
S. canis	M protein, Hemolysin
S.suis	Capsule, 136 and 100 kDa virulence proteins
S.porcinus	M protein
S.pneumoniae	Capsule, pneumolysin, IgA protease, neuraminidase
S.uberis	Capsule, hyaluronidase, antiphagocytic 65 kDa protein

Important diseases caused by *Streptococcal* species in animals are dealt here.

Streptococcus agalactiae

The organism is responsible for causing chronic, contagious bovine mastitis. Other animals namely dogs, cats, fish and hamsters are also affected. The polysaccharide capsule includes specific antigen types Ia, Ib, Ic, II & III. Type Ic is associated with a C protein antigen. About 25% of *S.agalactiae* strains are untypable.

The disease mastitis occurs wherever dairying is being practiced. *S. agalactiae* has been incriminated with *Staphylococcus aureus* as the major cause of bovine mastitis throughout the world. Palanivel *et al.* (2005) Isolated *S.agalactiae* from 4-5% of 155 buffaloes tested in Chennai area in India.

S.agalactiae possesses several virulence determinants on its surface. Type III capsular polysaccharide prevents deposition of C3 on its surface thereby escaping complement mediated killing. (Rainard and Boulard 1992). Protein X, a surface protein of *S.agalactiae* is frequently associated with bovine strains. It is a target for opsonins and, thus, probably a protective factor. Bovine complement S (Vitronectin) is thought to be important in the adherence of bacteria to bovine epithelial cells. R protein antigens are found on filamentous structures of the surface and might be associated with the virulence. *S. agalactiae* strains possess either R protein or C protein and R protein is a colonization factor (Kurl *et al.*, 1984). CAMP factor, aceramide binding protein may have a cytotoxic activity for mammary tissues. Besides haemolysin, neuraminidase and vasoactive extracellular toxin may be virulence factors. Lipoteichoic acid may act as adhesion molecule and potentiate the virulence.

Pathogenesis

While much work in this field has focused on the *S. agalactiae* polysaccharide capsule, which is an important virulence factor that elicits protective immunity, surface proteins have received increasing attention as potential virulence factors and vaccine components. These surface proteins have been implicated in interactions with human epithelial cells, binding to extracellular matrix components, and/or evasion of host immunity. Of note, several *S. agalactiae* surface proteins are related to surface proteins identified in other bacterial pathogens, emphasizing the general interest of the *S. agalactiae* proteins. Because some *S. agalactiae* surface proteins elicit protective immunity, they hold promise as components in a vaccine based only on proteins or as carriers in polysaccharide conjugate vaccines (Lindahl *et al.*, 2005). Fluegge *et al.* (2004) identified some major released proteins of *S. agalactiae*, including molecules known to be present on the surface of bacterial cells but not previously described as released proteins, such as CAMP factor, a phosphocarrier protein, aldolase, enolase, PcsB, and heat-shock protein 70. Serotype-specific differences in the protein patterns of extracellular products and immunoreactivity with human sera could be detected by SDS-PAGE and Western blot. The identification of unexpected released proteins may indicate secondary functions for these proteins. Fibrinogen (Fg) is often a common site for bacterial recognition. In Streptococcus agalactiae, two surface proteins that recognize Fg are FbsA and FbsB. FbsA and the N-terminal region of FbsB have been shown to bind to human Fg, while the C-terminal region of FbsB [FbsB(C)] has been speculated to bind to bovine Fg. This C-terminal region which is conserved in many of the S. agalactiae strains was tested for binding to bovine Fg. For this, FbsB(C) was cloned, expressed and purified. Dot blot, Western blot and ELISA experiments carried out with the purified protein showed that FbsB(C) has the ability to bind to bovine Fg. It was also observed that other than binding to the native form of Fg, FbsB(C) also has the ability to bind to the Fg subunits when reduced. On studying the influence of Ca(2+) on the FbsB(C)-bovine Fg binding it was observed that the addition of Ca(2+) in the assay experiment greatly stimulated the binding. When the primary structure of FbsB(C) was analyzed, it was seen that other than similarities with strains of the same organism, it does not have any similarity with any protein characterized so far. In addition to this, its secondary structure component analysis by circular dichroism revealed that it is composed mainly of alpha helices and random coils unlike other Fg-binding surface proteins where beta sheets are dominant. FbsB(C) indeed is a novel protein and understanding the mechanism of its interaction with Fg would be useful in developing strategies to fight against infections by Streptococcus (Devi and Ponnuraj 2010).

Telford *et al.*(2006) summarized that the recently discovered pili in gram-positive pathogens are formed by covalent polymerization of adhesive pilin subunits. Evidence from studies of pili in the three principal streptococcal pathogens of humans indicates that the genes that encode the pilin subunits and the enzymes that are required for the assembly of these subunits into pili have been acquired en bloc by the horizontal transfer of a pathogenicity island. In pathogenic streptococci the proteinaceous components of pili are covalently polymerized by the action of sortase enzymes similar to those involved in the covalent attachment of Gram-positive surface proteins to the peptidoglycan cell wall. With great relevance to the development of strategies to combat Gram-positive-associated infections, pilus components from pathogenic streptococci have been shown to induce protective immunity in mouse models of streptococcal disease (Soriani and Telford, 2010). In addition, recent papers have created new perspectives on the role of such organelles in streptococcal pathogenesis, from the involvement in colonization and biofilm formation to translocation of tissue barriers. *S.agalactiae* assembles two types of pili-pilus islands (PIs) 1 and 2-on its surface to adhere to host cells and to initiate colonization for pathogenesis. The GBS PI-1 pilus is made of one major pilin, GBS80, which forms the pilus shaft, and two secondary pilins, GBS104 and GBS52, which are incorporated into the pilus at various places. Vengadesan *et al* (2011) report the crystal structure of the 35-kDa C-terminal fragment from GBS80, which is composed of two IgG-like domains (N2-N3). The structure was solved by single-wavelength anomalous dispersion using sodium-iodide-soaked crystals and diffraction data collected at the home source. The N2 domain exhibits a cnaA/DEv-IgG fold with two calcium-binding sites, while the N3 domain displays a cnaB/IgG-rev fold. The authors have built a model for full-length GBS80 (N1, N2, and N3) with the help of available homologous major pilin structures, a model for the GBS PI-1 pilus shaft was proposed. The N2 and N3 domains are arranged in tandem along the pilus shaft, whereas the respective N1 domain is tilted by approximately 20° away from the pilus axis.A pilin-like motif in the minor pilin GBS52, which might aid its incorporation at the pilus base was also identified. The crystal structure of the pilin GBS52, reveals two IgG-like fold domains, N1 and N2. Each domain is comprised of seven antiparallel beta strands, an arrangement similar to the fold observed in the *Staphylococcus aureus* adhesin Cna. Consistent with its role as an adhesin, deletion of gbs52 gene significantly reduces bacterial adherence to pulmonary epithelial cells (Krishnan *et al.*, 2007). Moreover, latex beads linked to the GBS52 protein adhere to pulmonary but not to many other epithelial cells; binding to the former is specifically inhibited by antibodies against GBS52. Nonetheless, substantial binding is only observed with N2 domain-conjugated beads. This study presents the structure of a Gram-positive pilin that utilizes a distinct IgG fold variant to mediate pathogen adherence to a specific tissue.

Samen *et al.*(2011) describe the functional characterisation of a gene from *S. agalactiae*, designated rga, which encodes a protein with significant similarity to members of the RofA-like protein (RALP) family of transcriptional regulators. After deletion of the rga gene in the genome of *S. agalactiae*, the mutant strain exhibited a significantly reduced expression of the genes srr-1 and pilA, which encode a serine-rich repeat surface glycoprotein and a pilus protein, respectively, and a moderate increased expression of the fbsA gene, which encodes a fibrinogen-binding protein. Electrophoretic mobility shift assays demonstrated a specific DNA-binding of purified Rga to the promoter regions of pilA and fbsA, respectively, suggesting a direct control of pilA and fbsA transcription by Rga. Adherence assays revealed a significantly reduced binding of the delta-rga mutant to epithelial HEp-2 cells and to immobilized human keratin 4, respectively. In contrast, the adherence of the delta-rga mutant to A549 cells and its binding to human fibrinogen was significantly increased. Immunoblot and immunoelectron microscopy revealed a significantly reduced quantity of pili structures in the delta-rga mutant compared to the parental strain. The wild-type phenotype could be restored by a plasmid-mediated expression of rga, demonstrating that the mutant phenotypes resulted from a loss of Rga function.Gutekunst *et al.* (2003) suggests regulatory mechanisms that control the formation of specific virulence factors in these bacteria. The present study describes a gene from *S. agalactiae*, designated rogB, encoding a protein with significant similarity to members of the RofA-like protein (RALP) family of transcriptional regulators. Disruption of the rogB gene in the genome of S. agalactiae resulted in mutant strain RGB1, which was impaired in its ability to bind to fibrinogen and fibronectin. Mutant RGB1 also exhibited a reduced adherence to human epithelial cells but did not show an altered invasion of eukaryotic cells. By real-time PCR analysis, mutant RGB1 revealed an increased expression of the cpsA gene, encoding a regulator of capsule gene expression. However, strain RGB1 exhibited a reduced expression of the rogB gene and of two adjacent genes, encoding putative virulence factors in S. agalactiae. Furthermore, mutant RGB1 was impaired in the expression of the fbsA gene, coding for a fibrinogen receptor from *S. agalactiae*. The altered gene expression in mutant RGB1 could be restored by plasmid-mediated expression of rogB, confirming a RogB deficiency as the cause for the observed changes in virulence gene expression in *S. agalactiae*. Reporter gene studies with a promotorless luciferase gene fused to fbsA allowed a growth-dependent analysis of fbsA expression in *S. agalactiae*. These reporter gene studies also suggest that RogB exerts a positive effect on fbsA expression in *S. agalactiae*.

After the introduction of the infection into the teat, the invasion takes 1-4 days and appearance of inflammation takes 3-5 days. How the organisms adhere to the host is not known. Studies in human beings have shown that *S. agalactiae* adheres to a variety of epithelial cells. The work of Schubert *et al* (2004) demonstrates the importance of the fibrinogen receptor FbsA for the streptococcal adherence and invasion of epithelial cells. Deletion of the fbsA gene in various *S. agalactiae* strains substantially reduced their binding of soluble fibrinogen and their adherence to and invasion of epithelial cells, indicating a role of FbsA in these different processes. The adherence and invasiveness of an fbsA deletion mutant were partially restored by reintroducing the fbsA gene on an expression vector. Heterologous expression of fbsA in Lactococcus lactis enabled this bacterium to adhere to but not to invade epithelial cells, suggesting that FbsA is a streptococcal adhesin. Flow cytometry experiments revealed a dose-dependent binding of FbsA to the surface of epithelial cells. Furthermore, tissue culture experiments exhibited an intimate contact of FbsA-coated latex beads with the surfaces of human epithelial cells. Finally, host cell adherence and invasion were significantly blocked in competition experiments with either purified FbsA protein or a monoclonal antibody directed against the fibrinogen-binding epitope of FbsA. Taken together, studies demonstrate that FbsA promotes the adherence of S. agalactiae to epithelial cells but that FbsA does not mediate the bacterial invasion into host cells. These results also indicate that fibrinogen-binding epitopes within FbsA are involved in the adherence of *S. agalactiae* to epithelial cells.There is much variation depending on the integrity of the teat cistern and animals. There is a rapid multiplication of the organisms in the lactiferous ducts thereafter entering into the lymphatics and to the supramammary symph nodes. Gutekunst *et al.* (2004) describes the identification of the fbsB gene, encoding a novel fibrinogen-binding protein that plays a crucial role in the invasion of *S. agalactiae* into human cells. In Western blots and enzyme-linked immunosorbent assay (ELISA) experiments, the FbsB protein was demonstrated to interact with soluble and immobilized fibrinogen. Binding studies showed the N-terminal 388 residues of FbsB and the Aalpha-subunit of human fibrinogen to recognize each other. By reverse transcription (RT)-PCR, the fbsB gene was shown to be cotranscribed with the gbs0851 gene in *S. agalactiae*. Deletion of the fbsB gene in the genome of *S. agalactiae* did not influence the binding of the bacteria to fibrinogen, suggesting that FbsB does not participate in the attachment of *S. agalactiae* to fibrinogen. In tissue culture experiments, however, the fbsB deletion mutant was severely impaired in its invasion into lung epithelial cells. Bacterial invasion could be reestablished by introducing the fbsB gene on a shuttle plasmid into the fbsB deletion mutant. Furthermore, treatment of lung epithelial cells with FbsB fusion protein blocked *S. agalactiae* invasion of epithelial cells in a dose-dependent fashion. These results suggest an important role of the FbsB protein in the overall process of host cell entry by S. agalactiae.

The *S.agalactiae* rarely penetrates the epithelium, however, in some animals the organisms enters the lymphatics. This causes an influx of neutrophils in the mammary gland leading to the phagocytosis. Opsonization is probably carried out by C3 following activation of alternative complement pathway. The damage to the acinar and ductular epithelium results in sharp fall in inhibition and stasis of secretions due to development of a systemic reaction. This may lead to fibrosis of interalveolar tissues which may further increase leading to cell atrophy.

Bacterial count in milk rises during the early stage but falls when the cell count raises which later returns to normal. Death of PMNs and release of lysosomal enzymes cause tissue damage and inflammation. At this stage the mild fibril reaction is noticed with subsequent shedding of clots in the milk. The manner in which the organisms are recognized by monocytes and macrophages is poorly understood. In this study, The recognition of GBS and other Gram-positive bacteria by macrophages and monocytes relies on bacterial single-stranded RNA (ssRNA) (Deshmukh *et al.*2011). ssRNA interacts with a signalling complex, which comprises the Toll-like receptor adaptors MyD88 and UNC-93B, but not the established MyD88-dependent ssRNA sensors. The role of ssRNA in the recognition of Gram-positive bacteria—leading to the induction of inflammatory cytokines—has potential implications for sepsis pathogenesis, diagnosis and treatment.

At the stage of acute swelling, it is inflammed intra alveolar tissues combined with retained secretions in the alveoli which cause the swelling. Removal of the secretions may reduce the swelling. Local immunity probably does not occur but low grade of general immunity may develop. Immunity develops in milk and IgA and IgM type antibodies are chiefly responsible. Serum antibodies level has no role to play in the protection. The udder immunity is ineffective in clearance of the infection but the inflammatory reaction may subside.

Diagnosis

Gram positive cocci, single or in chains, can be demonstrated in milk samples. Culturally the organisms can be grown on serum or blood enriched medium. Colonies are small, round (dewdrops). On Lancefield testing, the organism should belong to group B. Several methods are used. Kits are available commercially for performing the test. Extraction method, the Latex agglutination test and slide co-agglutination test are available. The CAMP test may be used for the presumptive identification of *S.agalactiae*. In this reaction the partial haemolysis (beta toxin) caused by *S.aureus* is cleared by the haemolysin of *S.agalactiae* when grown on blood agar plates.Molecular techniques have been applied for diagnosis of *S.agalactiae* infection. McDonald *et al.* (2005) used 17 *S. agalactiae* and 26 S. dysgalactiae subsp. dysgalactiae strains which were was confirmed by RFLP. Use of a combination of restriction enzymes in a single tube enabled the rapid, accurate, cost effective and easily performed identification of all major streptococcal mastitis pathogens.

Treatment and Control

Antibiotics such as penicillin, erythromycin, cloxacillin & cephalosporin are effective and universally used as a mammary infusion. A mixture of penicillin and neomycin sulfate has a better efficacy, when infection with gram-negative pathogens is suspected or confirmed. Dry cow therapy is also recommended with these antibiotics. Penicillin resistant strains of bacteria may cause problem in the treatment.

Other drugs used for the treatment of *S.agalactiae* mastitis include tetracycline and cephalothin which have a wider antibacterial spectrum. Lincomycin combined with neomycin administered at 12 hours intervals also has a good record of treating the cases. The combination of cefalexin and kanamycin results in a fast initial killing of major mastitis pathogens at various concentration ratios (Maneke *et al.,* 2011).

Bacterial resistance to antibiotics is an issue that has led to the search for new antibacterial approaches. Drugs targeting virulence is an alternative approach to treat infections due to resistant bacteria. There is extensive literature and knowledge in the field of bacterial pathogenesis and genomic determinant of virulence. As therapeutic targets, virulence factors have been primarily addressed in the vaccine field to prevent infection by specific pathogens. Recently novel strategies to identify virulence inhibitors have been numerous and several new compounds were recently reported. It has been emphasized that the new virulence inhibitors that have shown a biological activity and have made a proof of concept that disarming bacteria lead to the inhibition of bacterial infection in experimental models in vivo. Moreover, some of these new antivirulence compounds are able to inhibit the virulence of different related pathogenic species, indicating that it is possible to target common virulence mechanisms. The progress reported recently with proof of concept for antivirulence molecules at the preclinical stages should allow the antivirulence concept to become a reality as a new antibacterial approach (Escaich 2008). A structure-activity relationship study from a screening hit and structure-based design strategy has led to the identification of bisarylureas as potent inhibitors of Streptococcus agalactiae Stk1. As this target has been directly linked to bacterial virulence, these inhibitors can be considered as a promising step towards antivirulence drugs (Oxoby *et al.*, 2010).

There is no satisfactory conventional or third generation vaccine available for the control of mastitis in cattle. Feasibility to use recombinant fragments of several GBS conservative proteins in vaccine for induction of protection against infections caused by different species of pathogenic streptococci including *S. agalactiae* exists.

Strepcoccus equi subsp. *equi*

S.equi subsp. *equi* is the causative agent of strangles in horses, mules, donkeys. It is a highly contagious disease of animals and morbidity may reach up to 100% in a typical outbreak of the disease. The disease is characterized by upper respiratory tract infection and abscessation of lymph nodes of head and neck, most typically submandibular lymph nodes. Horses pick up the infection from the contaminated pus or organisms shed in the nasal discharges. Infrequently, horses acts as carriers, however, horses occasionally develop encapsulated abscess in which organisms may survive for many months.

The incubation period varies from 4-15 days after exposure. Typical disease is marked by fever, lassitude, nasal discharge, slight cough and swelling of intermandibular areas. The abscesses are localized to submandibular areas, however metastasis of the disease may occur resulting in abscess formation through out the body. Non-encapsulated strains of *S.equi* subsp. *equi* expressing bacteriophage coded hyaluronidase have also been associated with clinically mild form of strangles.

During an outbreak of the disease mostly young foals are affected. The outbreaks appear soon after a large number of adult horses are transported to a long distance. If stabled together with other horses, the disease may appear in such horses also. The case fatality rate without treatment is 10-12% but with adequate early treatment it may be as low as 1-2%. Deaths are generally due to involvement of vital organs, endocarditis or purpura haemorrahagica. The disease is highly contagious, and produces high morbidity and low mortality in susceptible populations. Transmission occurs via fomites and direct contact with infectious exudates. Carrier animals are important for maintenance of the bacteria between epizootics and initiation of outbreaks on premises previously free of disease. Survival of the organism in the environment is dependent on temperature and humidity; it is susceptible to desiccation, extreme heat, and exposure to sunlight, and must be protected within mucoid secretions to survive. Under ideal environmental circumstances, the organism can survive 7-9 wk outside the host. Paddocks and barn facilities used by infected horses should be regarded as contaminated for ~2 mo after resolution of an outbreak.

Epidemiology

Strangles occurs throughout the world in countries where horses are maintained intensively. Outbreaks have been reported from horses, mules and ponies in several places in India. The disease is usually restricted to the animals of younger age group; however, adult animals are also affected. In old animals cases of complications of the disease are common. Disease usually occurs in cold wet weather but the movement of horses has more influence on the occurrence than the weather.

Abscessed draining pus and nasal discharges which contaminates the feed and water troughs are the source of infection. The organism is relatively resistant to the environmental conditions and the infection can remain viable at the pasture for at least a month after the infected animal has left. Inhalation and ingestion are the main routes of acquiring infection. The susceptible horse can carry the infection in the pharynx for up to 6-8 months. Such animals become source of infection to the susceptible population.

Virulence factors

Some of the factors that are assumed to be important in the virulence of *S. equi* subsp. *equi* include the hydrophobic antiphagocytic hyaluronic acid capsule, Streptokinase, peptidoglycan , IgG FC receptor binding protein the M-like proteins SeM and SzPSe , secreted toxins such as streptolysin S , and at least four pyrogenic mitogens along with the secreted pyrogenic superantigens SePE-I and H (Timoney, 2004). The initiation of *S. equi* infection is likely to involve several surface-anchored proteins (adhesins) binding to the tonsil epithelium of the host. Adhesins that could contribute to these interactions include the fibrinogen-binding proteins SzPSe and SeM; the immunoglobulin G (IgG)-, serum albumin-, and α_2-macroglobulin-binding protein ZAG; the collagen-binding protein CNE; and the collagen-like protein SclC.

A group of bacterial adhesins that have received much attention are proteins targeting fibronectin (Fn), a glycoprotein found in the extracellular matrix and body fluids of vertebrates. These proteins are found in *Streptococcus pyogenes* (SfbI/F1), *Staphylococcus aureus* (FnBPA and FnBPB), *Streptococcus dysgalactiae* (FnBA and FnBB), and other bacterial species . In *S. pyogenes* and *S. aureus,* these Fn-binding proteins have been reported to mediate the invasion of host cells without the need for other bacterial factors.

So far, two Fn-binding extracellular proteins of *S. equi* subsp. *equi* have been reported, FNE and SFS . Since neither of these contains cell wall-anchoring motifs and FNE has been found secreted in growth media, they are not likely to contribute to bacterial adherence.

Hyaluronic acid capsule is composed of repeating units of N-acetylglucosamine and glucoronic acid. Almost all strains of *S.equi* subsp. *equi* are encapsulated, however, a few strains with lower concentration of capsule do occur in nature (Matt variant). The matt variants have similar amount of M protein on the surface and stimulate protective antibodies in mice and horses (Timoney and Galan 1985).

Another virulence factor is Streptolysin O limited to Streptococci belonging to group A, C and G only. It is a membrane damaging enzyme that causes formation of hydrophilic channels in cholesterol rich membranes. It is a 53- kDa protein which is immunogenic and possess lytic activity of RBCs of different hosts. It is also toxic for other cells and cell components, such as PMNs, myocordial cells, platelets and lysosomes. It is not known whether in horses non-haemolytic strains possess any virulence, hence, the role of Streptolysin D as a virulence factor is not confirmed.

Another virulence factor is Streptokinase which causes lysis of fibrin which aid in spread and dispersion of bacteria in tissues. Probably the *in-situ* activation of complement and production of low molecular weight nitrogenous substrates may substantiate the virulence of *S.equi* subsp. *equi.*

Both Streptolysin O and Streptokinase may contribute in abscess formation and lysis by damaging cell membranes and activating the proteolytic properties of plasminogen.

The cell wall (peptidoglycan) is another virulence factor which actively activates alternative complement pathway and chemotactic factors such as

C3a & C4a. Peptidoglycan is also a potent pyrogen by inducing release of pyogenic cytokines from leucocytes (Mukhtar and Timoney 1988).

M protein on the bacterial surface is antiphagocytic, acid-resistant, dimeric fibrillar molecules projecting from cell wall surface. A typical M protein molecule of Group A Streptococci is about 50-60 nm long with a long, coiled central region flanked by a short, random coiled sequence at the N-terminus and by a specialized, highly conserved arrangement of hydrophobic and charged amino acids at the C-terminus that is anchored in cell wall (Robinson and Kehoe 1992). Unlike the M protein of Group A Streptococci the M protein of *S.equi* subsp. *equi* is highly conserved and shows no antigenic diversity. This property is useful in developing an M protein vaccine which could provide protection against all strains of *S.equi* subsp. *equi*. Studies have shown that M protein preparations are immunogenic in horses capable of inducing protective antibodies. Use of a *S.equi* subsp. *equi* strain rich in M protein could prove more immunogenic than strains deficient in M protein. *S.equi* subsp. *equi* cells passeged in equine blood have been demonstrated to have more M protein than normal cells (Srivastava *et al.,* 1985). Such passaged cells could then be used for preparation of vaccine. It is now possible to combine recent sequence data from the N-terminal region of the SeM protein and reassign the SeM alleles using the on-line database http://pubmlst.org/szooepidemicus/seM/.

Streptococcus equi possesses a haem-uptake system homologous to that of Streptococcus pyogenes and Streptococcus zooepidemicus. The system consists of two ligand-binding proteins (Shr and Shp) and proteins (HtsA-C) with homology to an ABC transporter (Meehan *et al* .2010). The haem-uptake system of S. equi differs from that of S. pyogenes and S. zooepidemicus in that Shr is truncated by two-thirds. This study focused on the SeShr, SeShp and SeHtsA proteins of S. equi. Analysis of shr, shp and shphtsA knockout mutants showed that all three proteins were expressed in vitro and that expression was upregulated under conditions of iron limitation. SeShr possesses no membrane-/cell wall-spanning sequences and was shown to be secreted. Both SeShp and SeHtsA were confirmed to be envelope-associated. Recombinant SeShp and SeHtsA proteins have been previously shown to bind haem and SeHtsA could capture haem from SeShp. This report extends these studies and shows that both SeShp and SeHtsA can sequester haem from haemoglobin but not from haemoglobin-haptoglobin complexes. Like full-length Shr, SeShr possesses haemoglobin and haemoglobin-haptoglobin binding ability but unlike full-length Shr, it lacks haem- or fibronectin-binding capabilities. Analysis of SeShr truncates showed that residues within and upstream of the near transporter (NEAT) domain are required for this ligand binding. Structural predictions suggest that truncation of NEAT1 in SeShr accounts for its impaired ability to bind haem. Haem and haemoglobin restored to almost normal the impaired growth rates of wild-type *S. equi* cultured under iron-limiting conditions. However, no difference in the growth rates of wild-type and mutants could be detected under the in vitro growth conditions tested.

Streptococcus equi subsp. *equi* possesses a 498-residue major cell-wall-associated protein (FgBP) which binds horse fibrinogen (Fg), reacts with convalescent horse serum and protects against lethal S. equi challenge in a small animal model. In one study, analysis of a panel of 17 purified N- and C-terminal FgBP truncates by ligand affinity blotting and SDS-PAGE revealed that the region required for maximum binding of Fg extended over the first half of the mature protein (Meehan *et al.*, 2000b). The C-terminal two-thirds of this domain is predicted to be alpha-helical coiled-coil and the N-terminal one-third to possess non-coiled-coil single strands. Residues at the extreme N-terminus and within the coiled-coil region are both required for ligand binding. A high incidence of alpha-helical coiled-coil structure also seems to be responsible in part for the aberrant mobility of FgBP on SDS gels. The efficiency with which FgBP binds Fg from different animal species decreases in the order horse > mouse, pig > rat > sheep, dog, bovine, human. Binding to horse Fg is inversely related to temperature over the range 45-4 degrees C and is independent of Ca2+ ions. MS analysis provided corroborative evidence that FgBP is covalently linked to the cell wall peptidoglycan. The major cell wall-associated protein (FgBP) of *Streptococcus equi* subsp. *equi* possesses two internal blocks of repeated sequence (A and B) and binds horse fibrinogen (Fg) avidly through residues located in the N-terminal half of the molecule. In a study, the roles of the two repeats blocks in Fg binding through construction of recombinant FgBP proteins containing defined internal deletions of sequence was investigated (Meehan *et al.*, 2000a). Ligand binding experiments clearly showed that neither repeat is essential for Fg binding. However, residues within the B repeats seem to play a major role in the aberrant mobility observed for FgBP following sodium dodecyl sulfate polyacrylamide gel electrophoresis. Fibrinogen-binding protein (FgBP, also termed SeM) is a cell-wall-associated anti-phagocytic M-like protein of the equine pathogen Streptococcus equi subsp. equi, and binds fibrinogen (Fg) and IgG. FgBP binds Fg avidly through residues located at the extreme N terminus of the molecule, whereas the IgG-binding site is more centrally located between the A and B repeats. FgBP binds equine IgG4 and IgG7 subclasses through interaction with the CH2-CH3 interdomain region of IgG-Fc, and possesses overlapping Fc-binding sites with protein A and protein G. In this study, FgBP truncates containing defined internal deletions were used to identify a stretch of 14 aa (residues 335-348) critical for IgG binding. Protein chimeras consisting of the non-IgG-binding alpha-helical coiled-coil M5 protein fused to FgBP sequences were used to identify a minimal equine IgG-binding domain consisting of residues 329-360. Competition ELISA tests suggested that IgG does not compromise Fg binding and vice versa (Meehan *et al.*, 2009). It is shown that FgBP additionally binds equine IgG-Fc. When tested against polyclonal IgG from ten other animal species, it was found that FgBP binds human, rabbit, pig and cat IgG, but does not bind mouse, rat, goat, sheep, cow or chicken IgG (Meehan *et al.*2001). Through the use of a panel of recombinant FgBP truncates containing defined deletions of sequence, it was shown that residues in the central regions of FgBP are important in IgG binding. An fbp knockout mutant which does not express FgBP on the cell surface was also constructed. Mutant cells failed to autoaggregate, bound no detectable equine Fg or IgG-Fc, were rapidly killed in horse blood, and showed greatly decreased virulence in a mouse model. Results suggest that FgBP is the major surface structure responsible for binding either Fg or IgG, that the molecule has pronounced antiphagocytic properties, and that it is a likely factor contributing to the virulence of wild-type *S. equi* subsp. *equi*.

Lannergard *et al.*(2005)describes the cloning and characterization of FNEB, a fibronectin-binding protein with cell wall-anchoring motifs. FNEB can thus be predicted as cell surface located, contrary to the two previously characterized fibronectin-binding proteins in *S. equi* subsp. *equi*, FNE and SFS. Assays of antibody titers in horses and in experimentally infected mice indicate that the protein is immunogenic and expressed in vivo during *S. equi* subsp. *equi* infection. Using Western ligand blotting, it was shown that FNEB binds to the N-terminal 29-kDa fragment of fibronectin, while SFS and FNE both bind to the adjacent 40-kDa fragment. *S. equi* subsp. *equi* is known to bind fibronectin to a much lower degree than the closely related *S. equi* subsp. *zooepidemicus*, but the binding is primarily directed to the 29-kDa fragment. Inhibition studies using *S. equi* subsp. *equi* cells indicate that FNEB mediates cellular binding to fibronectin in this species.

Se18.9, a novel H factor binding protein secreted by S. equi but not by S. zooepidemicus that reduces deposition of C3 on the bacterial surface and significantly reduces the bactericidal activity of equine neutrophils suspended in normal serum for both *S.equi* and *S. zooepidemicus* is described (Tiwari *et al.* 2007). Se18.9 is secreted abundantly by actively dividing cells and is also bound to the bacterial surface. Strong serum and mucosal antibody responses are elicited in *S. equi* infected horses. Although a gene identical to se18.9 was not detected in *S. zooepidemicus*, sequences encoding proteins of similar size with similar signal peptide sequences were found in 3 of 12 randomly selected strains. Lannegard *et al.* (2003) identified a gene denoted cne (gene encoding collagen-binding protein from *S. equi*) coding for a novel potential virulence factor of this species called protein CNE. The protein is composed of 657 amino acids and has the typical features found in cell surface-anchored proteins in Gram-positive bacteria. CNE displays amino acid sequence similarities to the previously well-studied collagen-binding protein CNA from *Staphylococcus aureus*, a proven virulence factor in septic arthritis. Based on similarity to CNA the structure of the mature CNE protein can be divided into an N-terminal A domain and a C-terminal B domain. The highest similarity between CNA and CNE is found in the A domains. The A domain in CNA is known to be the collagen-binding domain. Two parts of cne were amplified using polymerase chain reaction (PCR) and ligated into an expression vector, and recombinant CNE proteins were produced in Escherichia coli. The purified CNE proteins were shown to display collagen-binding activity in a Western ligand blot and to inhibit collagen binding to cells of subsp. equi and to CNE-coated microtitre wells. Furthermore, the A domain of CNE was sufficient for binding collagen, and was shown to compete for the same site on collagen as CNA in inhibition studies. Using PCR, the cne gene was detected in all studied strains of subsp. equi and *S. equi* subsp. *zooepidemicus.*

Pathogenesis

In order to study pathogenesis, previously unexposed horses and ponies were subjected to euthanasia 1, 3, 20 or 48 h following intranasal inoculation with biotin labelled or unlabelled S. equi CF32 (Timoney and Kunar 2008). Some ponies were inoculated with suspensions of equal numbers of CF32 and its mutants lacking capsule, *S. equi* M-like protein or streptolysin S. Others were infected by commingling exposure and subjected to euthanasia after onset of fever. Tonsils and lymph nodes were cultured for *S. equi* and tissues sectioned for histopathological examination and fluorescent microscopy. Tonsillar tissues of both the oro- and nasopharynx served as portals of entry. Entry was unexpectedly rapid but involved few bacteria. Small numbers of organisms were detected in tonsillar crypts, in adjacent subepithelial follicular tissue and draining lymph nodes 3 h after inoculation. By 48 h, clumps of S. equi were visible in the lamina propria. At onset of fever, tonsillar tissues and one or more mandibular and retropharyngeal lymph nodes were heavily infiltrated by neutrophils and long chains of extracellular *S. equi*. Mutant *S. equi* lacking virulence factors were not seen in draining lymph nodes. Although very small numbers of *S. equi* entered the lingual and nasopharyngeal tonsils, carriage to regional lymph nodes occurred within hours of inoculation. This observation, together with visual evidence of intracellular and extracellular multiplication of *S. equi* in tonsillar lymphoid tissue and lymph nodes over the following days, indicates involvement of potent antiphagocytic activity and failure of innate immune defences.

The organisms enters through the nasal route and bind to fibronectin of nasal, oral and pharyngeal mucosa through proteins found on the surface. It has been demonstrated that this adherence is mediated through structures most probably the M protein (Srivastava and Barnum 1983). Cell surface lipoteichoic acid may also be involved in the binding. Using shotgun phage display, cloned from *S. equi* subsp. equi and characterized a gene, called sfs, encoding a protein termed SFS, representing a new type of fibronectin (Fn)-binding protein. The sfs gene was found to be present in all 50 isolates of S. equi subsp. equi tested and in 41 of 48 S. equi subsp. zooepidemicus isolates tested (Lindmark and guss 1999). The sfs gene is down-regulated during growth in vitro compared to fnz, a previously characterized gene encoding an Fn-binding protein from *S. equi* subsp. *zooepidemicus*. Sequence comparisons revealed no similarities to previously characterized Fn-binding proteins, but high scores were obtained against collagen. Besides similarity due to the high content of glycine, serine, and proline residues present in both proteins, there was a nine-residue motif present both in collagen and in the Fn-binding domain of SFS. By searching the Oklahoma *S. pyogenes* database, Protein SFS was found to inhibit the binding between Fn and collagen in a concentration-dependent way.

Hamilton *et al.* (2006)investigated the contributions of a specific lipoprotein and the general lipoprotein processing pathway to the abilities of *S. equi* to colonize equine epithelial tissues in vitro and to cause disease in both a mouse model and the natural host *in vivo*. Colonization of air interface organ cultures after they were inoculated with a mutant strain deficient in the maturase lipoprotein (DeltaprtM [138-213]), with a deletion of nucleotides 138 to 213) was significantly less than that for cultures infected with wild-type *S. equi* strain 4047 or a mutant strain that was unable to lipidate preprolipoproteins (Deltalgt [190-685]). Moreover, mucus production was significantly greater in both wild-type-infected and Deltalgt (190-685)-infected organ cultures. Both mutants were significantly attenuated compared with the wild-type strain in a mouse model of strangles, although 2 of 30 mice infected with the Deltalgt (190-685) mutant did still exhibit signs of disease. In contrast, only the DeltaprtM (138-213) mutant was significantly attenuated in a pony infection study, with 0 of 5 infected ponies exhibiting pathological signs of strangles compared with 4 of 4 infected with the wild-type and 3 of 5 infected with the Deltalgt (190-685) mutant. These data suggest that the PrtM lipoprotein is a potential vaccine candidate.

The hyaluronic acid capsule resists phagocytosis by PMN cells and mononuclear cells in blood, lymphatics and tissue surfaces. Other virulence factors such as hyaluronidase also play a role in augmenting the pathogenicity of the organisms. Acute pharyngitis and rhinitis may occur. Drainage to local lymph nodes occurs and that causes abscessation. At this stage the animals experience high fever. Most commonly lymph nodes of head and neck including pharyngeal, submaxillary submadibular are involved. The infection may spread to other organs causing the development of lesions in kidneys, brain, liver, spleen, joint *etc.* Lymphatics may also be involved causing obstructive oedema. Metastasis spread to the lung which may cause the development of acute pneumonia and purulent meningitis. Cardiac involvement may also be observed. Purpura haemorrhagica may occur due to deposition of immune complexes in the blood which are deposited on the endothelial surface and also due to sensitivity to streptococcal proteins. During infection there is leucocytosis with neutrophilia reaching peak as the lymph node develop abscess. There may or may not be anaemia due to the haemolytic toxins of *S. equi* subsp. *equi.* A mild form of strangles may be caused by the matt types of *S.equi* strains characterized by fever, anorexia and profuse nasal discharge with moderate sub-mandibular lymph node swelling. Occasionally abscessation occurs.

Diagnosis

Smears of exudates are fixed and gram stained. Streptococci appear as gram-positive cocci in short and long chains. Streptococci have a tendency to lose their gram positive and some time stain weakly gram positive or gram negative.

Exudates, tissues, nasal swabs, pus and transtracheal aspirates are cultured directly on sheep blood agar and incubation at 37°C in 3% to 5% Co_2 is preferred. The smooth and mucoid colonies appear in 24-48 hours. Colonies are beta-haemolytic. Matt colonies producing lower amount of M protein may also be encountered. Identification requires Lancefield classification (*S.equi* subsp. *equi* belong to group C) and biochemical characterization.

The closely related streptococcal species Streptococcus equi subsp. zooepidemicus and *S. equi* subsp. *equi* are identified by polymerase chain reaction using oligonucleotide primers designed according to species-specific parts of the superoxide dismutase A encoding gene soda (Alber *et al.,* 2004). A further differentiation of both subspecies could be performed by amplification of the genes seeH and seeI encoding the exotoxins SeeH and SeeI, respectively, which could be detected for *S. equi* subsp. *equi* but not for *S. equi* subsp. *zooepidemicus.* A further simplification of the identification and differentiation of both subspecies was conducted by sodA-seeI multiplex polymerase chain reaction (Alber *et al.,* 2004).

Clinical strains of *S. equi* (n=24) and *Streptococcus equi* subsp. *zooepidemicus* (n=24) were genetically characterized by sequencing of the 16S rRNA and sodA genes in order to devise a real-time PCR system that can detect *S. equi* and *S. zooepidemicus* and distinguish between them (Baverud *et al.*, 2007). Sequencing demonstrated that all *S. equi* strains had the same 16S rRNA sequence, whereas *S. zooepidemicus* strains could be divided into subgroups. One of these (n=12 strains) had 16S rRNA sequences almost identical with the *S. equi* strains. Interestingly, four of the strains biochemically identified as *S. zooepidemicus* were found by sequencing of the 16S rRNA gene to have a sequence homologous with Streptococcus equi subsp. ruminatorum. However, they did not have the colony appearance or the biochemical characteristics of the type strain of *S. ruminatorum*. Classification of *S. ruminatorum* may thus not be determined solely by 16S rRNA sequencing. Sequencing of the sodA gene demonstrated that all *S. equi* strains had an identical sequence. For the *S. zooepidemicus* strains minor differences were found between the sodA sequences. The developed real-time PCR, based on the sodA and seeI genes was compared with conventional culturing on 103 cultured samples from horses with suspected strangles or other upper respiratory disease. The real-time PCR system was found to be more sensitive than conventional cultivation as two additional field isolates of *S. equi* and four of *S. zooepidemicus* were detected.

Treatment and Control

S.equi subsp. *equi* is sensitive to penicillin. Procaine penicillin is given twice daily. Horses given tetracycline often develop diarrhoea hence it is not recommended. During abscessation it is advisable to drain it for quick recovery or the abscesses enlarge and rupture. The open abscess is treated with a good disinfectant. The condition is painful to the horses. The treatment is followed for 5 days. Often there is recrudescence of the treatment after the infection has been discontinued. Application of trimethoprim/sulfonamide combinations for the initial therapy of equine respiratory tract infections can be recommended.

For controlling the infection, the affected animal should be immediately isolated and treatment continued. All affected animals may be housed together. The surrounding of stable should be thoroughly disinfected including the utensils. Management practices to prevent or control outbreaks of Streptococcus equi subsp. equi often include consideration of environment survival, but limited objective data are available. One study involved evaluation of S. equi persistence following inoculation of wood, metal, and rubber surfaces in an outdoor environment. Survival was short, ranging from < 1 to 3 d. There was no effect of rain ($P = 0.33$) or surface type ($P = 0.95$), but there was an effect of sunlight ($P = 0.002$) (Weese *et al.*, 2009). Outdoor survival of S. equi is poor, and prolonged quarantine of outdoor areas, particularly areas exposed to the sun, is probably unnecessary. The guttural pouches are the only detectable site of S. equi colonisation on endoscopic examination of horses S. equi was sometimes not detected by culture of nasopharyngeal swabs from carriers for up to 2 or 3 months before nasal shedding resumed sporadically. A more sensitive way of detecting S. equi on swabs from established guttural pouch carriers is therefore required. Conveniently selected 'strangles' outbreaks were investigated in detail using endoscopy, in order to develop and assess a suitable polymerase chain reaction (PCR) test (Newton *et al* . 2000). Of the infected horses, between 9 and 44% were identified as carrying S. equi by PCR after clinical signs had disappeared and the predominant site of carriage was the guttural pouch. Prolonged carriage of S. equi, which lasted up to 8 months, did not cease spontaneously before treatment was initiated to eliminate the infections. The detection and isolation of the carriers, in conjunction with strict hygiene measures, apparently resulted in the control of the outbreaks and allowed the premises to return to normal activity. Comparing PCR and culture, many more swabs were found to be positive using PCR (56 vs. 30% of 61 swabs). Similar results were obtained for guttural pouch samples from 12 established carriers (PCR 76% and culture 59%).

Vaccination of all horses, young and old, may be initiated with a yearly booster to provide immunity in all the animals at the farm, young animals of at least 12 weeks of age should be vaccinated. Exposed animals should not be vaccinated with the fear of developing hypersensitivity reactions. Use of M protein vaccine reduces the hypersensitivity reactions. Hypersensitivity reactions are higher with a whole killed cells vaccine because of the presence of several bacterial components in the vaccine.

For satisfactory results 3 doses of the vaccines are given. Immunity lasts for 12 months. Autogenic vaccine is always preferred over the commercial bacteria. However, the efficacy of strangles vaccination has always been in doubt as there have been many records of breakdown in immunity. This has encouraged workers to look for use of a more improved preparation as vaccines (Srivastava and Barnum 1985).

Vaccines so far improved for increasing the immunity have been whole cells and acid extract of *S.equi* subsp. *equi* administered three times at 10- day-intervals. Another vaccine consists of an enzymatic extract of *S.equi* subsp. *equi* added with an adjuvant. Only 2 doses of this vaccine are required (Wilson 1988). Partially purified M protein vaccine has been shown to confer only a partial protection in foals (Srivastava and Barnum 1985). However, purified M protein preparation when used to protect foals against strangles protected against challenge exposure but not when challenged by intranasal inoculation of *S.equi* subsp. *equi*. All the foals were given 3 doses of vaccine each containing

250μg of M – like protein vaccines. Studies suggested that M protein vaccine is a useful preparation for protecting animals against strangles (Srivastava and Barnum 1983). The ability of mucosally administered antigen to provide protection against Streptococcus equi ('Strangles') infections in horses was examined (Wallace *et al.*, 1995). Potential vaccine candidates were: (a) orally administered paraformaldehyde killed *S. equi*; (b) intraperitoneally (IP) administered paraformaldehyde killed *S. equi* in a non-inflammatory adjuvant; (c) orally administered live avirulent *S. equi*; (d) orally administered microencapsulated streptococcal M protein. The latter three preparations were first assessed in a rat model, using rate of lung bacterial clearance following intratracheal inoculation of live virulent bacteria as an indication of efficacy. Candidates (a) and (b) were then assessed in an equine model. IP immunisation of horses was shown to effectively induce production of specific antibody in mucosal and systemic sites. Four weeks after initial immunisation, horses were challenged intranasally with live virulent *S. equi*. Both groups of immunised horses demonstrated partial protection following vaccination. Of the IP immunised horses, only two out of four developed clinical signs of Strangles following live challenge. The orally immunised horses all developed submandibular abscesses containing *S. equi*. However, none of the immunised horses became as ill as the control horses in terms of fever, anorexia, loss of condition and general malaise.

A safe and effective vaccine against *S. equi* is highly desirable. A mouse model resembling Streptococcus equi subspecies equi infection in the horse, strangles, was used to assess the protective effect of vaccination with selected recombinant proteins from *S. equi* subsp. *equi*. After challenge the infection was monitored by weight loss and by nasal colonisation with *S. equi* subsp. equi (Flock *et al.*, 2006). Vaccination with a collagen-binding protein (CNE) and a collagen-like protein (SclC) resulted in protective antibodies, whereas a novel fibronectin-binding protein (FNEB) did not. Co-administration of CNE with EAG, a poorly immunogenic alpha2-macroglobulin-, albumin- and immunoglobulin G-binding protein, resulted in a significant synergistic effect and enhanced the protective immune response against EAG. Three recombinant antigens were used by Waller *et al.*(2007)to vaccinate horses, which were then experimentally challenged with Streptococcus equi, the causative agent for strangles. The vaccinated horses showed significantly reduced bacterial growth (p=0.02) and nasal discharge (p=0.0004), a typical symptom of strangles. Other clinical signs of strangles were also reduced and at post mortem examination, lower rate of empyaema or scarring of the guttural pouches was found in the vaccinated group (p=0.01). The antigens used were EAG (alpha2-macroglobulin, albumin, and IgG-binding protein), CNE (a collagen-binding protein), and SclC (a collagen-like protein). The adjuvant used was Abisco, a saponin derived matrix. No adverse effects were observed following vaccination with the antigens and adjuvant.

Florindo *et al.* (2010) developed and characterised stable surface modified poly(lactic acid) (PLA) nanoparticles, using polyvinyl alcohol (PVA), alginate (ALG) and glycolchitosan (GCS) containing a Streptococcus equi enzymatic extract adsorbed onto the surface. The characterisation of the preparations and a physicochemical study of the adsorption process were performed. The adsorption of S. equi proteins is a rapid process reaching, within 1h, maximum adsorption efficiency values of 75.2+/-1.9% (w/w) for PLA-PVA, 84.9+/-0.2% (w/w) for PLA-GCS and 78.1+/-0.4% (w/w) for PLA-ALG nanoparticles. No protein degradation was detected throughout the formulation procedures. As expected from a complex mixture of proteins, adsorption data suggest a Freundlich-type of equilibrium with regression coefficients (r(2)) of 0.9958, 0.9839 and 0.9940 for PLA-PVA, PLA-GCS and PLA-ALG, respectively. Desorption studies revealed a burst release within the first 6h, for all formulations, followed by a sustained release profile. Nanoparticle surface modification with GCS improved the sustained release profile, as 20% of protein remained attached to the particle surface after 30 days. The results show that adsorption is an alternative method for the production of S. equi antigen carriers for vaccination purposes.

The bacterium shows only limited genetic diversity and an effective vaccine could confer broad protection to horses throughout the world. Welsh mountain ponies (n = 7) vaccinated with a combination of seven recombinant *S. equi* proteins were significantly protected from experimental infection by *S. equi*, resembling the spontaneous disease. Vaccinated horses had significantly reduced incidence of lymph node swelling (p = 0.0013) lymph node abscessation (p = 0.00001), fewer days of pyrexia (p = 0.0001), reduced pathology scoring (p = 0.005) and lower bacterial recovery from lymph nodes (p = 0.004) when compared with non-vaccinated horses (n = 7). Six of 7 vaccinated horses were protected whereas all 7 non-vaccinated became infected. The protective antigens consisted of five surface localized proteins and two IgG endopeptidases. A second vaccination trial (n = 7+7), in which the IgG endopeptidases were omitted, demonstrated only partial protection against S. equi, highlighting an important role for these vaccine components in establishing a protective immune response (Guss *et al.*, 2009). Timoney *et al.* (2007) evaluated as vaccine components novel surface exposed or secreted *S. equi* proteins identified in an expression gene library with sera from resistant horses. Six proteins expressed by *S. equi* CF32 but not by *S. zooepidemicus* 631 were used to vaccinate one group of eight ponies. A second pony group was immunized with five adhesin and other proteins encoded by genes of Linkage Gr 1. All ponies made strong serum antibody responses to each protein as measured by ELISA but none were resistant to subsequent challenge with *S. equi* CF32. These results in combination with evidence that recovered horses rapidly clear intranasally inoculated *S. equi* and do not make detectable serum antibody responses to its surface proteins suggest that acquired immune-mediated tonsillar clearance and not serum antibody must be stimulated by an effective strangles vaccine.

Post exposure immunity is prolonged after natural disease in most horses, and protection is associated with local (nasal mucosa) production of antibody against the antiphagocytic M protein. The clinical attack rate of strangles is reduced by 50% in horses vaccinated with IM products that do not induce mucosal immunity. Local (mucosal) production of antibody requires mucosal antigen stimulation. An intranasal vaccine containing a live attenuated strain was designed to elicit a mucosal immunologic response. This attenuated strain is not temperature sensitive (inactivated by core body temperature), like the intranasal influenza vaccine. Reported complications include abscesses at subsequent IM injection sites (live culture), submandibular lymphadenophathy, serous nasal discharge, and purpura hemorrhagica.

Streptococcus suis

S.suis infection occurs more frequently in young pigs. The disease is characterized clinically by septicaemia, meningitis, arthritis, endocarditis, myocarditis and bronchopneumonia. Abortions are also observed. The organisms are carried principally in the palatine tonsils of pigs, however, many carriers do not exhibit the infection. These are strains of Lancefield group S (Type 1), R (Type 2) T and untypable strains. There are two types of *S.suis*, 1 & 2. Type 2 is of zoonotic importance. Infection with type 2 may occur at birth and both types are present in the nasal tract of all piglets of the infected herd by the time piglets attain the age of 4-6 weeks.

A sialic acid rich capsular material antigenic in nature, prevents deposition of C_3 on bacterial surface thereby obstructs in phagocytosis. There are 8 types of the capsular material based on the antigenicity. The capsular material from different serotypes has different morphologies. Another virulence factors are a 100 kDa protein which is required for the production of meningoencephalitis, polyserositis and polyarthritis (Vecht *et al.,* 1992) and a 136 kDa protein possibly binds to fibronectin (Smith *et al.,* 1992). The mechanism of action of these 2 proteins in exerting the virulence is not known. There are virulence differences between strains of the same serotype based on the muramidase release proteins. Fimbrae is present on cell surface and certain strains have haemagglutinating properties. Type 2 cells have the property to adhere to swine lungs which leads to multiplication of the organisms in the tonsils followed by invasion of the regional lymphatics from where it escapes and multiplies. A high level bacteremia is essential for the development of meningoencephalitis. It is easy to culture organisms from blood at this stage. *S.suis* cells are phagocytozed and survive in the circulating mononuclear cells and carried to joints and meninges subsequently invading the CNS via the choroid plexus and spread in the cerebrospinal fluid to cause the disease (Timoney 1993). The organisms are also present in vagina of sows.

Epidemiology

S.suis type 2 has been found in most swine rearing countries of the world. In India only a few cases have been recorded. The organisms are cultured from palatine tonsils collected at slaughter houses. In a study conducted in Australia 54% were infected with *S.suis* type 1 and 73% with type 2 (Robertson & Blackmore 1989). Cases are more in weaned pigs. After 10-14 days of weaning *S.suis* type 2 causes meningitis in pigs. Adult boars have also been known to suffer *S.suis* infection (Ravishankar *et al.,* 2005). Shome *et al.* (2006) isolated *S.suis* from nasal swabs of piglet showing respiratory symptoms in Meghalaya region of India. Earlier Chaturvedi and Srivastava (2004) had reported *S.suis* outbreaks in pigs. A case of pneumonitis has been reported in a boar in Kerala state (Ravishankar *et al.,* 2005). Padungtod *et al.* (2010) determined the incidence of Streptococcus suis infection in slaughtered pigs raised in industrial facility and backyard system in Chiang Mai City, Thailand. A total of 90 tonsils and submaxillary salivary gland/lymph node samples from slaughtered pigs raised in industrial facility and 122 samples from slaughtered pigs raised in backyard system were collected. Isolation and identification of *S. suis* were conducted using standard bacteriological methods. Farm management and risk factor data were collected by a questionnaire. Serotyping and presence of virulence factor genes, epf, mrp and sly, were determined by multiplex PCR assay. The overall incidence of *S. suis* in this study was 9% (n = 212) and the incidence is significantly higher in districts located at a greater distance south of Chiang Mai City. *S. suis* serotype 2 was present more in healthy pigs (43%) than ill pigs (10%). Every *S. suis* isolate carried mrp and sly and ill pigs carried epf (80%) more than healthy pigs (57%). However, the probability of *S. suis* serotype 2 with epf+ (0.245) detected in healthy pigs was higher than in ill pigs (0.08).

There are at least 28 serotypes of *S.suis* out of which type 2 is most prevalent in most countries except in Scandinavian countries where serotype 7 predominates. *S.suis* type 9 and *S.suis* type 2 have been isolated as the cause of septicaemia and meningitis in weaned pigs in Australia. There are differences in pathogenicity between serotypes. In UK type 1 causes less severe disease than type 2. World scenario is that the disease can occur in 0 to 15% cases in most of the countries. The incidence of the disease has increased markedly in United Kingdom since last 2 decades. Weaned carrier pigs transmit the infection to pigs after mixing following weaning. The organism can persist in the tonsil for more than one year in pigs given penicillin – medicated feed. Horse fly can carry the organism for at least 5 days and can contaminate feed for at least 4 days (Enright 1987). It is believed that strains of *S.suis* type 2 vary in pathogenicity and that occurrence of disease is dependent on both exposure to a pathogenic strain and several secondary factors such as inadequate ventilation, high population density and other stresses.

Pathogenesis

S.suis type 2 posses a capsule and resist phagocytosis. To study the role of the capsule of Streptococcus suis serotype 2 in virulence, Smith *et al* (1999) generated two isogenic mutants disturbed in capsule production. For that purpose, the authors first cloned and characterized a major part of the capsular polysaccharide biosynthesis (cps) locus of *S. suis* serotype 2. Based on the established sequence, 14 open reading frames (ORFs), designated Orf2Z, Orf2Y, Orf2X, and Cps2A to Cps2K, were identified. Twelve ORFs belonged to a single transcriptional unit. The gene products of 11 of these ORFs showed similarity to proteins involved in polysaccharide biosynthesis of other gram-positive microorganisms. Nonencapsulated isogenic mutants were generated in the cps2B and cps2EF genes by insertional mutagenesis. In contrast to the wild-type *S. suis* serotype 2 strain, the nonencapsulated strains were highly sensitive to ingestion by porcine alveolar lung macrophages *in vitro*. More importantly, the nonencapsulated mutant strains were completely avirulent in young germfree pigs after intranasal inoculation. These observations indicate that the capsule of *S. suis* serotype 2 plays an essential role in the pathogenesis of *S. suis* serotype 2 infections.

An unencapsulated *Streptococcus suis* mutant was used to investigate the pleiotropic effects resulting from capsule loss (Tanabe *et al.*, 2010). The capsule deficient mutant of *S. suis* acquired a biofilm-positive phenotype, which was associated with significantly increased cell surface hydrophobicity. Cell-associated fibrinogen-binding and chymotrypsin-like activities were decreased in the unencapsulated mutant. The mutant did not differ significantly from the encapsulated parent strain for minimal inhibitory concentrations to penicillin G, ampicillin, and tetracycline. However, while the encapsulated strain was highly resistant to the bactericidal action of penicillin G and ampicillin, the unencapsulated mutant was approximately 60-fold more sensitive. Compared with the parent strain, the unencapsulated mutant induced a much higher inflammatory response in monocyte-derived macrophages resulting in an increased secretion of tumor necrosis factor (TNF)-α, interleukin (IL)-1β, IL-6, and IL-8. The capsule appears to hinder important adhesins or hydrophobic molecules that mediate biofilm formation, as well as cell wall components capable of stimulating immune cells. After crossing of the epithelial barrier Streptococcus suis causes bacteraemia resulting in meningitis, endocarditis, and bronchopneumonia. Since the host environment seems to be an important regulatory component for virulence, related expression of virulence determinants of Streptococcus suis to glucose availability during growth and to the sugar metabolism regulator catabolite control protein A (CcpA) was studied (Willenborg *et al* 2011). It was found that expression of the virulence-associated genes arcB, representing arcABC-operon expression, cps2A, representing capsular locus expression, as well as sly, ofs, sao, and epf differed significantly between exponential to early stationary growth of a highly virulent serotype 2 strain. Deletion of ccpA altered expression of the surface associated virulence factors arcB, sao, eno as well as the two presently proven virulence factors in pigs, ofs and cps2A, at early exponential growth. A global expression analysis using a cDNA expression array revealed 259 differentially expressed genes at early exponential growth, of which 141 genes were higher expressed in the CcpA mutant strain 10ÄccpA and 118 genes were lower expressed. Interestingly, among the latter genes 18 could be related to capsule and cell wall synthesis. Correspondingly, electron microscopical characterisation of strain 10ÄccpA revealed a markedly reduced thickness of the capsule. This phenotype correlated with enhanced binding to porcine plasma proteins and a reduced resistance against killing by porcine neutrophils. Taken together, these data demonstrate that CcpA has a significant effect on capsule synthesis and virulence properties of Streptococcus suis.

Once phagocytozed they survive in the macrophages and make use of it in entering the cerebrospinal fluids. *S.suis* proteins, a 100 kDa protein, might have been associated with this entry. Once inside the brain the conditions such as meningitis may occur. Bacteremia also occurs resulting in septicaemia and bronchopneumonia. Arthritis may also develop. A novel virulence factor, termed opacity factor (OFs) has been identified which opacifies horses serum and binds fibronectin (Baum *et al.*, 2006). OFS deletion mutants of *S.suis* were found to be non-virulent. A fibronectin binding á – enolase of *S.suis* may have a role in pathogenesis similar to other fibronectin binding proteins (Esgleas *et al.*, 2008). In epidemics of type 2 meningitis sudden death occurs. Production of both IgM and IgG antibodies to surface components occur which are protective (Holt *et al.*, 1988). A 94 kDa antigen band, reactive with protective pig sera, stimulates antibodies that protect mice. This antigen may be part of the cell envelop 135 kDa protein (Smith *et al.*, 1992).

Vitrulent S.suis strains produce a suilysin, a Cholesterol Dependent Cytotoxin (CDC) suilysin does not require a host receptor for hemolytic activity;

yet the crystal structure of suilysin exhibits a similar conformation in the tryptophan rich motif to ILY. This observation suggests that the current view of the structure-function relationship between CDC proteins and membrane association is far from complete (Xu *et al* .2010). Autolysin is possessed by strains of *S.suis*. The autolysin gene was detected by PCR with genomic DNA of HA9801 (Jiangsu isolate), ZY05719 (Sichuan isolate), ATCC43765 (reference strain) other SS2 isolates from different regions, and strains of other different serotypes (such as serotype 1, 1/2, 7 and 9) in China (Gu and Lu 2008),. PCR results showed that all 27 SS2 virulent isolates harbored gene autolysin, but not in non-virulent SS2 strain. Among other serotypes, only serotype 7 strain had this gene. The complete autolysin genes of HA9801 and ZY05719 were respectively amplified by PCR and sequenced. Their putative protein sequences were analyzed through online software, results showed both had six repeated domain "GBS_Bsp-like" and one domain "N-acetylmuramoyl-L-alanine amidase". In addition, sequence similarity analysis demonstrated that autolysins of the two strains (HA9801 and ZY05719) showed high homologue to that of European strain P1/7 (99.8%), but obviously differed from Canada strain 89/1589, the latter lacked one domain "GBS Bsp-like". Software DNASTAR was used to analyze autolysin protein sequence and predicted its putative antigenicity. Then partial antigenic segment of autolysin was amplified, cloned and inserted into expression vector pET30a(+), and induced by IPTG to express recombinant autolysin. Its reactivity was analyzed by SDS-PAGE and western blot with swine convalescent sera, blot result showed that the recombinant protein had good reactivity and could be considered as a vaccine candidate.

Definition of virulent Streptococcus suis strains is controversial. One successful approach for identification of virulent European strains is differentiation of capsular serotypes (or the corresponding cps types) and subsequent detection of virulence-associated factors, namely the extracellular factor (EF, epf), the muramidase-released protein (MRP, mrp) and the hemolysin suilysin (SLY, sly). Silva *et al* (2006) presented a novel multiplex PCR (MP-PCR) and an mrp variant PCR for identification and characterization of virulent *S. suis* strains. The MP-PCR allowed identification of *S. suis* through detection of the housekeeping gene gdh, differentiation of four cps types (1, 2, 7 and 9), and detection of epf, mrp, sly and arcA (arginine deiminase from *S. suis*). Expression of the corresponding size variants of MRP was shown for four of the six mrp variants, but was undetectable for the two larger mrp variants in the particular strains investigated. The results of this study suggest that cps7 strains are associated with pneumonia and that variation of mrp is very pronounced among these strains. Gene profiles of invasive, pneumonia and carrier *S. suis* isolates by combination of PCR assays allowed differentiation of 24 different genotypes among cps1, 2, 7 and 9 strains. Forty-five percent of the invasive *S. suis* diseases investigated in this study were caused by only two of these genotypes, namely cps2/mrp+/epf+/sly+ and cps9/mrp(*)/epf-/sly+. In order to identify gene sequences unique to the virulent strains, suppression subtractive hybridization (SSH) was conducted using virulent *Streptococcus suis* type 2 (SS2) strain HA9801 and avirulent *S. suis* type 2 strain T15 (Jiang *et al.*, 2009). Thirty genomic regions were absent in T15, and the DNA sequences of these regions in HA9801 were determined. These DNA fragments, containing putative virulence genes, encoded 28 proteins that were homologous to proteins involved in various aspects of cellular surface structure, molecular synthesis, energy metabolism, regulation, transport systems and others of unknown function. According to the published SS2 genomic sequence of the Chinese strain 98HAH33, PCR primers for 14 significant DNA fragments were designed and used for detection of the distribution of these fragments in *S. suis* strains from different sources, serotypes, regions, groups and times. The results showed that these 14 DNA fragments were widely distributed in 37 detected SS2 strains, yet were absent among the avirulent strain T15. Moreover, these fragments could be detected in other serotypes of *S. suis*, but each serotype had a different distribution of the fragments. Zhu *et al.* (2008) identified the trag (transfer gene G) as one of the novel infection-related factors identified by *in vivo*-induced antigen technology (IVIAT) from Streptococcus suis type 2 expression libraries with swine convalesecent sera . The authors detected the distribution of trag in different *Streptococcus suis* isolates and identified the differential expression of the new infection-related factor between *in vivo* and *in vitro* condition. The trag was detected from virulent SS isolates but not from avirulent strain, which suggested that this gene may be related to the pathogenicity of SS. The special reactivity was only present with convalescent sera, and it indicated that TRAG might play a role during SS2 invasive course. Li *et al.* (2010) identified a novel virulence-related gene, virA, of *S. suis* 2. To investigate its role in pathogenesis, a virA deletion mutant of S. suis 2 wild-type strain ZY458, 458Deltavir, was constructed using suicide vector pSET4s, and a functionally complemented strain 458Deltavir(pvir) was constructed using shuttle plasmid pAT18 containing the virA gene. All rabbits infected with ZY458 and 458Deltavir(pvir) exhibited body weight loss and developed severe clinical symptoms. All 5 rabbits infected with ZY458, and 4 of 5 infected with 458Deltavir(pvir), died within 6 days of infection. In contrast, all 5 rabbits inoculated with 458Deltavir gained weight normally and none developed any clinical symptoms during the entire course monitored. These results indicate that virA plays an important role in the pathogenicity of *S. suis* serotype 2. To investigate the virA gene further, the authors compared and analyzed the sequences of virA from wild-type virulent and avirulent strains.

Results showed that functional virA appears to exist only in virulent strains and has been structurally mutated in avirulent strains. In conclusion, virA gene is a novel identified virulence-relate gene. It may play a key role in the evolution and pathogenicity of *S. suis* serotype 2.

Streptococcus suis 2 (SS2) is a zoonotic pathogen that can participate in biofilm formation to survive in hostile environments. Virulent SS2 strains HA9801 and ZY05719 displayed increased biofilm formation compared with SS2 avirulent strain T15 (Wang *et al.*, 2011). In addition, a 58% reduction in adherence to HEp-2 cells was observed for biofilm cells, compared with planktonic cells. The 50% lethal dose (LD(50)) of biofilm cells was 40-fold greater than that of planktonic cells. Quantification of expression levels of known virulence genes by real-time PCR revealed that the transcription levels of the gdh, cps2 and mrp genes in biofilm cells were downregulated, while the sly and gapdh genes were upregulated. HA9801 biofilm and planktonic vaccines provided 60% and 46% protection, respectively, when challenged with 50 times the (LD_{50}) of the HA9801 strain. These results suggest a possible connection between virulence and the ability of biofilm formation; cell adhesion, transcription levels and virulence properties are different between biofilm cells and planktonic cells. Furthermore, this work offers a novel insight into bacterium infection mechanisms, which suggests that a virulent strain may be able to decrease its virulence by forming a biofilm so that it can achieve persistent infection *in vivo*.

Diagnosis

Laboratory diagnosis depends on bacteriological and serological testing of clinical samples (blood, vaginal swabs, meningeal swab, cerebrospinal fluid, joint fluid etc.). Blood agar is used for the isolation. Gram - positive cocci can be demonstrated in smears from clinical materials after grams staining.

Colonies of *S.suis* are round, small, smooth and glistening with haemolysis. Freshly isolated colonies are more mucoid than those which have been subcultured.

Treatment and Control

S.suis shows a high degree of sensitivity to ampicillin, penicillin and resistance to lincomycin, erythromycin, neomycin, streptomycin and tetracyclines. Some strains may be resistant to trimethoprim - sulfamethoxazole. Some may be resistant to penicillins too, but not the derivatives.

Good management and hygienic techniques should be practiced at the farm. Mixing of newly purchased animals to the herd should be done following quarantine of the animals. Mass medication of individual pigs or medication of feed during periods of high risk way control the incidence. The feeding of oxytetracycline for 14 days before the onset of infection may control the occurrence of disease. Preventive chemotherapy is effective in suckling piglets. Oral prophylactic medication with either procaine penicillin G or a mixture of chlortetracycline, sulfadimidine and procaine penicillin G has been useful.

Tiamulin in the drinking water at 180mg/lit. of water for 5 days has significantly reduced the effect of experimentally induced *S.suis* type infections (Changappa *et al.*, 1990).

So far, no vaccine has been described which elicits protection against several serotypes. At the present time, vaccination of pigs against this infection is generally carried out with autogenous bacterins and results are equivocal. Application of *S. suis* serotype 2 bacterins to specific-pathogen-free (SPF) weaning piglets has been demonstrated to protect against the homologous serotype. However, autogenous *S. suis* bacterins are also applied to sows and suckling piglets in the field. Therefore, comparative evaluation of different bacterin immunization regimes, including sow vaccination, was performed in a study (Baum *et al.*, 2010). Experimental infection of 6- and 8-week-old weaning piglets was performed to elucidate protective efficacies. Humoral immune responses were investigated by an enzyme-linked immunosorbent assay (ELISA) measuring muramidase-released protein (MRP)-specific IgG titers and by opsonophagocytosis assays. Bacterin application elicited high MRP-specific IgG titers in the serum and colostrum of sows, as well as opsonizing antibodies. Piglets from vaccinated sows had significantly higher MRP-specific titers than respective piglets from nonvaccinated sows until 6 weeks postpartum. Vaccination of suckling piglets did not result in high MRP-specific titers nor in induction of opsonizing antibodies. Furthermore, neither vaccination of suckling nor of weaning piglets from immunized sows was associated with a prominent active immune response and protection at 8 weeks postpartum. However, protection was observed in respective 6-week-old weaning piglets, most likely because of protective maternal immunity. In conclusion, this study provides the first results suggesting protective passive maternal immunity for *S. suis* serotype 2 after bacterin vaccination of sows and a strong inhibitory effect on active immunization of suckling and weaning piglets, leading to highly susceptible growers.

An autogenous vaccine was developed, using sonicated bacteria, with a strain of Streptococcus suis capsular type ½ (Lapointe *et al.*, 2002). An enzyme-linked immunosorbent assay using the vaccine antigen was standardized. Results from a preliminary study indicated that all vaccinated pigs produced antibodies against 2 proteins of 34 and 43 kDa, respectively, and, in 3 out of

4 vaccinated pigs, against the 117-kDa muramidase-released protein. For the serologic profile, groups of 30 pigs from the infected herd were blood sampled at 2, 4, 6, 8, and 10 weeks of age. The lowest antibody level was observed between weeks 6 and 8, presumably corresponding to a decrease in maternal immunity. A marked increase was seen at 10 weeks of age, shortly after the onset of clinical signs in the herd. For the vaccination field trial, newly weaned, one-week-old piglets were divided into 2 groups of 200 piglets each (control and vaccinated); blood samples were collected from 36 piglets in each group at 2-week intervals for 12 weeks. A significant increase ($P < 0.05$) in antibody response was observed 4 weeks following vaccination and the level of antibodies stayed high until the end of the experiment. In the control group, the increase was only observed at 13 weeks of age, probably in response to a natural infection. The response to the vaccine varied considerably among pigs and was attributed, in part, to the levels of maternal antibodies at the time of vaccination.

Busque *et al.* (1997) studied the protective effect of a live avirulent *S. suis* type 2 strain (#1330) which had induced a good protection in mice, was evaluated in swine. The experiment was performed in triplicate using 4 week-old piglets. A total of 15 piglets were vaccinated 3 times, 15 others were vaccinated 2 times, and 15 piglets were injected 3 times with sterile Todd-Hewitt broth. Using an indirect ELISA, an increase in the IgG response to *S. suis* antigens was noted in 27 of the 30 vaccinated piglets. On day 21 post-vaccination, all animals were challenged intravenously with a virulent *S. suis* type 2 strain (#999). In the 2 vaccinated groups, 26 animals were fully protected. Only 1 out of the 15 piglets vaccinated 3 times developed mild clinical signs. In the group vaccinated twice, 3 piglets showed clinical signs and 1 of them died after the challenge. In the control group, 7 animals died out of the 11 with clinical signs of infection. In conclusion, a protective immunity was observed in swine when using strain 1330. However, more studies are needed to assess the use of a live *S. suis* strain in a vaccine for pigs.

Baum *et al.* (2009) determined the protective efficacy of a serotype 2 murein-associated protein (MAP) fraction subunit vaccine in comparison to that of a bacterin against experimental challenge with serotype 2 (containing muramidase-released protein [MRP], extracellular factor, and suilysin [SLY]) and serotype 9 (containing MRP variant MRP* and SLY) strains. MAP was shown to include different surface-associated proteins, such as the MRP and surface antigen one (SAO) expressed by both pathotypes used for challenge. The results of this study demonstrated that the serotype 2 bacterin induced protective immunity against homologous challenge. In contrast, the protective efficacy of the MAP subunit vaccine was low, though MAP immunization resulted in high serum immunoglobulin G2 titers against MRP and SAO.

Importantly, immunization with bacterin but not with MAP induced opsonizing antibody titers against the serotype 2 strain, and these antibody titers were found to correlate with protection. However, after absorption with a nonencapsulated isogenic mutant, the sera from bacterin-immunized piglets failed to facilitate neutrophil killing, indicating that antibodies directed against capsule may not have been essential for opsonophagocytosis. Furthermore, induction of opsonizing antibodies against serotype 9 was not detectable in the group receiving bacterin or in the group receiving the MAP vaccine. In agreement, protection against the heterologous serotype 9 strain was low in both groups. Thus, identification of an antigen protecting against these two important S. suis pathotypes remains an important goal of future studies. In a different study piglets were immunized with the attenuated S. suis serotype 2 strain 10Deltaofs2/12, which is deficient in expression of the serum opacity factor OFS (Kock *et al.*, 2009). Three weeks after intranasal application of 10Deltaofs2/12 piglets were challenged intravenously with two strains representing the most important S. suis pathotypes in Europe, the homologous MRP+ EF+ SLY+ serotype 2 strain and a heterologous MRP* SLY+ serotype 9 strain. Application of the live vaccine elicited significant serum IgG responses against muramidase-released protein (MRP), extracellular factor (EF) and, most prominently, suilysin. Seroconversion against suilysin was accompanied with an increase of suilysin-neutralization titers in the vaccinated group. Though mortality was lower in the vaccinated groups, significant protection was not observed, neither against the homologous nor against the heterologous challenge. This was in agreement with the finding that the vaccinated piglets had low opsonizing antibody titers insufficient to mediate elimination of the two challenge strains by porcine neutrophils. In conclusion, a single intranasal application of the S. suis serotype 2 strain 10Deltaofs2/12 elicited humoral immune responses against different *S. suis* antigens but failed to induce sufficient opsonizing antibody titers and protective immunity against systemic serotypes 2 and 9 challenges.

Streptococcus equi subsp. *zooepidemicus*

The organisms commonly reside on the mucosal surfaces of horses and produces disease as an opportunist pathogen in several animal species. Diseases produced in animal species include wound infections, joint ill, lymphatic abscesses, nasal catarrh and pneumonia of foals. It may be associated with mastitis and abortions in mares. It is a common cause of joint ill, endocarditis and meningitis in pigs. It also causes mastitis in cattle and goats, pneumonia, fibrinous pleuritis, septicaemia pericarditis and wound infection in lambs and dogs. *Streptococcus equi* subsp. *zooepidemicus* (*S. zooepidemicus*) has caused several outbreaks of haemorrhagic pneumonia in dogs in recent years. This highly contagious and often fatal disease is characterised by sudden onset of clinical signs including pyrexia, dyspnoea and haemorrhagic nasal discharge. Post mortem examination typically reveals pulmonary haemorrhage and pleural effusion. Histopathology demonstrates fibrino-suppurative, necrotising and haemorrhagic pneumonia in most cases. The pathogenesis of *S. zooepidemicus* infection in dogs is incompletely understood. Bacterial virulence factors as well as host factors may contribute to the severe outcome. *S. zooepidemicus* occasionally causes zoonotic infections with potentially serious consequences. Canine vaccines for *S. zooepidemicus* are currently not available and prevention of the disease therefore relies on limiting bacterial spread by implementing stringent control measures in kennels.

Many mares with typical sign of soreness of udder but with normal milk are first observed, which may turn as mastitis later. It is a causative agent of epididymitis in stallion and naval ill in foals. *Streptococcus equi* subsp. *zooepidemicus* has been linked to cases of acute fatal pneumonia in dogs in several countries. Outbreaks can occur in kenneled dog populations and result in significant levels of morbidity and mortality. This highly contagious disease is characterized by the sudden onset of clinical signs, including pyrexia, dyspnea, and hemorrhagic nasal discharge. The pathogenesis of *S. equi* subsp. *zooepidemicus* infection in dogs is poorly understood.

Pathogenesis

The organism possesses all the virulence factors described for *S.equi* subsp. *equi*, however, variability in the capsule production has been observed. Freshly isolated strains are encapsulated which become non-encapsulated. The capsule is an exopolysaccharide identified as hyaluronic acid (HA) based on IR and NMR spectroscopy while its Mw was found to be 5.38 × 10(5)Da. HA produced passed bacterial endotoxin test (Patil *et al.*, 2011). Somc strains produce copious amounts of hyaluronic acid, making *S. zooepidemicus* an important industrial microorganism for the production of this valuable biopolymer used in the pharmaceutical and cosmetic industry. Encapsulation by hyaluronic acid is considered an important virulence factor in other streptococci, though the importance in *S. zooepidemicus* remains poorly understood. Proteomics may provide a better understanding of virulence factors in *S. zooepidemicus*, facilitate the design of better diagnostics and treatments, and guide engineering of superior production strains. In bacteria, the HA synthase occurs in an operon (has) coding for enzymes involved in the production of HA precursors. Blank *et al.* (2008) reported two new members of the has operon family from *Streptococcus equi* subsp. *zooepidemicus* and *Streptococcus equi* subsp. *Equi*. The has operon of *S. zooepidemicus* contains, in order, hasA, hasB, hasC, glum, and pgi, whereas these genes are separated on two operons in *S. equi* (hasA, hasB, hasC and hasC, glmU, pgi). The transcription start site and a sigma (70) promoter were experimentally identified 50 bp upstream of hasA in *S. zooepidemicus*. The authors performed a phylogenetic analysis of each of the has operon genes to determine the evolutionary origin(s) of the streptococcal has operon. In contrast to other capsular and exopolysaccharide operons, has operons have undergone no detectable interspecies lateral gene transfers in their construction, instead relying on intragenome gene duplication for their assembly. Specifically, hasC and glmU appear to have been duplicated into the *S. zooepidemicus* has operon from remotely located but near-identical paralogues most likely to improve HA productivity by gene dosage in this streptococcus. The intragene rearrangements appear to be ongoing events and the two has operons of the *S. equi* subspecies represent two alternatives of the same gene arrangement.

The gain of four superantigens by *Streptococcus equi* is linked to the evolution of this host-restricted pathogen from an ancestral strain of the opportunistic pathogen *Streptococcus equi* subsp. *zooepidemicus*. A recent study determined that the culture supernatants of several *S. equi* subsp. *zooepidemicus* strains possessed mitogenic activity but lacked known superantigen-encoding genes. Paillot *et al.* (2010) reported the identification and activities of three novel superantigen-encoding genes. The products of szeF, szeN, and szeP share 59%, 49%, and 34% amino acid sequence identity with SPEH, SPEM, and SPEL, respectively. Recombinant SzeF, SzeN, and SzeP stimulated the proliferation of equine peripheral blood mononuclear cells, and tumor necrosis factor alpha (TNF-α) and gamma interferon (IFN-γ) production, in vitro. Although none of these superantigen genes were encoded within functional prophage elements, szeN and szeP were located next to a prophage remnant, suggesting that they were acquired by horizontal transfer. Eighty-one of 165 diverse *S. equi* subsp. *zooepidemicus* strains screened, including 7 out of 15 isolates from cases of disease in humans, contained at least one of these new superantigen-encoding genes. The presence of szeN or szeP, but not szeF, was significantly associated with mitogenic activity in the S. equi subsp. zooepidemicus population ($P < 0.000001$, $P < 0.000001$, and $P = 0.104$, respectively). It was concluded that horizontal transfer of these novel superantigens from and within the diverse *S. equi* subsp. *zooepidemicus* population is likely to have implications for veterinary and human disease. Priestnall *et al*(2010) recently described superantigen genes (szeF, szeN, and szeP) by PCR in 17/47 (36.2%) of the *S. equi* subsp. *zooepidemicus* isolates; however, there was no association between the presence of these genes and the histopathological score. The lungs of *S. equi* subsp. *zooepidemicus*-infected dogs with severe respiratory signs and lung pathology did however have significantly higher mRNA levels of the proinflammatory cytokines tumor necrosis factor alpha (TNF-α), interleukin 6 (IL-6), and interleukin 8 (IL-8) than in uninfected controls, suggesting a role for an exuberant host immune response in the pathogenesis of this disease.

The organisms belong to group C of Lancefield classification. Strains isolated from outbreaks of septicaemia in greyhounds are toxigenic (Sundbery *et al.*, 1981). *S. zooepidemicus* carry antigens with characteristics of the antiphagocytic M protein of the Lancefield group A and G streptococci; it was named M-like protein (SzP) . Cloning of the gene encoding SzP from an equine strain of subsp. *zooepidemicus* revealed a single open reading frame of 1,128 bp , whereas the SzP gene (GenBank accession number: AY263781from a pig strain of subsp. *zooepidemicus* showed a single open reading frame of 1,137 bp (GenBank accession number: U04620). M-like protein is similar to *S.equi* subsp. *equi,* but it shows great variability in antigenic specificity. M-like protein (SzP) of SEZ is a virulence factor with opsonin function. The N termini of M-like protein of strains of equine origin show variations in amino acid sequence which may account for the variation in the opsonic epitopes. M protein is composed of two predominantly α-helical protein chains assembled in a coiled-coil that extends from the bacterial cell surface. The M protein C terminus, which is anchored to the cell membrane and traverses the cell wall, is highly conserved, whereas the N terminus, which contacts the external environment, is highly variable and accounts for the type specificity. There are more than 100 known M protein serotypes of group A streptococci, and the serotype specificity is largely determined by epitopes located in the N-terminal 40 to 50 residues. SzP is similar in structure to M protein of group A streptococci. In addition to *S. zooepidemicus,* SzP have also been detected in other group C and G streptococci. SzP elicited protective antibodies and impaired deposition of C3 on the bacterial surface. *szp* gene has also been cloned from *S. zooepidemicus.* The predicted amino acid structure contains an alpha-helical repeat and shows highly homology to the C terminus of M proteins of group A, however the extensive A, B, C repeat regions found in M proteins of group A are absent. When compared to the SzP of *S. zooepidemicus* equine strain W60, the following N-terminal residues differ: S27G, S28V, V30A, and A32S; all of the swine strains shared the same signal peptide. The C terminus of SzP of *S. zooepidemicus* is rich in proline residues, and is composed primarily of PEPK repeats. The known swine strains shared 11 PEPK repeats with the SzP, whereas the equine strain W60 shared only 10 PEPK repeats.

Antibodies (IgA, IgG) against the M-like protein are present in the nasopharyngeal secretion of horses. There are 15 serotypes of *S.equi* subsp. *zooepidemicus.* Previous studies demonstrated that SzP is similar to M protein of group A Streptococcus in the structure and characteristics of antiphagocytosis. Similar to other streptococcal species, *S. zooepidemicus* binds to a number of host proteins, including immunoglobulin G , serum albumin , fibronectin, collagen , and á-macro-globulin through cell surface components. These host-parasite recognition components may function as virulence factors by acting as adhesions or antiopsonins.The M protein is an adhesin that can bind to the host cells, however it is not known whether the SzP of S. zooepidemicus also functions as an adhesin. The gene encoding SzP was expressed in E. coli, and the purified recombinant SzP (rSzP) was recognized by rabbit anti-S. zooepidemicus antibodies using immunoblot (Fan *et al.* 2008). Furthermore, the adherence of *S. zooepidemicus* to HEp-2 cells was inhibited by anti-rSzP antibodies in a dose-dependent manner. The authors employed a random 12-peptide phage display library for screening of immunodominant mimics of the SzP, which were recognized by an anti-SzP specific monoclonal antibody (mAb 2C8). Initial positive phage clones were identified by ELISA, followed by assays to determine the adherence-inhibiting ability of the peptide. Ten out of fourteen selected positive clones showed high reactivity that effectively inhibited the binding of mAb 2C8 to rSzP. The motif XSLSRX was highly conserved among six of the ten clones. Collectively, the findings suggest that the motif XSLSRX may represent an immunodominant mimic epitope of the SzP of *S. zooepidemicus* strain ATCC 35246, and that the same epitope may be used to mediate SzP binding to HEp-2 cells.

Diagnosis

Cultural methods as described for S.equi are suitable for the diagnosis. Besides, molecular techniques have been described for the diagnosis and identification of the isolates. In one study, clinical strains of S. equi (n=24) and *Streptococcus equi* subsp. *zooepidemicus* (n=24) were genetically characterized by sequencing of the 16S rRNA and sodA genes in order to devise a real-time PCR system that can detect *S. equi* and *S. zooepidemicus* and distinguish between them Baverud *et al.*, 2007). Sequencing demonstrated that all *S. equi* strains had the same 16S rRNA sequence, whereas *S. zooepidemicus* strains could be divided into subgroups. One of these (n=12 strains) had 16S rRNA sequences almost identical with the *S. equi* strains. Interestingly, four of the strains biochemically identified as *S. zooepidemicus* were found by sequencing of the 16S rRNA gene to have a sequence homologous with *Streptococcus equi* subsp. *ruminatorum*. However, they did not have the colony appearance or the biochemical characteristics of the type strain of *S. ruminatorum*. Sequencing of the sodA gene demonstrated that all S. equi strains had an identical sequence. For the *S. zooepidemicus* strains minor differences were found between the sodA sequences. The developed real-time PCR, based on the sodA and seeI genes was compared with conventional culturing on 103 cultured samples from horses with suspected strangles or other upper respiratory disease. The real-time PCR system was found to be more sensitive than conventional cultivation as two additional field isolates of *S. equi* and four of *S. zooepidemicus* were detected.

Vaccines

Several attempts have been made to develop a satisfactory immunizing preparation to control the *S. zooepidemicus* infection in mares. Widders *et al* (1995) immunised mares by the intramuscular and intrauterine administration of an antigen with adjuvant and they and unimmunised control mares were later challenged by the intrauterine instillation of pathogenic *Streptococcus zooepidemicus*; the response of all the mares was monitored clinically and bacteriologically for seven days. Significantly fewer *S zooepidemicus* were present in cervical swabs taken from the immunised mares than from the control mares ($P < 0.01$) and the degree of inflammation in the genital tract of the immunised mares was also significantly less ($P < 0.001$). This protective effect of immunisation was associated with the specific IgG response in the serum, and an IgG and IgA response in the uterine secretions. These results are the first demonstration that a previous immunisation with a suitable antigen can reduce an infection of the reproductive tract of mares. Hong-Jie *et al.* (2009) generated a szp-knockout strain by homologous recombination. Two fragments, upstream and downstream of the szp gene, were obtained by genome walking. The vector was then used to delete a 1090 bp segment of szp gene from a strain of SEZ (ATCC35246). The mutant strain had 1000-fold decrease in LD50 as compared with wild type, and provided 85% protection against challenge with a virulent strain when administered as a live vaccine. Semi-quantitative RT-PCR analysis showed a marked increased in levels of IL-4 and IFN-gamma mRNA in immunized mice. These data demonstrate that szp-knockout strain is a better candidate for vaccine development. Attenuated Salmonella enterica serovar Typhimurium MGN707, expressing the SzP protective protein of the MB9 serovar of Streptococcus equi subspecies zooepidemicus (SzP-MB9) was tested for its safety and efficacy as a nebulised intranasal vaccine against streptococcal uterine infections in mares (Causey *et al.* 2010). In a preliminary study, vaccinated mares (n=5) displayed serum, nasal and uterine responses ($P<0.05$) to S. Typhimurium lipopolysaccharide (St-LPS). Subsequently, vaccinated mares (expressor group, n=7), but not mares vaccinated with the vector only (control group, n=7), displayed significant increases in SzP-MB9 antibodies in serum, nasal and uterine washes ($P<0.05$). Assuming the uteri of all nine mares were free of streptococci prior to challenge with 6.3 x 10(9) colony forming units of S. e. zooepidemicus MB9, significantly fewer S. e. zooepidemicus were cultured from the uterine flushings of expressor-vaccinated mares (n=4) compared to control-vaccinated mares (n=5) ($P<0.001$). The only adverse reaction to vaccination was nasal haemorrhage in one mare.

Streptococcus dysgalactiae

Streptococcus dysgalactiae (SD) is comprised of two subspecies: *S. dysgalactiae subsp. equisimilis is* both a human commensal organism and a human pathogen, and *S. dysgalactiae subsp. dysgalactiae* is strictly an animal pathogen. Suzuki *et al.* (2011) presented complete genome sequences for both taxa, with analyses involving other species of Streptococcus but focusing on adaptation in the SD species group. We found little evidence for enrichment in biochemical categories of genes carried by each SD strain; however, differences in the virulence gene repertoire were apparent. Some of the differences could be ascribed to prophage and integrative conjugative elements. We identified approximately 9% of the nonrecombinant core genome to be under positive selection, some of which involved known virulence factors in other bacteria. Analyses of proteomes by pooling data across genes, by biochemical category, clade, or branch, provided evidence for increased rates of evolution in several gene categories, as well as external branches of the tree. Promoters were primarily evolving under purifying selection but with certain categories of genes evolving faster. Many of these fast-evolving categories were the same as those associated with rapid evolution in proteins. Overall, these results suggest that adaptation to changing environments and new hosts in the SD species group has involved the acquisition of key virulence genes along with selection of orthologous protein-coding loci and operon promoters.

During the infection caused by *S.dysgalactiae* there is severe swelling of the quarters with clots in milk and occasionally systemic reactions occur. It is most commonly associated with acute and severe mastitis. *S.equisimilis* is of human origin, and is generally carried in the mouth, vagina and skin lesions of udder. Relatively small numbers of the organisms are capable of producing mastitis following intramammary inoculation (Higgs *et al.*, 1980). In spite of its high prevalence, little is known about factors that contribute to the virulence of *S. dysgalactiae*. During the last decade, several cell-associated and extracellular factors of *S. dysgalactiae* have been identified; yet, the relative importance of these factors in the transmission and pathogenesis of mastitis caused by S. dysgalactiae has not been defined. *Streptococcus dysgalactiae* can interact with several plasma and extracellular host-derived proteins such as immunoglobulin G, albumin, fibronectin, fibrinogen, collagen, vitronectin, plasminogen, and alpha 2-macroglobulin. These interactions are mediated by bacterial surface proteins. This organism also produces hyaluronidase and fibrinolysin which may be involved in promoting dissemination of the organism into host tissue. *Streptococcus dysgalactiae* adheres to and is internalized by bovine mammary epithelial cells in vitro. Involvement of host cell kinases, intact microfilaments and de novo eukaryotic protein synthesis is required for internalization of *S. dysgalactiae* into bovine mammary epithelial cells; a process that appeared to occur by a receptor-mediated endocytosis mechanism. However, de novo bacterial protein synthesis was not required for epithelial cell internalization. Furthermore, *S. dysgalactiae* survived within mammary epithelial cells for extended periods of time without losing viability or damaging the eukaryotic cell. Further research on characterization of host-pathogen interactions that take place during the early stages of mammary gland infection will enhance our understanding of pathogenesis of intramammary infection which may contribute to development of methods to minimize production losses due to mastitis.

S.dysgalactiae possesses the property to adhere on bovine epithelial cells. The structure mediating this adherence has not been described in detail. Bacterial surface hydrophobicity (SH) plays a role in adhesion of bacteria to host surfaces and ingestion by phagocytic cells. Streptococcus dysgalactiae isolated from bovine intramammary infections were examined for expression of SH after growth in Todd-Hewitt broth (THB) and THB supplemented with skim milk, whey, lactose, and casein (Calvinho *et al.*1996). Strains were significantly more hydrophobic after growth in THB and THB plus whey and more hydrophilic after growth in THB plus skim milk. Both trypsin and proteinase K abolished SH in three strains tested. Mild pepsin treatment had little effect on SH, while heat treatment at 70 degrees or 80 degrees C abolished SH in two strains tested. A hydrophilic strain of S. dysgalactiae did not adhere as well to bovine mammary epithelial cells as a hydrophobic strain. Trypsin treatment significantly reduced adherence of a hydrophobic strain of S. dysgalactiae to epithelial cells while adherence of a hydrophilic strain remained unaltered. A hydrophilic strain of *S. dysgalactiae* was significantly more resistant to phagocytosis by bovine mammary gland macrophages than a hydrophobic strain. Differences in expression of SH may play an important role in determining the ability of *S. dysgalactiae* to establish successfully within the mammary gland.

Activity of tyrosine protein kinases, intact microfilaments and de novo eukaryotic protein synthesis was required for uptake of *S. dysgalactiae* by bovine mammary epithelial cells; a process that appeared to occur via receptor-mediated endocytosis. In contrast, de novo bacterial protein synthesis was not required for uptake of *S. dysgalactiae* by MAC-T cells. Studies have shown that *S. dysgalactiae* invaded epithelial cells, induced cellular damage, and was capable of persisting inside bovine mammary epithelial cells.The study of Calvinho and Oliver (1998) provides insight into bacterial and cellular mechanisms involved in early host-pathogen interactions, putting into perspective the role of mammary epithelial cells in the development and establishment of intramammary infections by S. dysgalactiae. The role of the

Mig protein of Streptococcus dysgalactiae in bacterial adhesion and internalization of bovine mammary gland epithelial cells (MAC-T) was investigated with the wild-type and isogenic mig mutant strains. While there was no difference in adhesion between the strains, the wild-type strain exhibited a significantly lower level of invasion than the mutants. The lower level of internalization of the Mig(+) strain is likely due to Mig-mediated interference with uptake of the microorganisms rather than the host protein binding properties of Mig. Avoidance of intimate interactions with the host cells might be an alternative strategy for S. dysgalactiae to survive and persist in the bovine mammary glands.

Infections with *S.dysgalactiae* artificially induced in goats are indistinguishable from *S.agalactiae* and the pathogenesis is probably similar with all streptococcal mastitides. Diagnosis depends on cultural examination of milk. Use of the real-time PCR-based test may be useful in diagnosing intramammary infections when milk samples with high somatic cell counts are culture-negative or when culturing results in the detection of minor pathogens (Bexiga *et al.*2011).

For treatment of mastitis antibiotics are used.Petrovsky *et al.*(2011) reported that Streptococcus uberis isolates demonstrated high overall susceptibility (>90.0%) to the majority of antimicrobial agents except ampicillin (81.7%), lincomycin (85.3%), trimethoprim/sulphonamide combination (88.6%), and, as expected, aminoglycosides (<4%). The susceptibility of S. dysgalactiae was similar to that of Strep. uberis, except for greater susceptibility to oxacillin (98.1%) and much lower susceptibility to tetracyclines (11.2%). The antimicrobial agents intended for treatment of bovine mastitis currently available in New Zealand generally demonstrated good in-vitro efficacy against streptococci and staphylococci, with the exception of aminoglycosides. Analysis of the results of antimicrobial susceptibility of bacterial isolates from milk samples from dairy cows in New Zealand provides useful data for surveillance purposes, and a baseline for identifying changes in antimicrobial sensitivity in this population. However, the variation in antimicrobial susceptibility between individual isolates means that these data are of limited value when determining treatment of mastitis at the farm level. On most dairy farms teat dips are applied to the teats of cows either before or after milking in order to prevent pathogens from gaining access to the mammary gland via the teat canal. In the present experiments (Klostermann *et al.*2010), a natural teat dip was developed using a fermentate containing the live bacterium Lactococcus lactis DPC 3251. This bacterium produces lacticin 3147, a two-component lantibiotic which was previously shown to effectively kill Gram-positive mastitis pathogens. Lacticin 3147 activity in the fermentate was retained at 53% of its original level following storage for 3 weeks at 4 degrees C. In the initial experiments in vitro, 105 colony-forming units/ml (cfu/ml) of either *Staphylococcus aureus, Streptococcus dysgalactiae* or *Streptococcus uberis* were introduced into the lacticin-containing fermentate. Neither Staph. aureus nor *S. dysgalactiae* could be detected after 30 min or 15 min, respectively, while *S. uberis* was reduced approximately 100-fold after 15 min. Following these trials, preliminary experiments were performed *in vivo* on teats of lactating dairy cows. In these experiments, teats were coated with each of the challenge organisms and then dipped with the lacticin-containing fermented teat dip. Following a dip contact time of 10 min, staphylococci were reduced by 80% when compared with the undipped control teat. Streptococcal challenges were reduced by 97% for *Str. dysgalactiae* and by 90% for Str. uberis. These trials showed that the teat dip is able to reduce mastitis pathogens on the teats of lactating cows. Current strategies aimed at reducing cases of mastitis include improved hygiene in the farm environment, particularly with regards to the health and cleanliness of teats. Once mastitis occurs, antibiotic therapy is a favoured option, and as a prophylactic tool, in the form of dry-cow therapy, has also shown value. Prevention of mastitis using immunological tools such as vaccines lags behind the major vaccine breakthroughs that have been achieved in preventing and/or reducing the severity of numerous infectious diseases in animals.

Sterptococcus uberis and *S.parauberis*

Streptococcus uberis is one of the more important environmental pathogens implicated in bovine mastitis, accounting for a significant proportion of subclinical and clinical intramammary infections in both lactating and nonlactating cows.*S.uberis* causes acute environmental mastitis as distinct from *S.agalactiae* which is a specific contagious mastitis. Both, *S.uberis* and parauberis are commensals to the epithelial cells of cattle and produces opportunistic infection in mammary gland under poor hygienic conditions. *S.uberis* is wide spread in environment so infection is produced quite frequently, particularly during the dry period especially during the month before parturition but most clinical cases occur during the first part of lactation. *S.uberis* is a common inhabitant of skin, lips and tonsils of cows in an infected herd, the skin of belly carrying largest population. Some cows shed the organisms in the feces. The genetically distinct but phenotypically similar, *S.uberis* and *S.parauberis* are differentiated by the ability of the latter to grow well at 10^0C and by DNA fingerprinting technique (Groschup *et al.,* 1991).

Epidemiology

An increasing prevalence of *S. uberis* mastitis has been reported throughout the world. Approximately 14 to 26% of clinical mastitis cases in Canada, the United States, The Netherlands, and the United Kingdom are caused by *S. uberis*. *S. uberis* is also one of the most significant causes of bovine mastitis in New Zealand and Australia, where the dairy industry is pasture based. Despite its high prevalence, the epidemiology of *S. uberis* mastitis is incompletely understood. *S. uberis* has been isolated from many sites on the cow including the skin surface, genital tract, intestinal tract, and tonsils. It can also be isolated in large numbers from bedding material, which is thought to be a major source for intramammary infections in housed cattle. Although many potential reservoirs have been identified, their significance and their association with the occurrence of mastitis in a herd are still unclear. A longitudinal observational study (18 months) was carried out in two Dutch dairy herds to explore clinical, epidemiological and molecular characteristics of *Streptococcus uberis* mastitis (Zadoks *et al.*, 2003). Bacterial isolates were characterized at strain level by random amplified polymorphic DNA (RAPD) fingerprinting. Persistent infections were usually attributable to one strain, while recurrent infections could be caused by different strains. When multiple quarters of a cow were infected, infections were mostly caused by one strain. In each herd, multiple strains were identified yet one strain predominated. The majority of all infections were subclinical, and infections attributed to predominant strains were more chronic than infections attributed to other strains. Epidemiological and molecular data suggest infection from environmental sources with a variety of *S. uberis* strains as well as within-cow and between-cow transmission of a limited number of *S. uberis* strains, with possible transfer of bacteria via the milking machine.

Pathogenesis

Transmission from quarter to quarter and cow to cow occurrs. Despite the great variation in *S. uberis* strains, persistent infection with the same strain within a lactation is observed in most cows. Predominant strains were present in problematic herds. The wide variety of *S. uberis* strains found is consistent with an environmental source of *S. uberis*. However, evidence of direct transmission, the persistence of infection, and the predominance of particular strains in some herds indicate that *S. uberis* infections are epidemiologically complex and that the relative importance of these factors in the occurrence of mastitis may differ between herds.

Virulence factors of *S.uberis* include a CAMP like factor similar to *S.agalactiae*. A trypsin resistant R- like antigen of 64 kDa capable of stimulating opsonic antibodies has also been reported (Timoney, 1993). Besides, *S.uberis* contain a hyaluronic acid capsule and its role in virulence specifically resistance against phagocytosis has been hypothesized. The frequency at which the genes responsible for capsule biosynthesis occurred in field isolates of *Streptococcus uberis* was determined (Field *et al.*, 2003). Of the two genotypes detected (hasABC and hasC), the capsular genotype (hasABC) was more common. This genotype was present at a higher frequency in a population isolated from mastitis cases than in a population isolated from cattle bedding. The virulence of a mutant strain of *S. uberis* (TRF0-6) that lacked the ability to produce a hyaluronic acid capsule due to an insertion within its single copy of hasA was compared to that of the capsular parental strain (0140J). Strains TRF0-6 and 0140J infected all mammary gland quarters following experimental challenge. The wild type and the mutant induced overt signs of disease in four out of four and in six out of eight mammary gland quarters, respectively. Both the wild type and the hasA mutant were resistant to killing by bovine neutrophils following cultivation in bovine milk. The ability to withstand the bactericidal action of neutrophils following growth in milk was therefore independent of the capsule and coincided with the ability of supernatants from such cultures to prevent the bactericidal action of neutrophils. This investigation revealed that, in the absence of the capsule, S. uberis is able to withstand the bactericidal effect of bovine neutrophils and induce mastitis in dairy cows.

The virulence factors associated with pathogenesis are not well understood. Reinoso *et al.*(2011) examined 11 putative and known virulence-associated genes by PCR in 78 *S. uberis* strains isolated from infected animals in Argentina. Additionally, the distribution of virulence patterns over various herds was determined. Not all genes were present in the strains but all of the detected virulence-associated genes were present in combination. Forty-seven (60.3%) isolates carried seven to 10 virulence-associated genes. Further analysis revealed 58 virulence patterns. Different patterns were found within the same herd and among herds, demonstrating that strains with different virulence patterns were able to cause mastitis. Despite the large number of strains with different virulence patterns, strains with identical patterns were found. Detection of virulence-associated genes in individual S. uberis strains isolated from infected animals revealed one to 10 virulence genes. This may indicate that other virulence factors could be involved. This study revealed the occurrence and distribution of 11 virulence-associated genes among S. uberis isolates from bovine mastitis in various herds and contributes to a better understanding of the pathogenicity of this bacterium. *Streptococcus uberis* also exibit biofilm growth. The transition from planktonic to biofilm growth in strain 0140J correlated with an upregulation of several gene products that have been shown to be important for pathogenesis, including a glutamine ABC transporter (SUB1152) and a lactoferrin binding protein (gene lbp; protein SUB0145) (Crowly *et al.*, 2011).

It is not clear how the organism enters the udder from the environment. It is possible that certain non-specific host specific factors are responsible for the entry. *S.uberis* most probably bind to epithelial cells and get internalized. Streptococcus uberis adhesion molecule (SUAM) in the pathogenesis of S. uberis mastitis has been studied. It has been demonstrated that bovine lactoferrin (LF), a whey protein present in milk and nonlactating cow mammary secretions, significantly enhanced adherence of *S. uberis* to mammary epithelial cells in culture. Bacteria were cultured with mammary epithelial cell monolayers for 1 hour. The culture supernatant was removed, and the epithelial cells were lysed. Adherence index was calculated as number of colony-forming units (CFU) in the cell lysate divided by number of CFU in the supernatant times 10,000. *S. uberis* were found to bind to purified LF and LF in milk. Addition of LF to the culture medium enhanced adherence of all 3 strains to mammary epithelial cells, whereas addition of milk enhanced adherence of 2 strains and decreased adherence of the third. Pretreatment of bacteria with LF or milk increased adherence of 1 of the strains but decreased adherence of the other 2. Increased adherence was antagonized by rabbit antibovine LF antibody. Results suggest that LF may function as a bridging molecule between *S. uberis* and bovine mammary epithelial cells, facilitating adherence of the bacteria to the cells(Fang *et al.*, 2000). *S. uberis* also expresses ligands with affinity for collagen that are up-regulated by collagen. Almeida and Oliver (2001) hypothesized that these ligands increase adherence by using collagen as a bridge between the bacterium and host cell and/or by direct interaction with host cell receptor(s). Subsequently Patel *et al.* (2009) identified *S. uberis* SUAM showing an affinity for LF. Interaction between SUAM, bovine LF, and a putative LF receptor on the bovine mammary epithelial cell surface could serve as a bridging molecule for internalization of *S. uberis* into mammary epithelial cells. When internalization assays were conducted using cell growth medium containing bovine LF, a significant increase in internalization of S. uberis into mammary epithelial cells was observed(Patel *et al.*, 2009). However, this effect was reversed when assays were conducted in the presence of antibodies to bovine LF suggesting that internalization of *S. uberis* into mammary epithelial cells, at least in part, was mediated by LF ligands. When *S. uberis* was pretreated with antibodies to SUAM, internalization in the presence of LF was reduced in the same manner as observed with antibodies to LF. Transmission and scanning electron microscopy results demonstrated that streptavidin-coated gold particles specifically localized on biotinylated LF receptors on *S. uberis* and mammary epithelial cell surfaces supporting the availability of LF receptors. Collectively, these results suggest that LF serves as a bridging molecule between SUAM located on the surface of *S. uberis* and LF receptors located on the surface of mammary epithelial cells thus enhancing internalization of *S. uberis* into host cells. Exploitation of LF as a molecular bridge for internalization of *S. uberis* into mammary epithelial cells may confer a significant advantage allowing mammary gland infection. The sua deletion in *S. uberis* UT888 was achieved by homologous recombination using a thermosensitive plasmid (Chen *et al.*, 2011). The deletion mutant was analyzed for sua deletion by PCR, southern blot and DNA sequencing, and was designated Äsua *S. uberis* UT888. As compared to the isogenic parent strain, Äsua *S. uberis* UT888 did not produce SUAM based on SDS-PAGE gel and western blot. Deletion of sua and lack of expression of SUAM by Äsua *S. uberis* UT888 markedly reduced the ability of the sua gene deletion mutant of *S. uberis* to adhere to and internalize into mammary epithelial cells. These results confirm the central role of SUAM in adherence to and internalization of *S. uberis* into host cells.

Luther *et al.*(2008) cloned and sequenced the SUAM gene (sua) from *S. uberis* UT888 and determined the prevalence of sua in strains of *S. uberis* isolated from geographically diverse locations. The 20 amino acid N-terminal sequence of purified SUAM was utilized to identify a single open reading frame (ORF) in the *S. uberis* O140J (ATCC BAA-854) genome database. Three sets of primers were identified from this sequence for amplification of sub-fragments and the complete gene encoding SUAM. Restriction fragment analysis of the largest polymerase chain reaction (PCR) product confirmed the desired fragment had been amplified. This 2970bp PCR fragment was cloned into plasmid pCR-XL-TOPO and sequenced. The S. uberis UT888 sua sequence (NCBI Accession no. DQ232760) was 99% similar to the *S. uberis* O140J database sequence. The three pairs of PCR primers were used in a subsequent experiment to identify sua in 12 strains of *S. uberis* isolated in milk from dairy cows with mastitis in Tennessee (n=6), Colorado (n=1), Washington (n=1), New Zealand (n=1) and from the American Type Culture Collection (n=3). Primer pairs yielded the expected 2970, 2639 and 2362bp PCR fragments in all strains evaluated. In conclusion, sua was detected in all strains of *S. uberis* evaluated suggesting that it is conserved.

Streptococcus uberis contains a single copy sortase A (srtA), encoding a transamidase capable of covalently anchoring specific proteins to peptidoglycan. Unlike the wild-type, an isogenic mutant carrying an inactivating ISS1 insertion within srtA was only able to infect the bovine mammary gland in a transient fashion. Data have demonstrated that a number of sortase anchored proteins each play a distinct, non-redundant and important role in pathogenesis of *S. uberis* infection within the lactating bovine mammary gland (Leigh *et al.*, 2010).

Diagnosis

Routine bacteriological methods are emploed for isolation and typing of strains from mastitis cases. Serological grouping of *S. uberis* reveal polysaccharide antigens of groups E, G, P and U. The biochemical properties of *S. uberis*, determined with the Strep-Zym identification system, differed clearly from those of *S. agalactiae* and S. dysgalactiae (Christ and Lammler 1992). Some cultures of *S. uberis* produce the enzymes hyaluronidase and neuraminidase. In addition *S. uberis* strains partly demonstrate CAMP-like synergistic hemolytic activities on sheep blood agar, reacted specifically with the lectins from Helix pomatia and Dolichos biflorus and produced bacteriocin-like inhibitors. These reactions, possibly of importance as virulence factors, as well as "DNA-fingerprinting" of *S. uberis*, might serve as individual markers of the respective cultures in epidemiological studies. Many clinical mastitis cases in which conventional culture failed to detect bacteria, mastitis pathogens are still present, often in substantial quantities. The clearly elevated N-acetyl-β-d-glucosaminidase activity values of the milk samples, together with clinical signs of the infected cows and quarters, confirm the diagnosis of clinical mastitis and indicat that real-time, PCR-based bacterial findings are able to reveal bacteriological etiology. All common mastitis bacteria can occur in large quantities in clinical mastitis samples that exhibit no growth in conventional culture, and that the real-time PCR assay is a useful tool for bacteriological diagnosis of such milk samples. The real-time PCR assay shows excellent analytical accuracy and holds much promise for use in routine bovine intraq mammary infection testing programs(Koskinen *et al.*, 2009).

Treatment and Control

Cases of mastitis respond well to penicillins, erythromycin, tetracyclines, cephalosporins and cloxacillin but are resistant to gentamicin, neomycin streptomycin, nitrofurazone and polymixin B. Recently high level resistance to streptomycin and kanamycin has been detected. *S. uberis* strains show elevated penicillin G MIC. All strains are susceptible to chloramphenicol and rifampicin.Treatment of sub-clinical cases are best left till the dry period. General methods described for control of *S.agalactiae* do not work with *S.uberis* infection because of the environmental origin. Because of this it is essential to treat the infected quarter vigorously. In herds where the disease is a problem in dry cows a second dry period treatment is recommended for 3-4 weeks after drying off. Dry cow therapy continues to lower significantly the rate of new dry period intramammary infection in herds with elevated somatic cell counts and a high prevalence of infection. More information on reservoirs and modes of transmission is needed for development of better control programs for this pathogen. Implementation of mastitis control programs based on improved milking practices, postmilking teat disinfection, therapeutic and prophylactic antimicrobial administration, and culling of persistently infected animals has effectively controlled intramammary infections caused by contagious pathogens. However, these measures have been less effective against environmental pathogens. Consequently, environmental mastitis has become a major problem, particularly in well-managed herds that have successfully controlled contagious pathogens. It has been hypothesized that the niche vacated by contagious mastitis pathogens becomes occupied by environmental mastitis pathogens, resulting in an increased prevalence of intramammary infection by environmental pathogens. Vaccination programmes have met with failure. However, live vaccines and, recently, crude sub-unit vaccines have shown promise against bovine mastitis due to *S. uberis*. A live vaccine in combination with an intramammary administration of a soluble cell surface extract was shown to induce protection of the mammary gland from experimental challenge with *S. uberis* (Leigh 2000). Protection was strain specific, but was achieved in the absence of opsonic activity and without a large influx of neutrophils. One hypothesis is that protection was achieved by reducing the rate of bacterial growth in vivo. This view has led to the identification and exploitation of a novel plasminogen activator as a vaccine antigen. Vaccines containing this antigen conferred cross strain protection. In another study, Finch *et al.* (1997) indicated that vaccination with live *S. uberis* protects against challenge with the homologous strain but was less effective against a heterologous strain. Reduced protection was also seen when the intramammary booster was omitted. For future development of vaccines it is argued that novel approaches must be considered to search for vaccine candidates, and vaccines need to be designed and constructed within the special framework of their uses, in the mammary gland which offers a unique immunological environment. In addition, effective vaccines against mastitis due to *S.uberis* may be more likely to emerge from strategies that target the cell-mediated arm of the immune response rather than strategies that target specific antibody responses.

Specific immune response in cows following infection is known to occur through production of opsonic antibodies in milk against *S.uberis* antigens. Immune modification of pathogenesis of S.uberis infection in cattle has been studied (Hill *et al.*, 1994). Two groups of 4 cows were vaccinated subcutaneously with live Streptococcus uberis strain 0140J or a surface extract derived from the same strain, at 14 days prior to the cessation of lactation (drying off) and at calving. Both groups also received an intramammary administration of the surface extract 7 days after drying off. A third group of unvaccinated animals acted as controls. Following intramammary challenge of two quarters per cow with the vaccine strain, all quarters on control cows and those vaccinated only with surface extract developed clinical mastitis. However, only 12.5% of challenged quarters on cows which were vaccinated with live bacteria developed clinical mastitis. In addition, the numbers of bacteria in the milk following challenge were 10(5) times higher from the control and extract vaccinated cows than those which received live vaccine.

Serum levels of *S. uberis* specific IgG2 were elevated in the animals vaccinated with the live organism when compared to that of either extract-vaccinates or controls, whilst S. uberis specific levels of IgG1 and IgM were similar in all groups throughout the experiment. Specific antibody levels in milk were unaffected by vaccination. Despite increased levels of IgG2, no increase in opsonic activity was detected in any serum or milk samples. Peripheral blood lymphocytes from animals vaccinated with live organisms showed a considerable increase in proliferative response to *S. uberis* antigen in vitro when compared with lymphocytes from control and extract-vaccinated animals. These results suggest that neutrophils and specific opsonising antibody may not form the major defence against infection with *S. uberis*.

Streptococcus pneumoniae

S.pneumoniae is the causative agent of pneumonia and mastitis in cows. It is of public health significance also. The organism has been associated with lower respiratory disease in young thoroughbred animals in training (Mackintosh *et al.*, 1988). *S.pneumoniae* is the apparent cause of septicaemia with sudden death in calves. Transmission of the pathogen from cases among calves to the attendants has been suggested. A severe form of mastitis is caused in cows as a result of *S.pneumoniae* infection. Disease in thoroughbred is characterized by fever and coughing with the involvement of bronchi and trachea, poor racing performance and nasal and ocular discharges. Respiratory infection in dogs, goats, monkeys, rabbits & rats are common.

Formerly known as *Diplocococcus pneumoniae,* it includes more than 80 serotypes that are identified on the basis of serological differences in the polysaccharide capsular antigen. It evolves the formation of opsonins which are protective.

Streptococcus pneumoniae, the pneumococcus, colonizes the nasopharynx and is a common etiologic agent of respiratory tract infection. In addition, infection with the pneumococcus frequently results in bacteremia and sepsis because of its capacity to invade the bloodstream. The ability to exist in these two host environments correlates with two distinct phenotypes observed in clinical isolates as compared in animal models of carriage and sepsis. There is spontaneous back-and-forth switching or phase variation among opaque, transparent, and in some isolates intermediate colony morphologies. The more transparent forms are more efficient at adherence to human epithelial cells and colonization of the nasopharynx while only the opaque forms are able to cause sepsis in mice.

The sialic acid capsule is also an antiphagocytic factor and also protects against complement by inhibiting the activation. However, phagocytosis in ponies by macrophages has been observed. The lysozyme-like protein, a new *Streptococcus pneumoniae* virulence factor, may regulate the proliferation and the capsular polysaccharides synthesis of *Streptococcus pneumoniae* to affect expression of virulence (Huang *et al.*, 2011). Comparison of cell surface factors that vary in association with opacity showed that transparent pneumococci have 2.1- to 3.8-fold more cell wall carbohydrate (C polysaccharide or teichoic acid). The pneumococcal teichoic acid has an unusual structure including choline which is derived from the growth medium and is a nutritional requirement. Choline in the form of phosphorylcholine (ChoP) on the teichoic acid has been implicated in direct adherence to host cells via the receptor for platelet-activating factor. In addition, a number of cell surface proteins, including several shown to contribute to the pathogenesis of pneumococcal infection, are anchored to the organism by noncovalent attachment to ChoP. The distribution of these choline-binding proteins differs in association with colony morphology and content of the ChoP anchor. ChoP is also a target for an acute-phase reactant in human serum, C-reactive protein (CRP), which has been shown to induce opsonophagocytic activity and to contribute to protection against invasive pneumococcal infection.

Opaque pneumococci, in contrast, have 1.2- to 5.6-fold-greater quantities of capsular polysaccharide, the major virulence determinant of the organism, than do related transparent organisms. The capsule acts to inhibit phagocytosis, the primary mechanism for clearance of the pneumococcus. Relatively small differences in the amount of capsular polysaccharide have been noted to be critical in the ability of the organism to cause experimental infection. The increased content of capsular polysaccharide in opaque pneumococci could account for the enhanced virulence associated with this phenotype in invasive infection in the mouse model.

Streptococcus pneumoniae undergoes spontaneous phase variation between a transparent and an opaque colony phenotype, the latter being more virulent in a murine model of sepsis. Opaque pneumococci have previously been shown to express lower amounts of *C polysaccharide* (cell wall teichoic acid) and were shown to have a higher content of capsular polysaccharide by immunoelectron microscopy. Kim *et al.* (1999) examined the relationship between expression of these two cell surface carbohydrate structures and their relative contribution to the increased virulence of opaque variants. Comparison of genetically related strains showed that the differential content of capsular polysaccharide did not affect the amount of teichoic acid as measured by a capture enzyme-linked immunosorbent assay (ELISA). In contrast, when the teichoic acid structure was altered by replacing choline in the growth medium with structural analogs, the quantity of capsular polysaccharide as measured by a capture ELISA was decreased, demonstrating a linkage in the expression of the two surface carbohydrate structures. A standardized assay was used to assess the relative contribution of cell surface carbohydrates to opsonophagocytosis. The opaque variants required 1.2- to 30-fold more immune human serum to achieve 50% opsonophagocytic killing than did related transparent variants (types 6B and 9V). The opsonophagocytic titer was proportional to the quantity of capsular polysaccharide rather than teichoic acid. The major factor in binding of the opsonin, C-reactive protein (CRP), was also the amount of capsular polysaccharide rather than the teichoic acid ligand. Only for the transparent variant (type 6B), which bound more CRP, was there enhanced opsonophagocytic killing in the presence of this serum protein. Increased expression of capsular polysaccharide, therefore, appeared to be the major factor in the decreased opsonophagocytic killing of opaque pneumococci.

Although closely related at the molecular level, the capsular polysaccharide (CPS) of serotype 10F Streptococcus pneumoniae and coaggregation receptor polysaccharide (RPS) of Streptococcus oralis C104 have distinct ecological roles. CPS prevents phagocytosis of pathogenic *S. pneumoniae*, whereas RPS of commensal S. oralis functions as a receptor for lectin-like adhesins on other members of the dental plaque biofilm community. Results from high resolution NMR identified the recognition region of *S. oralis* RPS (*i.e.* Galfbeta1-6GalNAcbeta1-3Galalpha) in the hexasaccharide repeat of S. pneumoniae CPS10F. The failure of this polysaccharide to support fimbriae-mediated adhesion of Actinomyces naeslundii was explained by the position of Galf, which occurred as a branch in CPS10F rather than within the linear polysaccharide chain, as in RPS. Carbohydrate engineering of *S. oralis* RPS with wzy from *S. pneumoniae* attributed formation of the Galf branch in CPS10F to the linkage of adjacent repeating units through sub terminal GalNAc in Galfbeta1-6GalNAcbeta1-3Galalpha rather than through terminal Galf, as in RPS. A gene (wcrD) from serotype 10A *S. pneumoniae* was then used to engineer a linear surface polysaccharide in *S. oralis* that was identical to RPS except for the presence of a beta1-3 linkage between Galf and GalNAcbeta1-3Galalpha. This polysaccharide also failed to support adhesion of A. naeslundii, thereby establishing the essential role of beta1-6-linked Galf in recognition of adjacent GalNAcbeta1-3Galalpha in wild-type RPS. These findings, which illustrate a molecular approach for relating bacterial polysaccharide structure to function, provide insight into the possible evolution of *S. oralis* RPS from *S. pneumoniae* CPS.

Beside the capsule, an alveolar necrosis producing toxin, including pneumolysin, a purpura - producing principle and autolysin, may play a role in disease pathogenesis (Boulnois *et al.*, 1991). This thiol activated toxin which is similar to streptolysin O, results in production of highly respiratory cellular exudates. It also slows the ciliary movement thus reduces the bacterial clearance from trachea. Neuraminidase produced by bacteria may expose the epithelial cell receptors by removing N-acetyl neuraminic acid residues of mucosal cells (Timoney 1993). It is believed that stress to the respiratory system play a role in development of the disease.

References

Alber J., El-Sayed A., Lämmler C., Hassan A.A., Weiss R. and Zschöck M.2004.Multiplex polymerase chain reaction for identification and differentiation of Streptococcus equi subsp. zooepidemicus and Streptococcus equi subsp. equi. J. Vet. Med. B. Infect. Dis. Vet. Public Health. **51:** 455-458.

Almeida R.A. and Oliver S.P. 2011.Role of collagen in adherence of Streptococcus uberis to bovine mammary epithelial cells. J. Vet. Med. B Infect. Dis. Vet. Public. Health. **48:** 759-763.

Baums, C.G., Kaim, U., Fulde, M., Ramchandran, G., Goethe, R. and Valentin – weigand, P. 2006. Identification of a novel virulence determinant with serum opacification activity in *Streptococcus suis*. Infect. Immun. **74:** 6154-6162.

Baums C.G., Brüggemann C., Kock C., Beineke A., Waldmann K.H.and Valentin-Weigand P.2010.Immunogenicity of an autogenous Streptococcus suis bacterin in preparturient sows and their piglets in relation to protection after weaning. Clin. Vaccine Immunol. **17:** 1589-1597.

Baums C.G., Kock C., Beineke A., Bennecke K., Goethe R., Schröder C., Waldmann K.H. and Valentin-Weigand .2009. Streptococcus suis bacterin and subunit vaccine immunogenicities and protective efficacies against serotypes 2 and 9. Clin. Vaccine Immunol. **16:** 200-208.

Båverud V., Johansson S.K. and Aspan A.2007.Real-time PCR for detection and differentiation of Streptococcus equi subsp. equi and Streptococcus equi subsp. zooepidemicus. Vet. Microbiol. **124:** 219-229.

Bexiga R., Koskinen M.T., Holopainen J., Carneiro C., Pereira H., Ellis K.A. and Vilela C.L.2011.Diagnosis of intramammary infection in samples yielding negative results or minor pathogens in conventional bacterial culturing. J. Dairy Res. **78:** 49-55.

Bhakdi, S.J., Tranum- Jensen, J. and Sziegoleit, A. 1985. Mechanism of damage by Streptolysin O. Infect. Immun. **47:** 5-60.

Blank L.M., Hugenholtz P. and Nielsen L.K..2008.Evolution of the hyaluronic acid synthesis (has) operon in Streptococcus zooepidemicus and other pathogenic streptococci. J. Mol. Evol. **67:** 13-22.

Boulnois, G.J., Mitchell, T.J., Saunders, K., Omen, R. *et al.*, 1991. In genetic and molecular biology of *Streptococci, Lactococci* and *Enterococci*. Ed. G.M. Dunny, P.P. Cleary and L.C. Mc Kary pp. 83-87. Washington DC, American Society for Microbiology.

Busque P., Higgins R., Caya F. and Quessy S.1997.Immunization of pigs against Streptococcus suis serotype 2 infection using a live avirulent strain. Can. J. Vet. Res. **61:** 275-279.

Calvinho L.F., Almeida R.A., Oliver S.P.1996.Influence of Streptococcus dysgalactiae surface hydrophobicity on adherence to mammary epithelial cells and phagocytosis by mammary macrophages. Zentralbl. Veterinarmed B. **43:** 257-266.

Calvinho L.F.and Oliver S.P.1998.Characterization of mechanisms involved in uptake of Streptococcus dysgalactiae by bovine mammary epithelial cells. Vet. Microbiol. **63:** 261-274.

Causey R.C., Artiushin S.C., Crowley I.F., Weber J.A., Homola A.D., Kelley A., Stephenson L.A., Opitz H.M., Guilmain S. and Timoney J.F.2010.Immunisation of the equine uterus against Streptococcus equi subspecies zooepidemicus using an intranasal attenuated Salmonella vector. Vet. J. **184:** 156-161.

Chaturvedi, V.K. and Srivastava, A.B. 2004. Paper presented in national symposium held at College of Animal Sciences, Palampur 176062, HP, India, October, 18-19 Abstract No. 1.21.

Chen X., Dego O.K., Almeida R.A., Fuller T.E., Luther D.A. and Oliver S.P.2011.Deletion of sua gene reduces the ability of Streptococcus uberis to adhere to and internalize into bovine mammary epithelial cells. Vet. Microbiol. **147:** 426-434.

Chengappa, M.M. *et al.*, 1990. J. Am. Vet. Med. Assoc. **197:** 1467.

Christ D.and Lämmler C. 1992. [Characterization of Streptococcus uberis with special consideration of supposed pathogenicity factors]. Berl. Munch. Tierarztl. Wochenschr. **105:** 224-30. [Article in German]

Crowley R.C., Leigh J.A., Ward P.N., Lappin-Scott H.M.and Bowler L.D.2011.Differential protein expression in Streptococcus uberis under planktonic and biofilm growth conditions. Appl. Environ. Microbiol. **77:** 382-384.

Deshmukh S.D., Kremer B., Freudenberg M., Bauer S., Golenbock D.T.and Henneke P.2011.Macrophages recognize streptococci through bacterial single-stranded RNA. EMBO Rep. **12:** 71-76.

Devi A..S.and Ponnuraj K.2010.Cloning, expression, purification and ligand binding studies of novel fibrinogen-binding protein FbsB of Streptococcus agalactiae. Protein Expr. Purif. **74:** 148-155.

Enright, M.R. *et al.*, 1987. Vet. Rec. **121:** 132.

Escaich S.2008. Antivirulence as a new antibacterial approach for chemotherapy. Curr .Opin. Chem. Biol. **12:** 400-408.

Esgleas, M., Liyuan, Yi, Hancock, M.A., Harel, J., Dubrecil, J.D. and Gottaschalk, M. 2008. Isolation and characterization of á-enolase, a novel fibronectin binding protein for *Streptococcus suis*. Microbiology (Reading). **154:** 2668-79].

Fan H., Wang Y., Tang F. and Lu C.2008.Determination of the mimic epitope of the M-like protein adhesin in swine Streptococcus equi subsp. zooepidemicus. BMC Microbiol. **8:** 170.

Fang W., Almeida R.A., and Oliver S.P.2000.Effects of lactoferrin and milk on adherence of Streptococcus uberis to bovine mammary epithelial cells. Am. J. Vet. Res. **61:** 275-279.

Field T.R., Ward P.N., Pedersen L.H. and Leigh J.A.2003.The hyaluronic acid capsule of Streptococcus uberis is not required for the development of infection and clinical mastitis. Infect. Immun. **71:** 132-139.

Finch J.M., Winter A., Walton A.W. and Leigh J.A.1997.Further studies on the efficacy of a live vaccine against mastitis caused by Streptococcus uberis. Vaccine. **15:** 1138-1143.

Flock M., Karlström A., Lannergård J., Guss B. and Flock JI.2006.Protective effect of vaccination with recombinant proteins from Streptococcus equi subspecies equi in a strangles model in the mouse. Vaccine. **24:** 4144-4151.

Florindo H.F., Pandit S., Gonçalves L.M., Alpar H.O. and Almeida A.J.2010.Surface modified polymeric nanoparticles for immunisation against equine strangles. Int. J. Pharm. **390:** 25-31.

Fluegge K., Schweier O., Schiltz E., Batsford S.and Berner R.2004.Identification and immunoreactivity of proteins released from Streptococcus agalactiae. Eur. J. Clin. Microbiol. Infect. Dis. **23:** 818-324.

Groschup, M.H., Hahn, G. and Timoney, J.F. 1991. Antigenic and genetic homogeneity of *Streptococcus uberis* strains from the bovine udder. Epidemiol. Infect. **107:** 297-310.

Gu H. and Lu C. 2008. [Identification and characterization of a novel infection-related factor (cell wall hydrolase/autolysin) of Streptococcus suis serotype 2]. Wei Sheng Wu Xue Bao. **48:** 68-72. [Article in Chinese]

Guss B., Flock M., Frykberg L., Waller A.S., Robinson C., Smith K.C. and Flock J.I.2009.Getting to grips with strangles: an effective multi-component recombinant vaccine for the protection of horses from Streptococcus equi infection. PLoS Pathog.5:e1000584. .

Gutekunst H., Eikmanns B.J.and Reinscheid D.J.2003.Analysis of RogB-controlled virulence mechanisms and gene repression in Streptococcus agalactiae. Infect. Immun. **71:** 5056-5064.

Gutekunst H., Eikmanns B.J. and Reinscheid D.J..2004.The novel fibrinogen-binding protein FbsB promotes Streptococcus agalactiae invasion into epithelial cells. Infect. Immun. 2004 **72:** 3495-3504.

Hamilton A., Robinson C., Sutcliffe I.C., Slater J., Maskell D.J., Davis-Poynter N., Smith K., Waller A. and Harrington D.J.2006.Mutation of the maturase lipoprotein attenuates the virulence of Streptococcus equi to a greater extent than does loss of general lipoprotein lipidation. Infect. Immun. **74:** 6907-6919.

Higgs, T.M., Neave, F.K. and Bramley, A.J. 1980. Differences in intramammary pathogenicity of four strains of *Streptococcus dysgalactiae*. J. Med. Microbiol. **12:** 393-399.

Hill A.W., Finch J.M., Field T.R. and Leigh J,A.1994.Immune modification of the pathogenesis of Streptococcus uberis mastitis in the dairy cow. FEMS Immunol, Med, Microbiol. **8:** 109-117.

Holt, M., Enright, M.R. and Alexander, T.J.L. 1988. Immunization of pigs with live cultures of *Streptococcus suis* type 2. Res. Vet. Sci. **45:** 349-352.

Hong-Jie F., Fu-yu T., Ying M., Cheng-ping L.2009. Virulence and antigenicity of the szp-gene deleted Streptococcus equi ssp. zooepidemicus mutant in mice. Vaccine. **27:** 56-61.

Huang J., Jiang X., Huang M., Yangi X., Liu M., Wang H. and Meng J.2011. [Influence of lysozyme-like protein on virulence and capsular polysaccharide synthesis of Streptococcus pneumoniae]. Wei. Sheng. Wu. Xue. Bao. **51:** 59-65.[Article in Chinese]

Jiang H., Fan H.J. and Lu C.P.2009.Identification and distribution of putative virulent genes in strains of Streptococcus suis serotype 2. Vet. Microbiol. **133:** 309-316.

Kim J.O., Romero-Steiner S., Sørensen U.B., Blom J., Carvalho M., Barnard S., Carlone G. and Weiser J.N.1999.Relationship between cell surface carbohydrates and intrastrain variation on opsonophagocytosis of Streptococcus pneumoniae. Infect. Immun. **67:** 2327-2333.

Klostermann K., Crispie F., Flynn J., Meaney W.J., Paul Ross R. and Hill C.2010.Efficacy of a teat dip containing the bacteriocin lacticin 3147 to eliminate Gram-positive pathogens associated with bovine mastitis. J Dairy Res. **77:** 231-238.

Kock C., Beineke A., Seitz M., Ganter M., Waldmann K.H., Valentin-Weigand P. and Baums C.G. 2009.Intranasal immunization with a live Streptococcus suis isogenic ofs mutant elicited suilysin-neutralization titers but failed to induce opsonizing antibodies and protection. Vet. Immunol. Immunopathol. **132:** 135-145.

Koskinen M.T., Holopainen J., Pyörälä S., Bredbacka P., Pitkälä A., Barkema H.W., Bexiga R., Roberson J., Sølverød L., Piccinini R., Kelton D., Lehmusto H., Niskala S. and Salmikivi L.2009.Analytical specificity and sensitivity of a real-time polymerase chain reaction assay for identification of bovine mastitis pathogens. J.Dairy Sci. **92:** 952-959.

Krishnan V., Gaspar A.H., Ye N., Mandlik A., Ton-That H. and Narayana S.V.2007.An IgG-like domain in the minor pilin GBS52 of Streptococcus agalactiae mediates lung epithelial cell adhesion. Structure. **15:** 893-903.

Kurl, D.N., Christensen, K.K. and Christensen, P. 1984. Colonization of the upper respiratory tract of mice with group B streptococci type III with reference to the R protein. J. Med. Microbiol. **17:** 347-351.

Lannergård J., Frykberg L. and Guss B.2003.CNE, a collagen-binding protein of Streptococcus equi. FEMS Microbiol. Lett. **222:** 69-74.

Lannergård J. Flock M., Johansson S., Flock J.I.and Guss B.2005.Studies of fibronectin-binding proteins of Streptococcus equi. Infect. Immun. **73:** 7243-7251.

Lapointe L., D'Allaire S., Lebrun A., Lacouture S. and Gottschalk M.2002.Antibody response to an autogenous vaccine and serologic profile for Streptococcus suis capsular type 1/2. Can. J. Vet. Res. **66:** 8-14.

Leigh J.A.2000.Vaccines against bovine mastitis due to Streptococcus uberis current status and future prospects. Adv. Exp. Med. Biol. **480:** 307-311.

Leigh J.A., Egan S.A., Ward P.N., Field T.R. and Coffey T.J. 2010.Sortase anchored proteins of Streptococcus uberis play major roles in the pathogenesis of bovine mastitis in dairy cattle. Vet, Res. **41:** 63.

.Li P., Liu J., Zhu L., Qi C., Bei W., Cai X., Sun Y. and Feng S.2010VirA: a virulence-related gene of Streptococcus suis serotype 2. Microb. Pathog. **49:** 305-310.

Lindahl G., Stålhammar-Carlemalm M. and Areschoug T.2005.Surface proteins of Streptococcus agalactiae and related proteins in other bacterial pathogens. Clin .Microbiol. Rev. **18:** 102-127.

Lindmark H. and Guss B.1999.SFS, a novel fibronectin-binding protein from Streptococcus equi, inhibits the binding between fibronectin and collagen. Infect. Immun. **67:** 2383-2388.

Luther D.A., Almeida R.A. and Oliver S.P.2008.Elucidation of the DNA sequence of Streptococcus uberis adhesion molecule gene (sua) and detection of sua in strains of Streptococcus uberis isolated from geographically diverse locations. Vet. Microbiol. **128:** 304-312.

.Mackintosh, M.E., Grant, S.T. and Buffel, M.H. 1988. Evidence for *Streptococcus pneumonia* as a cause of respiratory disease in young thoroughbred horses in training. In Equine Diseases V. Ed. D.G. Powell pp. 41-46, Lexington University of Kentucky Press.

Maneke E., Pridmore A., Goby L.and Lang L..2011.Kill rate of mastitis pathogens by a combination of cefalexin and kanamycin. J. Appl. Microbiol. **110:** 184-190.

McDonald W.L., Fry B.N.and Deighton M.A..2005.Identification of Streptococcus spp. causing bovine mastitis by PCR-RFLP of 16S-23S ribosomal DNA. Vet Microbiol. **111:** 241-246.

Meehan M., Lewis M.J., Byrne C., O'Hare D., Woof J.M. and Owen P.2009.Localization of the equine IgG-binding domain in the fibrinogen-binding protein (FgBP) of Streptococcus equi subsp. equi. Microbiology. **155:** 2583-2592.

Meehan M., Lynagh Y., Woods C., Owen P.2001.The fibrinogen-binding protein (FgBP) of Streptococcus equi subsp. equi additionally binds IgG and contributes to virulence in a mouse model. . Microbiology. **147:** 3311-3322.

Meehan M., Muldowney D.A., O'Meara F. and Owen P.2000 a.Neither the A- nor B-repeat regions of the fibrinogen-binding protein of Streptococcus equi subsp. equi are essential for fibrinogen binding. FEMS Microbiol; Lett. **190:** 317-321.

Meehan M., Muldowney D.A., Watkins N.J. and Owen P.2000 b.Localization and characterization of the ligand-binding domain of the fibrinogen-binding protein (FgBP) of Streptococcus equi subsp. equi. Microbiology. **146:** 1187-1194.

Meehan M., Burke F.M., Macken S. and Owen P.2010.Characterization of the haem-uptake system of the equine pathogen Streptococcus equi subsp. equi. Microbiology. **156:** 1824-1835.

Mukhtar, M.M. and Timoney, J.F. 1988. Chemotactic response of equine polymorphonuclear leucocytes to *Streptococcus equi*. Res. Vet. Sci. **45:** 225-229.

Newton J.R., Verheyen K., Talbot N.C., Timoney J.F., Wood J.L., Lakhani K.H. and Chanter N. 2000.Control of strangles outbreaks by isolation of guttural pouch carriers identified using PCR and culture of Streptococcus equi. Equine Vet. J. **32:** 515-526.

Oxoby M., Moreau F., Durant L., Denis A., Genevard J.M., Vongsouthi V., Escaich S. and Gerusz V.2010.Towards Gram-positive antivirulence drugs: New inhibitors of Streptococcus agalactiae Stk1. Bioorg. Med. Chem. Lett. 2010 May 7. [http://www.ncbi.nlm.nih.gov/pubmed/20580885].

Padungtod P., Tharavichitkul P., Junya S., Chaisowong W., Kadohira M., Makino S. and Sthitmatee N.2010.Incidence and presence of virulence factors of Streptococcus suis infection in slaughtered pigs from Chiang Mai, Thailand. Southeast Asian J. Trop. Med. Public. Health. **41:** 1454-1461.

Paillot R., Darby A.C., Robinson C., Wright N.L., Steward K.F., Anderson E., Webb K., Holden M.T., Efstratiou A., Broughton K., Jolley K.A., Priestnall S.L., Marotti Campi M.C., Hughes M.A., Radford A., Erles K. and Waller A.S.2010.Identification of three novel superantigen-encoding genes in Streptococcus equi subsp. zooepidemicus, szeF, szeN, and szeP. Infect. Immun. **78:** 4817-4827.

Palanivel, K.M., Thangathurai, R. and Ganesan, P.I. 2005. Prevalence of subclinical mastitis in buffaloes in and around Chennai (Madras) Buff. Jour. **21:** 127-133.

Patel D., Almeida R.A., Dunlap J.R. and Oliver S.P.2009.Bovine lactoferrin serves as a molecular bridge for internalization of Streptococcus uberis into bovine mammary epithelial cells. Vet. Microbiol. **137:** 297-301.

Patil K.P., Patil D.K., Chaudhari B.L. and Chincholkar S.B.2011.Production of hyaluronic acid from Streptococcus zooepidemicus MTCC 3523 and its wound healing activity. J. Biosci. Bioeng. **111:** 286-288.

Petrovski K., Laven R. and Lopez-Villalobos N.2011.A descriptive analysis of the antimicrobial susceptibility of mastitis-causing bacteria isolated from samples submitted to commercial diagnostic laboratories in New Zealand (2003-2006). N. Z. Vet. J. **59:** 59-66.

Priestnall S.L., Erles K., Brooks H.W., Cardwell J.M., Waller A.S., Paillot R., Robinson C., Darby A.C., Holden M.T. and Schöniger S.2010Characterization of pneumonia due to Streptococcus equi subsp. zooepidemicus in dogs. Clin. Vaccine Immunol. **17:** 1790-1796.

Rainard, P. and Boulard, C. 1992. Opsonization of *Streptococcus agalactiae* of bovine origin by complement and antibodies against group B polysaccharide. Infect. Immun. **60:** 4801-4808.

Ravishakar, C., Muthuramalingam, M., Shenoy, S.J. Min, M. and Jay prakasan, V. 2005. Isolation of *Streptococcus suis* from a fatal case of pneumonitis in a boar. Indian Vet. Jour. **82:** 910-911.

Reinoso E.B., Lasagno M.C., Dieser S.A., Odierno L.M.2011.Distribution of virulence-associated genes in Streptococcus uberis isolated from bovine mastitis. FEMS Microbiol. Lett. 2011 Mar 8. doi: 10.1111/j.1574-968.2011.02258.x.[http://www.ncbi.nlm.nih.gov/pubmed/21385204]

Robertson, I.D. and Blackmore, D.K. 1989. Vet. Rec. **124:** 391.

Robinson, J.H. and Kehoe, M.A. 1992. Group A *Streptococcal* M proteins. Virulence factors and protective antigen S. Immonol. Today **13:** 362-367.

Samen U., Heinz B., Boisvert H., Eikmanns B.J., Reinscheid D.J. and Borges F.2011.Rga is a regulator of adherence and pili formation in Streptococcus agalactiae. Microbiology. 2011 Feb 17. [http://www.ncbi.nlm.nih.gov/pubmed/21330442]

Schubert A., Zakikhany K., Pietrocola G., Meinke A., Speziale P., Eikmanns B.J. and Reinscheid D.J.2004.The fibrinogen receptor FbsA promotes adherence of Streptococcus agalactiae to human epithelial cells. Infect. Immun. **72:** 6197-6205.

Shome, R., Shome, B.R., Dev Sharma, S.P., Ashok Kumar and Rehman, H. 2006. Chronic respiratory infection in piglets caused by *Streptococcus suis*. Indian Vet. J. **83:** 94-95.

Silva L.M., Baums C.G., Rehm T., Wisselink H.J., Goethe R. and Valentin-Weigand P.2006.Virulence-associated gene profiling of Streptococcus suis isolates by PCR. Vet .Microbiol. **115:** 117-127.

Smith, H.E., Vecht, U., Gielkens, A.L.J. and Smits, M.A. 1992. Cloning and nuclotide sequencing of the gene encoding the 136 kDa surface protein (muramidase releasd protein) of *S.suis* type 2. Infect. Immun. **60:** 2361-2367.

Smith H.E., Damman M., van der Velde J., Wagenaar F., Wisselink H.J., Stockhofe-Zurwieden N. and Smits M.A.1999.Identification and characterization of the cps locus of Streptococcus suis serotype 2: the capsule protects against phagocytosis and is an important virulence factor. Infect. Immun. **67:** 1750-1756.

Soriani M.and Telford J.L..2010.Relevance of pili in pathogenic streptococci pathogenesis and vaccine development. Future Microbiol. **5:** 735-747.

Srivastava, S.K. and Barnum, D.A. 1983. Adherence of *Streptococcus equi* on tongue, cheek and nasal epithelial cells of ponies. Vet. Microbiol. **8:** 493-504.

Srivastava, S.K. and Barnum, D.A. 1983. Vaccination of pony foals with M like protein of *Streptococcus equi*. Am. J. Vet. Res. **44:** 41-55.

Srivastava, S.K. and Barnum, D.A. 1985. Studies on the immunogenicity of *Streptococcus equi* vaccines in foals. Can. J. Comp. Med. **49:** 351.

Srivastava, S.K., Barnum, D.A. and Prescott, J.F. 1985. Production and biological properties of M protein of *Streptococcus equi*. Res. Vet. Sci. **38:** 184-188.

Sundberg, J.P., Hill, D., Wyand, D.S. Ryan, M.I. and Baldwin, C.H. 1981. *Streptococcus zooepidemicus* as the cause of septicaemia in racing greyhounds. Vet. Med. Small Anim. Clin. **177:** 839-842.

Suzuki H., Lefébure T., Hubisz M.J., Pavinski Bitar P., Lang P., Siepel A. and Stanhope M.J.2011.Comparative Genomic Analysis of the Streptococcus dysgalactiae Species Group: Gene Content, Molecular Adaptation, and Promoter Evolution. Genome Biol. Evol. **3:** 168-185.

Tanabe, Shin-Ichi, Laetitia Bonifait, Nahuel Fittipaldi, Louis Grignon, Marcelo Gottschalk, and Daniel Grenier .2010.Pleiotropic effects of polysaccharide capsule loss on selected biological properties of *Streptococcus suis*. Can .J. Vet. Res. **74:** 65–70.

Telford J.L., Barocchi M.A., Margarit I., Rappuoli R. and Grandi G.2006.Pili in gram-positive pathogens. Nat. Rev. Microbiol. **4:** 509-519.

Timoney, J.F. 1993. Streptococcus. In pathogenesis of bacterial diseases in animals ed. C.L. Gyles and C.O. Thoen pp 3-20. International Book Distributing Co. Lucknow, India.

Timoney J.F.2004.The pathogenic equine streptococci. Vet. Res. **35:** 397-409.

Timoney, J.F. and Galan, J.E. 1985. The immune response of the horse to an virulent strain of *Streptococcus equi*. In Recent Advances in Streptococci and Streptococcal diseases. Ed. Y. Kimura, S. Kotami & Y. Shiokawa pp 294-95. Bracknell, UK, Reedbooks.

Timoney J.F. and Kumar P.2008.Early pathogenesis of equine Streptococcus equi infection (strangles). Equine Vet. J. **40:** 637-642.

Timoney J.F., Qin A., Muthupalani S. and Artiushin S.2007.Vaccine potential of novel surface exposed and secreted proteins of Streptococcus equi. Vaccine. **25:** 5583-5590.

Tiwari R., Qin A., Artiushin S. and Timoney JF.2007.Se18.9, an anti-phagocytic factor H binding protein of Streptococcus equi. Vet. Microbiol. **121:** 105-115.

Vengadesan K., Ma X., Dwivedi P., Ton-That H.and Narayana S.V.2011.A Model for Group B Streptococcus Pilus Type 1: The Structure of a 35-kDa C-Terminal Fragment of the Major Pilin GBS80. J. Mol. Biol. **407:** 731-743.

Vecht, U., Wisselink, H.J., Van Dizk, J.E. and Smith, H.E. 1992. Virulence of *Streptococcus suis* type 2 strain in new born germfree pigs depends on phenotype. Infect. Immun. **60:** 550-556.

Wallace F.J., Emery J.D., Cripps A.W. and Husband A,J.1995.An assessment of mucosal immunisation in protection against Streptococcus equi ('Strangles') infections in horses. Vet, Immunol, Immunopathol.**48:** 139-154.

Waller A., Flock M., Smith K., Robinson C., Mitchell Z., Karlström A., Lannergård J., Bergman R., Guss B. and Flock J.I. 2007.Vaccination of horses against strangles using recombinant antigens from Streptococcus equi. Vaccine. **25:** 3629-3635.

Wang Y., Zhang W., Wu Z., Lu C..2011.Reduced virulence is an important characteristic of biofilm infection of Streptococcus suis. FEMS Microbiol. Lett. **316:** 36-43.

Weese J.S., Jarlot C.and Morley P.S.2009.Survival of Streptococcus equi on surfaces in an outdoor environment. Can. Vet. J. **50:** 968-970.

Widders P.R., Warner S. and Huntington P.J.1995.Immunisation of mares to control endometritis caused by Streptococcus zooepidemicus. Res. Vet. Sci. **58:** 75-81.

Willenborg J., Fulde M., de Greeff A., Rohde M., Smith H.E., Valentin-Weigand P. and Goethe R.2011.Role of glucose and CcpA in capsule expression and virulenceof Streptococcus suis. Microbiology. 2011 Feb 24. [http://www.ncbi.nlm.nih.gov/pubmed/21349980].

Wilson, W.D. 1988. Equine Pract. **10:** 12.

Xu L., Huang B., Du H., Zhang X.C., Xu J., Li X. and Rao Z.2010.Crystal structure of cytotoxin protein suilysin from Streptococcus suis. Protein Cell. **1:** 96-105.

Zadoks R.N., Gillespie B.E., Barkema H.W., Sampimon O.C., Oliver S.P. and Schukken Y.H.2003.Clinical, epidemiological and molecular characteristics of Streptococcus uberis infections in dairy herds. Epidemiol. Infect. **130:** 335-349.

Zhu H., Gu H. and Lu C.2008. [Identification and detection of trag: a new infection-related gene expressed in vivo from isolates of Streptococcus suis]. Wei. Sheng. Wu. Xue. Bao 4; **48:** 1642-8. [Article in Chinese].

□□□

Chapter 7

Diseases Caused by *Shigella* spp.

Dr. S.K. SRIVASTAVA
Former, Division of Bacteriology & Mycology
Indian Veterinary Research Institute, Izatnagar-243122
Bareilly (U.P.)

Members of the genus *Shigella* are responsible for causing shigellosis, which exclusively occurs in captive primates and appears to be related to stressful situation. In India shigellosis is a major cause of diarrhoea in human beings (Taneja 2007). Shigella dysentery may account for as much as 80% of all deaths among newly imported monkeys. Shigella flexneri was isolated from feces of lion-tailed macaques. Shigella sonnei was isolated from feces of grey-cheeked mangabeys, celebes macaques, and spider monkeys in zoological park sample collection in USA(Banish *et al*.1993)..The Shigella species are occasionally associated with dysentery in puppies. *Shigella* species are classified by seven serogroups:

- Serogroup *A*: *S. dysenteriae* (12 serotypes)
- Serogroup *B*: *S. flexneri* (6 serotypes)
- Serogroup *C*: *S. boydii* (23 serotypes)
- Serogroup *D*: *S. sonnei* (1 serotype)

Group *A–C* are physiologically similar; *S. sonnei* (group *D*) can be differentiated on the basis of biochemical metabolism assays. Three *Shigella* groups are the major disease-causing species: *S. flexneri* is the most frequently isolated species worldwide and accounts for 60% of cases in the developing world; *S. sonnei* causes 77% of cases in the developed world, compared to only 15% of cases in the developing world; and *S. dysenteriae* is usually the cause of epidemics of dysentery, particularly in confined populations such as refugee camps.

There are several serovars of these species, respectively, identified by Arabic numerals and 2 serovars of *S.flexneri* that are identified as X and Y. Four of the serovars (1-4) of *S.flexneri* are divided into 9 subserovars, Ia, Ib, 2a, 2b, 3a, 3b, 3c, 4a and 4b. Identification of species is based on O-repeat units of lipopolysaccharide. Humans are affected by all four species of *Shigella* whereas non-human primates are affected by all except *S.dysenteriae*. The genus is named after Kiyoshi Shiga, who first discovered it in 1898. In primates a subclinical carrier state is common and overt disease may be precipitated by stress. Signs include watery to bloody diarrhea,weakness, and edema of the face and neck. Rectal prolapse is common. High mortality can result from Shigellosis in NHP. Recovered animals often are carriers and serve as a reservoir of infection. Post mortem lesions include ulcerative colitis, distended hyperemic large intestine with mucus and blood in lumen, and enlarged mesenteric lymph nodes.

Shigella are gram-negative, non-motile, non-capsulated, lactose negative members of the family Enterobacteriaceae. Shigellosis is characterized by frequent passage of low volume of stool that contains blood, mucus and inflammatory cells. Disease caused by *S.dysenteriae* is more severe than caused by other species. Shigella dysenteriae serotype 1 causes deadly epidemics but Shigella boydii is restricted to the Indian subcontinent, while Shigella flexneri and Shigella sonnei are prevalent in developing and developed countries respectively. To begin to explain these distinctive epidemiological and pathological features at the genome level, Yang *et al.* (2005) carried out comparative genomics on four representative strains. Each of the Shigella genomes includes a virulence plasmid that encodes conserved primary virulence determinants. The Shigella chromosomes share most of their genes with that of E. coli K12 strain MG1655, but each has over 200 pseudogenes, 300 approximately 700 copies of insertion sequence (IS) elements, and numerous deletions, insertions, translocations and inversions. There is extensive diversity of putative virulence genes, mostly acquired via bacteriophage-mediated lateral gene transfer. Hence, via convergent evolution involving gain and loss of functions, through bacteriophage-mediated gene acquisition, IS-mediated DNA rearrangements and formation of pseudogenes, the *Shigella* spp. became highly specific human pathogens with variable epidemiological and pathological features.

The organisms invade the colonic epithelium and induce an inflammatory response that leads to formation of colonic abscesses. A mannose resistant adhesin is responsible for colonic pathology. Under anaerobic conditions of the intestine *S.flexneri* expresses its pathogenic effect or system that facilitates entry to intestinal epithelium (Baxt and Goldberg 2010). Shigellosis may be accompanied with number of complications, most commonly the haemolytic uraemic syndrome which is very serious. Organisms as low as 10 to 100 in number can cause the disease.

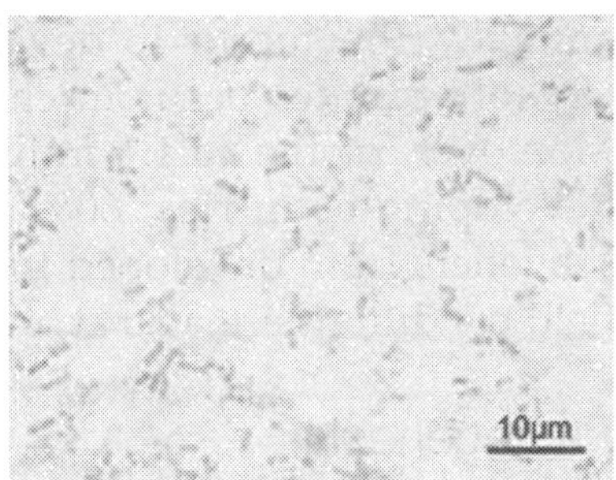

Shigella flexneri gram stained

Epidemiology

Shigellosis is endemic in developing countries were sanitation is poor. Typically 10 to 20 percent of enteric disease, and 50% of the bloody diarrhea or dysentery of young children, can be characterized as shigellosis, and the prevalence of these infections decreases significantly after five years of life. In developed countries, single-source, food or water-borne outbreaks occur sporadically, and pockets of endemic shigellosis can be found in institutions and in remote areas with substandard sanitary facilities.

Epidemics in man have been reported in Central American countries, Bangladesh, Sri Lanka, Maldives, Nepal, Bhutan, Myanmar and several states of India.

The epidemiology and antibiotic sensitivity of Shigella species is changing worldwide. Yurdakok *et al.* (1997) surveyed the changing clinical and epidemiological characteristics and antibiotic susceptibility of Shigella gastroenteritis in Hacettepe University Ihsan Dogramaci Children's Hospital Diarrhoea Training and Treatment Unit between 1987 and 1994. Among 19,812 diarrheal admissions, 618 (3.2%) patient files with Shigella gastroenteritis were reviewed retrospectively. Shigella soneii has been the commonest isolate (64%) since 1987 followed by S. flexineri (30%), S. boydii (5%) and S. dysenteriae (1%), the latter having not been isolated since 1990. The isolate rate of *S. sonnei* has increased whereas the isolation rate of S. flexineri has decreased concomitantly since 1987 ($r = -0.94$; $P < 0.001$). The majority of cases (365/618, 59%) were between 1 and 5 years of age. On admission bloody diarrhea was present in 36%, seizures in 3% and mild-moderate dehydration in 11% of cases. No case had severe dehydration. Only six patients (1%) were hospitalized. No deaths were recordedChanging Shigella sp. over the years may be the reason for the mild course of Shigella gastroenteritis. Further regional epidemiological studies are necessary to develop more appropriate management guidelines, especially in developing countries. Of the estimated 165 million cases of Shigella diarrhoea that occur annually, 99% occur in developing countries, and in developing countries 69% of episodes occur in children under five years of age (Niyogi, 2005). Moreover, of the ca.1.1 million deaths attributed to Shigella infections in developing countries, 60% of deaths occur in the under-five age group. Travellers from developed to developing regions and soldiers serving under field conditions are also at an increased risk to develop shigellosis.

Pathogenesis

Several proteins are responsible for expression of virulence by *Shigella* following their entrance and multiplication in the small intestine which results in a toxin mediated diarrhoea. The organism has the ability to resist gastric acidity. With in 2-3 days the organisms leave the small intestine and establish in the colon. RNA polymerase containing Rpous gene is responsible for acid tolerance allowing safe transit through the stomach. The organisms adhere on the colonic cell surface most possibly through a 38 kDa protein, Ipa D. The intestinal epithelium undergoes a rapid turnover in addition to rapid exfoliation in response to bacterial infection, thus acting as an intrinsic defense against microbial intruders. It has long been questioned how mucosal pathogens can circumvent the intestinal defense systems. Shigella delivers OspE via the type III secretion system during multiplication within epithelial cells (Kim *et al.* 2010). This effector protein reinforces epithelial adherence to the basement membrane by interacting with integrin-linked kinase (ILK), a unique intracellular Ser/Thr kinase that links the cell-adhesion receptors, integrin, and growth factors to the actin cytoskeleton. The interaction between OspE and ILK increased formation of focal adhesions (FAs) and surface levels of b1-integrin, while suppressing phosphorylation of FAK and paxillin, thus suppressing rapid turnover of FAs, reducing cell motility and promoting cell adhesion to extracellular matrix. The impact of this OspE-ILK interplay was demonstrated both in vitro and in vivo by infecting polarized epithelial cell monolayers and guinea pig colons with Shigella possessing or lacking the ospE gene. This findings thus establish a new class of virulence-associated factors, and provide new insight into the functioning of the intestinal barrier and bacterial strategies for circumventing it.

The organisms invade epithelium through M cells and this up take is initiated by 2 proteins, Ipa B and Ipa C. The organisms multiply in the vacuole and the protein Ipa B causes lysis of vacuole resulting in escape of the organisms. The organisms multiply rapidly in cytoplasm which is associated with cells protrusions and intracellular spread is facilitated by another protein Ics A. Initially, the bacteria express organelle like movement along actin of the cell cytoskeleton (Vasselon *et al.*, 1991) and subsequently become covered with filamentous actin, whose movement propels the bacteria in the cells resulting in intercellular spread. This intercellular spread is also caused by Ics B. This results in cell death due to blockage of respiration and infection of the adjacent cells. The mechanism responsible for shutdown of host cell respiration is due to non-functionality of mitochondria. A drop in intracellular ATP is seen. An *S.flexneri* outer membrane protein Ics P has been identified which cleaves the actin based motility protein IsA from the bacterial surface (Hensley *et al.*, 2011), and consequently modulates Shigella actin based motility and cell to cell spread. Ics A is an outer membrane protein which is localized to the old pole of bacterium and is both necessary and sufficient for actin assembly (Steinhauer *et al.*, 1999). Ics A is a 120 kDa outer membrane protein necessary for actin based motility and is located on a single pole of the bacterium (Goldberg and Thariot, 1995). These proteins which act as important virulence factors are present on large plasmids, termed invasion plasmids. These genes for the most part are regulated by at least 6 chromosomal genes. The plasmid gene products encode proteins, Mxi and Spa proteins that are responsible for excretion of virulence proteins. The organisms then invade submucosa and damage blood vessels resulting in dysentery. A toxin is responsible for the production of dysentery. Two enterotoxins have been described, ShET1 (Chromosomal Shigella enterotoxin) and a 63 kDa product of the sen gene (Invasion plasmid Shigella enterotoxin). The exact mechanism of their function is yet to be explored.

Another major factor in the virulence is the ability of Shigella to penetrate and multiply within the epithelial cells of colon. Type III secretion system encoded on a large plasmid is a key virulence factor of *Shigella flexneri*. The powerful weapon of Shigella spp. is Type Three Secretion System, which remains the focus of pathogenic research.This secretion system determines the interaction of *S.flexneri* with intestinal cells by consecutively translocating 2 sets of effector proteins into the target cells. Thus *S.flexneri* control invasion into cells, inter and intra-cellular spread, macrophage cell death and host inflammatory responses. Some of the translocated effector proteins show novel biochemical activities by which they intercept host cell signal transduction pathways (Schroeder and Hilbi 2008). Some 25-30 effectors are injected into host cells by the type III secretion system (Parsot 2009). Two different set of effectors are involved in inducing actin cytoskeleton reorganization to promote epithelial all entry. Research performed over the last 25 years revealed that a type III secretion system (T3SS) encoded on a large plasmid is a key virulence factor of Shigella flexneri. The T3SS determines the interactions of S. flexneri with intestinal cells by consecutively translocating two sets of effector proteins into the target cells. Thus, S. flexneri controls invasion into EC, intra- and intercellular spread, macrophage cell death, as well as host inflammatory responses. Some of the translocated effector proteins show novel biochemical activities by which they intercept host cell signal transduction pathways.

The type III secretion system is composed of a basal body and an exposed needle with invasive plasmid antigen D forming a tip complex that control secretion. The bile salt deoxycholate (DOC) stimulates recruitment of the translocator protein Ipa B into the maturing type III secretion system needle tip complex. This process appears to be triggered by a direct interaction between DOC and Ipa D (Dickenson *et al.*, 2010).

The type III secretion system is essential for cell invasion and virulence in anaerobic environment of gastrointestinal tract. The type III secretion system is primed for invasion and expresses extended needles while reducing Ipa effector system. This is mediated by fumarate and nitrate reduction, a regulator of anaerobic metabolism that represses transcription of Spa 32 and Spa33 virulence genes that regulate secretion through the type III secretion system. Marteyn *et al.* (2010) demonstrated a zone of relative oxygenation adjacent to the gastrointestinal tract mucosa, caused by diffusion from the capillary network at the tips of villi. This reverses the anaerobic block of Ipa secretion, allowing type III secretion system activation at its precise site of action, enhancing invasion and virulence. Experimental infections (oral) in monkeys with S. flexneri 2a develop severe colitis with diarrhoea or dysentery or both. However, more studies have shown that dysenteriae is the essential feature of shigellosis and that the early diarrhoeal phase often seen in some animals is due to fluid disturbances in the jejunum, associated with the presence of bacteria in that part of the intestine. Diarrhoea is probably brought about by the activation of phospholipase C leading to increase in intracellular calcium ions, activation of protein kinase C and subsequent phosphorylation of protein of the chloride ion channels and those of the membrane associated ion transport proteins involved in Nacl absorption.

In the pathogenesis of shigellosis the organism penetrate the epithelial cells. This internalization occurs by a phagocytosis like (endocytosis) process in the epithelial cells. It involves polymerization of actin and accumulation of myosin. This endocytosis requires energy production by the bacterium and the epithelial cells. The cellular inflammatory reaction is confined to the mucosa and the submucosa is involved by edema only. It has been postulated that the bacteria enters through apical surface of colonic epithelial cells but evidences are there which support the view that *S.flexneri* enters through M cells in the colon and spread to villus epithelial cells (Mounier *et al.*, 1992; Hale and keren 1992). The enteric glial cells and cell derived *S-nitrosoglutathione* play important protective function in the intestinal epithelial barrier against *S.flexneri* attack (Flamant *et al.*, 2010).

The lipopolysaccharide (LPS) of *Shigella* organisms is required for the virulence. LPS may contribute to the systemic disturbances in shigellosis. Rough strains devoid of LPS are unable to spread to neighboring cells and are readily eliminated from the host (Hale 1991). Changes in the LPS core can alter virulence, possibly due to its affect on the outer membrane organization. Heterogeneity of LPS occurs in several mutants of *Shigella sonnei* due to phosphate and fatty acid composition (Kilar *et al.*, 2011). Table 1 show the bacterial products implicated in virulence of *Shigella*. The structure of the repeating unit of the O-antigen polysaccharide from Shigella flexneri provisional serotype 88-893 has been determined (Foster *et al.*, 2011).. The carbohydrate part of the hexasaccharide repeating unit is identical to the previously elucidated structure of the O-polysaccharide from *S. flexneri* prov. serotype Y394. The O-antigen of *S. flexneri* prov. serotype 88-893 carries 0.7mol O-acetyl group per repeating unit located at O-2 of the 3-substituted rhamnosyl residue, as identified by H2BC and BS-CT-HMBC NMR experiments. The O-antigen polysaccharide is composed of hexasaccharide repeating units with the following structure: >2)-α-l-Rhap-(1>2)-α-l-Rhap-(1>3)-α-l-Rhap2Ac-(1>3)[α-d-Glcp-(1>2)-α-d-Glcp-(1>4)]-β-d-GlcpNAc-(1>. Serological studies showed that type antigens for the two provisional serotypes are identical; in addition 88-893 expresses *S. flexneri* group factor 6 antigen.

Shigella posses the property to produce a congo red binding protein, genes of which are carried on a large virulence plasmid. Congo red binding appears to be affected by a 101 kDa haeme-binding protein on the bacterial surface and hemin can substitute for congo red in binding studies. Role of congo red binding property with the virulence is not known but it has been found that binding to congo red can induce expression of *Shigella* virulence genes (Maurelli *et al.*, 1992).

Toxins

Shigella dysenteriae is the only member of the group that has the gene (Chromosomal) necessary for production of shiga toxin. The toxin is cytotoxic, enterotoxic and lethal and inhibits protein synthesis, leading to cell death. Toxin binds to the glycolipid receptor, globotriosylceramide and is internalized by receptor mediated endocytosis. The toxin containing vesicle probably fuses with lysosomes and is transported to the golgi apparatus before release into cytosol. The toxin is a 70,000 MW protein composed of A subunit (32,000 MW) and five identical B subunits (each about 7700 MW). The toxins act on the endothelial cells of the blood vessels. B subunits mediated binding on specific receptors and the A subunit affects the elongation factor-1 dependent process which inhibit elongation of peptide chains at the level of the ribosomes, leading to the cell death. This toxin is the important virulence factor. Shigatoxin appears to increase the severity of dysentery by damaging small blood vessels of large intestine, resulting in oedema haemorrhage and an increased inflammatory response (Fontaine *et al.,* 1988). Toxin inhibits Na^+, Cl^- absorption and promotes premature expulsion of mature, absorptive villus epithelial cells in rabbit small intestine (Kandel *et al.,* 1989). Shigella has been reported to produce a protein termed Shigella enterotoxin 2 (Farfan *et al.,* 2011). This enterotoxin induces rise in short circuit current in rabbit ileum. It has been postulated that this toxin may be secreted by the Shigella type III secretion system. The toxin might also participate in the *Shigella* induced inflammation of epithelial cells.

Spent medium from *S flexneri* or EIEC cultures elicits fluid accumulation in rabbit ligated ileal loops and ion secretion in isolated ileal tissue. Using these assays, enterotoxins designated ShET1 and ShET2 have been identified, and the genetic loci encoding these toxins have been localized to the chromosome and plasmid, respectively. ShET1 is neutralized by convalescent sera from volunteers challenged with *S flexneri* 2a, suggesting that this toxic moiety is expressed by *shigellae* growing in the human intestine. The ShET1 locus is present on the chromosome of *S flexneri*2a, but it is only occasionally found in other serotypes. In contrast, ShET2 is more widespread and detectable in 80% of *shigellae* representing all four species. These enterotoxins may elicit the diarrheal prodrome that often precedes bacillary dysentery; however, their role in the disease process remains to be defined by controlled challenge studies using toxin-negative mutants.

S dysenteriae serotype 1 expresses Shiga toxin, an extremely potent, ricin-like, cytotoxin that inhibits protein synthesis in susceptible mammalian cells. This toxin also has enterotoxic activity in rabbit ileal loops, but its role in human diarrhea is unclear, since shigellae apparently express a number of enterotoxins. Experimental infection of rhesus monkeys with *S dysenteriae* 1, and with a Shiga toxin-negative mutant, suggests that this cytotoxin causes capillary destruction and focal hemorrhage that exacerbates dysentery . More importantly, Shiga toxin is associated with the hemolytic-uremic syndrome, a complication of infections with *S dysenteriae* 1. Closely related toxins are expressed by enterohemorrhagic *E coli* (EHEC) including the potentially lethal, food-borne O157-H7 serotype.

Table 1 : Several bacterial products associated with the virulence of *Shigella*

Bacterial Products	Virulence Effect
Plasmid encoded products	
Congo red binding (101 kDa protein)	Binds hemin; induces expression of virulence genes
Invasion protein antigens	Uptake of *Shigella* and lysis of vacuoles
IpB (62 kDa)	Invasin, Cytolysin
IpaC (42 kDa)	Invasin
Ics A (Vir G) (120 kDa)	Positive sereny test; intracellular survival and multiplication
Ics B	Lysis of cellular protrusions
Mxi A, Mxi B	Export of invasion protein
Vir B	Positive regulator of invasion genes
Vir F (30 kDa)	Positive regulator of plasmid virulence genes.
Ipa D	Induces Shigella - host cell interaction
Chromosomal Products	
Hydroxamate siderophore system	Promotes multiplication in tissues
Kcp A	Positive sereny test
LPS	Required for invasion
Omp B	Modulation of expression of plasmid virulence genes
Superoxide dismutase	Resistance to killing by leukocytes and macrophages
Shiga toxin (*S.dysenteriae I*)	Vascular damage in the intestine; systemic effects
Vir R	Repressor of plasmid virulence genes

Source : Gyles, 1993

Expression of *Shigella* virulence is regulated by the temperature at which the organisms are grown. Strains which are phenotypically virulent when grown at 37 °C are phenotypically avirulent at 30 °C. The chromosomal gene virR, which is required for the temperature - dependent regulation of *Shigella* species (Gyles 1993), has been identified.

Shigella organisms produce different proteins when the organism is intracellular compared with extra-cellular environment. Headley and Payne (1990) reported a high expression of a 140 kDa protein and an 80 kDa protein

(IpaA) during intracellular growth of *S.flexneri* compared with earlier stages of infection of Hella cells.

Host Defense

Shigellae are remarkably infectious enteric pathogenes that can cause disease after the ingestion of as few as 10 organisms. Nonetheless, shigellosis is normally an acute, self-limiting disease that exemplifies the regenerative capacity of the intestinal epithelium. *Shigella* virulence probably reflects both the efficient uptake by the follicle associated epithelium (M cells) and the amplifying effect of the inflammatory cascade generated by apoptic macrophages. Tenesmus and evacuation of mucus by intestinal goblet cells may effectively eliminate both extracellular *shigellae* and infected enterocytes from the intestinal lumen, but this defensive response, in conjunction with PMN infiltration, also constitutes the definitive sign of bacillary dysentery. The host response to primary infection is characterized by the induction of an acute inflammation, which is accompanied by the polymorphonuclear cell (PMN) infiltration, resulting in massive destruction of the colonic mucosa. However, PMN play a major role in the recovery from primary infection, by restricting the bacterial infection at the intestinal mucosa. Le-Barillec *et al.* (2005) assessed the roles for T and NK cells in the control of primary *S. flexneri* infection, using an alymphoid mouse strain (Rag null gamma(c) null) devoid of B, T, and NK cells. Using the mouse pulmonary model of Shigella infection, it was showed that alymphoid Rag null gamma(c) null mice were highly susceptible to S. flexneri infection in comparison with wild-type (wt) mice. Whereas PMN recruitment upon infection was similar, macrophage recruitment and production of proinflammatory cytokines were significantly decreased in Rag null gamma(c) null mice compared with wt mice. Upon selective engraftment of Rag null gamma(c) null mice with polyclonal alphabeta T cells, but not with alphabeta T cells from IFN-gamma null, *S. flexneri* infection could be subsequently controlled. Rag null mice devoid of B and T cells but harboring NK cells could control infection. Local IFN-gamma production by T and NK cells recruited to the lung was demonstrated in *S. flexneri*-infected wt mice. These data demonstrate that both alphabeta T cells and NK cells contribute to the early control of *S. flexneri* infection through amplification of an inflammatory response. This cellular lymphocyte redundancy assures IFN-gamma production, which is central to innate immunity against *Shigella* infection.

To identify immune effectors associated with protection of the naive host during infection, the susceptibility to pulmonary *Shigella* infection of each of various mouse strains that have a targeted deletion in a specific aspect of the immune system was evaluated (Way *et al.*, 1998). The results demonstrate that mice deficient in gamma interferon are 5 orders of magnitude more susceptible to Shigella than are wild-type mice, whereas mice deficient in B and T lymphocytes or in T lymphocytes alone exhibit no difference in susceptibility. Significantly lower numbers of shigellae were recovered from immunocompetent compared with gamma-interferon-deficient mice after infection. While immunocompetent mice were able to clear a sublethal *Shigella* inoculum by day 5 postinfection, progressively increasing numbers of *shigellae* were cultured from the lungs of gamma interferon-deficient mice over the same period. Histopathology of the lungs from immunocompetent mice infected with a sublethal *Shigella* inoculum showed mild inflammatory changes, whereas the lungs from gamma interferon-deficient mice demonstrated progressively worsening acute bronchiolitis with ulceration. Further, the time to death in gamma interferon-deficient mice correlates inversely with the size of the *Shigella* inoculum. To identify the cellular source of gamma interferon, the authors infected SCID mice, T-cell-receptor-deficient mice, beige mice (a mouse strain deficient in natural killer [NK] cell activity), and mice depleted of NK cells using anti-asialo-GM1. Each NK cell-deficient mouse strain exhibited a 10-fold-greater susceptibility to *Shigella* infection than immunocompetent mice. To test the protective effects of gamma interferon in vitro, survival of intracellular *Shigella* was examined in primary macrophages from wild-type mice, primary macrophages from gamma interferon-deficient mice, a macrophage cell line, and a fibroblast cell line. Following activation with gamma interferon, each cell type eradicated intracellular *Shigella*, while nonactivated macrophages fostered *Shigella* replication and nonactivated fibroblast cells fostered both *Shigella* replication and intercellular spread. Taken together, these data establish that NK cell-mediated gamma interferon is essential to resistance following primary *Shigella* infection.

In endemic areas, shigellosis is essentially a childhood disease, and the incidence decreases drastically in the indigenous population over 5 years of age. Controlled volunteer challenge studies in North American adults also indicate that prior infection with *S flexneri* protects against reinfection with the homologous serotype (70% efficacy). Serotype-specific immune protection against shigellosis suggests that antibody recognizing the O-polysaccharide of LPS protects against clinical symptoms. Ingested bovine colostrum containing antibody recognizing the O-polysaccharide of *S. flexneri* 2a passively protects volunteers challenged with the homologous *Shigella* serotype. These observations have encouraged the development of a number of parenteral and mucosally administered O-polysaccharide vaccines that are currently in safety and/or efficacy trials. Boullier *et al.* (2009) explored the mechanisms of protection mediated by *Shigella* LPS-specific secretory IgA

(SIgA), the major mucosal Ab induced upon natural infection. Bacteria, SIgA, or SIgA-*S. flexneri* immune complexes were administered into rabbit ligated intestinal loops containing a Peyer's patch. After 8 h, localizations of bacteria, SIgA, and SIgA-S. flexneri immune complexes were examined by immunohistochemistry and confocal microscopy imaging. It was found that anti-Shigella LPS SIgA, mainly via immune exclusion, prevented *Shigella*-induced inflammation responsible for the destruction of the intestinal barrier. Besides this luminal trapping, a small proportion of SIgA-*S. flexneri* immune complexes were shown to enter the rabbit Peyer's patch and were internalized by dendritic cells of the subepithelial dome region. Local inflammatory status was analyzed by quantitative RT-PCR using newly designed primers for rabbit pro- and anti-inflammatory mediator genes. In Peyer's patches exposed to immune complexes, limited up-regulation of the expression of proinflammatory genes, including TNF-alpha, IL-6, Cox-2, and IFN-gamma, was observed, consistent with preserved morphology. In contrast, in Peyer's patches exposed to *Shigella* alone, high expression of the same mediators was measured, indicating that neutralizing SIgA dampens the proinflammatory properties of *Shigella*. These results show that in the form of immune complexes, SIgA guarantees both immune exclusion and neutralization of translocated bacteria, thus preserving the intestinal barrier integrity by preventing bacterial-induced inflammation. These findings add to the multiple facets of the noninflammatory properties of SIgA. A type III secretion system that delivers effector proteins into target eukaryotic cells is largely responsible for cell and tissue invasion. However, the respective role of this invasive phenotype and of lipid A, the endotoxin of the Shigella LPS, in eliciting the inflammatory cascade that leads to rupture and destruction of the epithelial barrier, was unknown. D'Hauteville *et al.* (2002) investigated whether genetic detoxification of lipid A would cause significant alteration in pathogenicity. It was showed that S. flexneri has two functional msbB genes, one carried by the chromosome (msbB1) and the other by the virulence plasmid (msbB2), the products of which act in complement to produce full acyl-oxy-acylation of the myristate at the 3' position of the lipid A glucosamine disaccharide. A mutant in which both the msbB1 and msbB2 genes have been inactivated was impaired in its capacity to cause TNF-alpha production by human monocytes and to cause rupture and inflammatory destruction of the epithelial barrier in the rabbit ligated intestinal loop model of shigellosis, indicating that lipid A plays a significant role in aggravating inflammation that eventually destroys the intestinal barrier. In addition, neutralization of TNF-alpha during invasion by the wild-type strain strongly impaired its ability to cause rupture and inflammatory destruction of the epithelial lining, thus indicating that TNF-alpha is a major effector of epithelial destruction by *Shigella*.

Laboratory diagnosis

Fecal material is collected and examined directly under the microscope. It contains inflammatory cells, cellular debris and red blood cells. The presence of gram-negative rods in abundance is suggestive of shigellosis. Neutrophils in fecal smears is also a strongly suggestive sign. Nonetheless, watery, mucoid diarrhea may be the only symptom of many *S sonnei* infections, and any clinical diagnosis should be confirmed by cultivation of the etiologic agent from stools.

Culturing the stool samples using selective/differential agar media is carried out. *Shigella* spp. are highly fragile organism and considerable care must be exercised in collecting faecal specimens, transporting them to the laboratories and in using appropriate media for isolation. The sample is inoculated on a selective medium such as MacConkey agar, XLD agar and Hektoen Enteric medium. Salmônella *Shigella* agar is also used but it is inhibitory to some strains of *Shigella*. GN both is used for enrichment of the samples. After 2-3 days of incubation at 37 ºC the colonies appear which are non-lactose fermenting on lactose containing medium, although some species (*S.sonnei* and *S.boydii* 9) ferment this sugar. Suspicious colonies are tested directly with *Shigellae*-specific antisera or inoculated into differential media and then tested with antisera. Biochemical tests can also be performed for identification. *Shigella* species are negative for motility and are non-lactose fermenters. (However, *S. sonnei* can ferment lactose). They typically do not produce gas from carbohydrates (with the exception of certain strains of *S. flexneri*) and tend to be overall biochemically inert. *Shigella* should also be Urea Hydrolysis negative. When inoculated to a Triple Sugar Iron slant they react as follows: K/A, gas -, H2S -. Indole reactions are mixed, positive and negative, with the exception of *S. sonnei* which is always indole negative.

PCR technique has been developed for amplification of *Shigella flexneri* plasmid DNA in food for identifying the presence of the organism (Lampel *et al.*, 1990). Islam and Lindberg (1992) described an immunomagnetic isolation and PCR in fecal specimens from diarrhoeic patients. The technique proved better than conventional methods. Often the testing procedure is able to isolate *Escherichia coli* from the clinical samples. Identification of these invasive organisms is carried out with the Sereny test, chicken embryo lethality and invasion to culture cells assays, DNA probe hybridization, polymerase chain reaction, ELISA, Congo red binding, and biochemical and serological tests. Cristea *et al.* (2009) optimized an in vitro pathogenicity model, as an alternative to Sereny test (on Guinea pigs). The investigation implied the comparative evaluation between the Sereny test and Cravioto's adapted method for the assessment of the adherence and invasion capacity of the studied bacterial strains on HeLa cells, as well as the PCR detection of ipaH gene presence. The Sereny test was positive for all the strains tested. All strains adhered to the cellular layer, with a prevalent diffuse pattern for EIEC and an aggregative diffuse one for *Shigella* strains. The quantitative assessment of the invasion potential proved a high intracellular multiplication rate in 100% of the tested strains, with a progressive increase correlated with the incubation time. The present study has proven the existence of a good correlation between *in vivo* Sereny test and in vitro determination of the invasive capacity on eukaryotic HeLa cells, pleading for the utility of this test in identifying the invasive strains, taking into consideration the rigid regulations concerning the use of laboratory animals.

Polymerase chain reaction (PCR) diagnostic methods have rarely been used in epidemiologic studies of *Shigella* infections. As the sensitivity of the conventional techniques for identifying Shigella spp. and enteroinvasive Escherichia coli (EIEC) causing dysentery cases is low, a PCR assay was evaluated by Dutta *et al.* (2001). Analytical sensitivity (2 x 10(2) cfu) of the PCR technique was obtained by artificially spiking negative stool samples with a standard strain of S. flexneri type 2, then determining the detection limit. Specificity (100%) of the method was determined by testing a number of known Shigella and EIEC strains and organisms other than *Shigella* spp. A total of 300 stool samples collected from children with acute diarrhoea was plated on to two selective agar media after enrichment in Luria broth. *Shigella* spp. were isolated from 7.7% (23 of 300) and EIEC from 1% (3 of 300) patients. All enriched stool samples were subjected to PCR to amplify the target sequence of invasive plasmid antigen (ipa)H locus, a multicopy element found on the chromosome and invasion plasmid. The stool PCR was positive in 24 of the 26 culture-positive and in 22 culture-negative stools, thus detecting the presence of Shigella spp. or EIEC in 15.3% (46 of 300) of diarrhoea cases. When an ial probe was used for colony hybridistion with enriched stool cultures blotted on to membranes, 9.6% (29 of 300) of dysentery cases were identified as being caused by *Shigella* spp. or EIEC. Thus the sensitivity of enriched stool culture, colony hybridisation and enriched stool PCR was found to be 54%, 60% and 96%, respectively, when each of the methods was compared to the total microbiologically confirmed cases of dysentery. It was also observed that only 38% (48 of 126) of acute bloody dysentery cases actually had *shigella* or EIEC infection, as confirmed by laboratory methods. Moreover, this PCR assay could identify a number of untypable *Shigella* strains (Sh OUT), which would have remained undiagnosed had this assay not been used.

In one study, amplification of the invasion plasmid antigen H (ipaH) gene by PCR and standard culture methods was used to identify *Shigella* species or enteroinvasive *E. coli* among 154 patients with dysentery, 154 age-matched controls, and family contacts in Thailand (Gaudio *et al.*, 1997). The ipaH PCR system increased the detection of *Shigella* species and EIEC from 58% to 79%

among patients with dysentery and from 6% to 22% among 527 family contacts; 75% of infections in family members were asymptomatic. Detection of the ipaH gene was statistically associated with dysentery. Household contacts of patients with shigellosis diagnosed only by PCR had significantly higher rates of shigellosis than household contacts of patients who did not have *Shigella* or EIEC infections. Detection of the ipaH gene by PCR is far more sensitive than detection by standard culture and is highly correlated with evidence of *Shigella* transmission among family contacts.Polymerase chain reactions can also be performed to differentiate *E.coli* from *Shigella* spp. (Yamazaki and Fukasawa 2010).Wang *et al.*(2010) applied real-time PCR to detect Shigella infection in parallel with routine culture, to investigate the true burden of disease caused by *Shigella* spp. Rectal swab specimens of 39 *Shigella* culture positive and 298 *Shigella* culture negative patients from a population-based surveillance study were selected randomly. Real-time PCR targeting the invasion plasmid antigen H gene sequence (ipaH) was used to detect DNA sequences characteristic for *Shigella* spp. ipaH were detected in 174 of 298 (58%) randomly selected Shigella culture negative specimens and in 38 of 39 (97%) *Shigella* culture positive specimens ($p < 0.001$). Among 10 variables, culture results was the strongest predictive factor (OR = 15.5; 95% CI: 2.0-119.0), followed by a clinical presentation of diarrhea with fever (OR = 2.8; 95% CI: 1.2-6.2), epidemic season (OR = 2.4; 95% CI: 1.4-4.3), and female gender (OR = 1.8; 95% CI: 1.1-3.0). The high detection rate of ipaH in culture negative specimens through use of real-time PCR suggests that earlier estimates of shigellosis burden measured by conventional culture may have underestimated the true disease burden.

Treatment and Control

Antimicrobials are used in primates affected with Shigellosis. Trimethoprim- sulfonamides or a fluoroquinolone are effective and preferred since these do not effect the normal microflora. In India, *S.flexneri* continue to be the major species isolated and Ciprofloxacin resistance among strains is emerging (Taneja 2007). Multidrug resistance is also increasing in India (Taneja *et al.,* 2005). Folster *et al.,* (2011) reported a decreased resistance of *Shigella* strains to fluoroquinolones. The rise in antimicrobial resistance may necessitate the increased use of extended spectrum Cephalosporins or macrolides in some patients. Emergence of multidrug-resistant strains of *Shigella* is a growing concern across the globe. Third-generation cephalosporins are used for treating infections caused by multidrug-resistant Shigellae. However, resistance to these cephalosporin antibiotics due to extended-spectrum ß-lactamases, has emerged as a new problem. Iversen *et al.* (2003) investigated antimicrobial resistance, plasmids and class 1 integrons in 150 Shigella strains isolated from patients with diarrhea in Vietnam. Most isolates were resistant to the majority of antimicrobial agents used for treatment in the isolation areas and 90% were resistant to three or more antibiotics. A total of 20 strains yielded class 1 integrons, which harbored oxa1, dfrA, orfF, and aadA gene cassettes. The most common gene cassette, aadA2, was always located closest to the 3' conserved segment of the integrons and oxa1 and dfrA closest to the 5' end. Plasmid profiles of the 20 class 1 integron-positive strains all contained more than one plasmid, and 14 different profiles were found. No correlation was found between species, antibiograms, plasmid profiles, or presence of class 1 integrons. Conjugation resulted in 25 transconjugants, which all were resistant to four or more antimicrobial agents and all harbored at least one plasmid (>60 kb). Class 1 integrons were detected in 64% of the transconjugants. Phenotypic resistance pattern and plasmid profiles of the transconjugants seemed independent of the presence of an integron. Class 1 integrons seemed of less importance in phenotypic antibiograms and in transfer of resistance genes than conjugative plasmids. Ninety *Shigella* strains (83 S. *flexneri* and 7 *S. sonnei*) were isolated from the stools of patients in China. Susceptibility to 8 antimicrobials was tested for all isolated strains. PCR, RFLP and sequencing analysis of integrons were applied to all of them (Zhu *et al* 2011). High prevalence of multi-drug resistance (95.6%) was identified. Of the isolates 79 (87.8%) carried integrase genes of class 1 integron (3.3%), class 2 integron (10.0%) or both (74.4%). No intI3 was detected in the tested isolates. The prevalence of intI2 was significantly higher in isolates with multi-drug resistance to at least 3 antibiotics than that in isolates with resistance to 2 and less antibiotics ($P<0.05$). Gene cassettes dfrA17-aadA5, dfrA12-orfF-aadA2 of class 1 integron and dfrA1-sat1-aadA1 of class 2 integron were identified. The class 2 integron may play a role in the emergence of multi-drug resistance in *Shigella* spp.

Fluid therapy is carried out in severe cases of diarrhoea and dysentery.

Since the 1940s vaccines for *S.flexneri* have been developed for human beings with little success (Jennison and Verma 2004). Parenterally administered vaccines have been ineffective, however, vaccines give orally have been found to confer type - specific protection. Because immunity to *Shigella* is serotype-specific, the priority is to develop vaccine against S. dysenteriae type 1 and S. *flexneri* type 2a. Owing to the wide range of *Shigella* serotypes and subtypes, there is a need for a multivalent vaccine representing prevalent species and serotypes. Virulent strains of *Shigella flexneri* 1b, S. flexneri 3, and S. sonnei I were mated with an Hfr strain of Escherichia coli K-12, and hybrids were selected for the xylose marker (Formal *et al.*, 1966). One hybrid strain of each of the serotypes was chosen for study of their biological characteristics. Their capacity to cause a fatal enteric infection in starved guinea pigs was reduced, they failed to cause dysentery when fed to monkeys, they caused keratoconjunctivitis in the guinea pig eye, and they penetrated HeLa cells. Two doses of a polyvalent oral vaccine composed of *S. flexneri* 1b, 2a, and 3, and *S. sonnei* I hybrid strains were fed to groups of monkeys at an interval of 4 to 7 days, and they, together with controls, were challenged 10 days after the last dose with one or another of the virulent parent dysentery strains. A significant degree of protection was afforded in all vaccinated groups with the exception of one group challenged with *S. flexneri* 6, a component not included in the vaccine. When animals were challenged with virulent *S. flexneri* 2a 1 month after oral vaccination, they were also protected. The vaccine produced a rise in serum antibody, but we were not able to detect coproantibody in saline extracts of feces from animals which received the vaccine. Dzhikidze *et al.* (1988) immunized monkeys with *S. sonnei* ribosomal vaccine and all control monkeys fell ill as the result of oral challenge with *S. sonnei* virulent strain. The immunized monkeys stopped excreting Shigellae earlier than the control monkeys. Antibody to lipopolysaccharide (LPS) in the serum and saliva of the monkeys were studied in the enzyme immunoassay with monospecific antibodies to human IgA, IgG and IgM. A single injection of the ribosomal vaccine in a dose of 600 micrograms was shown to lead to a considerable increase in the levels of IgA, IgG and IgM antibodies to LPS in saliva. In parenteral immunization with the ribosomal vaccine the stimulation of secretory IgA system is similar to that resulting from oral challenge with Shigella virulent strain introduced in a dose of 50 X 10(9) microbial cells. No difference in the response of monkeys to primary and booster immunization was noted.

The presence of type-specific somatic antigens and ability to penetrate the intestinal epithelium are associated with ability of organisms to induce protection. Antibodies to LPS appear to be ineffective but a combination of antibodies against the O antigen on the surface plus cell mediated immunity against infected host cells is effective (Hale and Karen 1992). Because immunity to *Shigella* is serotype - specific the priority is to develop vaccine against *S.dysenteriae* type 1 and *S.flexneri* type 2a. Certain live attenuated cultures have been found to confer cross-protection. *S.flexneri* serotype Y, attenuated by inactivation of aroD gene, induced protection against challenge with *S.flexneri* serotype Y, 2a and Ib in orally vaccinated monkeys (Lindberg *et al.*, 1990). Live attenuated strains of *S. flexneri* 2a, S. sonnei and *S. dysenteriae* 1 containing deletions in guaBA biosynthetic pathway genes as well as in genes encoding enterotoxins, were constructed(Barry *et al.*, 2006). Each strain was subsequently used as a live vector for the expression of one or two critical ETEC antigens. The resulting three *Shigella* derivative strains were tested for immunogenicty and protective capacity alone or as mixtures in the guinea pig model. *S. flexneri* strain CVD 1208 (pCFA/I-CS3), S. sonnei strain CVD

1233(pCS4-LThK63) and *S. dysenteriae* 1 strain CVD 1252(pCS2) were able to elicit serum and mucosal antibody responses against the live vector as well as the guest ETEC antigens. Vaccination with combinations of two or three of these strains was able to elicit specific immune responses against each live vector as well as each ETEC antigen represented in the mixture. These studies demonstrate the potential of the use of mixtures of live *Shigella* derivatives expressing ETEC antigens to serve as an immunogenic multivalent vaccine.

Barrett *et al.* (2010) presented formulation and immunogenicity studies for the three type III secretion system (TTSS) needle proteins MxiH(Ä5), PrgI(Ä5), and BsaL(Ä5) (each truncated by five residues at its C terminus) as potential candidates for vaccine development. These antigens are found to be thermally stabilized by the presence of carbohydrates and polyols. Additionally, all adsorb readily to aluminum hydroxide apparently through a combination of hydrogen bonds and/or Van der Waals forces. The interaction of these proteins with the aluminum-based adjuvant changes with time resulting in varying degrees of irreversible binding. Peptide maps of desorbed protein, however, suggest that chemical changes are not responsible for this irreversible association. The ability of MxiH(Ä5) and PrgI(Ä5) to elicit strong humoral immune responses was tested in a murine model. When administered intramuscularly as monomers, the needle components exhibited dose dependent immunogenic behavior. The polymerized version of MxiH was exceptionally immunogenic even at low doses. The responses of both monomeric and polymerized forms were boosted by adsorption to an aluminum salt adjuvant.

References

Banish L.D., Sims R., Sack D., Montali R.J., Phillips L. Jr and Bush M.1993.Prevalence of shigellosis and other enteric pathogens in a zoological collection of primates. J. Am. Vet. Med. Assoc. **203:** 126-132.

Barry E.M., Wang J., Wu T., Davis T., Levine M.M.2006.Immunogenicity of multivalent Shigella-ETEC candidate vaccine strains in a guinea pig model. Vaccine. **24:** 3727-3734.

Barrett B.S., Markham A.P., Esfandiary R., Picking W.L., Picking W.D., Joshi S.B. and Middaugh C.R.2010.Formulation and immunogenicity studies of type III secretion system needle antigens as vaccine candidates. J. Pharm. Sci. **99:** 4488-4496.

Baxt, L.A. and Goldberg, M.B. 2010. Anaerobic environment of the intestine primes pathogenic Shigella for infection. Expert Rev. Antiinfect. Ther. **8:** 1225-1229.

Boullier S., Tanguy M., Kadaoui K.A., Caubet C., Sansonetti P., Corthésy B. and Phalipon A.2009.Secretory IgA-mediated neutralization of Shigella flexneri prevents intestinal tissue destruction by down-regulating inflammatory circuits. J. Immunol. **183:** 5879-5885.

Cristea D., Ceciu S., Chitoiu D.T., Bleotu C., Lazăr V. and Chifiriuc M.C.2009.Comparative study of pathogenicity tests for Shigella spp. and enteroinvasive Escherichia coli strains. Roum. Arch. Microbiol. Immunol. **68:** 44-49.

Dickenson, N.E., Zhang, L., Epler, C.R., Adam, P.R., Picking, W.L. and Picking, W.D. 2010. Conformational changes in Ipa D from *Shigella flexneri* upon binding bile salts provide insight into the second step of type III secretion. Biochemistry Dec. 15 [http://www.ncbi.nlm.nih.gov/pubmed/21126091].

D'Hauteville H., Khan S., Maskell D.J., Kussak A., Weintraub A., Mathison J., Ulevitch R.J., Wuscher N., Parsot C. and Sansonetti P.J.2002. Two msbB genes encoding maximal acylation of lipid A are required for invasive Shigella flexneri to mediate inflammatory rupture and destruction of the intestinal epithelium. J. Immunol. **168:** 5240-5251.

Dutta S., Chatterjee A., Dutta P., Rajendran K., Roy S., Pramanik K.C. and Bhattacharya S.K..2001.Sensitivity and performance characteristics of a direct PCR with stool samples in comparison to conventional techniques for diagnosis of Shigella and enteroinvasive Escherichia coli infection in children with acute diarrhoea in Calcutta, India. J. Med. Microbiol. **50:** 667-674.

Dzhikidze E.K., Stasilevich Z.K. and Salamatova S.A.1988. [Stimulation of the secretory IgA system in monkeys by parenteral immunization with a ribosomal Sonne dysentery vaccine]. Zh. Mikrobiol. Epidemiol. Immunobiol. 8 Sep;(9):66-70. [Article in Russian].

Farfan, M.J., Toro, C.S., Barry, E.M. and Nataro, J.P. 2011. *Shigella enterotoxin*-2 is a type III effector that participates in Shigella induced interleukin-8 secretion by epithelial cells. FEMS Immunol. Med. Microbiol. Han10, doi 10:1111.1574-695. [http://www.ncbi.nlm.nih.gov/pubmed/21219446].

Flamant, M., Aubert, P., Rolli-Derkinderen, M., Bourreille, A., Neunlist, M.R., Mahe, M.M., Meurette, G., Marteyn, B., Savidge, T., Galmiche, J.P., Sansonetti, P.J. and Neunlist, M. 2010. Enteric glia protects against *Shigella flexneri* invasion in intestinal epithelial cells: a role for S-nitroglutathione. Gut. [http://www.ncbi.nlm.nih.gov/pubmed/21139062].

Folster, J.P., Pecic, G., Bowen, A., Rickert, R., Caratolli, A. and Whichard, J.M. 2011. Decreased susceptibility to ciprofloxacin among Shigella isolated in United States 2006-2009. Antimicrob. Agents Chemother. 10: [http://www. ncbi.nlm.nih.gov/pubmed/21220535].

Fontaine, A., Arondel, J. and Sansonetti, P.J. 1988. Role of Shiga toxin in the pathogenesis of shigellosis as studied using a Tox mutant of *Shigella dysenteriae* 1. Infect. Immun. **56:** 3099-3109.

Formal S.B., Kent T.H., May H.C., Palmer A., Falkow S. and LaBrec E.H.1966. Protection of monkeys against experimental shigellosis with a living attenuated oral polyvalent dysentery vaccine. J. Bacteriol. **92:** 17-22.

Foster R.A., Carlin N.I., Majcher M., Tabor H., Ng L.K. and Widmalm G.2011.Structural elucidation of the O-antigen of the Shigella flexneri provisional serotype 88-893:

structural and serological similarities with S. flexneri provisional serotype Y394 (1c). Carbohydr. Res. **346:** 872-876.

Gaudio P.A., Sethabutr O., Echeverria P. and Hoge C.W. 1997.Utility of a polymerase chain reaction diagnostic system in a study of the epidemiology of shigellosis among dysentery patients, family contacts, and well controls living in a shigellosis-endemic area. J.Infect.Dis. **176**(4): 1013-1018.

Goldberg, M.B. and Theriot, J.A. 1995. *Shigella flexneri* surface protein IcsA is sufficient to direct actin-based motility. Proc. Natt. Acad. Sci. USA. **92:** 6572-6576.

Gyles, C.L. 1993. Shigella. In Pathogenesis of Bacterial infections in animals pp. 104-163 Ed. Carlton, L. Gyles and Charles, O. Thoen. Iowa State University Press, Ames., USA.

Hale, T.L. 1991. Genetic basis of virulence in *Shigella* species. Microbiol. Rev. **55:** 206-224.

Hale, T.L. and Karen, D.F. 1992. Pathogenesis and immonology in Shigellosis: Applications for vaccine development. Curr. Top. Microbiol. Immunol. **180:** 117-137.

Headley, V.L. and Payne, S.M. 1990. Differential protein expression by *Shigella flexneri* in intracellular and extracellular environments. Proc. Natl. Acad. Sci. USA **87:** 4179-4183.

Hensley, C.T., Kamneva, O.K., Levy, K.M., Labahn, S.K., Africa, L.A. and Wing, H.J. 2011. Two promoters and two translation starts outer membrane protease IcsP. Arch. Microbiol. 12:[http://www.ncbi.nlm.nih.gov/pubmed/ 21225241].

Islam, D. and Lindberg, A.A. 1992. Detection of *Shigella dysenteriae* type 1 and *Shigella flexneri* in feces by immunomagnetic isolation and polymerase chain reaction. J. Clin. Microbiol. **30:** 2801-2806.

Iversen J., Sandvang D., Srijan A., Cam P.D. and Dalsgaard A.2003.Characterization of antimicrobial resistance, plasmids, and gene cassettes in Shigella spp. from patients in vietnam. Microb. Drug. Resist. 9 Suppl **1:** 517-524.

Jennison, A.V. and Verma, N.K. 2004. *Shigella flexneri* infection: pathogenesis and vaccine development FEMS Microbiol. Rev. **28:** 43-58.

Kandel, G., Donohue-Rolfe, A., Donowitz, M. and Keusch, G.T. 1989. Pathogenesis of *Shigella diarrhoea* 16. Selective targetting of Shiga toxin to vilus cells of rabbit jejunum explain the effect of the toxin on the intestinal electrolyte transport. J. Clin. Invest. **84:** 1509-1517.

Kilar, A., Dornyei, A., Bui, A., Szabo, Z., Kocsi, S.B. and Kilar, F. 2011. Structural variability of endotoxins from R-type isogenic mutants of *Shigella sonnei*. J. Mass. Spectrom. **46:** 61-70.

Kim M.,Ogawa M., Mimuro H. and Sasakawa C.2010. Reinforcement of epithelial cell adhesion to basement membrane by a bacterial pathogen as a new infectious stratagem. Virulence. **1:** 52-55.

Lambel, K.A., Jagow, J.A., Truckgess, M. and Hill, W.E. 1990. Polymerase chain reaction for detection of *Shigella flexneri* in food. App. Environ. Microbiol. **56:** 1536-1540.

Le-Barillec K., Magalhaes J.G., Corcuff E., Thuizat A., Sansonetti P.J., Phalipon A. and Di Santo JP.2005.Roles for T and NK cells in the innate immune response to Shigella flexneri. J. Immunol. **175:** 1735-1740.

Lindberg, A.A., Karnell, A., Pal, T., Sweiha, H., Hultenby, K. and Stocker, B.A.D. 1990. Construction of an auxotrophic *Shigella flexneri* strain for use as live vaccine. Microb. Pathog. **8:** 433-440.

Marteyn, B., West, N.P., Browning, D.F., Cole, J.A., Shaw, J.G., Palm, F., Mounier, J., Prevost, M.C., Sansonetti, P. and Tang, C.M. 2010. Modulation of Shigella virulence in response to available oxygen in vivo. Nature **465:** 355-358.

Maurelli, A.T., Hromockyj, A.E. and Bernardini, M.L. 1992. Environmental regulation of *Shigella* virulence. Curr. Top. Microbiol. Immunol. **180:** 95-116.

Mounier, J., Vasselon, T., Hellio, R., Lesourd, M. Ad Sansonetti, P.J. 1992. *Shigella flexneri* enters human caco-2 epithelial cells through the basolateral pole. Infect. Immun. **60:** 237-248.

Niyogi S.K. 2005. Shigellosis. J. Microbiol. **43:** 133-143.

Schreder, G.N. and Hilbi, H. 2008. Molecular pathogenesis of Shigella spp.: Controlling host cell signaling, invasion and death by type III secretion. Clin. Microbiol. **21:** 134-156.

Steinhauer, J., Agha, R., Pham, T., Varga, A.W. and Goldberg, M.B. 1999. The unipolar Shigella surface protein IcsA is targeted directly to the bacterial old pole: IcsP cleavage of Ics A occur over the entire bacterial surface. Mol. Microbiol. **32:** 367-377.

Taneja, N. 2007. Changing epidemiology of *shigellosis* and emergence of Ciprofloxacin-resistant Shigellae in India. J. Clin. Microbiol. **45:** 678-679.

Taneja, N., Lyngdoh, V., Vermani, A., Mohan, B., Rao, P., Singh, M., Dogra, A., Singh, M.P. and Sharma, M. 2005. Re-emergence of multi-drug resistant *Shigella dysenteriae* with added resistance to Ciprofloxacin in north India and their plasmid profile. Indian J. Med. Res. **122:** 348-354.

Vasselon, T., Mounier, J., Prevost, M.C., Hellio, R. and Sansonetti, P.J. 1991. Stress fiber-based movement of *Shigella flexneri* within cells. Infect. Immun. **59:** 1723-1732.

Wang S.M., Ma J.C., Hao Z.Y., Zhang Z.Y., Mason C., Sethabutr O., von Seidlein L., Wang X.Y. and Xu Z.Y.2010.Surveillance of shigellosis by real-time PCR suggests underestimation of shigellosis prevalence by culture-based methods in a population of rural China. J. Infect. **61:** 471-475.

Way S.S., Borczuk A.C., Dominitz R. and Goldberg M.B.1998.An essential role for gamma interferon in innate resistance to Shigella flexneri infection. Infect. Immun. **66:** 1342-1348.

Yamazaki, Y. and Fukasawa, A. 2010. Multiplex polymerase chain reaction method discriminating *Escherichia coli* and *Shigella* spp. Arch. Microbiol. 9 [http://www.ncbi.nlm.nih.gov/pubmed/21060994].

Yang F., Yang J., Zhang X., Chen L., Jiang Y., Yan Y., Tang X., Wang J., Xiong Z., Dong J., Xue Y., Zhu Y., Xu X., Sun L., Chen S,. Nie H., Peng J., Xu J., Wang Y., Yuan Z., Wen Y., Yao Z., Shen Y., Qiang B., Hou Y., Yu J. and Jin Q.2005.Genome dynamics and diversity of *Shigella* species, the etiologic agents of bacillary dysentery. Nucleic Acids Res. **33:** 6445-6458.

Yurdakök K., Sahin N., Ozmert E. and Berkman E.1997.Shigella gastroenteritis: clinical and epidemiological aspects, and antibiotic susceptibility. Acta. Paediatr. Jpn. **39:** 681-684.

Zhu J., Duan G., Yang H., Fan Q. and Xi Y.2011.Multi-drug Resistance and Characteristic of Integrons in *Shigella* spp.Isolated from China. Biomed. Environ. Sci. **24:** 56-61.

□□□

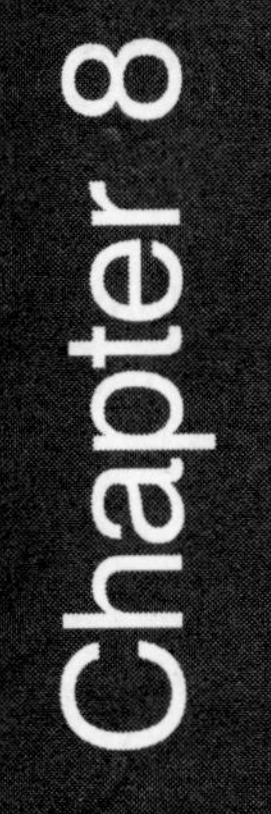

Anthrax

Dr. S.K. SRIVASTAVA
Former, Division of Bacteriology & Mycology
Indian Veterinary Research Institute, Izatnagar-243122
Bareilly (U.P.)

Anthrax is primarily associated with domesticated and wild herbivorous animals. Among domestic animals, cattle and sheep appear most susceptible whereas horses and goats are slightly less. Carnivores are relatively resistant. In swine, it is relatively less but mortality is high. This is also are important zoonotic problem though the frequency of transmission to man is less. Anthrax is characterized by septicaemia and sudden death accompanied by the exudation of dark blood from natural orifices of the dead animals. The blood fail to clot and splenomegaly is the most important post-mortem finding.

Etiology

The disease is caused by *Bacillus anthracis,* a large, gram-positive, endospore forming bacterium. It was shown to cause disease by Robert Koch in 1876. Like many other members of the genus *Bacillus, Bacillus anthracis* can form dormant endospores (often referred to as "spores" for short, but not to be confused with fungal spores) that are able to survive in harsh conditions for decades or even centuries. Such spores can be found on all continents, even Antarctica. When spores are inhaled, ingested, or come into contact with a skin lesion on a host they may reactivate and multiply rapidly.The spores are highly resistant to physical and chemical treatments and remain viable for a long period in animal by products, contaminated soil and on surgical equipments used for performing necropsy. In contaminated soil anthrax spores can survive for 48 years. Aerobically, *B.anthracis* grows as a long chain of rod-shaped cells in rough colonies with slightly serrated edges. On magnification the colonies may display the classic medusa head appearance around their periphery. Growth in 5-10% Co_2 on media containing 0.5% sodium bicarbonate or serum virulent strains produce a poly-D-glutamic acid capsule which gives rise to smooth, mucoid, convex colonies.

The virulent Ames strain, which had been used in the 2001 anthrax attacks in the United States, has received the most news coverage of any anthrax outbreak. The Ames strain contains two virulence plasmids, which separately encode for a three-protein toxin, called anthrax toxin, and a poly-glutamic acid capsule. Nonetheless, the Vollum strain, developed but never used as a biological weapon during the Second World War, is much more dangerous. The *Vollum* (also incorrectly referred to as *Vellum*) strain was isolated in 1935 from a cow in Oxfordshire, UK. This is the same strain that was used during the Gruinard bioweapons trials. A variation of Vollum known as "Vollum 1B" was used during the 1960s in the US and UK bioweapon programs. Vollum 1B is widely believed to have been isolated from William A. Boyles, a 46-year-old scientist at the U.S. Army Biological Warfare Laboratories at Camp (later Fort) Detrick (precursor to USAMRIID) who died in 1951 after being accidentally infected with the Vollum strain. The *Sterne* strain, named after the Trieste-born immunologist Max Sterne, is an attenuated strain used as a vaccine, which contains only the anthrax toxin virulence plasmid and not the poly-glutamic acid capsule expressing plasmid.

Epidemiology

Until the twentieth century, anthrax infections killed hundreds and thousands of animals and people each year in Australia, Asia, Africa, North America, and Europe, particularly in the concentration camps during WWII French scientist Louis Pasteur developed the first effective vaccine for anthrax in 1881. Thanks to over a century of animal vaccination programs, sterilization of raw animal waste materials and anthrax eradication programs in North America, Australia, New Zealand, Russia, Europe, and parts of Africa and Asia, anthrax infection is now relatively rare in domestic animals, with only a few dozen cases reported every year. Anthrax is especially rare in dogs and cats, as is evidenced by a single reported case in the USA in 2001. Anthrax typically does not cause disease in carnivores and scavengers, even when these animals consume anthrax-infected carcasses. Anthrax outbreaks do occur in some wild animal populations with some

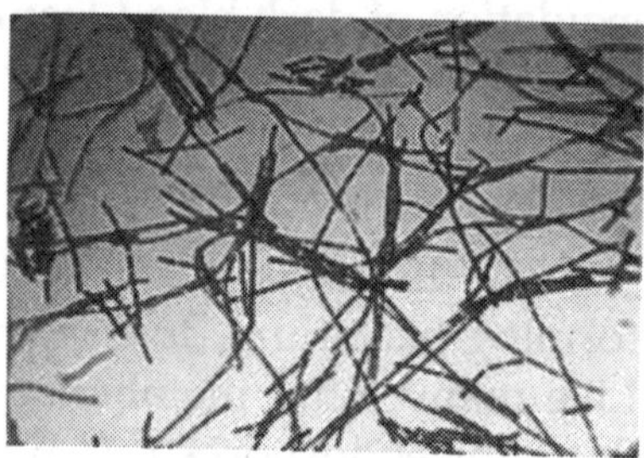

Bacillus anthracis cells

regularity. The disease is more common in developing countries without widespread veterinary or human public health programs.

Anthrax is worldwide in occurrence including India. Most cases have been observed in southern and central part of the country. There appear anthrax belts where it is enzootic. In such belts many deaths occur without any observed illness. The source of infection is usually the soil in which cases occur during rainy seasons. In some countries the cases occur every summer. In temperate cool climate only sporadic outbreaks occur.

Between January and February 1997, there was a severe outbreak of anthrax on 83 properties in north-central Victoria, Australia. Vaccination was used as a major tool to control the outbreak by establishing a vaccination buffer zone 30 km by 20 km. In all, 78, 649 cattle in 457 herds were vaccinated in a three week program. In the face of the outbreak, there was a delay before vaccination was able to stop deaths. In the 10 days following vaccination 144 cases of confirmed anthrax occurred and 38 cases occurred more than 10 days after vaccination. When all cattle on at-risk properties were revaccinated in October and early November 1997, there were only two confirmed cases of anthrax in vaccinated seven and nine month old calves in the following anthrax season. Investigations into the epidemiology of the outbreak were unable to establish a single major association for the spread of the disease by flies, biting insects, carrion scavengers, wind, manufactured feed, milk factory tanker routes, veterinary visits, animal treatments, movements of personnel between farms or burning of carcases. The weather conditions in the outbreak area were part of a long dry spell with periods of high daily and night temperatures, continuing high humidity over the period and higher than normal soil temperatures. It is possible that extensive earth works in the district involving irrigated pasture renovation and water channel and drainage renovation could have disturbed old anthrax graves. It is postulated that these works released spores that were dispersed in the preceding wet winter across poorly drained areas that formed the axis for the outbreak. The earth moving renovations establishing irrigation in the area were conducted in the late 1890s, and before the occurrence of anthrax outbreaks were recorded. The axis of the outbreak was the major stock route for cattle and sheep moving from southern Victoria to northern Victoria and southern New South Wales, and undoubtedly there would have been extensive anthrax outbreaks before vaccine became available in the 1890s. In respect of other outbreaks, the events in Victoria most resembled outbreaks of anthrax recorded in the United States of America in the 1950s, 1960s and 1970s.

The disease occurs in 2 forms; cutaneous and septicaemic (Lincoln and Fish 1970). The cutaneous form is characterized by a dark, relatively painless edematous eschar which heals readily following antibiotic therapy. The septicemic form is characterized by various initial sites of infection such as wound, cutaneous lesions or gastro-intestinal or pulmonary infections. The initial site of infection and the susceptibility of the animal species determine the course of the disease. An atypical form of disease has been observed in pigs in Papua-New Guinea. Severe outbreaks with heavy mortality occur in pigs.

The morbidity rate may be high among all farm animals although susceptibility is highest among farm ruminants followed by horses and swine.

Anthrax spores are picked up directly from the soil, from contaminated bone meal or from infected excreta, blood or other material by the susceptible animals which later succumb to the disease. Water can be contaminated by the effluent from tanneries, infected carcasses and by flooding and the deposition of the anthrax-contaminated soil, which later becomes source of infection for animals. Introduction of infection into a new area is usually through contaminated animal by products such as fertilizers, bone meal, hides, hair and wool. In many countries most outbreaks of the disease are caused by feeding infected feed usually bone meal. Wound infection occasionally could be the source of infection.

In man there are three forms of disease caused by anthrax: cutaneous (skin) anthrax, inhalation anthrax, and gastrointestinal (bowel) anthrax.

Cutaneous Anthrax

The cutaneous (skin) form of anthrax starts as a red-brown raised spot that enlarges with considerable redness around it, blistering, and hardening. The center of the spot then shows an ulcer crater with blood-tinged drainage and the formation of a black crust called an eschar. There are swollen glands (lymph nodes) in the area. Symptoms include muscle aches and pain, headache, fever, nausea, and vomiting. The illness usually resolves in about six weeks, but deaths may occur if patients do not receive appropriate antibiotics.

Inhalation Anthrax

The first symptoms are subtle, gradual and flu-like (influenza). In a few days, however, the illness worsens and there may be severe respiratory distress. Shock, coma, and death follow. Inhalation anthrax does not cause a true pneumonia. In fact, the spores get picked in the lungs up by scavenger cells called macrophages. Most of the spores are killed. Unfortunately, some survive and are transported to glands in the chest called lymph nodes. In the lymph nodes, the spores that survive multiply, produce deadly toxins, and spread throughout the body. Severe hemorrhage and tissue death (necrosis) occurs in these lymph nodes in the chest. From there, the disease spreads to the adjacent lungs and the rest of the body. Inhalation anthrax is a very serious disease, and unfortunately, most affected individuals will die even if they get appropriate antibiotics. Why is this so? The antibiotics are effective in killing the bacteria, but they do not destroy the deadly toxins that have already been released by the anthrax bacteria.

Gastrointestinal Anthrax

Now rare, anthrax of the bowels (gastrointestinal anthrax) is the result of eating undercooked, contaminated meat. The symptoms of this form of anthrax include nausea, loss of appetite, bloody diarrhea and fever followed by abdominal pain. The bacteria invade through the bowel wall. Then the infection spreads throughout the body through the bloodstream (septicemia) with deadly toxicity.

Transmission

Cattle, sheep & swine contract anthrax primarily through ingestion of contaminated feedstuffs; however, parenteral introduction is often non-fatal, except sheep. Following ingestion the disease is evident after an incubation period of 3-7 days. The first indication of a disease in a herd is sudden death. After death blood discharges out from natural orifices. Incomplete rigor mortis with un-clotted blood is typical of anthrax.

An acute disease usually develops in horses except when infection originates with insect bite. Rapidly progressing subcutaneous edema of neck, throat, abdomen and mammary glands is characteristic. Goats and human may also become infected through insect bites which carry organisms subsequent to feeding on carcasses died on anthrax.

Inhalation of organism or spores does not seem to play a major role in acquiring the infection in animals. Wool sorter disease in human is due to the inhalation of anthrax spores by workers in wool and hair industries but in such industries, cutaneous anthrax is more common. Anthrax spores have not been found to germinate in lung tissues after they have been inhaled. Anthrax spores can be produced in vitro and used as a biological weapon. Anthrax does not usuallyspread directly from one infected animal or person to another; it is spread by spores. These spores can be transported by clothing or shoes. The body of an animal that had active anthrax at the time of death can also be a source of anthrax spores.

If disease is caused by inhalation in herbivores (and occasionally humans), the spores are transported through the air passages into alveoli in the lungs where they are phagocytozed by macrophages and transported through lymphatics to the adjoining lymph nodes of mediastinum. Chest pain and difficult breathing in human are common at this stage. Germination of the spores occurs in the macrophages and following multiplication the vegetative cells spread in the body and produce toxins and lethal factors, primarily causing tissue destruction, bleeding & death of the host. At this stage even if the antibiotics are administered, it has no effect because the toxins are responsible for the damage.

Pathogenesis

The anthrax bacilli is known to posses 2 virulence factors, a poly–D-glutamate capsule and a mixture of 3 protein factors (Beall *et al.*, 1962; Beall and Daldorf 1966; Fish *et al.*, 1968) composed of Edema factor (EF), protective antigen (PA) and lethal factor (LF). Both PF and LF require PA for activity, which transports the former 2 protein toxins to the target cells (Leepla 1982; 1984, Brossier *et al.*, 2000). None of the 2 factors is active individually. The synergistic effects of the lethal and edema toxins results purely from their enzymatic activity. The genes coding for toxin production and capsule production are carried on 2 plasmids PX 01 (110 Mdal) and PX 02 (60 Mdal), respectively. (Uchida *et al.*, 1985) Leepla (1982; 1984) established that EF is an active adenylate cyclase which is activated by eukaryotic host cell calmodulin. In tissue culture, PA-EF combinations increase cyclic AMP concentrations in several cell lines. LF is a metalloprotease. O' Brien *et al* (1985) reported PMN phagocytosis and oxidative metabolism to be inhibited by PA+EF but not by other combinations.

EF can be implicated in many pathophysiological implications during the course of systemic anthrax infections.

Observed progressive hyperglycemia accompanied by marked reduction in liver glycogen followed by severe terminal hypoglycemia (Fish *et al.*, 1968) may reflect alterations in cAMP concentrations in hepatic tissues and possibly other tissues as well (Ezzell, 1986).

Lethal factor appears to inhibit macrophage function since PA+LF are highly toxic to mouse macrophages *in vitro*. LF probably alters membrane integrity and increase capillary permeability (Ezzell 1986).

Fisher rats inoculated LF die following administration of the toxin. It is postulated that the death is attributable to respiratory distress resulting from fluid loss into the lungs and to circulatory distress due to pressure from fluid loss into the mediastinum (Smith and Stoner 1967). These complications in addition to oxygen utilization by the massive number of circulating bacilli contribute to the extreme anoxia observed in dying animals.

Edema factor inactivates neutrophils and induce production of TNF - alpha and interleukin I - beta from macrophages, used to induce an inflammatory reaction, ultimately leading to septic shock and death. Recent studies have shown that anthrax also targets endothelial cells causing vascular leakage of fluid and cells and ultimately hypovolumic shock and septic shock. On Calmodulin binding, the edema factor helical domain of relative molecular mass 15000 under goes a structural change which leads to enzyme activation (Drum *et al.*, 2002).

PA may interact with LF before binding to cell receptor (Brossier *et al.*, 2000). Firoved *et al.* (2005) reported that B.anthracis edema toxin (ET) is an adenylyl cryclase and an important virulence determinant. It causes intestinal intralumenal fluid accumulation in dead mice followed by focal haemorrhages of ileum and adrenal glands with histophathological lesions in several organs. Several cytokines released are granulocyte colony stimulating factor, toxin, and keratinocyte derived cytokine, Il-6, IL-10 & 1 L-1B. Studies have shown that *B.anthracis* poly-gamma-D-glutamate capsule is essential for virulence. It impedes phagocytosis and protects bacilli from immune system, thus promoting systemic dissemination. It also helps in mediating the trapping of the bacteria with in the liver thus affecting the pathogenesis (Piris-Gimenez *et al.*, 2009). The capsule may bind the LF and exhert LT protease activity (Ezzell *et al.*, 2009).

Yoo HanSang *et al.* (1999) reported that PA did not induce inflammatory response, but sonicated cellular antigens and whole cell antigens induced production of nitric oxide, interleukin - 6 and TNF - alpha in a time and dose dependent manner. It is suggested that in addition to major virulence factors other cellular antigens are also involved in the initial stage of disease by inducing inflammatory mediators.

It is the production of two powerful exo-toxins and *lethal toxin* by the bacteria that causes death. Veterinarians can often tell a possible anthrax-induced death by its sudden occurrence, and by the dark, non-clotting blood that oozes from the body orifices. Most anthrax bacteria inside the body after death are out-competed and destroyed by anaerobic bacteria within minutes to hours postmortem. However, anthrax vegetative bacteria that escape the body via oozing blood or through the opening of the carcass may form hardy spores. One spore forms per one vegetative bacterium. The triggers for spore formation are not yet known, though oxygen tension and lack of nutrients may play roles. Once formed, these spores are very hard to eradicate.

The infection of herbivores (and occasionally humans) via the inhalational route normally proceeds as follows: Once the spores are inhaled, they are transported through the air passages into the tiny air particles sacs (alveoli) in the lungs. The spores are then picked up by scavenger cells (macrophages) in the lungs and are transported through small vessels (lymphatics) to the lymph nodes in the central chest cavity (mediastinum). Damage caused by the anthrax spores and bacilli to the central chest cavity can cause chest pain and difficulty breathing. Once in the lymph nodes, the spores germinate into active bacilli that multiply and eventually burst the macrophages, releasing many more bacilli into the bloodstream to be transferred to the entire body. Once in the blood stream, these bacilli release three proteins named *lethal factor*, *edema factor*, and *protective antigen*. All three are non-toxic by themselves, but the combination is incredibly lethal to humans.[12] Protective antigen combines with these other two factors to form lethal toxin and edema toxin, respectively. These toxins are the primary agents of tissue destruction, bleeding, and death of the host. If antibiotics are administered too late, even if the antibiotics eradicate the bacteria, some hosts will still die of toxemia. This is because the toxins produced by the bacilli remain in their system at lethal dose levels.

In order to enter the cells, the edema and lethal factors use another protein produced by *B. anthracis* called *protective antigen*. Protective antigen binds to two surface receptors on the host cell. A cell protease then cleaves PA into two fragments: PA_{20} and PA_{63}. PA_{20} dissociates into the extracellular medium, playing no further role in the toxic cycle. PA_{63} then oligomerizes with six other PA_{63} fragments forming a heptameric ring-shaped structure named a prepore. Once in this shape, the complex can competitively bind up to three EF or LF forming a resistant complex.[12] Receptor-mediated endocytosis occurs next, providing the newly formed toxic complex access to the interior of the host cell. The acidified environment within the endosome triggers the heptamer to release the LF and/or EF into the cytosol.[13] It is unknown how exactly the complex results in the death of the cell.

Edema factor is a calmodulin-dependent adenylate cyclase. Adenylate cyclase catalyzes the conversion of ATP into cyclic AMP (cAMP) and pyrophosphate. The complexation of adenylate cyclase with calmodulin removes calmodulin from stimulating calcium-triggered signaling, thus inhibiting the immune response.[12] To be specific, LF inactivates neutrophils (a type of phagocytic cell) by the process just described so that they cannot phagocytose bacteria. Throughout history, it was believed that lethal factor caused macrophages to make TNF-alpha and interleukin 1, beta (IL1B). TNF-alpha is a cytokine whose primary role is to regulate immune cells as well as to induce inflammation and apoptosis or programmed cell death. Interleukin 1, beta is another cytokine that also regulates inflammation and apoptosis. The over-production of TNF-alpha and IL1B ultimately leads to septic shock and death. However, recent evidence indicates that anthrax also targets endothelial cells (cells that line serous cavities such as the pericardial cavity, pleural cavity, and the peritoneal cavity, lymph vessels, and blood vessels), causing vascular leakage of fluid and cells, and ultimately hypovolemic shock (low blood volume), and septic shock.

In order to initiate a productive infection, *B. anthracis* needs to circumvent the innate protective response of the host. It has been shown that the pathogen employs a number of strategies against the immune cells using secreted pathogenic factors. For example, lethal and edema toxins secreted along with other virulence factors such as hemolysins within the phagosomal compartment of macrophages allow the bacteria to resist being killed and to escape from the phagocytes. Cleavage of mitogen-activated protein kinase kinases by lethal toxin seems to play a central role in the immunosuppressive capacity of *B. anthracis* to induce necrosis or apoptosis of macrophages and to inhibit responses of dendritic and T cells. The pore-forming hemolysin anthrolysin O is able to damage membranes of different immune cell types and to sensitize macrophages to lethal toxin. However, interference of *B. anthracis* with the innate immune system through specific interaction of the spore surface with the host proteins such as the complement system has heretofore attracted little attention.

The complement system facilitates bactericidal activity of normal human serum (NHS) in early clearance of pathogens. The complement system can be activated through three different pathways: classical, lectin, and alternative. Deposition of complement C3b onto the bacterial surface is a crucial step in eliminating the pathogen. To escape complement-mediated killing, pathogens use a common evasion strategy by acquiring the fluid-phase complement factor H, complement factor H-related proteins (FHRs), complement factor H-like proteins (FHLs), the complement C4-binding protein from host serum. It has also been observed that *B. anthracis* can directly infect non-phagocytic cells and invade tissues of the nasopharynx after spore inhalation without needing to be transported by alveolar macrophages to the lymphatics . Since functional complement proteins are present in the bronchoalveolar lavage fluid (BALF), complement C3-dependent opsonization is expected to play an important role in the early stages of inhalational *B. anthracis* infection. In fact, C3b can bind to *B. anthracis* spores opsonized by the normal human serum (NHS) and thus enhance phagocytosis by human macrophages. Complement-deficient A/J mice are highly susceptible to the attenuated *B. anthracis* Sterne strain, and the resistant C57BL/6 mice acquire susceptibility to challenge with the attenuated Sterne strain after depletion of complement by cobra venom injection.

In order to assess the mechanisms by which B. anthracis evades the defense system, Chung et al.(2011) employed a proteomic analysis to identify human serum proteins interacting with B. anthracis spores, and found that plasminogen (PLG) is a major surface-bound protein. PLG efficiently bound to spores in a lysine- and exosporium-dependent manner. The authors identified α-enolase and elongation factor tu as PLG receptors. PLG-bound spores were capable of exhibiting anti-opsonic properties by cleaving C3b molecules in vitro and in rabbit bronchoalveolar lavage fluid, resulting in a decrease in macrophage phagocytosis. These findings represent a step forward in understanding the mechanisms involved in the evasion of innate immunity by B. anthracis through recruitment of PLG resulting in the enhancement of anti-complement and anti-opsonization properties of the pathogen. Research by other groups has indicated that anthrax toxin kills macrophages by inducing a runaway reaction called an oxidative burst. It has been speculated that this kinesin protein might be transporting either the elements that are part of this oxidative burst, or the actual oxidative compounds themselves. Or, the protein may be ensuring the prompt and appropriate delivery of compounds that protect the macrophage against its own oxidative bursts. So, while the subtle mutations that we see in *Kif1C* gene probably don't affect the macrophages in their normal functioning, the decrease in efficiency during the stress of intoxication by the anthrax toxin can mean the difference between death and survival of the macrophage.

To evaluate the pathogenic potential of Bacillus anthracis-secreted proteases distinct from lethal toxin, two neutral zinc metalloproteases were purified to apparent homogeneity from the culture supernatant of a non-virulent delta Ames strain (pXO1-, pXO2-) (Chung et al.2006). The first (designated Npr599) is a thermolysin-like enzyme highly homologous to bacillolysins from other Bacillus species. The second (designated InhA) is a homolog of the Bacillus thuringiensis immune inhibitor A. These proteases belong to the M4 and M6 families, respectively. Both enzymes digested various substrates, including extracellular matrix proteins, endogenous inhibitors, and coagulation proteins, with some differences in specificity. In addition, InhA accelerated urokinase-mediated plasminogen activation, suggesting that InhA acts as a modulator of plasmin in the host inflammatory system. Relevant to epithelial barrier function, Npr599 and InhA significantly enhanced syndecan-1 shedding from cultured normal murine mammary gland cells without affecting their viability through stimulation of the host cell ectodomain shedding mechanism. In addition, Npr599 and InhA directly cleaved recombinant syndecan-1 fused to glutathione S-transferase. Mass spectrometric analysis suggested that the cleavage sites of Npr599 and InhA are the Asp(39)-Asp(40) and Gly(48)-Thr(49) bonds, respectively. It was proposed that Npr599 and InhA from B. anthracis are multifunctional pathogenic factors that may contribute to anthrax pathology through direct degradation of host tissues, increases in barrier permeability, and/or modulation of host defenses.

The fibrinolytic system is often the target for pathogenic bacteria, resulting in increased fibrinolysis, bacterial dissemination, and inflammation (Chung *et al.* 2011a). The purpose of this study was to explore whether proteases NprB and InhA secreted by Bacillus anthracis could activate the host's fibrinolytic system. NprB efficiently activated human pro-urokinase plasminogen activator (pro-uPA), a key protein in the fibrinolytic cascade. Conversely, InhA had little effect on pro-uPA. Plasminogen activator inhibitors (PAI)-1, 2 and the uPA receptor were also targets for NprB in vitro. InhA efficiently degraded the thrombin-activatable fibrinolysis inhibitor (TAFI) in vitro. Mice infected with B. anthracis showed a significant decrease in blood TAFI levels. In another mouse experiment, animals infected with isogenic inhA deletion mutants restored TAFI levels, while the levels in the parent strain decreased. It was propose that NprB and InhA may contribute to the activation of the fibrinolytic system in anthrax infection.

Jenkins *et al.* (2011) hypothesized that an intact purine biosynthetic pathway is required for the virulence of B. anthracis in guinea pigs.

Diagnosis

Diagnosis is often difficult to arrive at due to sudden death of the animals. Presence of black uncoagulated blood oozing out of the nose, mouth and anus of dead animals is indicative of anthrax. Other than Gram Stain of specimens, there are no specific direct identification techniques for identification of *Bacillus species* in clinical material. These organisms are Gram-positive but with age can be Gram-variable to Gram-negative. A specific feature of *Bacillus species* that makes it unique from other aerobic microorganisms is its ability to produce spores. Although spores are not always evident on a Gram stain of this organism, the presence of spores confirms that the organism is of the genus *Bacillus*.

To confirm the diagnosis an ear or portion of spleen should be sent to a laboratory for conducting Ascoli Precipitation Test and for culture of the causative bacteria using 5% sheep blood agar and other routine culture media. Selective medium can be used for isolation from contaminated medium. *B.anthrax* will grow with in 24 hours at 35-37ºC in air or in 5% Co_2. If carbonate agar is used for isolation then the bacterium must be grown at 5% Co_2. Colonies are non-haemolytic on sheep blood and produce "medusa head". Experimental animal inoculation may be carried out using guinea pigs. Utmost care is required while handling the suspected material. Microscopic examination of blood reveals large numbers of encapsulated bacilli either in single or short chains. Wrights, methylene blue or Giemsa staining of blood smear is suitable. In wet smears the organisms are non-motile. Confirmatory testing to identify

B.anthracis includes gamma bacteriophage testing, indirect haemagglutination and ELISA to detect antibodies.

Duriez *et al.* (2009) have developed a sensitive enzymatic assay to be able to monitor functional EF in human and animal plasma. Samples containing EF are incubated in the presence of calmodulin and ATP, which is converted to cAMP. After oxidation and derivatization, cAMP is monitored by competitive enzyme immunoassay. Because of the high turnover of EF and the sensitivity of cAMP detection, EF can be detected at concentrations of 1 pg/mL (10 fM) in 4 h in plasma from humans or at 10 pg/mL in the plasma of various animal species using only a blood volume of 5 microL. The assay has good reproducibility with intra- and interday coefficients of variation in the range of 20% and is not subject to significant interindividual matrix effects. In an experimental study performed in mice infected with the Berne strain, the authors were able to detect EF in serum and ear tissues. This simple and robust combination of enzymatic reaction and enzyme immunoassay for the diagnosis of anthrax toxemia could prove useful in biological threat detection as well in research and clinical practice.

Treatment and Control

There is no effective antibiotic for treatment of septicaemic anthrax. Respiratory anthrax,can be cured which in the absence of early antibiotic treatment, is a fatal disease. One study aimed to test the efficiency of antibiotic therapy in curing infected animals and those sick with anthrax has been reported (Weiss et al 2011) . Postexposure prophylaxis (24 h postinfection [p.i.]) of guinea pigs infected intranasally with Bacillus anthracis Vollum spores with doxycycline, ofloxacin, imipenem, and gentamicin conferred protection. However, upon termination of treatment, the animals died from respiratory anthrax. Combined treatment with antibiotics and active vaccination with a protective antigen-based vaccine leads to full protection even after cessation of treatment. Delaying the initiation of antibiotic administration to over 24 h post -infection resulted in treatment of animals with anthrax exhibiting various degrees of bacteremia and toxemia. Treatment with doxycycline or ciprofloxacin cured sick guinea pigs and rabbits exhibiting bacteremia levels up to 10(5) CFU/ml. Addition of anti-protective antigen (PA) antibodies augmented the efficiency of protection, allowing the cure of guinea pigs and rabbits with 10- to 20-fold-higher bacteremia levels, up to 7 × 10(5) CFU/ml and 2 × 10(6) CFU/ml, respectively. Treatment with ciprofloxacin and a monoclonal anti-PA antibody rescued rabbits with bacteremia levels up to 4 × 10(6) CFU/ml. During antibiotic administration, all surviving animals developed a protective immune response against development of a fatal disease and subcutaneous challenge with Vollum spores. In conclusion, antibiotic treatment can prevent the development of fatal disease in respiratory-anthrax-infected animals and can cure animals after disease establishment. A therapeutic time window of 40 h to 48 h from infection to initiation of efficient antibiotic-mediated cure was observed.

During an outbreak adoption of strict quarantine measures is the first priority. This also includes prohibition of movement of milk and meat from the farm. As such hygiene is the biggest single factor in the prevention of spread of the disease. Careful disposal of infected material is most important. Infected carcasses should not be opened but immediately burnt or buried. Deep burial is preferred with quicklime or be incinerated. Suspected animals should be segregated. Prophylactic administration of a single dose of long acting antibiotic is preferred. Washing of floor especially the abattoir floor with any disinfectant is useful to prevent formation of spores from the vegetative cells. Strong solutions of formalin or sodium hydroxide (5-10%) are most effective especially when formation of spores is suspected. Infected clothing should be sterilized by soaking in 10% formaldehyde. Destruction of discharges is advocated and shoes, clothes etc. should be exposed to germicidal substances for proper disinfection.

Special care must be taken to avoid human contact with infected material and accidentally if contact occurs, the contaminated skin should be thoroughly disinfected. Prophylactic experiments for treatment of respiratory anthrax have been conducted in monkeys, guinea pigs, mice, and sheep. Treatment of infected rhesus monkeys with penicillin for 20 or 30 days protected the animals, but upon cessation of treatment only approximately 70% of the animals survived. Treatment with doxycyline and ciprofloxacin for 30 days provided protection during treatment, and after termination of antibiotic injections approximately 90% of the animals survived. The surviving animals did not develop protective immune responses, and following rechallenge, 85 to 100% of the animals developed fatal disease. Full protection was achieved by combination of treatment with penicillin or doxycycline together with active immunization with protective antigen (PA)-based vaccines, which include components of the lethal and edema toxins Lincoln et al. (1964) described a successful treatment that protected 84% of septicemic monkeys by administration of antibiotics together with anti-Sterne antisera and the PA-based vaccine. Successful treatment of sheep that were infected via inhalation with Vollum spores was achieved by 5 days of injections of penicillin or tetracycline with and without coadministration of the PA-based vaccine. Experiments with infected guinea pigs were performed with penicillin and doxycycline and ciprofloxacin. In the latter experiment, the antibiotic treatment was begun 2 days prior to infection. During treatment the infected animals survived. However, after cessation of treatment, 14% of the penicillin-treated animals survived, compared to 92.5 and 90% of the animals treated with doxycycline and ciprofloxacin, respectively. Similar experiments with mice indicated that penicillin and streptomycin could provide either partial or full protection. Chloramphenicol failed to protect the animals. Altboum et al.(2002) tested the efficiency of postexposure prophylaxis against Bacillus anthracis infection in guinea pigs infected intranasally with either Vollum or strain ATCC 6605 spores (75 times the 50% lethal dose [LD(50)] and 87 times LD(50,) respectively). Starting 24 h postinfection, animals were treated three times per day for 14 days with ciprofloxacin, tetracycline, erythromycin, cefazolin, and trimethoprim-sulfamethoxazole (TMP-SMX). Administration of cefazolin and TMP-SMX failed to protect the animals, while ciprofloxacin, tetracycline, and erythromycin prevented death. Upon cessation of treatment all erythromycin-treated animals died; of the tetracycline-treated animals, two of eight infected with Vollum and one of nine infected with ATCC 6605 survived; and of the ciprofloxacin group injected with either 10 or 20 mg/kg of body weight, five of nine and five of five animals, respectively, survived. To test the added value of extending the treatment period, Vollum-infected (46 times the LD(50)) animals were treated for 30 days with ciprofloxacin or tetracycline, resulting in protection of eight of nine and nine of nine animals, respectively. Once treatment was discontinued, only four of eight and five of nine animals, respectively, survived. Following rechallenge (intramuscularly) of the survivors with 30 times the LD(50) of Vollum spores, all ciprofloxacin-treated animals were protected while none of the tetracycline-treated animals survived. In an attempt to confer protective immunity lasting beyond the termination of antibiotic administration, Vollum-infected animals were immunized with a protective antigen (PA)-based vaccine concurrently with treatment with either ciprofloxacin or tetracycline. The combined treatment protected eight of eight and nine of nine animals. Following cessation of antibiotic administration seven of eight and eight of eight animals survived, of which six of seven and eight of eight resisted rechallenge. These results indicate that a combined treatment of antibiotics together with a PA-based vaccine could provide long-term protection to prevent reoccurrence of anthrax disease.

Passive immunization with antitoxin antibodies that neutralize the activity of the lethal toxin may be an effective adjunct or alternative treatment. Passive immunization may also be efficient as preexposure treatment when the prolonged vaccination schedule is not applicable and antibiotic treatment is not efficient, as in the case of infection with antibiotic-resistant strains or in immunocompromised persons.At the beginning of the previous century, prior to the antibiotic era, people infected with anthrax were treated with antiserum obtained from animals that were immunized with virulent strains. However, the use of antianthrax serum for human treatment was abandoned years ago in most Western countries as being of negligible value.

The efficacy of passive immunization as a postexposure prophylactic measure for treatment of guinea pigs intranasally infected with Bacillus anthracis spores was evaluated (Kobiler et al.2002). Antisera directed either against the lethal toxin components (PA or LF) or against a toxinogenic strain (Sterne) were used for this evaluation. All antisera exhibited high enzyme-linked immunosorbent assay titers against the corresponding antigens, high titers of neutralization of cytotoxicity activity in an in vitro mouse macrophages cell line (J774A.1), as well as in vivo neutralization of toxicity when administered either directly to Fisher rats prior to challenge with the lethal toxin or after incubation with the lethal toxin. In these tests, anti-LF antiserum exhibited the highest neutralization efficiency, followed by anti-Sterne and anti-PA. The time dependence and antibody dose necessary for conferring postexposure protection by the various antibodies of guinea pigs infected with 25 50% lethal doses of Vollum spores was examined. Rabbit anti-PA serum was found to be the most effective. Intraperitoneal injections of anti-PA serum given 24 h postinfection protected 90% of the infected animals, whereas anti-Sterne and anti-LF were less effective. These results further emphasize the importance of anti-PA antibodies in conferring protection against B. anthracis infection and demonstrated the ability of such antibodies to be effectively applied as an efficient postexposure treatment against anthrax disease.

In May 1881 Louis Pasteur performed a public experiment to demonstrate his concept of vaccination. He prepared two groups of 25 sheep, one goat and several cows. The animals of one group were injected with an anthrax vaccine prepared by Pasteur twice, at an interval of 15 days; the control group was left unvaccinated. Thirty days after the first injection, both groups were injected with a culture of live anthrax bacteria. All the animals in the non-vaccinated group died, while all of the animals in the vaccinated group survived. The human vaccine for anthrax became available in 1954. This was a cell-free vaccine instead of the live-cell Pasteur-style vaccine used for veterinary purposes. An improved cell-free vaccine became available in 1970.

Duverger et al. (2010) have shown that intranasal coapplication of Bacillus anthracis protective Ag (PA) together with a B. anthracis edema factor (EF) mutant having reduced adenylate cyclase activity (i.e., EF-S414N) enhances anti-PA Ab responses, but also acts as a mucosal adjuvant for coadministered unrelated Ags. To elucidate the role of edema toxin (EdTx) components in its adjuvanticity, the authors examined how a PA mutant lacking the ability to bind EF (PA-U7) or another mutant that allows the cellular uptake of EF, but fails to efficiently mediate its translocation into the cytosol (PA-dFF), would affect EdTx-induced adaptive immunity. Native EdTx promotes costimulatory molecule expression by macrophages and B lymphocytes, and a broad spectrum of cytokine responses by cervical lymph node cells in vitro. These effects were reduced or abrogated when cells were treated with EF plus PA-dFF, or PA-U7 instead of PA. We also intranasally immunized groups of mice with a recombinant fusion protein of Yersinia pestis F1 and LcrV Ags (F1-V) together with EdTx variants consisting of wild-type or mutants PA and EF. Analysis of serum and mucosal Ab responses against F1-V or EdTx components (i.e., PA and EF) revealed no adjuvant activity in mice that received PA-U7 instead of PA. In contrast, coimmunization with PA-dFF enhanced serum Ab responses. Finally, immunization with native PA and an EF mutant lacking adenylate cyclase activity (EF-K346R) failed to enhance Ab responses. In summary, a fully functional PA and a minimum of adenylate cyclase activity are needed for EdTx to act as a mucosal adjuvant.

Vaccination with an avirulent spore vaccine using Stern strain is now used for large animals in India. This vaccine produces strong immunity for up to 1-2 years in cattle & sheep. Although one dose is sufficient to induce immunity 2 vaccinations are necessary in some situation (Salmon and Ferrier, 1992). A febrile reaction occurs following the vaccination which is characterized by the drop in milk production and abortion in pregnant sows. Localized subcutaneous edema often occurs with in 24 hours at the site of injection but is rarely severe. In enzootic areas, annual revaccination of animals is recommended. In case of occurrence of disease in otherwise clean areas, all in contact animals should be treated. Vaccination in clean areas is not recommended with the fear of introduction of infection at the farm. Milk from vaccinated cows is discarded for 3 days after the inoculation of the vaccine although ordinarily the organisms of stern strain are not excreted in milk. Antibiotics should not be administered soon after the vaccination since the spores in the vaccine germinate to vegetative cells to induce immunity.

References

Altboum Z., Gozes Y., Barnea A., Pass A., White M. and Kobiler D.2002.Postexposure prophylaxis against anthrax: evaluation of various treatment regimens in intranasally infected guinea pigs. Infect Immun. **70:** 6231-6241.

Beall, F.A. and Daldorf, F.G. 1966. The pathogenesis of the lethal effect of anthrax toxin in rats. J. Infect. Dis. **116:** 377-389.

Beall, F.A., Taylor, M.J. and Thorne, C.B. 1962. Rapid lethal effect in rats of a third component found upon functioning of the toxin of *Bacillus anthracis*. J. Bacteriol. **83:** 1274-1280.

Brossier, F., Weber, Levy, M., Mock, M. and Sirad, J.C. 2000. Role of toxin functional domains in anthrax pathogenesis. Infect. Immun. **68:** 1781-1786.

Chung M.C., Jorgensen S.C., Tonry J.H., Kashanchi F., Bailey C. and Popov S.2011a Secreted Bacillus anthracis proteases target the host fibrinolytic system. FEMS Immunol. Med Microbiol.doi:10.1111/j.1574-5X.2011.00798.x[http://www.ncbi.nlm.nih.gov/pubmed/21395696].

Chung M.C., Popova T.G., Millis B.A., Mukherjee D.V., Zhou W., Liotta L.A., Petricoin E.F., Chandhoke V., Bailey C. and Popov S.G.2006.Secreted neutral metalloproteases of Bacillus anthracis as candidate pathogenic factors. J. Biol. Chem. **281:** 31408-31418. Epub 2006 Aug 22.

Chung M.C., Tonry J.H., Narayanan A., Manes N.P., Mackie R.S., Gutting B., Mukherjee D.V., Popova T.G., Kashanchi F., Bailey C.L. and Popov S.G.2011.Bacillus anthracis Interacts with Plasmin(ogen) to Evade C3b-Dependent Innate Immunity. PLoS One. 6:e18119.

Drum, C.L., Yan, S.Z., Bard, J., Shen, Y.Q., Lu, D., Soeleima, S., Grabarek, Z., Bohm, A., and Tang, W.J. 2002. Structural basis for the activation of anthrax adenylyl cyclase exotoxin by calmodulin. Nature, **415:** 396-402.

Duriez E., Goossens P.L., Becher F. and Ezan E.2009.Femtomolar detection of the anthrax edema factor in human and animal plasma. Anal. Chem. **81:** 5935-5941.

Duverger A., Carré J.M., Jee J., Leppla S.H., Cormet-Boyaka E., Tang W.J., Tomé D. and Boyaka P.N. 2010.Contributions of edema factor and protective antigen to the induction of protective immunity by Bacillus anthracis edema toxin as an intranasal adjuvant. J. Immunol. **185:** 5943-52. Epub 2010 Oct 15.

Ezzell, J. 1986. *Bacillus anthracis*. In pathogenesis of bacterial infections in animals, ed. Gyles, C.L. and Thoen, C.O. pp. 21-25. Iowa: Iowa State Univ. Press.

Ezzell, J.W., Abshire, T.G., Panchal, R., Chabot, D., Bavari, S., Leffel, E.K. and Purcell, B. 2009. Association of *B.anthracis* capsule with lethal toxin during experimental infection. Infcct. Immun. **77:** 749-755.

Firoved, A.M., Miller, G.F., Mouyeri, M., Kakkar, R., *et al.*, 2005. *B.anthracis* edema toxin causes extensive tissue lesions and rapid lethality in mice. Am. J. Pathol. **167:** 1309-1320.

Fish, D.C:, Klein, F., Lincoln, R.E., Walker, J.S. and Dobbs, J.P. 1968. Pathophysiological changes in the rat associated with anthrax toxin. J. Infect. Dis. **118:** 114-124.

Jenkins A., Cote C., Twenhafel N., Merkel T., Bozue J. and Welkos S. 2011.Role of purine biosynthesis in Bacillus anthracis pathogenesis and virulence. Infect. Immun. **79:** 153-166. Epub 2010 Nov 1.

Kobiler D., Gozes Y., Rosenberg H., Marcus D., Reuveny S. and Altboum Z.2002.Efficiency of protection of guinea pigs against infection with Bacillus anthracis spores by passive immunization. Infect. Immun. **70:** 544-560.

Leepla, S.H. 1982. Anthrax toxin edema factor: A bacterial adenylal cyclase that increases cyclic AMP concentrations in eukaryotic cells. Proc. Natl. Acad. Sci. **79:** 3162-3166.

Leepla, S.H. 1984. *Bacillus anthracis* calmodulin dependent adenycate cyclase: Chemical and enzymatic properties and interaction with eukaryotic cells. In Advances in cyclic Nucleotide and protein phosphorylation research. Vol 17, ed. P. Greengard and G.A. Robinson. pp 189-98 New York: Raven Press.

Lincoln, R. E., Klein F. , J. S. Walker, B. W. Haines, W. I. Jones, B. G. Mahlandt, and R. H. Friedman. 1964. Successful treatment of monkeys for septicemia anthrax. Antimicrob. Agent. Chemother. **4:** 759-763.

Lincoln, R.E. and Fish, D.C. 1970. Anthrax toxin. In Microbial Toxins Vo. 3 ed. T. Monte, S. Kadis, and S. Ajl. Pp 361-419. New York, Academic Press.

O'Brien, J., Friedlander, A., Dreier, T., Ezzell, J. and Leepla, S. 1985. Effects of anthrax toxin components on human neutrophils. Infect. Immun. **47:** 306-310.

Piris - Gimenez, A., Corre, J.P., Jourion, G., Candela, T., Khun-Hout and Goossens, P.L. 2009. Encapsulated *B.anthracis* interacts closely with liver endothelium. J. Infect. Dis. **200:** 1381-1389.

Salmon, DD and Ferrier, G.R. 1992. Vet. Rec. 130, 14a

Uchida, I., Sekizaki, T., Hashimoto, K. and Terakado, N. 1985. Association of the encapsulation of *Bacillus anthracis* with a 60 megadalton plasmid. J. Gen. Microbiol. **131:** 363-367.

Yoo HanSang, Kim - JaeWook and Cho-YuuSang. 1999. Production of nitric oxide, interleukin 6 and TNF-á from mouse peritoneal macrophages in response to *B.anthracis* antigens. Korean J. Vet. Res. **39:** 301-310.

Weiss S., Kobiler D., Levy H., Pass A., Ophir Y., Rothschild N., Tal A., Schlomovitz J. and Altboum Z.2011.Antibiotics cure anthrax in animal models. Antimicrob. Agents Chemother. **55:** 1533-1542. Epub 2011 Jan 24.

□□□

Chapter 9

Leptospirosis

Dr. S.K. SRIVASTAVA
Former, Division of Bacteriology & Mycology
Indian Veterinary Research Institute, Izatnagar-243122
Bareilly (U.P.)

Leptospirosis

Leptospirosis is an important zoonotic disease responsible for septicaemia, interstitial nephritis, Jaundice, abortions and reproductive problems in most animal species. In older cattle, signs vary greatly and diagnosis is more difficult. Enzootic infections of naive cattle with serovar *hardjo* , which usually result in abnormal milk, are more obvious in dairy cattle. Signs usually are restricted to a sudden drop in milk production; a hemolytic crisis does not occur. The milk is thick, yellow, and blood-tinged, with thick clots and a high somatic cell count; milk production can drop 10-75%, depending on the infecting strain. The udder is typically soft and flabby, which is unique for leptospirosis. Milk production can return to normal in 10-14 days even in the absence of treatment; however, cows with a severe drop in production may not recover to full production during that lactation cycle.

The chronic forms of leptospirosis manifest as abortion and stillbirths, and occur with infections of serovars *Pomona* and *Hardjo* . Abortion generally occurs 6-12 wk after initial infection and is more common during the third trimester. Stillbirths and birth of premature or weak infected calves also occur. An abortion storm in a breeding herd is often the first indication of leptospirosis infection, because the mild initial signs often pass unnoticed. In endemically infected herds, abortions occur mostly in younger animals and are sporadic. Calves reared by previously infected cows are protected by colostral antibodies for up to 6 mo. The calves generally have an antibody titer similar to that of their dams. Infertility may also be a problem in endemically infected herds, possibly as a consequence of localization of infection in the uterus and oviducts.

In the acute form, anemia, icterus, hemoglobinuria, and submucosal hemorrhages are prominent. The kidneys are swollen and dark, with multifocal petechial and ecchymotic hemorrhages, and later develop pale foci of interstitial cell infiltrates. The liver may be swollen, pale, and friable, with minute areas of focal necrosis. Petechiae in other organs are seen in fulminating cases; however, in the more prevalent serovar *hardjo* infections, the lesions are primarily restricted to the kidneys.

Among dogs there is no age or gender predilection, although German Shepherds may be at increased risk compared with other breeds. The incubation period is 4-12 days but may be as short as 2 days. Acute renal failure occurs in 80-90% of dogs that develop clinically significant disease. Early findings are nonspecific and include fever, depression, lethargy, anorexia, arthralgia or myalgia, and oculonasal discharge. This may progress within a few days to a uremic crisis characterized by vomiting, dehydration, lumbar pain from renomegaly and nephritis, and tongue-tip ulceration and necrosis. Icterus and bilirubinuria, suggestive of cholestasis and/or hepatic necrosis, develop in ~20% of these cases and may be present without renal failure. In dogs that develop milder forms of renal failure, polyuria and polydipsia may be the primary sign. Other syndromes reported in dogs include intussusception, pulmonary hemorrhage, uveitis, pneumonitis, chronic hepatitis, and reproductive failure.

The most common hematologic abnormality is a mild to moderate neutrophilic leukocytosis without a left shift, although a normal WBC count may be seen. A mild anemia is seen in 25-35% of cases, often as a result of subclinical hemolysis. Thrombocytopenia occurs in only 10-20% of dogs but is rarely severe enough to be a source of bleeding. Vasculitis is typically the cause of hemorrhage associated with leptospirosis. Azotemia is the most common finding on a serum biochemistry profile. When liver values are abnormal, elevations in serum alkaline phosphatase are typically more pronounced than elevations in ALT and AST. Serum bilirubin is elevated in ~20% of cases. Isosthenuria or hyposthenuria is typically present on the urinalysis, and hematuria, proteinuria, and granular casts are identified in ~30% of cases. Pyuria is less frequently seen, and glycosuria may be identified on occasion as a result of renal tubular damage. Leptospirosis in horses is most commonly associated with uveitis or abortions. The disease is typically seen as a self-limiting mild fever with anorexia, although in severe forms hemolysis and vasculitis can result in petechial hemorrhages on mucosal surfaces, hemoglobinuria, anemia, icterus, conjunctival suffusion, depression, and weakness. Renal failure has been documented in foals. Recurrent uveitis (moon blindness) develops anytime from 2-8 mo following the initial infection. Leptospirosis appears to be a significant cause of recurrent uveitis in horses, accounting for up to 67% of the cases. Serovar *pomona* and an unidentified serovar have been isolated from the aqueous humor of horses with uveitis. It is not clear whether the uveitis is due to intraocular infection or is immune-mediated. Leptospirosis is responsible for 3-4% of all equine abortions annually, although flooding and other environmental catastrophes may result in abortion outbreaks. In the USA, serovar *Pomona* type Kennewicki appears to be the most significant cause of abortion. The prevalence of leptospirosis in horses is unknown, but serologic evidence indicates a higher incidence than is apparent clinically. In the USA, seroconversion to serovar Bratislava is reported in up to 40% of horses in large population studies; horses may be a reservoir host for serovar Bratislava.

The disease has a worldwide distribution and in India more cases have been reported in southern coastal regions of the country than other areas. In general, the disease is more common in areas or seasons when the climate is warm and humid, where soil is lightly alkaline and water is in abundance. Thus, leptospirosis usually follows in area after heavy rain.

Seroprevalence of leptospirosis was investigated in animals from various states of India during a period of 10 years beginning 1990. Most of these animals had suffered with fever, jaundice, abortions, repeat breeding etc. A total of 15.8% of sera from cattle were found to posses diagnostic levels of anti - Leptospira agglutinins. Most of these were from various regions of Andhra Pradesh and Gujarat. In addition 2.8% of the buffalo sera from Gujarat were positive. Goat, sheep, equine and swine sera were also found positive in various regions of the country. Wild animals viz; Sambhar, Cheetal, Tiger and Elephant were found positive up to 12.5%. Most of the Leptospira serovars which reacted with the positive sera were in decreasing order, Icterohaemorrhagiae, Hardjo, Patoc, Australis, Canicola, Grippotyphosa, Pyrogenes, Pomona, Tarassovi & Ballum. The finding has very well established the prevalence of various *Leptospira* serovars in animal population in the country.

Leptospirosis in human beings is caused by accidental infections. The prevalence of *Leptospira* serovars in human populations generally is a reflection of the prevalence in the animal population with which those people have contact. Infection with Icterohaemorrhagiae is the most commonly diagnosed leptospiral infection in human beings. Distinct high risk groups for leptospirosis are workers on livestock farms and in slaughterhouses who are exposed to other serovars, especially Pomona and Hardjo. In India, percent seropositivity of leptospirosis among pet owners, sewage workers and farmers is higher than other groups. The cases of the disease recorded in man are more than those in women because the former are more involved in outward activities.

Etiology

Leptospires are long, spiral, filamentous, motile organisms that measure 0.2 to 0.3 μm in diameter and up to 10 μm in length. The ends are hooked in most of the cells.

Traditionally, two species have been described in the literature. The pathogenic species, *Leptospira interrogans* and a saprophytic, *L. biflexa. L. interrogans* with more than 230 serovars has been grouped into 23 serogroups (Estaroyer *et al.*, 2001). Differentiation of serovars belonging to serogroup is based on the cross agglutinin absorption test. Two strains are considered different if after cross absorption with heterologous antigen, 10% or more of the homologous titers always remain in one of the paired sera samples tested. Presently, finger printing technique of bacterial DNA has been used as a genotyping taxonomic tool (Zuerner *et al.*, 1990). In genotypic classification 12 genospecies and 5 unclassified genospecies has been described. These genospecies do not correspond to previously described 2 species. Some of the pathogenic species are *L.interrogans, L.borgpetersenii, L.inadai, L.myeri, L.noguchii, L.sanatarosai, L.weilli, L.wolbachii, L.fainei, L.alexanderi, L.parva* & *L.kirchneri. L.biflexa* is the saprophytic species. Interestingly many animal & human sera are found to react with this *L.biflexa* species indicating an antigenic relatedness among these species (Brenner *et al.*, 1999; Levett *et al.*, 2001).

All Leptospira cells posses an outer envelop (outer membrane) consisting of proteins and lipopolysaccharide. Several OM protein have been identified of which 32 kD & 41 kDa proteins are immunodominant. The outer envelop cytoplasmic components contain a structure called cytoplasmic cylinder, which has a peptidoglycan layer and a protoplasmic membrane. Leptospires possess 2 flagella that are modified into a structure called axial filament that is embedded between the outer envelop and the cytoplasmic cylinder. The leptospires can pass through the 0.2 m membrane filters. This property is utilized in purification of the Leptospira from the culture contaminated with bacterial population.

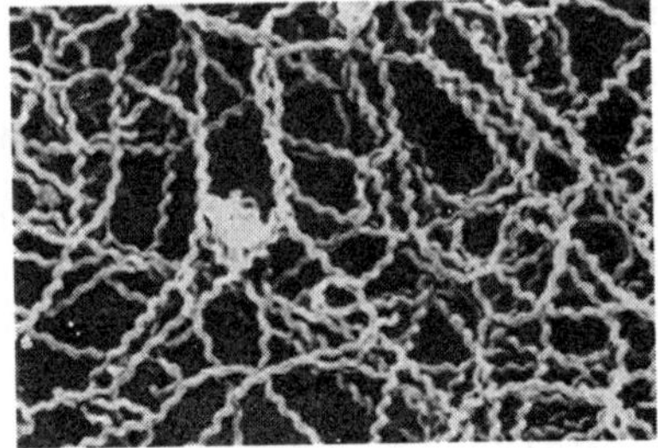

Scanning micrograph of Leptospira cells

Epidemiology

Field rats and other rodents are the important natural carriers of most of the *Leptospira* serovars; however, there is some host specificity (Table 1). Some of the *Leptospira* serovars viz; Pomona, Tarassovi and Hardjo are adapted to large animals. Combined culture and immunofluorscence studies in USA have shown that 2010 of cattle to be renal carriers (Miller *et al.*, 1999). These carrier animals play an important role in transmission and occurrence of the disease in natural host. The maintenance of cycle in nature is also based on the role these animals play as carriers of the pathogen.

Leptospirosis is endemic in many countries of the world. *L.interrogans* serovars Pomona, Canicola, Icterohaemorrhagiae, Tarassovi, Bataviae, Australis and Autumnalis are the commonest serovars prevalent in many countries. The number of serovars identified in many countries of the world is increasing.

L.interrogans serovar Pomona infection has been identified in cattle, pigs and horses and ovine as well. Serovar Hardjo has become a very common infection in cattle in many countries of the world including U.K., USA and Australia (Kmety & Dikken 1988; Silbreck & Davies, 1989). There are at least 2 distinct genotypes of serovar Hardjo present in many countries, *Hardjo bovis* and *Hardjo prajitno*. In addition there are at lease two variants of *hardjo prajitno* genotype. The degree of cross-protection conferred by these genotypes in vaccines is not known.

L.interrogans serovar Hardjo, although an important pathogen of cows but its significance in other ruminants is not well established. In India, serovar Hardjo as a major pathogen of cattle has not been identified.

L.interrogans serovar Icterohaemorrhagiae is rarely isolated from large animals but has been reported in cattle and pigs in many countries. Serological evidence is present in horses. Similarly serovars Hyos has been isolated from cattle and pigs & Grippotyphosa from cattle and goats. Similarly sejroe, Hebdomadis & Australis infection has been observed in cattle. Seroprevalence of leptospirosis has been observed in several species of animals including cattle in various regions of the country (Mariya *et al.*, 2007; Anju Singh *et al.*, 2005). Available data on animal leptospirosis in ten tropical islands: Barbados, Martinique, Guadeloupe, Grenada, Trinidad, New Caledonia, Hawaii, French Polynesia, La Réunion and Mayotte reveals that Leptospirosis is endemic in these insular wild and domestic fauna. Each island presents a specific panel of circulating serovars, closely linked with animal and environmental biodiversity, making it epidemiologically different from the mainland. Rats, mongooses and mice are proven major renal carriers of leptospires in these areas but dogs also constitute a significant potential reservoir. In some islands seroprevalence of leptospirosis in animals evolves with time, inducing changes in the epidemiology of the human disease (Desvars *et al.*, 2011).

Serovars and host susceptibility

There is some degree of host susceptibility among *Leptospira* serovars although they may cause disease in any mammalian host. A serovar behave, differently within its maintenance host species than it does in others; incidental or accidental host. Serovars *Bratislava* and *Hardjo* bovis are maintained in pigs and cattle, respectively, whereas for serovar kennewicki cattle are the incidental host.

Table 1 : The common serovars and their maintenance hosts are as follows:

Serovar	Maintenance host
Hardjo bovis (North America)	Cattle
Hardjo prajitno (Europe)	Cattle
Bratislava	Pig, Horse
Kennewicki	Pig, Skunk, raccoon, opossum
Grippotyphosa	Racoon, opssum, squirrels
Icterohaemorrhagiae	Brown rat

Some common leptospiral serovars and their accidental hosts:

Serovar	Accidental Hosts
Hardjo	Sheep, man
Pomona	Sheep, cattle
Grippotyphosa	Sheep, cattle
Icterohaemorrhagiae	Cattle, pig

Mariya *et al.* (2007) reported that serovar sejroe was most prominent in causing sero-positivity in cattle and buffalo in Uttranchal, Tamil Nadu and Uttar Pradesh. This was followed by serovars *Hardjo, Pomona, Pyrogenes, Ballum, Icterohaemorrhagiae, Javanica* and *Tarassovi*. Anju Singh (2005) collected sera from apparently healthy equines from Haryana, Vijaywada, Andhra Pradesh and Maharashtra. A total of 25.8% of animals were seropositive with highest prevalence recorded for serovar Javanica, followed by *Hardjo* bovis, *Hebdomadis, Canicola, Pomona, Sejroe, Grippotyphosa* & Australis.

Environmental Factors

Environmental factors contribute significantly in the maintenance and spread of infection among animals and man. The organisms present in the infected urine or in other material such as aborted foetus, vaginal discharge, contaminated milk become a source of infection. The urine may mix with water and mud where leptospires may remain viable for a long time. Optimum conditions for the survival of organisms are a warm and wet environment with neutral or slightly alkaline water; however, they may survive in cold water provided that it does not freeze. Because of environmental conditions Leptospira infection in tropical and subtropical regions occur through out the year. In temperate regions such infections are seasonal i.e. more common during rainy and warm months . Flood helps dissemination of infection from one place to other. Swimming pools, open tanks and fishing tanks can be contaminated and may serve as a source of infection. Rice field workers, sugarcane workers, miners, plantation workers, veterinarians, pet owners, slaughter house workers, thus are more exposed to infection. The prevalence and pattern of infection in human population at risk may shift from one professional group to other under certain epidemiological conditions .

In Guadeloupe (French West Indies) in 2003-2004 compared to data in 1994-2001, leptospirosis incidence in humans increased fourfold during 2002-2004, a period with two El Niño events whereas the main risk factors were unchanged (male gender, occupational exposure, contact with cattle or pigs). A major role of rodent exposure emerged (52%, P=0.02, multivariate analysis). Interestingly, mean age of cases shifted to the older population (51.7 years vs. 43 years, P<0.05). Moreover, the Ballum serogroup rose dramatically (36% of incidence) competing with the Icterohaemorragiae serogroup (62%): However, severe forms were less recorded. Data suggest that the changes in leptospirosis features could be related to exceptional meteorological events and their consequences on rodent populations.

Transmission

Leptospira serovars are maintained for long term in urine of reservoir hosts (Babudieri, 1958). Such urine from the infected animals or reservoir hosts contaminates the pasture, drinking water and feed. Aborted foetus may also contaminate. Uterine discharge may also contribute in the contamination. A contaminated foetus may carry the infection for as long as seven weeks after birth (Giles *et al.*, 1983). The semen of an infected bull may carry leptospires and transmit to heifers by coitus or artificial insemination.

Transmission from natural carriers to the susceptible hosts is a possibility. *L. interrogans* serovar Canicola has been shown to be transmitted from dogs and Jackals to cattle. Pigs may carry the organisms in the urine for a long duration after recovery from infection, as long as for 2 months. They may act as a common source of infection for calves which are housed together with pigs. Similarly cattle have been shown to have leptospiruria for months with the highest excretion rate in the first half of the period. Sheep and goats may not act as a source of infection for other animal species and man because of intermittent and low grade leptospiruria.

L. interrogans serovar Hardjo is excreted from the genital tract of aborting cows for more than a week after abortion or calving and is detectable in the genital tract for up to 90 days after experimental infection, and in naturally infected cows. Changes in soil pH and moisture play an important role in the survival of leptospires in the environment. The organisms are susceptible to acidic pH and drying. A pH lower than 6 and greater than 8 is inhibitory. Temperature lower than 8-10^{0}C and higher than 35-37^{0}C is detrimental to the organisms. Moisture is most important for the survival of microorganisms in the soil. In a well moist land it can survive for as long as 180 day but survives for only 30 minutes in dried soil. In average conditions the survival is for 42 days for *L.interrogans* serovar Pomona.

The organism remain alive in stagnant than flowing water. The ability of the organism to survive for a long period in wet land enables it to cause higher incidence of disease in high rainfall, and temperate climate zones, in marshy fields and muddy paddocks or feed lots. New cases most likely occur in wet seasons and low lying areas.

The organisms enter the body through cutaneous or mucosal abrasions. Motility of the microorganism seems to be helping in the entrance of the organisms in the host. Tran-placental transmission is not common but *in-vitro* neonatal infection has been recorded. Transmission through tick bites or carrion feeding is possible. Swimming of the susceptible hosts in the contaminated ponds or rivers facilitates entrance of the pathogen through mucous membrane.

The role of bats as potential sources of transmission to humans or as maintenance hosts of leptospires is poorly understood. Matthias et al.(2005) quantified the prevalence of leptospiral colonization in bats in the Peruvian Amazon in the vicinity of Iquitos, an area of high biologic diversity. Of 589 analyzed bats, culture (3 of 589) and molecular evidence (20 of 589) of leptospiral colonization was found in the kidneys, yielding an overall colonization rate of 3.4%. Infection rates differed with habitat and location, and among different bat species. Bayesian analysis was used to infer phylogenic relationships of leptospiral 16S ribosomal DNA sequences. Tree topologies were consistent with groupings based on DNA-DNA hybridization studies.

A diverse group of leptospires was found in peri-Iquitos bat populations including *Leptospira interrogans* (5 clones), *L. kirschneri* (1), *L. borgpetersenii* (4), *L. fainei* (1), and two previously undescribed leptospiral species (8). Although *L. kirschenri* and *L. interrogans* have been previously isolated from bats, this report is the first to describe *L. borgpetersenii* and *L. fainei* infection of bats. A wild animal reservoir of *L. fainei* has not been previously described. The detection in bats of the *L. interrogans* serovar Icterohemorrhagiae, a leptospire typically maintained by peridomestic rats, suggests a rodent-bat infection cycle. Bats in Iquitos maintain a genetically diverse group of leptospires. These results provide a solid basis for pursuing molecular epidemiologic studies of bat-associated *Leptospira*, a potentially new epidemiologic reservoir of transmission of leptospirosis to humans.

The biodiversity of potential leptospiral reservoir hosts is lower in urban than in rural environments. Previous data indicate the potential for bats to act as carriers of Leptospira in regions such as the Amazon of South America and in Australia (Bessa *et al.*, 2010). Yet, little is known about the contribution of bats to leptospirosis in urban environments in South America. This study aimed to test the hypothesis that bats infected with *Leptospira* are sources of leptospirosis transmission to humans in São Paulo City, Brazil. Six of 343 bats caught in different districts within the city of Sao Paulo (182 insectivorous, 161 frugivorous or nectarivorous) were polymerase chain reaction (PCR) positive for pathogenic *Leptospira*; no seropositive bats were found. That few renal carriers of Leptospira were found in the city of Sao Paulo suggests that bats are not important in the transmission of leptospirosis to humans in this, and possibly other urban settings.

Virulence factors

Several bacterial cell factors have been associated with the virulence of leptospires. The evidence of the association of virulence factors with the severity of the diseases has been amply proven with most of the serovars of *Leptospira*. Endotoxins are incriminated with extensive damage caused to several organs with most of the serovars. A sphingomyelinase like cytotoxin factor has been associated with the extensive vascular lesions in animals (Chaperon *et al.*, 1979). Motility appears to be helpful in entrance of organisms into the host through the mucous membrane. Endotoxins are potent inducer of interlukin-1 from macrophages which reset the hypothalamus to produce fever & TNF from phagocytes which induces severe shock & tissue damage. However, purified endotoxin has not been shown to be cytotoxic (Srivastava 2002).

Yang *et al.* (2009) described a pore forming haemolysin from serovar Lai strain 56601 also possessing the ability to cause damage and inducing apoptosis on the membrane of human L-02 liner cells. Earlier, nine haemolysin genes have been identified in *L.interrogans* serovar Icterohaemorrhagiae serotype lai. These genes were classified into 2 groups: sphingomyelinase [sphingomyelin phosphodiesterase] gene and non-sphingomyclinase gene. Studies revealed that haemolysins are the important virulence factors of *Leptospira* serotypes (Zhang *et al.*, 2005).

Outer membrane proteins are also considered to be important virulence factors as they act as adhesins, porins and renders *Leptospira* cells resistant to complement (Cullen *et al.*, 2004). Several OMPs have been identified performing different function . Nicholson and Prescott (1993) investigated outer membrane proteins of seven reference strains of pathogenic Leptospira (*L. alstoni* serovar grippotyphosa, *L. borgpetersenii* serovar *hardjo*, and *L. interrogans* serovars *autumnalis, bratislava, canicola, icterohaemorrhagiae,* and *pomona*) to identify common surface-exposed outer membrane proteins. Sodium dodecyl sulfate-polyacrylamide gel electrophoresis of sodium-N-lauroylsarcosinate-insoluble outer membrane enriched fractions of the reference serovars and two field isolates of serovars hardjo and pomona revealed six common protein bands with approximate molecular masses of 77, 66, 42, 35.5, 24, and 18 kDa. At times the 35.5 kDa endoflagellar band resolved into two distinct bands, 35.5 kDa and 34 kDa. Immunoblotting of the same fractions using rabbit leptospiral antibodies showed six bands to be common (66, 59.5, 44, 42, 35.5, and 18 kDa). The 44 kDa band stained poorly with Coomassie blue but prominently by immunoblotting. Four reference strains (serovars bratislava, canicola, icterohaemorrhagiae, pomona), and two field isolates of serovar pomona and one of serovar *bratislava* were grown in low iron media to which the iron chelators 2,2'-dipyridyl or ethylenediaminehydroxyphenylacetic acid were added. No iron-dependent expression of outer membrane proteins was observed. The only difference observed between the outer membrane proteins when reference serovars of canicola or pomona were grown in dialysis bags in the peritoneum of swine or in vitro was the loss of the 77 kDa band from in vivo grown organisms. Treatment of whole leptospires with proteinase K did not remove the 77, 66, 59.5, or 42 kDa protein; these proteins may not be surface expressed or are inaccessible to the proteinase K. The 44 kDa band could not be evaluated by this method and the 18 kDa band was proteinase K resistant. Leptospiral outer membrane proteins (OMPs) are highly conserved in different species, and play an essential role in the development of new immunoprotection and serodiagnosis strategies.Cullen *et al.* (2003) identified the gene encoding pL21 and found it to encode a putative lipoprotein; accordingly, the protein was renamed LipL21. Southern hybridization analysis revealed the presence of lipL21 in all of the pathogenic species but in none of the saprophytic species examined. Alignment of the LipL21 sequence from six strains of Leptospira revealed 96 to 100% identity. When specific polyclonal antisera to recombinant LipL21 were used, LipL21 was isolated together with other known leptospiral OMPs by both Triton X-114 extraction and sucrose density gradient membrane fractionation. All nine strains of pathogenic leptospires investigated by Western blotting, whether culture attenuated or virulent, were found to express LipL21. In contrast, the expression of LipL21 or an antigenically related protein could not be detected in nonpathogenic *L. biflexa*. Infected hamster sera and two of eight human leptospirosis sera tested were found to react with recombinant LipL21. Native LipL21 was found to incorporate tritiated palmitic acid, consistent with the prediction of a lipoprotein signal peptidase cleavage site. Biotinylation of the leptospiral surface resulted in selective labeling of LipL21 and the previously known OMPs LipL32 and LipL41. These findings show that LipL21 is a surface-exposed, abundant outer membrane lipoprotein that is expressed during infection and conserved among pathogenic *Leptospira* species.

The genes encoding LipL21, LipL32 and OmpL1 were cloned from the complete genome sequence of *Leptospira* interrogans serovar lai strain Lai and expressed *in vitro* (Zhang *et al.*, 2005). Sequence comparison analysis revealed that the three genes were highly conserved among distinct epidemic leptospires, including three major epidemic species Leptospira interrogans, Leptospira borgpetersenii and Leptospira weilii, in China. Immunoblot analysis was further performed to scrutinize 15 epidemic Leptospira reference strains using the antisera of the recombinant OMPs. Both immunoblot assay and reverse transcription-polymerase chain reaction demonstrated that these three OMPs were conservatively expressed in pathogenic *L. interrogans* strains and other pathogenic leptospires. Additionally, the use of these recombinant OMPs as antigens in enzyme-linked immunosorbent assay (ELISA) for serodiagnosis of leptospirosis was evaluated. The recombinant LipL32 and OmpL1 proteins showed a high degree of ELISA reactivity with sera from patients infected with *L. interrogans* strain Lai and other pathogenic leptospires. These results may contribute to the identification of candidates for broad-range vaccines and immunodiagnostic antigens in further research. Adaptation to a wide variety of environmental conditions has required leptospires to acquire a large genome and a complex outer membrane with features that are unique among bacteria. The most abundant surface-exposed outer membrane proteins are lipoproteins that are integrated into the lipid bilayer by amino-terminal fatty acids. In contrast to many spirochaetes, the leptospiral outer membrane also includes lipopolysaccharide and many homologues of well-known beta-barrel transmembrane outer membrane proteins. Research on leptospiral transmembrane outer membrane proteins has lagged behind studies of lipoproteins because of their aberrant behaviour by Triton X-114 detergent fractionation. For this reason, transmembrane outer membrane proteins are best characterized by assessing membrane integration and surface exposure. Not surprisingly, some outer membrane proteins that mediate host-pathogen interactions are strongly regulated by conditions found in mammalian host tissues. For example, the leptospiral immunoglobulin-like (Lig) repeat proteins are dramatically induced by osmolarity and mediate interactions with host extracellular matrix proteins. Development of molecular genetic tools are making it possible to finally understand the roles of these and other outer membrane proteins in mechanisms of leptospiral pathogenesis.

Transmission of leptospirosis occurs through contact of mucous membranes and abraded skin with freshwater contaminated by pathogenic Leptospira spp. Exposure to physiological osmolarity induces leptospires to express high levels of the Lig surface proteins containing imperfect immunoglobulin-like repeats that are shared or differ between LigA and LigB. Choy *et al.* (2007) reported that osmotic induction of Lig is accompanied by 1.6- to 2.5-fold increases in leptospiral adhesion to immobilized extracellular matrix and plasma proteins, including collagens I and IV, laminin, and especially fibronectin and fibrinogen. Recombinant LigA-unique and LigB-unique repeat proteins bind to these same host ligands. It was found that the avidity of LigB in binding fibronectin is comparable to that of the Staphylococcus aureus FnBPA D repeats. Both LigA- and LigB-unique repeats interact with the amino-terminal fibrin- and gelatin-binding domains of fibronectin, which are also recognized by fibronectin-binding proteins mediating the adhesion of other microbial pathogens. In contrast, repeats common to both LigA and LigB do not bind these host proteins, and nonrepeat sequences in the carboxy-terminal domain of LigB show only weak interaction with fibronectin and fibrinogen. A functional role for the binding activity of LigA and LigB is suggested by the ability of the recombinants to inhibit leptospiral adhesion to fibronectin by 28% and 21%, respectively. The binding of LigA and LigB to multiple ligands present in different tissues suggests that these adhesins may be involved in the initial colonization and dissemination stages of leptospirosis. Leptospira immunoglobulin-like (Lig) proteins including LigA and LigB are adhesins that bind to fibronectin, collagen, laminin and elastin. In addition, Lig proteins are fibrinogen (Fg)-binding proteins, although the physiological role of the Lig-Fg interaction is unclear. In this study, a previously identified Fg-binding region, LigBCen2 (amino acids 1014-1165 of LigB), has been further localized to LigBCen2R, which consists of the partial 11th and entire 12th Ig-like domain (amino acids 1014-1119). LigBCen2R was found to bind to the C-terminal αC domain of Fg (FgαCC; amino acids 392-644 in Fg α chain; isothermal titration calorimetry, K(D) = 0.375 μM;

fluorescence spectrometry, K(D) = 0.364 μM). The quenching and blue shift observed for the maximum wavelength intensities of the tryptophan fluorescence spectra for FgαCCY570W upon LigBCen2RW1073C binding suggested an RGD motif close to the sole tryptophan on FgαCCY570W was buried in LigBCen2R upon saturation with FgαCC. A conformational change in LigBCen2R when bound to the FgαCC RGD motif blocked further binding to integrin α(IIb) β3 on platelets, thus preventing their aggregation. LigBCen2R binding to FgαCC reduced clot formation but did not affect plasminogen and tissue-type plasminogen activator interactions with FgαCC (Lin et al.2011). This study is the first to report that a spirochaetal protein binds to the C-terminal αC domain of Fg, which regulates thrombosis and fibrinolysis, and may help explain the pulmonary haemorrhage and thrombocytopenia seen in clinical cases of leptospirosis.

Leptospires display a rich repertoire of adhesins endowed with multifunctional biological activities such as adhesion to host tissue components, plasminogen activation, resistance to complement. These adhesins are proteins or liproteins located on the outer membrane. Some of them (LenA) escape innate defence such as complement killing and some escape phagocytosis.

Pathogenesis

The disease in different animal species varies. Further, the serovar involved in causation of the disease is also a deciding factor in the pathogenesis. For example *L. interrogans* serovar Pomona causes intravascular haemolysis and interstitial nephritis whereas serovar Hardjo is capable of growing only in the pregnant uterus and lactating mammary glands so that it produces only septicaemia, mastitis accompanied with abortion. The various form of disease as caused by *L.interrogans* serovar Pomona in various animal species varies considerably from acute form in most of the animal species to subacute to chronic form. During acute phase the organisms multiply rapidly in the liver and then migrate to peripheral blood for several days accompanied with fever. This is followed by generation of immune response in animals. At the early stage sufficient haemolysin production may lead to haemoglobinuria, especially in young cattle. Following this, the organisms lodge in the kidneys and form micro colonies particularly in the proximal convoluted tubules. The haemolysis of red blood cells is visible microscopically. Capillary damage is common to all serotypes and during the septicaemic phase petechial haemorrhages in mucosae are commonly observed. If the haemolysis is severe, anemic anoxia and haemoglobinuria with nephrosis are visible. The infection localizes in the renal parenchyma and causes interstitial nephritis and persistence of leptospires in these lesions leads to prolonged leptospiruria.

The animal may die of the disease due to acute septicaemia, haemolytic anaemia and uremia. The attachment of *Leptospira* is considered to be an initial step of infection. Virulent strains attach to collagen and fibronectin. Usually, the attachment is through one end then becoming lateral (Ito and yanagawa 1988).

Pathogenic leptospires possess the capability to cause bacteraemia characterized by fever, myalgia and shivering. The hallmark of *Leptospira* pathogenesis is the ability of these bacteria to penetrate skin and mucous membranes and to disseminate rapidly to other tissues shortly after infection. Deposition of the cells is mostly in liver, lungs and in other organs causing jaundice, hepatitis, pneumonia, meningitis. In chronic cases kidneys are affected causing nephropathy. Gravid uterus is also affected resulting in abortions and reproductive failure. Infected bull exhibit oxidative damage along with inflammation which might take part in the pathogenesis of bovine leptospirosis.

Bacterial lipopolysaccharide and Outer membrane protein components may be the virulence attributes. However, potential determinant of leptospirosis severity could include the dose of *Leptospira* inoculated during environmental exposure. It has been demonstrated that most of the Leptospira strains can form biofilms in vitro. The formation of biofilms is consistent with the life of saprophytic strains in water and may facilitate the pathogenic strains to survive in environmental niches and colonize the host. Biofilm-like structures of *L. interrogans* have been observed in rat kidney tubules. The presence of biofilms in proximal kidney tubules may play an important role in maintaining chronic carriage in rats. The genome sequences of *Leptospira* suggest that these bacteria possess several iron acquisition systems. An analysis of *L. biflexa* mutants obtained by random and targeted mutagenesis allowed the characterization of genes involved in iron uptake systems, such as TonB-dependent receptors, ABC transporters, and a two-component system.

Leptospirosis is an important cause of sepsis in tropical areas, and pulmonary hemorrhage associated with thrombocytopenia is the major cause of death, but the coagulopathy in severe leptospirosis has not been well characterized. Activation of the coagulation system is an important feature of leptospirosis. Disseminated intravascular coagulation (DIC) is common among patients with sepsis.

The discrepancy between infection and symptomatic and severe disease remains a central mystery. Possible explanations include considerations of both the pathogen and the human host. It has long been thought that certain leptospiral serovars are particularly pathogenic. For example, serovars Copenhageni and Lai, whose whole genome sequences have been determined, have been associated with severe human *leptospirosis*. These serovars do not cause disease in their natural mammalian reservoirs (*Rattus* spp. and *Apodemus* mice, respectively) but cause severe disease in experimental models of infection such as in hamsters or guinea pigs or in accidental hosts such as dogs. In fact most people infected with these serovars probably do not develop severe disease, possible no disease at all. Conversely, a wide variety of *Leptospira* have been shown to cause severe disease, including the 'intermediate' *Leptospira fainei* serovar Hurstbridge, even though, most infections are probably inapparent. Therefore, intrinsic virulence properties of pathogenic or intermediate *Leptospira* cannot be the sole explanation of severe human or animal disease.

Renal involvement is common in *leptospirosis* characterized by tubulo-interstitial nephritis, and tubular dysfunction. Leptospira outer membrane proteins (OMPs) may elicit tubular injury and inflammation through Toll-like receptors (TLRs)-dependent pathway followed by activation of nuclear transcription factor kappa B and mitogen-activated protein kinases and a differential induction of chemokines and cytokines relevant to tubular inflammation. Leptospira OMP may also induce activation of the transforming growth factor-/Smad-associated fibrosis pathway leading to accumulation of extra cellular matrix. Thus, *leptospirosis* renal disease is a model for understanding the pathogenesis and initiation of pathogen-induced tubulo-interstitial nephritis and fibrosis. In particular, TLRs may be important mediator.

An in vivo murine model of severe leptospirosis in which a single gene, TLR4, determines the clinical outcome of infection as well as tissue burden of leptospires in sub lethal infection has been described. A lack of antibody and B and T lymphocytes does not prevent jaundice or pulmonary hemorrhage, suggesting that these arms of the immune system are not involved in *Leptospira*-induced immunopathology. In *in-vitro* assays, *Leptospira*-stimulated proinflammatory cytokines and chemokines are dependent on TLR4 and MD-2 present in the TLR4 signaling complex but independent of CD14. These observations indicate that a CD14-independent, TLR4-dependent pathway of the innate immune response contributes an unexpectedly important component of protection against death in severe murine *leptospirosis* and in controlling leptospiral proliferation during chronic infection.

Experimental infection of calves with serovar *Pomona* may follow this course of infection. Signs appear usually after 4-9 days of incubation period. During the acute febrile phase there is leukocytosis and transitory anaemia, hemoglobinuria and jaundice due to intravascular haemolysis without any biochemical indication of renal or hepatic insufficiency. Experimental infection with *L.interrogans* serovars *Hebdomadis* and *Hardjo* in heifers cause fever but infection with the latter serovar alone produce no clinical illness. In Canicola infection there is no haemoglobinuria or jaundice and there is usually no significant renal or hepatic impairment. Infection with serovar Hardjo occurs only in pregnant or lactating cows because of the predilection of the organisms to pregnant uterus and lactating mammary gland. The udder is flabby, has no heat or pain and all quarters are equally affected. Almost 50% of the animals in a herd may be affected with the drop in milk. The leukocytes count in affected milk may increase which subside later within a fortnight.

During chronic stage abortions may occur in pregnant animals following the initial systemic invasion. Dead fetus may be aborted without placental degeneration. Abortion occurs most commonly during the 3rd quarter of the pregnancy. Abortion storms may occur in cattle herd resulting in greater loss to the farmer. Often observance of abortion without any clinical illness is common. It may be because the mild clinical symptoms may go unnoticed and abortion is the only clinical sign noticed by the veterinarians. Occurrence of still birth and repeat breeding is a continuous problem at many farms in India. In whatever the case, leptospires are rarely present in the aborted fetus. However, if the aborted fetuses have survived the infection long enough to produce antibodies, these may be detected (Radostitis *et al.*, 1994).

In sub acute from the disease is less severe. This form is more common in adult cattle and horses however; other animals may also show this form of the disease. In many cases rise in antibody titre is the only indication of the infection. Horses may develop periodic opthalmia. This is due to the reaction caused by anti outer membrane protein agglutinins present in the greater concentration in aqueous humor with corneal cells. A 90 kDa protein of *L.interrogans* has been shown to cross react with equine corneal protein by Western blotting. Antibodies against this protein recognize a 66 kDa equine corneal protein (Cucchesi and Parma, 1999). Serovar Pomona is associated with anterior uveitis in the USA. Not all leptospires are able to penetrate the eyes. Majority of cases of recurrent uveitis associated with Grippotyphosa (78.2%) have been found among equines belonging to various European countries. This is followed by Australis (14.2%) group, sejroe group (3.6%) the Pomona group (2.5%) and javanica group (1.5%) (Hartskeerl *et al.*, 2004). Encephalitis may also be caused by *Leptospira* organisms in most of the animal species as a result of localization of the organisms in the nervous tissues. Similarly localization of leptospires in lung tissues gives rise to pneumonia. Yan et al.(2010) determined serologic, hematologic responses of horses to Leptospira interrogans serovar *Kennewicki* infection. Four adult horses seronegative for leptospirosis were used for the experimental and observational study. Horses were challenged with an equine isolate of L. interrogans serovar

Kennewicki at 2 different doses and different inoculation sites. After challenge, the horses were monitored for 60 days. Blood, urine, and aqueous humor samples were collected at intervals until euthanasia 60 days after infection. Pyrexia (39.3-40 degrees C) occurred as early as 1 day after challenge with 10x10(8)Leptospira divided equally between topical ocular and intraperitoneal injection in 2 horses. Leptospires were recovered from the blood and urine but not from the aqueous humor of the 2 febrile horses. The sera of all 4 challenged horses developed microscopic agglutination test antibody after challenge and remained relatively constant for 21 days. Titer to cross-reacting strains declined earlier than titer to the challenge strain. It is concluded that clinical disease in experimentally infected horses can be mild or inapparent in Leptospira infected horses. Repeated serologic testing can allow recognition of the infecting serovar. In febrile horses, *Leptospira* can be isolated from blood while isolation from the urine can occur after fever has subsided.

The more severe clinical signs include marked malaise, intense muscular pain, jaundice & encephalitis in all the animal species. The combination of jaundice and severe nephritis, as indicated by high blood urea nitrogen (BUN) and anuria are indication of a severe disease. Jaundice occurs due to occlusion of bile ducts by hepatic debris.

Experimental infection of goats using *L.interrogans* serovars Hebdomadis and Icterohaemorrhagiae have revealed weight loss, unthriftiness, moderate biphasic pyrexia along with decrease in PCV and haemoglobin up to 4th week post infection in all the animals but was of low grade in Hebdomadis infected animals. Leukocytosis was observed up to 3rd week post infection in both the groups. (Kiem *et al.*, 1995). Biochemical parameter revealed an increased serum total protein by Ist week, increased levels of serum cholesterol, serum bilirubin, blood urea nitrogen suggestive of hepatic damage. The increase in Asparate amino transferare (AST) and alanine amino transferase (ALT) suggested hepato cellular degeneration. The changes were more pronounced in Icterohaemorrhagiae infected group.

Experimental infection of calves with serovar Hardjo bovis have produced varied results. Animals do not show a rise in body temperature (Singh *et al.*, 2007). These animals showed initially leukocytosis followed by leucopoenia upto 4th week post infection. AST & ALT levels also slightly changed suggestive of heptorenal damage. Finding revealed a mild chronic form of disease which occurred in animals. Similar finding were observed in goats infected with serovar Hardjo (Srivastava & Sharma 1990).

The leptospiral lifecycle involves interactions with host tissues at multiple stages of infection, including: (i) entering the host, (ii) evading its immune response, and (iii) adhering to tissues. Identification and characterization of novel proteins that mediate the stage-specific interactions with the host are essential for the understanding of leptospiral pathogenesis, and in the development of diagnostic and protective antigens for leptospirosis. Pathogenic leptospires have been shown to bind to a variety of host ligands, including fibronectin, fibrinogen, collagen, laminin, elastin, and proteoglycans, indicating that cell surface and extracellular matrix (ECM)-binding OMPs, or adhesins, are likely to be expressed by the spirochetes. It is possible that leptospires express distinct adhesins at different stages of infection, including initial attachment, dissemination, and colonization. Many leptospiral proteins, including LigA/B, Lsa21, Lsa27, Lsa63, Lsa24 (LfhA/LenA), LenB to F, LipL32, Lp95, TlyC, and LipL53, have been shown to have affinity for host ligands *in vitro*. However, it is unclear to what extent these putative adhesins mediate interactions of leptospires with cell surface and ECM proteins. Only Lsa24, LigA/B, and Lsa63 have been tested for their capacity to inhibit leptospiral adherence to ECM proteins. In each case, only partial inhibition was observed, suggesting that additional fibronectin-, laminin-, collagen-, and elastin-binding proteins likely exist in *Leptospira*. Leptospira infection involves the adhesion of the bacteria followed by invasion of the host crossing the extracellular matrix barrier. In an effort to understand the molecular mechanism of this process, the possibility of occurrence of matrix degrading enzymes from *Leptospira* was investigated (Madathiparambil *et al.*, 2011). Zymographic analysis showed that the outer membrane of Leptospires contains a gelatinase of average molecular size of 46 kDa. The gelatinase exhibited maximum activity at neutral pH and was inhibited by metal chelators such as EGTA, EDTA, and Orthophenanthroline and was activated by calcium, magnesium, zinc, and copper, suggesting that it is a membrane-associated neutral matrix metalloproteinase. Analysis of the production of the enzyme by various serovars showed that the pathogenic serovars expressed significant amount of this enzyme while nonpathogenic forms either did not express or showed only very low activity, suggesting that this enzyme may be associated with pathogenesis of leptospirosis.

Pathogenic Leptospira spp. shed in the urine of reservoir hosts into freshwater can be transmitted to a susceptible host through skin abrasions or mucous membranes causing leptospirosis(Pinne *et al.*, 2010). The infection process involves the ability of leptospires to adhere to cell surface and extracellular matrix components, a crucial step for dissemination and colonization of host tissues. Therefore, the elucidation of novel mediators of host-pathogen interaction is important in the discovery of virulence factors involved in the pathogenesis of leptospirosis. In this study, the functional roles of transmembrane outer membrane proteins OmpL36 (LIC13166), OmpL37 (LIC12263), and OmpL47 (LIC13050) was assessed which the authors recently identified on the leptospiral surface. The authors determined the capacity of these proteins to bind to host tissue components by enzyme-linked immunosorbent assay. OmpL37 binds elastin preferentially, exhibiting dose-dependent, saturating binding to human skin (K(d), 104±19 nM) and aortic elastin (K(d), 152±27 nM). It also binds fibrinogen (K(d), 244±15 nM), fibrinogen fragment D (K(d), 132±30 nM), plasma fibronectin (K(d), 359±68 nM), and murine laminin (K(d), 410±81 nM). The binding to human skin elastin by both recombinant OmpL37 and live Leptospira interrogans is specifically enhanced by rabbit antiserum for OmpL37, suggesting the involvement of OmpL37 in leptospiral binding to elastin and also the possibility that host-generated antibodies may promote rather than inhibit the adherence of leptospires to elastin-rich tissues. Further, it was demonstrated that OmpL37 is recognized by acute and convalescent leptospirosis patient sera and also by Leptospira-infected hamster sera. Finally, OmpL37 protein is detected in pathogenic Leptospira serovars and not in saprophytic Leptospira. Thus, OmpL37 is a novel elastin-binding protein of pathogenic *Leptospira* that may be promoting attachment of *Leptospira* to host tissues.

The interaction of leptospires with pathogen recognition receptors is a fundamental issue in leptospiral immunity as well as in immunophatology. Pathogenic but not saprophytic leptospires are able to evade the host complement system, circulate in the blood and spread into tissues. The target organs in human leptospirosis include the kidneys and the lungs. The association of an autoimmune process with these pathologies has been explored and diverse mechanisms that permit leptospires to survive in the kidneys of reservoir animals have been proposed. However, despite the intense research aimed at the development of a leptospirosis vaccine supported by the genome sequencing of Leptospira strains, there have been relatively few studies focused on leptospiral immunity. The knowledge of evasion strategies employed by pathogenic leptospires to subvert the immune system is of extreme importance as they may represent targets for the development of new treatments and prophylactic approaches in leptospirosis. Barbosa et al.(2009) analyzed the serum resistance of six *Leptospira* strains. It was demonstrated that the pathogenic strain isolated from infected hamsters avoids serum bactericidal activity more efficiently than the culture-attenuated or the nonpathogenic Leptospira strains. Moreover, both the alternative and the classical pathways of complement seem to be responsible for the killing of leptospires. Serum-resistant and serum-intermediate strains are able to bind C4BP, whereas the serum-sensitive strain Patoc I is not. Surface-bound C4BP promotes factor I-mediated cleavage of C4b. Accordingly; we found that pathogenic strains displayed reduced deposition of the late complement components C5 to C9 upon exposure to serum. We conclude that binding of C4BP contributes to leptospiral serum resistance against host complement.

Diagnosis

The organisms can easily be identified as coiled, filamentous motile organisms under dark field microscope in urine, blood or other fluids. Clinical material viz. urine, foetal tissues, blood etc. collected from the infected animals can be directly visualized under dark field microscope for the presence of long, motile, coiled leptospires. The materials under examination may be centrifuged to concentrate the *Leptospira* cells in the deposit. More preferably the preparations can be stained using silver impregnation technique of Fontana and viewed. Serovar identification of clinical isolates of Leptospira is generally not performed on a routine basis, yet the identity of an infecting serovar is valuable from both epidemiologic and public health standpoints. Only a small number of reference laboratories worldwide have the capability to perform the cross agglutinin absorption test (CAAT), the reference method for serovar identification. Pulsed-field gel electrophoresis (PFGE) is an alternative method to CAAT that facilitates rapid identification of leptospires to the serovar level. Galloway and Levett(2010) employed PFGE to evaluate 175 isolates obtained from humans and animals submitted to the Centers for Disease Control and Prevention (CDC) between 1993 and 2007. PFGE patterns for each isolate were generated using the NotI restriction enzyme and compared to a reference database consisting of more than 200 reference strains. Of the 175 clinical isolates evaluated, 136 (78%) were identified to the serovar level by the database, and an additional 27 isolates (15%) have been identified as probable new serovars. The remaining isolates yet to be identified are either not represented in the database or require further study to determine whether or not they also represent new serovars. PFGE proved to be a useful tool for serovar identification of clinical isolates of known serovars from different geographic regions and a variety of different hosts and for recognizing potential new serovars.

For applying immunofluorescent technique on routine basis, preparation of conjugates in the laboratory for the specific purpose is recommended against the commercial conjugates. Additional newer techniques for demonstrating leptospires in tissue materials and urine include detection of leptospiral antigens using monoclonal antibodies. Sharma et al [37] reported that a rapid sandwich dot-ELISA appeared more advantageous over PCR in being simple, rapid, field based, and economical for detection of antigens in infected animals.

EMJH medium is used for isolating the cells from up to 10 fold diluted samples. At least 6 weeks may be required for the organism to grow in artificial medium.

Microscopic agglutination test (MAT) is the most widely utilized test for serological diagnosis of leptospirosis (Cole *et al.*, 1973; WHO 1967). A titer of at least 1:100 is considered positive. In paired sera a four fold increase in the titer is indicative and quite specific, however, its use is limited owing to the difficulty in maintaining the *Leptospira* strains used for serology. In recent years Enzyme linked Imunosorbant assay has been routinely used for diagnosing leptospirosis (Thierman & Garett 1983). The test can be standardized as the serovar specific or the organism specific depending on the antigen used. Recently, recombinant proteins belonging to outer membrane of pathogenic leptospires has been used as genus specific antigen for conducting the test. The recombinant leptospiral outer membrane protein LipL32 was evaluated for use in the diagnosis of bovine leptospirosis by enzyme-linked immunosorbent assay (rLipL32 IgG ELISA)(Bonfim et al. 2005). The microscopic agglutination test (MAT) of 150 serum samples from cattle suspected of leptospirosis showed that 125 (83.3%) samples had positive reciprocal agglutination titres, which ranged from 100 to 1600. The highest titres were observed for the serovars Hardjoprajitno and Bratislava. In the rLipL32 IgG ELISA, 83.3% of the samples were positive. The sensitivity of IgG ELISA for 125 bovine sera, which had MAT titres of greater than or equal to 100, was 100%. ELISA showed a specificity of 100% with 58 bovine sera, which were negative at a 1:50 dilution in the MAT for Leptospira interrogans serovars. When analytical specificity of the IgG ELISA was evaluted using 60 bovine serum samples from animals showing serum antibodies to other pathogens that cause abortion in cattle, such as Babesia sp., Anaplasma sp. and Brucella sp. and no cross-reaction was observed. The recombinant LipL32 IgG ELISA can be an alternative to the MAT for diagnosis of leptospiral infection in cattle. The efficacy of a recombinant leptospiral lipoprotein LipL41 as an antigen for conducting enzyme-linked immunosorbent assay (ELISA) for diagnosis of bovine leptospirosis was evaluated (Mariya et al.2006). Using known positive and known negative cattle sera the recombinant antigen was found to be highly reactive in the concentration of 100 ng/well. Using a total of 321 field cattle sera the sensitivity of ELISA as compared to microscopic agglutination test (MAT) was calculated to be 100% whereas the specificity was 85.3%. The seropositivity of leptospirosis among bovine population was found to be 21.18% having the predominance of serovars Sejroe and Pomona. It was concluded that rLipL41 protein could be a putative diagnostic candidate for serodiagnosis of bovine leptospirosis. A recombinant leptospiral lipoprotein, LigB, was evaluated for use in the diagnosis of bovine leptospirosis by enzyme-linked immunosorbent assay (rLigB IgG ELISA)(Sankar et al.2010). The standard reference test (Microscopic agglutination test, MAT) of 200 serum samples from cattle suspected of leptospirosis showed that 95 (47.5%) samples had positive agglutination titres, which ranged from 100 to 1600. In rLigB IgG ELISA, 49% of the samples were positive. Sensitivity of IgG ELISA for 95 bovine sera, which had MAT titres of greater than or equal to 100, were

100%. ELISA showed a specificity of 97.1% with 105 bovine sera, which were negative at a 1:50 dilution in MAT for Leptospira interrogans serovars. The results of ELISA and MAT corresponded very good. When analytical specificity of IgG ELISA was evaluated using bovine serum samples from animals showing the serum antibodies to other pathogens, no cross-reaction was observed.

Leptospira kirschneri serovar Grippotyposa strain Moskva V was chosen to be a target for cloning the conserved region of Lig gene (La-Ard et al.2011). This assay was evaluated with canine sera (n = 91) that were MAT-negative (< 1:100 dilution) and sera (n = 103) that were MAT-positive (> or = 1:100 dilution) using 24 serovars. The ELISA showed a relative sensitivity as compared to MAT of 84.5% whereas the specificity was 76.9%. This assay is simple and can be routinely prepared in large amounts. It was concluded that the GST.Lig recombinant protein-based ELISA could be used as a screening test for serodiagnosis of canine leptospirosis with also for confirmation of MAT-positive test results.

A recombinant LipL 32 antigen-based dipstick ELISA was developed as a screening test for the detection of leptospiral antibodies in serum samples from dogs (Dey *et al.*, 2007). The antibodies were detected by a change in the colour of the substrate solution when the recombinant antigen-coated dipsticks were dipped into it. The relative sensitivity, specificity and accuracy of the test, compared with the standard microscopic agglutination test, were 95.9 per cent, 93.8 per cent and 94.8 per cent, respectively, suggesting that it could be a useful and rapid test for the diagnosis of leptospirosis.

Chirathaworn et al.(2011) demonstrated that gold nanoparticles can be used to facilitate *Leptospira* detection. Gold nanoparticles were coated with rabbit antibody specific to *Leptospira* interrogans serovar Bratislava and these coated particles were used to detect *Leptospira* in urine. Agglutination of gold particles indicated the presence of *Leptospira* in samples tested. The sensitivity of detection was 10 leptospires/ml. No agglutination was observed when anti-*Leptospira*-coated particles were tested with urine containing the organisms commonly found in urine such as *Klebsiella pneumoniae, Escherichia coli* and *Enterococcus faecalis*. This assay is very easy to perform and results could be observed with the naked eyes. Fresh or frozen urine samples could be used. The stability of antibody-coated particles was at least 2 months when kept at 4°C. In conclusion, we have demonstrated that the technique using antibody-coated gold nanoparticles is a promising tool for further validation as a rapid assay for Leptospirosis diagnosis.

Molecular techniques such as polymerase chain reaction have been standardized to demonstrate leptospires in blood, urine, tissue material *etc.*

The DNA of leptospires present in clinical samples in small concentration (1-10 cell/ml) may be detected after amplification. Gravekemp *et al.* (1993) derived 2 sets of primers G1 and G2 from genomic libraries of serovar Icterohaemorrhagiae and Bim and enabled amplification by PCR of DNA of several other serovars in serum samples collected from patients. Polymerase chain reaction assay (PCR) amplifying a fragment of the Leptospira rrs gene was compared with culture and microagglutination test (MAT) for the diagnosis of leptospirosis in a study of 200 patients with various clinical syndromes compatible with leptospirosis (Merien *et al.,* 1995). For the first group of samples tested, PCR identified the 14 cases that later were unequivocally confirmed to be leptospirosis. Thirteen other systemic cases presenting decreasing leptospiral antibody titers were also detected by PCR. The average persistence of leptospiral DNA in serum was estimated at 12 days, with a maximum of 56 days in a culture-confirmed case. The possibility of detecting leptospires in aqueous humor during the ocular complications of the disease was confirmed. The results suggest that PCR is an efficient tool for early diagnosis of leptospirosis during the first 10 days of the disease, especially when the clinical expression of the disease is confusing.

A PCR assay with the best combination of specificity (100%) and sensitivity (91%) was selected for comparison with the other diagnostic tests. Sensitivity for nucleic acid hybridization was 55%, whereas sensitivity for bacteriologic culture and immunofluorescence was 89 to 93% (Wagenaar *et al.* 2000). Bacteriologic culture, PCR, and immunofluorescence were sensitive for detection of L borgpetersenii serovar hardjo type hardjo-bovis in urine specimens of cattle, but a single technique was not the most sensitive for each animal tested. Therefore, the use of 2 techniques in combination is warranted for maximal sensitivity for diagnosis. Bomfim and Koury (2006) evaluated the use of low-stringency single specific primer PCR (LSSP-PCR) for genetically typing *Leptospira* directly from urine samples of cattle with clinical suspicion of leptospirosis. Urine samples obtained from 40 cattle with clinical suspicion of leptospirosis were amplified by specific PCR using the following primers: Internal 1/Internal 2 and G1/G2. The internal primers were designed from the gene sequence of the outer membrane lipoprotein Lip32 from Leptospira kirschneri, strain RM52. The PCR products were amplified with these two pairs of primers, which had approximately 497 and 285bp, respectively, and were subsequently used as a template for LSSP-PCR analysis. The genetic signatures from the leptospires which were present in the urine samples allowed us to make a preliminary identification of the leptospires by comparing the LSSP-PCR profiles obtained directly from urine samples with those from reference leptospires. The LSSP-PCR profiles obtained with the Internal 1 primer or with the G1 primer allowed the grouping of the leptospires into serogroups. LSSP-PCR was found to be a useful and sensitive approach capable of identifying leptospires directly from biological samples without the need for prior bacterial isolation. In conclusion, the LSSP-PCR technique may still be helpful in discriminating serogroups of Leptospira from different animal reservoirs, since the early identification of carrier animals and information on the shedding state are crucial to prevent the spread of leptospiral infection to other animals and humans. A multiplex polymerase chain reaction (PCR) was developed for diagnosing leptospirosis and differentiating pathogenic and saprophytic leptospires. Specific primers were designed to amplify 23S rDNA from pathogenic Leptospira and saprophytic Leptospira spp. PCR products from 27 pathogenic and 5 (including 1 intermediate) saprophytic serovars were 615 and 316 base pairs (bp), respectively. After the restriction enzyme's digestion of PCR products, the fragments by SacI of pathogenic serovars and by PstI of saprophytic serovars were 339 and 276 bp and 202 and 114 bp, respectively. The PCR primers enabled amplification of DNA from L. meyeri serovar Ranarum as a pathogenic Leptospira spp. The PCR assay could detect 1 to 2 cells of leptospires and not amplify DNA from other 18 bacterial species. The sensitivity and specificity of this PCR in rat kidney, using isolation as gold standard, were 98.6% and 100%, respectively. The most appropriate sample preparation of blood for detecting DNA was buffy coat. Among the sample preparations from 7 laboratory-confirmed leptospirosis cases, leptospiral DNA was detected in all 7 buffy coat preparations, whereas leptospiral DNA was detected in only 3 plasma or serum samples. The PCR assay may be useful as a diagnostic tool for leptospirosis (Kositanont *et al.* 2007).

Hermandez-Rodriguez *et al.* (2011) compared polymerase chain reaction (PCR) with microbiological culture and dark field microscopy for the diagnosis of leptospirosis. Microbiological and molecular techniques were performed on 83 samples of urine taken from bovines in the savannahs surrounding Bogotá in Colombia, with presumptive diagnosis of leptospirosis. 117 samples of urine taken from healthy bovines were used as negative controls. 83 samples were MAT positive with titers = 1:50; 81 with titers = 1:100; and 66 with titers = 1:200. 36% of the total samples (73/200) were Leptospira positives by microbiological culture, 32% (63/200) by dark field microscopy and 37% (74/200) by PCR. Amplicons obtained by PCR were 482 base pair long which are Leptospira specific. An amplicon of 262 base pairs typical of pathogenic Leptospira was observed in 71 out of the 74 PCR positive samples. The remaining 3 samples showed a 240 base pair amplicon which is typical of saprophytic Leptospira. PCR as a Leptospira diagnosis technique was 100% sensitive and 99% specific in comparison to microbiological culture. Kappa value of 0.99 indicated an excellent concordance between these techniques.

Sensitivity and specificity reported for MAT when compared to microbiological culture was 0.95 and 0.89 with a = 1:50 cut off. PCR was a reliable method for the rapid and precise diagnosis of leptospirosis when compared to traditional techniques. Bedir *et al.* (2010) developed a rapid and simple assay for specific detection and differentiation of pathogenic *Leptospira* spp. by multiplex real-time PCR (TaqMan) assay using primers and probes targeting *Leptospira* genus specific 16S ribosomal RNA gene, the pathogen specific lig A/B genes and nonpathogen *Leptospira biflexa* specific 23S ribosomal RNA gene. Sixteen reference strains of Leptospira spp. including pathogenic and nonpathogenic and ten other negative control bacterial strains were used in the study. While the 16S primers amplified target from both pathogenic and non-pathogenic leptospires, the ligA/B and the 23S primers amplified target DNA from pathogenic and non-pathogenic leptospires, respectively. The multiplex real-time PCR (TaqMan) assay detection limit, that is, the sensitivity was found approximately 1 x 10(2) cells/ml for ligA/B gene and 23S ribosomal RNA gene, and 10 cells/ml 16S ribosomal RNA. The reaction efficiencies were 83-105% with decision coefficients of more than 0.99 in all multiplex assays. The multiplex real-time PCR (TaqMan) assay yielded negative results with the ten other control bacteria. In conclusion, the developed multiplex real-time PCR (TaqMan) assay is highly useful for early diagnosis and differentiation between pathogenic and non-pathogenic leptospires in a reaction tube as having high sensitivity and specificity.

Conventional classification of leptospires with the serovar as the basic taxon, based on serological recognition of lipopolysaccharide (LPS) composition does not correlate well with species determination, based on general genomic features. Bezerra da Silva *et al.*, 2011) investigated the selective amplification of polymorphic regions from the LPS biosynthesis loci (rfb) as a potential tool for serovar typing of Leptospira interrogans species. Eight pairs of primers were designed to target six ORFs from the rfb operon with varying levels of sequence polymorphism. They were tested both separately and multiplexed. Half of these primer pairs produced serovar-specific amplicons, allowing the identification of some specific serovars and also groups of serovars. It was shown that the serovar classification of *Leptospira* can be accessed by selective amplification of rfb operons in some cases, which may permit a parallel between the serological and the genomic classifications of *Leptospira*. As a conclusion, the selective amplification of rfb generated promising and already useful results, but it appears necessary to characterize a larger variety of Leptospira genomes or rfb operons to fully develop this method.

Treatment

The microorganisms are susceptible to most of the broad spectrum antibiotics. Treatment of most of the domestic animals is carried out by injecting dihydrostreptomycin. Often use of only the penicillin is effective. Supportive therapy is also advocated. For elimination of leptospiruria in cattle and pigs a single injection of streptomycin (25 mg/kg body weight) is recommended. Dihydrostreptomycin is not an effective treatment for serovar Hardjo infection. Other antibiotics may also be effective. Alt et al.(@001) evaluated antibiotics for treatment of cattle with leptospirosis caused by Leptospira borgpetersenii serovar Hardjo in a randomized controlled trial using 42 healthy mixed-breed cattle. The animals were inoculated via conjunctival instillation with *L. borgpetersenii* serovar *hardjo*. After infection and urinary shedding of *L. borgpetersenii* were confirmed, cattle were treated with various antibiotics. To determine effectiveness of antibiotic treatment, urinary shedding of *L. borgpetersenii* was monitored for 4 to 6 weeks after administration of antibiotics, using darkfield microscopic examination, microbial culture, immunofluorescence testing, and a polymerase chain reaction assay. ll inoculated cattle developed leptospirosis and shed leptospires in their urine. The following antibiotic treatments resulted in elimination of urinary shedding of leptospires: a single injection of oxytetracycline (20 mg/kg 19 mg/lb] of body weight, IM), tilmicosin (10 mg/kg [4.5 mg/lb], SC), or a combination product that contained dihydrostreptomycin-penicillin G (25 mg/kg [11.4 mg/lb], IM) or multiple injections of ceftiofur sodium (2.2 or 5 mg/kg [1 or 2.3 mg/lb], IM, once daily for 5 days, or 20 mg/kg, IM, once daily for 3 days). Successful resolution of leptospirosis in cattle by administration of dihydrostreptomycin-penicillin G confirms results obtained by other investigators. Three other antibiotics (oxytetracycline, tilmicosin, and ceftiofur) also were effective for resolving leptospirosis and may be useful substitutes for dihydrostreptomycin, an antibiotic that is no longer available for use in food-producing animals in the United States. Cost, safety, and withdrawal times of these various treatment options need to be considered.

Control

Since carriers play an important role in the maintenance of the disease for ultimate transmission to the susceptible host, the control at the carrier level is of utmost significance. Rodent control or the inaccessibility of wild life at the animal farm is of significance. This should be accompanied with the elimination of the reactors from the herd is essential since many reactors may be the urinary shedder of the leptospires. The reactors may also be treated with suitable antibiotics in order to eliminate the shedder state. In groups of pigs it is advisable to consider the infection to be herd-wide and to treat all the animal rather than the individual pigs. In case of cattle this approach is not advisable. Bulls and cows should be individually treated. Infected bulls should not be used for artificial insemination or natural service even though the advocated concentration of penicillin and streptomycin in the semen is effective in killing of the organisms.

Febrile cases of leptospirosis should be immediately segregated and treated till they return to normal conditions. Cows which have aborted or shown still birth should immediately be segregated and treated. It should be ensured that urine shedder stage does not develop. Newly purchased animals should not be introduced in the herd without proper testing to ensure that by both serologically and clinically, these animals are free of leptospires. Timely testing of all the animals by Microscopic Agglutination test for the development of reactors is useful in identifying the cases of leptospirosis particularly those which have failed to develop any clinical sign and symptoms.

Animals should not be allowed to graze on pasture where communal grazing is practiced due to the fear of picking up the infected from any infected animal.

Vaccines have been shown to be effective in preventing the disease in susceptible animals providing they have been prepared using serovars which are endemic in the area in which they are to be used. Vaccines used in the past have been bacterins. The initial vaccination regimen has been inoculation of 2 doses administered 4 weeks apart. It is an accepted practice to revaccinate with one dose annually. The vaccination schedule remains unchanged with polyvalent vaccines. In an open herd revaccination every 6 months is advised. During episodes of clinical leptospirosis vaccination along with the antibiotic therapy is useful. Vaccination should be practiced, if a suitable vaccine is available, every 6-9 months and should be continued for 2-3 years. Vaccination of animals less than 3 months of age is unlikely to be effective but vaccination of cows in late pregnancy gives effective immunity to their calves. This procedure is not effective in cows (Kingscote 1986). In India suitable vaccines are not available. However, there can be imported from USA, New Zealand, Australia or UK. The vaccine generally comprise of formalin killed whole cells of a few serovars of leptospires. Vaccination with the whole-cell vaccines may lead to incomplete, short-term immunity as well as serious side effects. A universal vaccine against leptospirosis is not available yet, making the identification of genus-specific protein antigens (GP-Ag) that display extensive cross-immunity very valuable for developing new vaccines and serodiagnostic methods.The choice of serovars in the vaccine depends on the prevalence of such serovars in the zone or herd to be vaccinated. The immunity provided is serovar specific hence choice of the vaccine is very critical. The bacterins stimulate low antibody titres as detected using microscopic agglutination test (MAT) and decline early. Bolin and Alt (2001) conducted a study to determine whether a monovalent Leptospira borgpetersenii serovar hardjo (type hardjobovis) vaccine commercially available in Australia, New Zealand, Ireland, and the United Kingdom would protect cattle from renal colonization and urinary shedding when exposed to a US strain of Leptospira borgpetersenii serovar hardjo. 24 Hereford heifers that lacked detectable antibodies against serovar Hardjo were used. Heifers received 2 doses, 4 weeks apart, of the commercial hardjo vaccine (n = 8) or a monovalent US reference hardjo vaccine (8) or were not vaccinated (controls; 8). Heifers were challenged 16 weeks later by intraperitoneal inoculation or conjunctival instillation. Serum antibody titers were measured weekly, and urine samples were examined for leptospires. Heifers were euthanatized 11 to 14 weeks after challenge, and kidney tissue was examined for evidence of colonization. All 8 heifers vaccinated with the reference vaccine were found to be shedding leptospires in their urine and had evidence of renal colonization. All 4 control heifers challenged by conjunctival instillation and 2 of 4 control heifers challenged by intraperitoneal inoculation shed leptospires in their urine, and all 8 had evidence of renal colonization. In contrast, leptospires were not detected in the urine or tissues of any of the 8 heifers that received the commercial hardjo vaccine. Heifers that received the commercial hardjo vaccine had significantly higher antibody titers than did heifers that received the reference vaccine. Results suggest that cattle that received 2 doses of the commercial hardjo vaccine were protected against renal colonization and urinary shedding when challenged with L borgpetersenii serovar hardjo strain 203 four months after vaccination.

Virtually all bovine leptospiral vaccines contain the reference strain *hardjo-prajitno,* however, North American cattle are predominantly infected with serovar *hardjo-bovis* (Radostitis *et al.,* 1994). DNA probe techniques can be used to identify animals infected with serovar *hardjo bovis*. The hardjo component of whole cell leptospiral vaccines is a weak immunogen, as evidenced by low serum agglutinating antibody titres in vaccinated cattle and short duration immunity. It is not clear in Indian context as to which vaccine is useful for vaccination, the vaccine containing *hardjo bovis* or *hardjo prajitno*. Vaccines containing Australis, Autumnalis, Grippotyphosa, Autumnalis, Pomona, Canicola, Tarassovi, Pyrogenes should be useful in Indian context. A hamster model was used to determine the efficacy of commercially prepared canine vaccines against Leptospira serovars circulating in Trinidad and to assess the effectiveness of killed whole-cell vaccines prepared from local isolates (Suepaul et al.2010). The local isolates used for vaccine preparation and challenge were isolates of serovars Copenhageni and Mankarso obtained from a local dog and rodent. Their estimated lethal dose-50 LD (50)) were 5 and 10 organisms, respectively and clinical signs observed on infection were consistent with leptospirosis. An unvaccinated control group of hamsters and other groups of hamsters that had been vaccinated with 3 doses of (i) in-house whole-cell Copenhageni vaccine, (ii) in-house whole-cell Mankarso vaccine, (iii) commercial vaccine Brand A or (iv) commercial vaccines Brand B were challenged with 1000 times the LD(50) of the respective challenge serovar. The most commonly used commercial vaccine (Brand A) did not offer protection to challenged hamsters, whereas Brand B facilitated the renal carrier state of the *Leptospira* organism. In contrast the whole-cell vaccines developed from local strains of serovars *Copenhageni* and *Mankarso*, protected all hamsters tested from both clinical disease and renal carrier states.

References

Alt D.P., Zuerner R.L. and Bolin C.A. 2001. Evaluation of antibiotics for treatment of cattle infected with Leptospira borgpetersenii serovar hardjo. J. Am. Vet. Med. Assoc. **219:** 636-639.

Anju Singh, Manoj Kumar & S.K. Srivastava. 2005. A report on seroprevalence of leptospirosis among equines. Indian Vet. Med. J. **29:** 197-198.

Anju Singh, Manoj Kumar, J.P. Varsheney & S.K. Srivastava 2007. Haematobiochemical changes in calves experimentally infected with Leptospira borgpetersenii serovar Hardjo. Indian Vet. J. **84:** 458-60.

Babudieri, B. 1958. Animal reservoirs of leptospires Ann. NY Acad. Sci. **70:** 393-413.

Barbosa A.S., Abreu P.A., Vasconcellos S.A., Morais Z.M., Gonçales A.P., Silva A.S. , Daha M,R, and Isaac L.2009.Immune evasion of leptospira species by acquisition of human complement regulator C4BP. Infect. Immun. **77:** 1137-43. Epub 2008 Dec 29.

Bedir O., Kilic A., Atabek E., Kuskucu A.M., Turhan V. and Basustaoglu A.C. 2010. Simultaneous detection and differentiation of pathogenic and nonpathogenic Leptospira spp. by multiplex real-time PCR (TaqMan) assay. Pol. J. Microbiol. **59:** 167-73.

Bessa T.A., Spichler A., Chapola E.G., Husch .AC., de Almeida M.F., Sodré M.M., Savani E.S., Sacramento D.R. and Vinetz J.M.2010.The contribution of bats to leptospirosis transmission in Sao Paulo City, Brazil. Am. J. Trop. Med. Hyg. **82:** 315-317.

Bezerra da Silva J., Carvalho E., Hartskeerl R.A. and Ho P.L. 2011.Evaluation of the use of selective PCR amplification of LPS biosynthesis genes for molecular typing of leptospira at the serovar level. Curr. Microbiol. **62:** 518-524. Epub 2010 Aug 19.

Brenner, D.J., Kauffman, A.F., Sulzer, K. R. *et al.*, 1999. Further determination of DNA relatedness between serogroups and serovars in the family Leptospiracea with a proposal for *L.alexanderi* sp. Nov. and 4 new Leptospira genomospecies. Int. J. Syst. Bact. **49:** 839-858.

Bolin C.A. and Alt D.P. 2001.Use of a monovalent leptospiral vaccine to prevent renal colonization and urinary shedding in cattle exposed to Leptospira borgpetersenii serovar hardjo. Am. J. Vet. Res. **62:** 995-1000.

Bomfim M.R., Ko A. and Koury M.C.2005.Evaluation of the recombinant LipL32 in enzyme-linked immunosorbent assay for the serodiagnosis of bovine leptospirosis. Vet. Microbiol. **109:** 89-94.

Bomfim M.R. and Koury M.C.2006.Evaluation of LSSP-PCR for identification of Leptospira spp. in urine samples of cattle with clinical suspicion of leptospirosis. Vet. Microbiol. **118:** 278-288. Epub 2006 Aug 1.

Chaperon, K.M., Davis, R.B. & Miller, N.G. 1979. Effect of a plasma cytotoxic factor in leptospirosis on platelets in vivo. Thrombosis Research **14:** 975-980.

Chirathaworn C., Chantaramalai T., Sereemaspun A., Kongthong N. and Suwancharoen D.2011.Detection of Leptospira in urine using anti-Leptospira-coated gold nanoparticles. Comp. Immunol. Microbiol. Infect. Dis. **34:** 31-34. Epub 2009 Dec 16.

Choy H.A., Kelley M.M., Chen T.L., Møller A.K., Matsunaga J. and Haake D.A. 2007. Physiological osmotic induction of Leptospira interrogans adhesion: LigA and LigB bind extracellular matrix proteins and fibrinogen. Infect. Immun. 2007 **75:** 2441-2450. Epub 2007 Feb 12.

Cole J.R. Jr, Sulzer C.R. and Pursell A.R. 1973.Improved microtechnique for the leptospiral microscopic agglutination test. Appl. Microbiol. **25:** 976-980.

Cullen, P.A., Haake, D.A. and Adler, B. 2004. Outer membrane proteins of pathogenic spirochetes. FEMS Microbiology Reviews. **25:** 291-318.

Cullen P.A., Haake D.A., Bulach D.M, Zuerner R.L. and Adler B.2003. LipL21 is a novel surface-exposed lipoprotein of pathogenic Leptospira species. Infect. Immun. **71:** 2414-2421.

Desvars A., Cardinale E. and Michault A.2011.Animal leptospirosis in small tropical areas. Epidemiol. Infect. **139:** 167-188. Epub 2010 Sep 28.

Dey S., Mohan C.M., Ramadass P. and Nachimuthu K.2007.Recombinant antigen-based dipstick ELISA for the diagnosis of leptospirosis in dogs. Vet. Rec. **160:** 186-188.

Estaroyer, J.M., Tran, T.A. and Hoen, B. Leptospirosis review practice 2001; **51:** 2086-2090.

Galloway R.L. and Levett P.N.2010.Application and validation of PFGE for serovar identification of Leptospira clinical isolates. PLoS Negl. Trop. Dis. 4. pii: e824.

Giles N., Hathaway S.C. and Stevens A.E.1983 Isolation of Leptospira interrogans serovar hardjo from a viable premature calf. Vet Rec. **113:** 174-176.

Gravekemp, C., Vanderkamp, H., Frozeri, M., Carrengton, D., Schoon, G.J., Van, Eys, G.J.J.M. and Everard, C.O.R. 1993. Detection of 7 species of pathogenic leptospires by PCR using 2 sets of primers. J. Gen. Microbiol. **139:** 1691-1700.

Hartskeerl, R.A., Goris, M.G.A., Brem, S., Meyer, P., Kopp, H. Gerhards, H. and Wollanke, B. 2004. Classification of Leptospira from the eyes of horses suffering for recurrent uveitis. Jour. Vet. Med. Ser. B. **51:** 110-115.

Hernández-Rodríguez P., Díaz C.A., Dalmau E.A., Quintero G.M.. 2011.A comparison between polymerase chain reaction (PCR) and traditional techniques for the diagnosis of leptospirosis in bovines. J. Microbiol. Methods. **84:** 1-7. Epub 2010 Oct 31.

Ito, T., and Yanagawa, R. 1988. Two types of attachments of leptospires. Israil J. Vet. Med. **44:** 9-14.

Kiem, N.T., Charan, K., Srivastava, S.K., Parihar, N.S. & Bisht, G.S. 1995. Haematological, Biochemical and serological studies on experimental leptospirosis in goats. Indian Vet. J. **72:** 229-232.

Kingscote B.F. 1986.Leptospirosis: an occupational hazard to veterinarians. Can Vet J. **27:** 78-81.

Kmety, E. and Dikken, H. (1988). Revised list of Leptospira serovars. Groningen. The Netherlands Univ. Press.

Kositanont U., Rugsasuk S., Leelaporn A., Phulsuksombati D., Tantitanawat S. and Naigowit P.2007.Detection and differentiation between pathogenic and saprophytic Leptospira spp. by multiplex polymerase chain reaction. Diagn. Microbiol. Infect. Dis. **57:** 117-122. Epub 2006 Oct 3.

La-Ard A., Amavisit P., Sukpuaram T. and Wajjwalku W.2011.Evaluation of recombinant Lig antigen-based ELISA for detection of leptospiral antibodies in canine sera. Southeast Asian J Trop Med Public Health. **42:** 128-137.

Levett, P.N., Branch, S.L., Whittengton, C.U. *et al.*, 2001. Leptospirosis. Clin. Diag. Lab. Immunol. **18:** 349-351.

Lin Y.P., McDonough S.P., Sharma Y. and Chang Y.F.2011..Leptospira immunoglobulin-like protein B (LigB) binding to the C-terminal fibrinogen áC domain inhibits fibrin clot formation, platelet adhesion and aggregation. Mol. Microbiol. **79:** 1063-1076. Epub 2011 Jan 10.

Lucchesi, PMA and Parma, A.E. 1999. A DNA fragment of *L.interrogans* encodes a protein which shares epitopes with equine cornea. Vet. Immunol. Immunopathol. **71:** 173-179.

Madathiparambil MG., Cattavarayane S., Perumana S.R., Manickam G.D. aqnd Sehgal S.C.2011. Presence of 46 kDa Gelatinase on the Outer Membrane of Leptospira. Curr. Microbiol. **62:** 1478-1482. Epub 2011 Feb 9.

Mariya R., Chaudhary P., Kumar A.A., Thangapandian E., Amutha R. and Srivastava S.K. 2006.Evaluation of a recombinant LipL41 antigen of Leptospira interrogans serovar canicola in ELISA for serodiagnosis of bovine leptospirosis. Comp. Immunol. Microbiol. Infect. Dis. **29:** 269-277. Epub 2006 Sep 18.

Mariya, R., Srivastava, S.K. and Thangapandian, E. 2007. Seroprevalence of leptospiral antibodies in bovines. Indian Vet. J. **84:** 547-548.

Matthias M.A., Díaz M.M., Campos K.J., Calderon M., Willig M.R., Pacheco V., Gotuzzo E., Gilman R.H. and Vinetz J.M.2005.Diversity of bat-associated *Leptospira* in the

Peruvian Amazon inferred by bayesian phylogenetic analysis of 16S ribosomal DNA sequences. Am. J. Trop. Med. Hyg. **73:** 964-974.

Merien F., Baranton G. and Perolat P.1995.Comparison of polymerase chain reaction with microagglutination test and culture for diagnosis of leptospirosis. J. Infect. Dis. **172:** 281-285.

Miller D.A., Wilson M.A. and Beran G.W. 1991.Survey to estimate prevalence of Leptospira interrogans infection in mature cattle in the United States. Am. J. Vet. Res. **52:** 1761-1765.

Nicholson V.M. and Prescott J.F. 1993.Outer membrane proteins of three pathogenic Leptospira species. Vet. Microbiol. **36:** 123-138.

Pinne M., Choy H.A. and Haake D.A.2010.The OmpL37 surface-exposed protein is expressed by pathogenic Leptospira during infection and binds skin and vascular elastin. PLoS Negl. Trop. Dis. 4:e815.

Radostitis, O.M., Blood, D.C., Gay, C.C. 1994. Veterinary Medicine. A text book of the diseases of cattle, sheep, pigs, goats & horses. ELBS with Bailliere Tindall, London.

Sankar S., Harshan H.M., Somarajan S.R. and Srivastava S.K. 2010.Evaluation of a recombinant LigB protein of Leptospira interrogans serovar Canicola in an enzyme-linked immunosorbent assay for the serodiagnosis of bovine leptospirosis. Res. Vet. Sci. **88:** 375-8. Epub 2009 Dec 22.

Sharma, R, Tuteja U.,Khushiramani, R. et al.2008. A simple technique for diagnosis of leptospirosis. Hybridoma (Larchmt) Apr. **27:** 113-121.

Silbreck, N.W. and Davies, W.D. (1989). Aust. Vet. J. **64:** 1

Srivastava, S.K. 2002. Properties of Lipopolysaccharide antigen of *L. interrogans* serovar pyrogens. Indian Vet. J. **79:** 1201-1202.

Srivastava, S.K. and Kumar, A. 2003. Seroprevalence of leptospirosis in animals and human beings in various regions of the country. Indian J. Comp. Microbiol. Immunol. Infect. Dis. **24:** 155-159.

Srivastava, S.K. and Sharma, M.C. 1990. Some observations on goats following administration of *Leptospira interrogans* serovar hardjo. Current Sci. **59:** 171-173.

Suepaul S.M., Carrington C.V., Campbell M., Borde G. and Adesiyun A.A.2010.Study on the efficacy of Leptospira vaccines developed from serovars isolated from Trinidad and comparison with commercial vaccines using a hamster model. Vaccine. **28:** 5421-5426. Epub 2010 Jun 19.

Wagenaar J., Zuerner R.L., Alt D.and Bolin C.A.2000.Comparison of polymerase chain reaction assays with bacteriologic culture, immunofluorescence, and nucleic acid hybridization for detection of Leptospira borgpetersenii serovar hardjo in urine of cattle. Am. J. Vet. Res. **61:** 316-320.

Yan W., Faisal S.M., Divers T., McDonough S.P., Akey B. and Chang Y.F.2010.Experimental *Leptospira* interrogans serovar Kennewicki infection of horses. J. Vet. Intern. Med. **24:** 912-917.

Yang-yang, Qing-Jin Hang, Zhang Yi, He Ping, Hu-Baoyu, Guo-Xiaokui. 2009. A novel pore forming haemolysin protein in *Leptospira* species. Chinese J. Zoonoses. **25:** 831-836.

Zhang-Yi, Guo, X, Wn-C. & Zhao, G. 2003. Characteristic analysis of haemolysin gene in *Leptospira interrogans*. Chinese J. Zoonoses. **19:** 10-16.

Zhang X.Y., Yu Y., He P., Zhang Y.X., Hu B.Y., Yang Y., Nie Y.X., Jiang X.G., Zhao G.P. and Guo X.K. 2005.Expression and comparative analysis of genes encoding outer membrane proteins LipL21, LipL32 and OmpL1 in epidemic leptospires. Acta. Biochim. Biophys. Sin (Shanghai). **37:** 649-656.

Zuerner R.L. and Bolin C.A. 1990.Nucleic acid probe characterizes *Leptospira interrogans* serovars by restriction fragment length polymorphisms. Vet. Microbiol. **24:** 355-366.

□□□

Chapter 10

Diseases Caused by *Actinobacillus* spp.

Dr. S.K. SRIVASTAVA
Former, Division of Bacteriology & Mycology
Indian Veterinary Research Institute, Izatnagar-243122
Bareilly (U.P.)

Diseases caused by *Actinobacillus* spp.

Species of *Actinobacillus* are gram-negative, non motile, small rods and coccobacilli. They are non-sporing, faultatively anaerobic, fermentative and require complex nutrients for growth. They have a low G+C ratio (38-44mol %) and a relatively small genome. The taxonomy of the members of the genus Actinobacillus associated with animals has been reviewed with focus on classification and identification including molecular based characterization, typing and identification. Out of the 22 species or species like taxa reported as Actinobacillus, 19 are associated with animals. When classified on the basis of 16S rRNA sequence based phylogenetic analysis, DNA-DNA hybridizations and phenotypic analysis, Actinobacillus sensu stricto is restricted to include *A. lignieresii, A. pleuropneumoniae, A. equuli* subsp. *equuli, A. equuli* subsp. *haemolyticus* (taxon 11 of Bisgaard), *A. hominis, A. suis, A. ureae, A. arthritidis* (taxon 9 of Bisgaard), *Actinobacillus* genomospecies 1 and 2 and the taxa 8 and 26 of Bisgaard. The remaining 11 species of *Actinobacillus* are unrelated to *A. sensu* stricto and should consequently be grouped with other genera or be renamed as new genera depending on new data. Identification of members of Actinobacillus at species level is possible through phenotypic characterization combined with information on host of isolation. PCR tests are available for specific detection of *A. pleuropneumoniae*. Only A. pleuropneumoniae is presently considered as a primary pathogen. Based on different types of RTX genes it is possible to PCR type *A. pleuropneumoniae* to serotype level. PCR might also be used for the specific detection of *A. equuli* subsp. haemolyticus. Epidemiological investigations and surveillance have so far included serotyping, multilocus enzyme electrophoresis (MLEE), ribotyping and restriction fragment length profiling.

The following species cause important diseases in animals.

1. *Actinobacillus lignieresii* - causes wooden tongue in cattle and suppurative lesion of skin and lungs in swine.
2. *Actinobacillus equuli* - causes foal septicaemia or joint ill.
3. *Actinobacillus pleuropneumonia* - causes contagious pleuropneumonia of pigs.
4. *Actinobacillus suis* - causes septicaemia and other infectious disease in pigs.
5. *Actinobacillus capsulatus* - causes arthritis in rabbits.
6. *Actinobacillus seminis* - epididymitis in young rams and purulent arthritis in sheep.

Except *A.pleuroneumonia* all are present in the animals as part of the normal microflora and give rise to endogenous as well as exogenous infections. These organisms share significant biochemical characteristics and electrophoretic patterns.

Actinobacillus lignieresii

It is a normal inhabitant of oral cavity and rumen of ruminants. The organism is the causative agent of wooden tongue in cattle where the infection is caused due to damage to the oral mucosa, as a result of ulcerating and penetrating lesions to the sulcus of the tongue and laceration to the side of the body of the tongue caused by the teeth. *Actinobacillus lignieresii* is a commensal of the oropharynx and rumen in cattle and sheep and has also been found in the oral cavity of healthy horses. The disease is fairly acute, with swelling in the affected part, under the jaw and in the regional lymph nodes. The clinical symptoms are excess salivation, difficult mastication and inappetance. The condition is seen either as an outbreak in several animals simultaneously or as an individual case in a single animal, often in association with a diet change

In cattle, 'wooden tongue' is the most commonly recognised, acute presentation of actinobacillosis, but the bacteria can affect soft tissues anywhere in the gastrointestinal tract (including the rumen and reticulum) and may present as a chronic condition of up to six months duration. Additionally, cutaneous actinobacillosis has been reported where it is important to differentiate this condition from cutaneous lymphosarcoma.

Carmalt *et al.* (1999) first reported mastitis and chronic nasal cellulitis caused by A lignieresii infection in horses.In bovine and ovine hosts the organism may cause pyogranulomatous inflammation, especially of the upper alimentary tract. In horses it has been found in association with pyemic processes of soft tissues and cases of stomatitis. A human infection following the horse bite has been reported (Benaoudia *et al.*, 1994). Concurrent infection with *Actinobacillus lignieresii* and Mycobacterium farcinogenes was detected in slaughtered cattle (Tageldin *et al.*, 1988). The lesions were confined to the retropharyngeal, mandibular and parotid lymph nodes. The *actinobacillus granulomas* were seen either inside the caseous lesions or between the caseous part and the epithelioid zone of bovine farcy granuloma. In concomitant infections, actinobacillosis was always in the early active phase, whereas in actinobacillosis alone, active as well as healed stages were encountered.

Phenotypic characterization of bacteria from diseased and healthy horses identified 18 isolates as Bisgaard taxon 9 and 11 isolates as *Actinobacillus lignieresii* (Christensen *et al.*, 2002). All strains of taxon 9 were alpha-galactosidase- and raffinose-positive and showed variable fermentation of (+) L-arabinose and (-) D-sorbitol. Strains of *A. lignieresii* were negative for these characteristics, with the exception of raffinose. Two strains from the (-) D-sorbitol-negative group of taxon 9 showed a 16S rRNA similarity of 99-6%, while 99.5% similarity was found between two strains of the (-)D-sorbitol-positive group. DNA-DNA hybridization between the two strains representing the (-)D-sorbitol-negative group showed 98% binding, and their closest relationship was to a strain of A. lignieresii (64%). The two strains of the (-)D-sorbitol-positive group showed 83% binding and were related to the (-)D-sorbitol-negative group at a 76% DNA binding level. Actinobacillus arthritidis sp. nov. is proposed for 12 strains of the (-)D-sorbitol-positive group. Actinobacillus genomospecies 2 is suggested for the six strains of the (-)D-sorbitol-negative group. Phenotypically, strains of A. arthritidis and Actinobacillus genomospecies 2 differ in (-)D-sorbitol fermentation and can be separated from Actinobacillus equuli by being trehalose-negative, while a positive reaction for alpha-galactosidase separates the taxa from A. lignieresii. The type strain of A. arthritidis, CCUG 24862T, was isolated from a joint of a horse. Three equine isolates of *A. lignieresii* that could not be separated from the type strain by means of phenotypic characteristics showed 98.6-100% 16S rRNA similarity, but only 96.4-96.7% similarity to the type strain. DNA-DNA hybridization between two strains of this group showed 92% binding but only 70% binding to the type strain of A. lignieresii. Consequently, these equine isolates of A. lignieresii represent a new genomospecies of Actinobacillus, suggested as genomospecies 1 because phenotypic characteristics are not presently available to separate it from the type strain of *A. lignieresii*.

The virulence factors of *A. lignieresii* remain unknown. Different strains may vary in their ability to induce disease, but little progress has been made to identify reliable markers that will allow their epidemiological tracing. In addition, there is also limited information concerning genetic diversity in the natural population of the species.

The disease in cattle is worldwide in distribution with sporadic occurrence at individual farms. Copper deficiency predisposes the animals to actinobacillosis. High incidence of the disease has been recorded when they graze on tough, dry, course fodder or 'burnt over' pastures. Occasionally, the granuloma may occur at unusual sites such as the external nares or jugular furrow following the infection of the traumatic lesions. They are pliable on palpation, red and bleed easily. Lesions usually consist of multiple granulomatous abscesses. In cattle and sheep, these occur most frequently around the head and neck region. The lesions commences as a small nodule which later become suppurative and ulcerates and release white to green pus containing greenish white granules of less than 1mm in diameter. Pus from the abscesses may contain microcolonies surrounded by clublike spicules of calcium phosphate giving the appearance of sulphur granules.

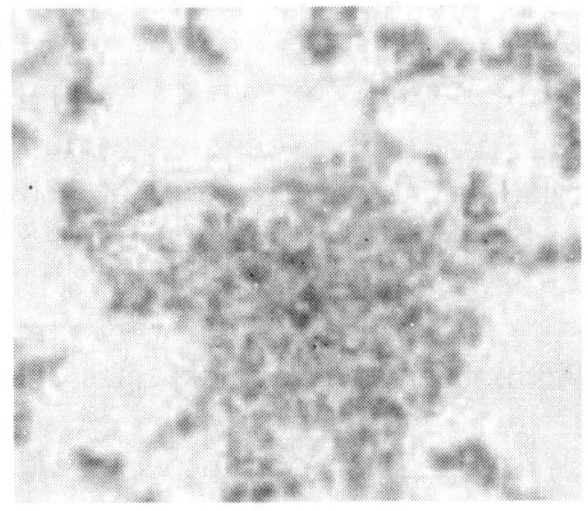

Actinobacillus lignieresii
Gram stained

Genetic diversity detected by analysis of amplified fragment length polymorphisms (AFLPs) of 54 Actinobacillus lignieresii isolates from different hosts and geographic localities is described (Kokotovic *et al.*2011). On the basis of variances in AFLP profiles, the strains were grouped in two major clusters; one comprising strains isolated from horses and infected wounds of humans bitten by horses and another consisting of strains isolated from bovine and ovine hosts. The present data indicate a comparatively higher degree of genetic diversity among strains isolated from equine hosts and confirm the existence of a separate genomospecies for *A. lignieresi*-like isolates from horses. Among the isolates from bovine and ovine hosts some clonal lines appear to be genetically stable over time and could be detected at very distant geographic localities. Although all ovine strains investigated grouped in a single cluster, the existence of distinct genetic lineages that have evolved specificity for ovine hosts is not obvious and needs to be confirmed in other studies.

Pathogenesis

The spread of the infection is via lymphatics. Lungs and other organs are involved. The onset is usually acute and the affected animal is unable to eat for 2-3 days. The tongue is swollen and hard particularly at the base. In the later stage the acute inflammation is replaced by fibrous tissues with tongue showing hardness. Lymphadenitis is common. The lymph nodes show swelling which often rupture with the discharge of pus. Healing of the lesions is slow.

A.lignieresii possesses a gene encoding an RTX membrane active toxin. This toxin kills macrophages and neutrophils at high concentration and stimulates an oxidative burst at lower concentration. Very small amount of this toxin is produced as a result, the colonies growing on blood agar plates do not show clear cut haemolysis. The organisms are not leukocytoxic as compared to other organisms that produce this class of toxin. This toxin is involved in chemotaxis of neutrophils as a result formation of pus is common. The RTX toxin induced oxidative burst leads to the damage to surrounding cells that in turn cause inflammation.

Actinobacillus is gram-negative, therefore, probably the lipopolysaccharide in outer membrane induces an inflammatory response with subsequent release of pro-inflammatory Cytokines, IL-1 and TNF. The antiphagocytic capsule has not been demonstrated in *A.lignieresii* to play a role in pathogenesis.

Lesions produced in wooden tongue are suppurative to granulomatous resembling actinomycosis. In wooden tongue, the lesion has a center which has *A.lignieresii* ringed by eosinophilic, club like "rosette", surrounded by polymorphonuclear cells and granulation. Macrophages, plasma cells, lymphocytes, giant cells and fibroblasts are also present. The infection may spread to lymph nodes. Superficial lesions are often produced at other organs which often ulcerate. In sheep, the head and neck is involved along with skin and mammary glands. Tongue involvement is not typical.

Diagnosis

Actinobacilli can be demonstrated in lesions. They grow best under increased Co_2 tension. Colonies are often sticky. Cultural and biochemical identification of the species is required. The organisms are Gram-negative. Catalase- and oxidase-positive. Non-motile and attacks sugars by fermentation

The organisms grows on MacConkey and are usually non-haemolytic on blood agar. They are catalase and urease positive.

Treatment and Control

Administration of iodides is advocated which are very effective in curing the disease almost permanently. Sulfonamides are also effective. It is probable that iodides exert their effect by reducing the severity of the fibrous tissue reaction. The broad spectrum antibiotics are generally used these days to treat the cases of wooden tongue. The iodides are given orally or intravenously. Treatment is continued until iodism develops characterized by lacrimation, anorexia, coughing and appearance of dandruff. One course of potassium iodide is usually sufficient for soft tissue lesions. At least one or 2 more treatments are required for bony lesions.

Subcutaneous infection of sodium iodide in sheep causes severe imitation and local swelling immediately.

Restriction of the spread of actinobacillosis is best implemented by quick treatment of affected animals and the prevention of contamination of pasture and feed troughs. The affected animals should be immediately segregated.

Actinobacillus equuli

A.equuli is responsible for fatal septicaemia in new born foals. Localization in various organs is seen in foals which have survived the disease. The organism is normally found in the intestinal tract of horses. Isolation of *A.equuli* from oral cavity of healthy horses has been reported (Stemberg, 1998).Aalbaek *et al.* (2007) first reported an etiological association between A. equuli subsp. equuli and equine endocarditis. *Actinobacillus equuli,* a gram-negative, rod-shaped bacterium that naturally occurs as a commensal on the mucosal membranes of adult horses, is commonly the cause of fatal septicemia in newborn foals. Foals are thought to be directly infected by the mare through the mouth or respiratory tract during or immediately following birth. Case of fatal pulmonary hemorrhage in a 6-year-old American Paint mare with a 2-week history of intermittent coughing, fever, and epistaxis is described (Pusteria *et al* 2008). Significant macroscopic abnormalities at postmortem examination were restricted to the respiratory system, and microscopically, severe pulmonary hemorrhage with suppurative bronchopneumonia was found. Actinobacillus equuli subsp. haemolyticus was cultured from a transtracheal wash performed antemortem as well as from the lungs at necropsy. The presence of airway-associated hemorrhage in conjunction with bacterial bronchopneumonia suggested endothelial damage caused by a locally elaborated bacterial toxin, possibly produced by the A. equuli strain isolated from the lungs. The objective of this report was to indirectly document the presence of hemolysin repeat in structural toxin (RTX) in the lungs of the reported mare. Matthews *et al* (2001) reviewed the clinical findings, diagnosis and treatment of 51 horses with peritonitis attributed to Actinobacillus equuli. Breed, age and gender of horse, history, physical examination findings, treatment and outcome were determined from the hospital records of 51 horses in which a diagnosis of peritonitis attributed to *A. equuli* was made between January 1993 and June 1999. Results of abdominal fluid cytology and bacteriology, antimicrobial sensitivity patterns, haematology and faecal egg counts, when performed, were also retrieved.There was a variety of breeds of horses affected. There were 35 male and 17 female horses, aged from 9 months to 22 years, presented. Lethargy, signs of depression with mild to moderate signs of abdominal pain and inappetence were the most common reasons for presentation. Most horses had elevated heart and respiratory rates, an elevated rectal temperature and reduced intestinal borborygmi heard on auscultation of the abdomen. Abnormal colour with an elevated protein were features of an abdominal fluid sample in 98% of horses and a marked elevation in nucleated cell count was present in all samples. Pleomorphic gram-negative rods were seen on cytology in 53% of samples and a positive culture of *A. equuli* was returned in 72% of samples. Other laboratory findings in some horses included mild haemoconcentration, hypoproteinaemia, an elevated circulating nucleated cell count with a left shift, an elevation in fibrinogen concentration and an elevated faecal egg count. All horses demonstrated a rapid response to treatment with procaine penicillin alone, or a combination of procaine penicillin and gentamicin sulphate. Where antimicrobial sensitivity tests were performed, all but two isolates were sensitive to procaine penicillin. All horses responded to antimicrobial and supportive therapy and were discharged from hospital. Horses with *A. equuli* peritonitis present with similar clinical signs as horses with other causes of abdominal pain. However, these signs, when evaluated in conjunction with the results of abdominal fluid analysis and response to treatment, are characteristic of *A. equuli* peritonitis. Pleomorphic gram-negative bacteria may be seen on a cytological preparation of the abdominal fluid sample, and a positive bacterial culture may be obtained in some, but not all, cases. Most isolates are sensitive to procaine penicillin, so treatment with procaine penicillin and gentamicin sulphate is recommended until antimicrobial sensitivity is known.

On rare occasions, *A. equuli* has been reported to be an opportunistic pathogen of pigs. The infection of pigs is typically associated with abortion, septicemia, and polyarthritis. The death of over 300 sows in 2 months on a 3000 sow farrow-to-isowean operation in Manitoba (Canada)was attributed to infection with *Actinobacillus equuli*. This pathogen commonly infects foals, and is rarely reported in swine. Our report is the second recently published case of this pathogen in North American swine (Thompson *et al.*, 2010).

The bacterial species has been recently divided into *A.equuli* subsp. *equuli* and the haemolytic, *A.equuli* subsp. haemolyticus. Of these the latter species contain the gene aqx and other toxin genes (Kuhnert *etal.,* 2003). It has also been isolated from retropharyngeal infections and other lesions in the gastrointestinal tract of the horse. Usually new born foals are the most susceptible, however, older animals can also be infected. Occasionally it can be of zoonotic importance (Ashhurst-smith *etal.,* 1988). Usually it is a secondary invader in animals showing concurrent infection. The mare is not clinically affected but can transmit the infection to the foals in utero, however infection through the naval is also possible. The following manifestations can be seen in older horses; lameness caused by purulent arthritis, infrequent abortions, nephritis, peritonitis and endocarditis. It occasionally causes septicaemic disease or enteritis in pigs and calves. The disease is prevalent throughout the world. In India during 1985-88, several cases have been describe from stud farm in Karnataka state (Varshney & Uppal 1993). The disease is enzootic at certain farms and causes the infection episodes. Many foals develop *A.equuli* infection with in hours of days of birth. Those dying with in 24 hrs. of life show a severe enteritis. Those living for several days develop a purulent nephritis, meningitis, pneumonia or septic arthritis.

In foals dying of acute septicaemia without showing specific symptoms, in such animals adrenal cortical deficiency may be a major factor in causing the death. Foals which survive the illness for more than 24 hours develop suppurative lesions in the renal cortex in joints and intestine. Facial cellulitis due to *A.equuli* is caused in neonatal foal (Castognetti *etal.,* 2008). Rarely metritis, vascular endocarditis and septicaemia have been reported in gilt by Ramos-Vare *etal* (2008) as confirmed by histological examination and polymerase chain reaction.

Pathogenesis

To date little is known about the virulence factors of *A.equuli.* Recent data indicate that *A.equuli* may possess toxins similar to AqX toxin family of *A.pleuropneumonia* which may play a role in pathogenesis. The presence of pneumonia associated with haemorrhagic pulmonary fluid and the culture of large numbers of haemolytic *A.equuli* with endothelial damage is indicative of role of AqX toxins (Pusterla *etal.,* 2008). This toxin is membrane active and very small amount of this toxin is produced. Strains are antigenically heterogenous. By screening hemolytic A. equuli strains with specific gene probes, a hemolysin, designated Aqx (A. equuli RTX (repeats in the structural toxin)) was identified (Berthhoud *et al.*2002). This hemolysin was shown to be an RTX type of toxin by characterization of the aqxCABD operon. All hemolytic A. equuli isolates contained a functional aqxCABD operon and expressed the Aqx hemolysin as shown by genetic and phenotypic assays. The structural toxin AqxA is the hemolysin of *A. equuli* as shown by expression of recombinant aqx constructs in *E. coli*. Its hemolytic activity can be inhibited by specific antibodies raised against AqxA. Sequence analysis of the 16S rRNA gene (rrs) of the taxonomically diffuse group of *A. equuli* and related strains defined two phylogenetically distinct groups. The presence of the Aqx operon is not correlated with this phylogenetic grouping. The operon is found in both groups of *A. equuli* strains where it specifies the hemolytic activity and is supposedly to be a determinative virulence factor. The aqx operon was not found in closely related members of the Pasteurellaceae family. The Aqx protein of A equuli, belonging to the RTX family of pore-forming toxins, is also cytotoxic to horse lymphocytes. The presence of antibodies to Aqx was investigated in sera from individual horses from different regions; the sera from adult horses and foals 24 hours after birth reacted with Aqx, and sera from foals sampled shortly after an intake of colostrum also reacted with Aqx, but sera from foals taken before an intake of colostrum did not react with Aqx (Berthhoud *et al.* 2004).Kuhnert *et al.* 2003a) assessed and compared host cell specificity of the haemolytic and cytotoxic activity of the RTX toxins from Actinobacillus equuli, an equine pathogen, and Actinobacillus suis, which is pathogenic for pigs. The two bacterial species are closely related, phenotypically as well as phylogenetically, sharing the same 16S rRNA gene sequence. Both species contain specific protein toxins from the family of pore-forming RTX toxins, however, the two species differ in their RTX toxin profiles. Haemolytic *A. equuli* contains the operon for the Aqx toxin, whereas *A. suis* harbours genes for ApxI and ApxII. We tested the toxic activity of the corresponding proteins on erythrocytes as well as on lymphocytes isolated from horse and pig blood. The strength of the haemolytic activity for each of the toxins was independent of the origin of erythrocytes. When testing cytotoxic activity, the Aqx protein showed a higher toxic effect for horse lymphocytes than for porcine lymphocytes. On the other hand, ApxI and ApxII showed a strong cytotoxic effect on porcine lymphocytes and a reduced toxicity for horse lymphocytes; the toxicity of ApxII was generally much lower than ApxI. These results indicate a host species specificity of the toxic activity of RTX toxins Aqx of *A. equuli* and ApxI and ApxII of A. suis. A real-time polymerase chain reaction (PCR) assay targeting the recently described aqx gene of *A. equuli* subsp. *haemolyticus* was established and validated. Transcriptional activity of the aqx gene was used as a surrogate method to document toxin production. Real-time PCR analysis of the transtracheal fluid and lung tissue of the affected mare confirmed the presence and the transcriptional activity of the aqx gene at the genomic (gDNA) and complementary DNA (cDNA) levels, respectively.

Diagnosis

Clinical samples such as affected tissues, feces, purulent material and blood are subjected to bacteriological analysis. The colonies of fresh isolates are rough and mucoid appearance probably because of mucinous capsule. On subculture mucoid character is lost. The organism is catalase negative and urease positive and beta haemolytic property is seen with only some strains. A polymerase chain reaction is available for specific detection of *A.equuli* subsp. haemolyticus. For epidemiological purpose serotyping, multilocus enzyme electrophoresis, ribotyping & RFLP have been used (Christensen and Bisgaard 2004).

Treatment and Control

Prophylactic treatment of all the foals shortly after birth with penicillin or tetracyclines is very effective. Drug of choice for treating cases of *A.equuli* infection in foals are chloramphenicol, tetracycline, third generation cephalosporins and trimethoprin- sulfonamide combination.

Cefquinome has been shown to be effective against A.equuli strains (Thomas *etal.,* 2006). There is no vaccine against this disease.

Meternal antibodies in the colostrums are important in protecting foals against the disease. These antibodies are against the whole cells, outer membrane proteins and AqX toxins. By day 30, these antibodies decline significantly in foals (Holyoak *etal.,* 2007). New born foals show phagocytosis of *A.equuli* by the serum as indicated by opsonization of the cells. This opsonic activity increase after feeding of colostrum with predominance of IgG sub-isotypes switched from IgGb to 2gGa. Complement activation was necessary for opsonization of *A.equuli* as well as *E.coli* tested (Grondahl *etal.,* 2001).

Actinobacillus pleuropneumoniae

Actinobacillus pleuropneumoniae is the causative agent of a contagious disease of pigs characterized by a short course of disease with dyspnea cyanosis, fever and a high case fatality rate. The acute form of disease is characterized by extensive haemorrhages and fibrin deposition in the lungs. In chronic cases there is sequestration of organisms in the lungs in necrotic tissues covered with a thick capsule of connective tissue. It is of great economic importance in all those countries where intensive swine husbandry is practiced. The disease is seen more frequently in pigs of 2-6 months of age. In India, there is no evidence of this disease, however, in North Eastern region of the country, pleuropneumonia- like disease has been reported. Risk factors involved confinement rearing, crowding, inadequate ventilation, close contact and excessive humidity. Limited evidence shows that *A.pleuropneumoniae* may interact with *Pasteurella multocida* to produce a severe from of disease. Transportation of pigs to and from the barn exposes the animals to the risk of exposure leading to the outbreaks. The highest risk is associated with the introduction of new pigs.

The organism comprise of 15 serotypes and 2 biotypes (Nielsen 1990). Biotyping is based on the requirement of necotinamide adenine dinucleotide (NAD): biotype 1 isolates require the NAD whereas biotype 2 isolates are NAD independent. Serotyping is based on capsular antigen whereas the cell membrane lipopolysaccharide is commonly shared by some serotype. The outer membrane proteins are common to all the serotypes. Only a limited number of clones are associated with disease (Moller *etal.*, 1992). In particular, the genetic heterogeneity of serotypes 1, 2, 5 and 6 is limited whereas diversity has been recorded among serotypes 7, 8 and 12. Variation in the virulence among the serotypes has also been recorded. The prevalence of serotypes among different geographical locations varies considerably. Serovars 1, 5 & 7 are common in North America, serovars 2 and 9 are common in continental Europe while serovar 3 is common in England. Serovars 1, 2, 3, 5, & 7 are present in Australian pigs with serovar 5 & 7 being the most common. Two distinct antigenic subtypes of Actinobacillus pleuropneumoniae serotype 1 were identified via coagglutination (Co-A) and designated as 1A and 1B(Jolie *et al.*1994). The reference strains, ATCC 27088 (1A) and ISU 158 (1B), were used to prepare hyperimmune rabbit sera for Co-A reagents. Of 75 serotype 1 field isolates tested by Co-A, 35 isolates typed as 1A, 12 as 1B and 28 as 1A/1B. Significant cross-reactivity between the 2 subtypes was found in the Co-A and was eliminated in 20/28 1A/1B strains by using Co-A reagents prepared with rabbit sera absorbed with the heterologous reference strain. However, twelve isolates (5 1A and 7 1A/1B; 16%) showed no reaction with Co-A reagents prepared with absorbed sera. Immunoblots of outer membranes (OM) prepared from APP 1A or 1B reference strains and field isolates indicated that antigenic differences between subtypes 1A and 1B were located within the high molecular weight (MW) region of the gels (40-100 kDa). Hyperimmune rabbit sera against 1A or 1B and sera from pigs vaccinated with whole-cell, formalin inactivated 1A or 1B bacterins reacted with the high MW region only in strains of the homologous subtype. In contrast, 4 of 5 sera from 1B infected pigs and 2 of 5 sera from 1A infected pigs reacted with all APP serotype 1 strains regardless of subtype. Apparently, infection exposed cross-reactive antigenic determinants that were not exposed by immunization with killed bacteria preparations. SDS-PAGE gels with LPS purified from APP 1A, 1B, 9 and 11 showed that 1A, 9 and 11 LPS O-antigens had an identical smooth ladder pattern, while 1B LPS was distinctly different. In immunoblots with OM or LPS and in dot-immunobinding assays with LPS, rabbit antiserum against APP 1A reacted with 1A, 9 and 11. In contrast, rabbit antiserum against APP 1B only reacted with APP 1B and weakly with APP 9 in the OM immunoblot and with LPS from APP 1B, 9 and 11 in the LPS immunoblot and dot-immunobinding assay. We conclude that 2 subtypes of APP serotype 1 can be distinguished based on their antigenic differences. These differences are located, at least in part, within the LPS O-antigens. LPS O-antigens from APP 1B appear more antigenically similar to APP 9 LPS than to either APP 1A or APP 11 LPS. There may also be antigenic differences in the capsular polysaccharides of APP 1A and 1B strains.

Pathogenesis

In acute infections the organism enters the lung and multiplies rapidly. *A.pleuropneumoniae* synthesize fimbriae adhesion molecules that help in attachment to tonsillar crypts. The natural route of infection is aerogenous. Experimentally by aerosol exposure of pigs to the organism a severe fibrinous haemorrhagic necrotizing pleuropneumonia develops as seen in the natural infection. Pulmonary oedema develops with multifocal petechial haemorrhages and a diffuse neutrophilic bronchilitis. Intratracheally, occurrence of blood coagulation and cyclooxyenase- dependent variable lung lesions are common. The ability of haemolysin to affect the pulmonary macrophages may enhance the multiplication of organisms. Ultrastructurally, there is marked capillary dilatation and mild degeneration of endothelial cells and fibrin thrombi. Inflammatory cells are primarily macrophages and a few neutrophils are present due to the release of cytotoxins and other cellular factors. Once at the site of infection, the neutrophils are lysed by one or more of the cytolysins. After this period, few intact neutrophils can be found. Lysis of neutrophils is responsible for massive and rapid tissue damage.

Several virulence factors have been described which help in progress of the disease in the host. These include cytotoxins, haemolysins, outer membrane proteins, capsule and lipopolysaccharide (Inzana 1991). Capsule renders the bacteria resistant to complement activity and opsonization. Capsular strains are antiphagocytic and virulent whereas non-capsulated mutant cells can provide good protection against subsequent challenge with virulent organisms. The capsule antigen (polysaccharide) divides the organisms into a number of serotypes.

The lipopolysaccharide (LPS) molecule of *A.pleuropneumoniae* is unique in exerting its typical effect on host cells. LPS as antigen is cross-reactive among several serotypes of *A.pleuropneumoniae*. Similar to the LPS from other gram-negative bacteria, it is a good mitogen, activate the alternative complement pathway and produce a positive Shwartzman reaction (Fenwick 1990). LPS causes marked inflammatory cell activation via activation of complement and induction of cytokines such as IL-1, IL-6 and tumor necrosis factor in alveolar macrophages. The haemorrhagic and necrotic lesions are due to the release of lytic enzymes and reactive oxygen radicals produced by the cytotoxin induced damaged macrophages and neutrophils. LPS is also an adhesive factor in capsule deficient strain (Belanger *etal.,* 1992). This structure binds to treacheal epithelium of hosts. The LPS antibody complexes damage blood vessel epithelium and result in vasculitis, thrombosis with odema, necrosis, infarction and haemorrhages. *A.pleuropneumoniae* is piliated and may be responsible for specific adhesion to alveolar epithelium and the cilia of terminal bronchioles. It is also responsible for biofilm formation.

Actinobacillus pleuropneumonia outer membrane protein (OMP) is also a virulence factor. OMP contain 3-5 major proteins and approximately 15 minor ones (Inzama 1991). It is also a protective factor. This structure binds porcine transferring-iron complexes (a source of iron needed for growth). This trait is associated with host species specificity of the organism. A periplasmic iron-binding protein, AfuA is involved in iron transport. This protein (TbpA and TbpB) is a 60 kDa transforrin binding protein. Immunization with OMP provides partial protection against *A.pleuropneumonia* infection. The bacteria receptors directly bind the host transferrin and aquire the iron. *A.pleuropneumoniae* expresses receptors for porcine haemoglobin and ferrichrome isolates.

A.pleuropneumoniae isolates produce 3 different cytotoxins, ApXIA, ApXIIA and ApXIIIA, of 105, 103 & 120 molecular weight, respectively. These belong to RTX family of toxins. ApXIA & ApXIIA are strongly cytotoxic whereas ApXIIA produces a weakly cytotoxic toxin. In addition, ApXIA and ApXIIIA toxins are strongly haemolytic. The toxins are heat labile, immunogenic and thought to be responsible for severe lesions. All serotypes except serotype 10 produce ApXIIA toxin whereas serotype 10 produce ApXIIA toxin whereas serotypes 1, 5, 9, 10 & 11 produce ApXIA and serotypes 2, 3, 4 & 8 produce ApXIIIA toxin (Macinnes and Smart, 1993). The toxins act by forming pores in the cell membrane. It is because of the presence of a domain in the amino terminal half comprising of 4 hydrophobic regions. At sublytic concentrations, the toxin has effect on oxidative metabolism of phagocytic cells alongwith other biological effects (Udez and Kadis 1992). The C-terminal portion of the ApXAII contains the cytolytic activity and is separate from haemolytic region. Lysis of host cells is essential for the bacterium to obtain nutrients through several mechanisms (Chiers *etal.,* 2010). In addition to persistence in lung lesions, colonization of the upper respiratory tract and the tonsils in particular may also be important for long term persistent asymptomatic infection.

The *A.pleuropneumoniae* cells also produce various cytotoxins: camp factor toxin (Devenish *et al.*, 1992) and a RTF (apx) toxin IV. Genes for all the RTF toxins have been characterized and expressed to produce vaccines using recombinant products (Shao *etal.*, 2010).

Biofilm formation is an important ability possessed by numerous bacterial pathogens including *A. pleuropneumoniae*. Biofilm formation is an important virulence trait of many bacterial pathogens. Biofilms are composed of bacterial cells embedded in an extracellular polysaccharide matrix. A major component of the Escherichia coli biofilm matrix is PGA, a linear polymer of N-acetyl-D-glucosamine residues in beta (1,6) linkage. PGA mediates intercellular adhesion and attachment of cells to abiotic surfaces. Kaplan *et al.* (2004) presented genetic and biochemical evidence that PGA is also a major matrix component of biofilms produced by the human periodontopathogen Actinobacillus actinomycetemcomitans and the porcine respiratory pathogen Actinobacillus pleuropneumoniae. The authors showed that PGA is a substrate for dispersin B, a biofilm-releasing glycosyl hydrolase produced by *A. actinomy-*cetemcomitans, and that an orthologous dispersin B enzyme is produced by A. pleuropneumoniae. Further , A. actinomycetemcomitans PGA cross-reacts with antiserum raised against polysaccharide intercellular adhesin, a staphylococcal biofilm matrix polysaccharide that is genetically and structurally related to PGA. These findings confirm that PGA functions as a biofilm matrix polysaccharide in phylogenetically diverse bacterial species and suggest that PGA may play a role in intercellular adhesion and cellular detachment and dispersal in A. actinomycetemcomitans and *A. pleuropneumoniae* biofilms.Most field isolates of the swine pathogen Actinobacillus pleuropneumoniae form tenacious biofilms on abiotic surfaces *in vitro*. Izano *et al.* (2007) purified matrix polysaccharides from biofilms produced by A. pleuropneumoniae field isolates IA1 and IA5 (serotypes 1 and 5, respectively), and determined their chemical structures by using NMR spectroscopy. Both strains produced matrix polysaccharides consisting of linear chains of N-acetyl-D-glucosamine (GlcNAc) residues in beta(1,6) linkage (poly-beta-1,6-GlcNAc or PGA). A small percentage of the GlcNAc residues in each polysaccharide were N-deacetylated. These structures were nearly identical to those of biofilm matrix polysaccharides produced by Escherichia coli, Staphylococcus aureus and Staphylococcus epidermidis. PCR analyses indicated that a gene encoding the PGA-specific glycoside transferase enzyme PgaC was present on the chromosome of 15 out of 15 A. pleuropneumoniae reference strains (serotypes 1-12) and 76 out of 77 A. pleuropneumoniae field isolates (serotypes 1, 5 and 7). A pgaC mutant of strain IA5 failed to form biofilms in vitro, as did wild-type strains IA1 and IA5 when grown in broth supplemented with the PGA-hydrolyzing enzyme dispersin B. Treatment of

IA5 biofilms with dispersin B rendered them more sensitive to killing by ampicillin. These findings suggest that PGA functions as a major biofilm adhesin in *A. pleuropneumoniae*. Biofilm formation may have relevance to the colonization and pathogenesis of *A. pleuropneumoniae* in pigs.

Two biofilm-producing mutants were identified from the transposon mutagenesis mutant pools of *A. pleuropneumoniae* strain 4074 of serovar 1 (a non-biofilm forming strain) (Dalai *et al.*, 2009). Inverse PCR and sequencing analysis revealed that the hns gene encoding the histone-like nucleoid structuring protein (H-NS) was inactivated by the mini-Tn10 transposon in both mutant strains. Further analysis revealed that the virulence was attenuated in the mutant strains when their haemolytic activity and 50% lethal doses in mice were compared with the parental strain. Real-time RT-PCR analysis suggested that the down-regulation of the exotoxin genes in the hns mutants may partly contribute to the virulence attenuation. These data indicate that H-NS plays important roles in regulating biofilm formation and virulence in *A. pleuropneumoniae*. It has been reported in the literature that only two of the reference strains of the swine pathogen Actinobacillus pleuropneumoniae, representing serotypes 5b and 11, were able to form biofilm *in vitro*. Labrie *et al.* (2010) compared biofilm formation by the serotype 1 reference strain S4074 of A. pleuropneumoniae grown in five different culture media. It was observed that strain S4074 of A. pleuropneumoniae is able to form biofilms after growth in one of the culture conditions tested brain heart infusion (BHI medium, supplier B). Confocal laser scanning microscopy using a fluorescent probe specific to the poly-N-acetylglucosamine (PGA) polysaccharide further confirmed biofilm formation. In accordance, biofilm formation was susceptible to dispersin B, a PGA hydrolase. Transcriptional profiles of A. pleuropneumoniae S4074 following growth in BHI-B, which allowed a robust biofilm formation, and in BHI-A, in which only a slight biofilm formation was observed, were compared. Genes such as tadC, tadD, genes with homology to autotransporter adhesins as well as genes pgaABC involved in PGA biosynthesis and genes involved in zinc transport were up-regulated after growth in BHI-B. Interestingly, biofilm formation was inhibited by zinc, which was found to be more present in BHI-A (no or slight biofilm) than in BHI-B. We also observed biofilm formation in reference strains representing serotypes 3, 4, 5a, 12 and 14 as well as in 20 of the 37 fresh field isolates tested. Our data indicate that *A. pleuropneumoniae* has the ability to form biofilms under appropriate growth conditions and transition from a biofilm-positive to a biofilm-negative phenotype was reversible. Grasteau *et al.* (2011) identified and characterized biofilm mutants of *A. pleuropneumoniae* serotype 1 strain S4074 created using a mini Tn-10 transposon. The transposon library was screened to identify mutants with a modified ability to form biofilms in polystyrene microtiter plates. A total of 1200 mutants were screened and the analysis identified 24 mutants that exhibited abnormal biofilm formation, at least 16 unique genes were identified. Most genes identified in the enhanced-biofilm mutants encoded proteins with unknown functions, whereas most genes identified in the biofilm-reduced mutants encoded proteins related to transport, protein synthesis and nucleic acid synthesis. Approximately 50% of genes, including hns, potD2, ptsI, tig and rpmF, identified in our screen have been previously associated with biofilm formation in *A. pleuropneumoniae* and other bacterial species, and thus validated the screening method. The rest of genes identified, such as APL_0049, APL_0637 and APL_1572, have not been previously associated with biofilm formation. Interestingly, gene APL_0049 was previously seen among the genes differentially expressed during a natural infection of pig lungs. Preliminary characterization of the mutants was also initiated by assessing their hydrophobicity, their biofilm matrix composition and their ability to adhere to a polystyrene surface or NPTr cells. Based on the preliminary characterization, some of the mutants identified appear to have deficiencies during the initial attachment or growth of the biofilm. In conclusion, transposon mutagenesis analysis allowed the identification of new genes associated with biofilm formation in *A. pleuropneumoniae*.

Diagnosis

The clinical material is subjected to bacteriological analysis using blood or serum enriched agar. Isolation of the organisms from the tonsils and upper respiratory tract of swine is useful for detection of carrier pigs and complements serological screening (Sidibe *etal.*, 1993). Most strains require the V factor (NAD) which can be provided by yeast extract or *Staphylococcus* streak. Strain requiring V factor grow only along with the *Staphylococcus* streak. Strains not requiring V factor are usually non-haemolytic and are not involved in the causation of the disease. Upon incubation for 2-3 days, 2 colony types are seen; a haemolytic round "waxy" type and a soft, glistening haemolytic variety. A positive CAMP reaction is seen with a â-toxin producing Staphylococcus strain. *A.pleuropneumoniae* strains possess V factor requirement and show CAMP positive reaction. Definitive identification is generally based on various biochemical characteristics. A rapid latex agglutination test has been developed for rapid identification of serotypes involved in the disease.

Serology involves complement fixation, 2-mercapto ethanol agglutination and enzyme linked immunosorbent assay to detect the infection in swine. These tests are serotype specific. Commercial ELISA tests are available for testing of animals (Costa *et al.*, 2010). Multiplex PCR assays were developed to identify Actinobacillus pleuropneumoniae serotypes 1, 2, and 8. Primers designed for the conserved capsular polysaccharide (CP) export region amplified a 489-bp DNA fragment from all serotypes. Primers specific to the CP biosynthesis regions of serotypes 1, 2, and 8 amplified fragments of 1.6 kb, 1.7 kb, and 970 bp from only their respective serotypes(Schuchert *et al*, 2004).

Multiplex PCR has been developed for parallel identification of *Actinobacillus pleuropneumoniae, Pasteurella multocida* and *Haemophilus* parasuis, important pathogens of swine, responsible for considerable economic losses in swine industry. Multiplex PCR and bacteriological cultivation was used to analyze lung samples from slaughterhouse pigs. From a total of 219 lung samples, 164 (74.9%) were positive for P. multocida, 45 (20.5%) for *A. pleuropneumoniae* and 4 (1.83%) for H. parasuis. Bacteriological examination revealed that 145 samples (66.2%) were positive for P. multocida, 31 (14.2 %) for *A. pleuropneumoniae* and 2 (0.91%) for H. parasuis (Hricinova *et al.*, 2010). Ito 2010) developed a cps-based multiplex PCR for typing of *Actinobacillus pleuropneumoniae* serotypes 1, 2 and 5. This method was considered to be specific and practical in Japan where more than 88% of isolates are serotypes 1, 2 or 5.

A DNA microarray composed of 18 DNA polymerase chain reaction amplicons printed on glass slides and arranged in 3 sub arrays was developed. The result showed that the micro array system proved to be a valuable tool for identifying and typing isolates of *A. pleuropneumoniae* (Xiao *et al.*, 2009).

Treatment and Control

Treatment is usually disappointing because of the severity of the acute disease. Many antimicrobial drugs including tetracycline, chloramphenicol, spectinomycin, erythromycin, ampicillin, gentamycin & penicillin G are effective which may be tried against the disease. Tiamulin in the drinking water for 5 days after an initial treatment of individual animals is recommended. The anti microbial sensitivities of isolates should be monitored. Plasmid mediated antimicrobial resistance has been found in the isolates of the organisms which are resistant to certain antimicrobials. Prolonged treatment of acute cases is required. Chronic cases are difficult to treat. Treated animals continue to harbour the organism and are source of infection.

For control of the infection, segregation and isolation of affected animals is required. Isolation and preventive treatment of newly introduced animals is essential. Recovered pigs carry the organism and become source of infection. The farmer should depopulate all the animals before newly purchased animals are brought to the farm. The all in/all out system of purchasing, feeding and marketing pigs in a finishing operation should be adopted. Quarantine of newly purchased animals is another method of eliminating cases of the *pleuropneumonia*. An approach to control the infection consists of identification of seroreactors and elimination. Following this mass medication is effective. The polyvalent bacterins with adjuvant only elicit serotype specific antibodies as against natural infection which provides cross-serotypes immunity. Use of subunit vaccines containing purified or partially purified antigen is protective. Capsular antigens, LPS, OMPs and soluble toxic factors, all have been tested in pigs but only capsular antigen is protective. Other confers partial protection. Live antigen vaccine and recombinant vaccines are available.

Cross-protection experiments were conducted to determine whether antigenic differences located within the lipopolysaccharides (LPS) of *Actinobacillus pleuropneumoniae* subtypes 1A and 1B were important with respect to the efficacy of whole cell, formalin-inactivated bacterins (Jolie *et al.* 1995). Based on clinical signs, lung lesions scores and mortality rates, pigs immunized with *A. pleuropneumoniae* subtype 1A were partially protected against severe challenge with both subtypes 1A and 1B. In contrast, 1B vaccinated pigs were not protected against severe challenge with subtype 1A but were partially protected against 1B challenge. Cross-reactive serum antibody levels were measured with an ELISA using outer membranes of subtype 1A or 1B as the coating antigen. Serum antibodies were detected against both subtypes within 2 weeks after the first immunization. Antibody levels increased with time and were generally higher against the homologous subtype coating antigen. We conclude that antigenic variation within a capsular serotype, due to antigenic variation within LPS, can result in the failure of whole cell bacterins to provide protection against challenge with the same capsular serotype. This lack of cross-protection within a capsular serotype provides partial explanation for vaccination failures observed under field conditions.

Pigs immunized with *Actinobacillus pleuropneumoniae* ghosts or a formalin-inactivated bacterin were found to be protected against clinical disease in both vaccination groups, whereas colonization of the lungs with *A. pleuropneumoniae* was only prevented in ghost-vaccinated pigs (Huter *et al*, 2000). Bacterial ghosts are empty cell envelopes created by the expression of a cloned bacteriophage lysis gene and, unlike formalin-inactivated bacteria, suffer no denaturing steps during their production. This quality may lead to a superior presentation of surface antigens to the immune system. Analysis by SDS-PAGE and immunoblotting of the two vaccine preparations revealed different contents of antigenic proteins. In order to better understand the immunogenic properties of *A. pleuropneumoniae* ghosts and formalin-inactivated bacteria, the authors compared the serum antibody response induced in both treatment groups. Immune sera were tested on whole cell antigen or purified virulence factors including outer membrane protein preparations (OMPs), outer membrane lipoprotein OmlA1, transferrin binding proteins (TfbA1, TfbA7 and TfbB) and Apx toxins (ApxI, II and III). SDS-PAGE and immunoblots revealed no specific antibody response against the single virulence factors tested in any vaccinated animal. The two vaccination groups showed different recognition patterns of whole cell antigen and OMP-enriched preparations. A 100 kDa protein was recognized significantly stronger by ghost-vaccinated pigs than convalescent pigs. This unique antibody population induced by ghosts could play a determining role in the prevention of lung colonization. The same 100 kDa antigen was recognized by ghost-sera in homologous as well as heterologous serotype *A. pleuropneumoniae* protein preparations. Indications for a crossprotective potential in the ghost vaccine were supported by studies on rabbit hyperimmune sera.

The role of antibodies to the outer membrane protein PalA of *Actinobacillus pleuropneumoniae* in protective immunity was studied in pigs vaccinated with purified PalA alone and PalA in combination with toxoids of the RTX toxins ApxI and ApxII using an established challenge model with the virulent serotype 1 of *A. pleuropneumoniae* (Van den Bosch and Frey, 2003). Pigs that developed antibody titers against PalA after immunization were more significantly affected by challenge with *A. pleuropneumoniae* serotype 1. Following challenge, pigs that were immunized with PalA showed more severe respiratory symptoms, had a higher mortality rate and died faster. They also displayed much more severe lung lesions after necropsy than animals not immunized with PalA. Pigs that were immunized with toxoids of the two cytotoxins ApxI and ApxII were protected against challenge with *A. pleuropneumoniae*. In contrast, the protective efficacy of the ApxI and ApxII vaccine was completely lost when it was supplemented with PalA. Hence, antibodies induced against the outer membrane protein PalA of *A. pleuropneumoniae* aggravated the consequences of infection and counteracted the protective effect of anti-ApxI and anti-ApxII antibodies.

Shao *et al.*, (2010) conducted studies in BALB mice on the efficacy of a multicomponent recombinant vaccine containing all the 3 toxins and OMP and concluded that effective protection can be conferred. A neutralizing epitope fragment of ApXIIa toxin from a Korean strain of the organism was expressed and immunolitized on *Saccharomyces cerevisae* for use as a vaccine in mice. Immunoassay revealed the presence of antibodies in the sera of mice which were antigen-specific. These mice were protected against challenge with *A.pleuropneumoniae* (Kim *et al.*, 2010). Studies on immunogenic proteins of *A.pleuropneumoniae* serotype 3 have revealed 30 immunogenic proteins of which 24 were novel immunogenic proteins which could be used to develop subunit vaccines (Liao *et al.*, 2009). Whole OMP confers protection in pigs when given alongwith all the 4 cytotoxins. In a vaccine containing all the cytotoxins, higher antibodies are detected against ApXIV but ApXIV vaccine alone does not protect pigs against the challenge infection (Wang *et al.*, 2009).

Protection of pigs by vaccination against *Actinobacillus pleuropneumoniae*, the causative agent of *porcine pleuropneumonia*, is hampered by the presence of 15 different serotypes. A DIVA subunit vaccine comprised of detergent-released proteins from *A. pleuropneumoniae* serotypes 1, 2 and 5 has been developed and shown to protect pigs from clinical symptoms upon homologous and heterologous challenge (Buettner *et al.*, 2011). This vaccine has not been characterized in-depth so far. Thus the authors performed i) mass spectrometry in order to identify the exact protein content of the vaccine and ii) cross-serotype 2-D immunoblotting in order to discover cross-reactive antigens. By these approaches it was expected to gain results enabling the authors to argue about the reasons for the efficacy of the analyzed vaccine. The authors identified 75 different proteins in the vaccine. Using the PSORTb algorithm these proteins were classified according to their cellular localization. Highly enriched proteins are outer membrane-associated lipoproteins like OmlA and TbpB, integral outer membrane proteins like FrpB, TbpA, OmpA1, OmpA2, HgbA and OmpP2, and secreted Apx toxins. The subunit vaccine also contained large amounts of the ApxIVA toxin so far thought to be expressed only during infection. Applying two-dimensional difference gel electrophoresis (2-D DIGE) we showed different isoforms and variations in expression levels of several proteins among the strains used for vaccine production. For detection of cross-reactive antigens we used detergent released proteins of serotype 7. Sera of pigs vaccinated with the detergent-released proteins of serotypes 1, 2, and 5 detected seven different proteins of serotype 7, and convalescent sera of pigs surviving experimental infection with serotype 7 reacted with 13 different proteins of the detergent-released proteins of *A. pleuropneumoniae* serotypes 1, 2, and 5. This detergent extraction-based subunit vaccine of *A. pleuropneumoniae* was characterized by mass spectrometry. It contained a large variety of immunogenic and virulence associated proteins, among them the ApxIVA toxin. The identification of differences in expression as well as isoform variation between the serotypes implied the importance of combining proteins of different serotypes for vaccine generation. This finding was supported by immunoblotting showing the induction of cross-reactive antibodies against several surface associated proteins in immunized animals.

DNA vaccines encoding ApXIA and ApXIIA have been successfully use in mice and opens up a new field for development of third generation vaccines against *A.pleuropneumoniae* infection in animal. The mortality rate is lower in vaccinated animals but they become carrier of the organism. Serotype 8 is closely related to serotype 3 and 6 and parenteral revaccination with serotype 8 provides immunity against serotype 3 and 6. Bacterins elicit local reactions resulting in abscesses and granulomas due to mineral oil adjuvants, however, high antibody titers are produced than vaccine containing aluminum hydroxide gel, which is less irritating. Immunity against swine pleuropneumonia is chiefly humoral. Material immunity protects neonates for 5-9 weeks.

Actinobacillus suis

Actinobacillus suis is prevalent in many parts of the world. Wilson and McOrist (2000) made first report of the isolation of Actinobacillus suis in association with significant disease among preweaned pigs in Australia. Sudden deaths occurred in preweaned piglets at one facility and enlarged joints, particularly the stifles and tarsi, occurred at another. Isolates with the biochemical phenotype and apx genotype profile of A suis were cultured from affected piglets. Both facilities were of high health status and one had undergone a recent depopulation, disinfection and sow repopulation process. Reviewing initial reports of A suis disease overseas, it is apparent that outbreaks occurred sporadically in various locations, with disease occurring among the herds involved for some months only, before development of immunity.The swine are highly susceptible to the infection particularly those having high health status (MacInnes and Desrosiers 1999). In such high-health-status herds, however, *A. suis* may be a considerable threat either when the organism is introduced or when high-health-status animals are mixed with conventionally reared swine. In very young pigs, *A. suis* infection is characterized by an acute septicemia with a high mortality rate. Cyanosis, respiratory distress, neurological disturbances, and arthritis can also be seen. The course of the disease in mature animals in conventional herds may be less severe and can include erysipelas-like lesions, abortion, metritis, and meningitis. In grow/finish and adult animals in high-health-status herds, however, *A. suis* can cause septicemia with lung lesions that superficially resemble *Actinobacillus pleuropneumoniae* pleuropneumonia. *Actinobacillus suis* has been isolated from the lungs of 9-month-old cat (Daignault *et al.*, 1999).

Actinobacillus pleuropneumoniae is a significant respiratory pathogen of swine causing a severe and often fatal fibrinous hemorrhagic bronchopneumonia with significant economic losses resulting from chronic as well as acute infections.It normally resides in the upper respiratory tract and tonsils and causes endogenous infection in animals of all ages. Using PCR-based signature-tagged transposon mutagenesis, 13 genes belonging to 9 different functional classes have been identified that were necessary for *A. suis* colonization of the upper respiratory tract of swine. Sheehan *et al.* (2003)

used signature-tagged mutagenesis (STM) to identify genes required for survival of the organism within the pig. A total of 2,064 signature-tagged Tn10 transposon mutants were assembled into pools of 48 each, and used to inoculate pigs by the endotracheal route. Out of 105 mutants that were consistently attenuated *in vivo*, only 11 mutants showed a >2-fold reduction in growth in vitro compared to the wild type, whereas 8 of 14 mutants tested showed significant levels of attenuation in pig as evidenced from competitive index experiments. Inverse PCR was used to generate DNA sequence of the chromosomal domains flanking each transposon insertion. Only one sibling pair of mutants was identified, but three apparent transposon insertion hot spots were found—an anticipated consequence of the use of a Tn10-based system. Transposon insertions were found within 55 different loci, and similarity (BLAST) searching identified possible analogues or homologues for all but four of these. Matches included proteins putatively involved in metabolism and transport of various nutrients or unknown substances, in stress responses, in gene regulation, and in the production of cell surface components. Ten of the sequences have homology with genes involved in lipopolysaccharide and capsule production. The results highlight the importance of genes involved in energy metabolism, nutrient uptake and stress responses for the survival of *A. pleuropneumoniae* in its natural host: the pig.

A.suis has been isolated from other animals also. Twenty-four *Actinobacillus suis* isolates obtained from several species of non-porcine mammals were compared to the representative porcine strains, ATCC 15557 (serotype O1) and H89-1173 (serotype O2), by O serotyping (Jeannotte *et al.* 2002), DNA fingerprinting, PCR amplification of apxICA, apxIICA and apxIIICA toxin genes and by rrs (16S rRNA) gene sequencing. Only two strains, both equine, reacted with O1 antiserum while two others, one canine and the other feline, reacted with O2 antiserum. One equine strain reacted weakly with both antisera. No amplification of apx genes was found with the non-porcine O1 or the "not O1/O2" strains but amplification of the apxICA and apxIICA genes was observed with the two O2 strains. In addition, these two O2 strains had both BamHI and BglII fingerprints that were very similar to the porcine O2 reference strain, H89-1173 and rrs gene sequences that were identical to the *A. suis* reference strain ATCC 15557. Taken together, these data suggest that although many non-porcine *A. suis* isolates are not *A. suis* (sensu stricto), some isolates are genotypically as well as phenotypically similar to *A. suis*.

Polymerase chain reaction has been tested to detects ApXII gene for *A.suis* (MacInnes *et al.*, 2008). It is also present on mucous membrane of genital tract of pigs. A serious disease is produced in young animals. In neonatal pigs, it can cause a rapidly fatal septicaemia. The organism has also been implicated in arthritis, pneumonia, pericarditis, nephritis, meningitis and metritis in older pigs. Other lesions include various types of pneumonia, mastitis, fluid in body cavities and whitish foci of hepatic necrosis and lymphadenopathy (Sanford *et al.*, 1990). Affected animals may show signs of cyanosis, petechial haemorrhages, fever, respiratory distress, abortion, neurological disturbances and arthritis. Mortality is generally very low.

Pathogenesis

The pathogenicity of the *A. suis* disease is not well understood, although it is likely that two RTX toxins ($ApxI_{var.\ suis}$ and $ApxII_{var.\ suis}$, urease, capsular polysaccharide (CPS), and lipopolysaccharide (LPS) contribute to virulence. Although early studies suggested that *A. suis* isolates from Canada were homogeneous, the present work has shown that there are at least two serologically distinct groups. Consistent with this finding, chemical characterization of the major surface polysaccharides of selected *A. suis* strains revealed two different lipopolysaccharide O-antigen types; the O1 antigen, which is a homopolymer with the structure >6)-β-D-Glc-(1>6)-β-D-Glc-(1γ, and the O2 antigen, which contains a [Glc, Gal_2, GlcNAc] branched tetrasaccharide

Following entry of organisms in the host, it enters the blood stream and lodge in different organs. Microcolonies are formed on vessel walls leading to regions of haemorrhages and necrosis. Capsule and LPS may play a role in pathogenesis similar to *A.pleuropneumoniae*. The chemical nature of both LPS and capsule is 1-6 β- D glucan. Additionally, capsule contains sialic acid. *A.suis* produce enterobacterial common antigen similar to *Salmonella* but its role in virulence is not known (Bottger *et al.*, 1987). The chemical and antigenic properties of the cell-surface lipopolysaccharides (LPSs) and capsular polysaccharides (CPSs) of seven representative strains of Actinobacillus suis from healthy and diseased pigs were investigated (Monteiro *et al.*, 2000). Four strains produced a linear (1 → 6)-β-D-glucan homopolymer, β-D-Glcp-(1-[→ 6)-β-D-Glcp-(1-]n →, as a LPS-O-chain (O1) and as a CPS (K1). Polyclonal antisera prepared against a (1 → 6)-β-D-glucan-containing strain showed a positive reaction against both LPSs and CPSs derived from the above strains (designated serotype O1/K1). One strain carried the (1 → 6)-β-D-glucan solely as a LPS-O-chain (serotype O1) and two strains did not express the (1 → 6)-β-D-glucan, but, instead, produced a different O-chain (designated serotype 02); these three strains expressed their own characteristic CPSs. (1 → 6)-β-D-Glucan structures are common cell wall components of yeast, fungi and lichens. Conformational and nuclear magnetic resonance analyses showed that the beta-D-Glcp-(1 → 6)-β-D-Glcp linkage was flexible and two distinct glycosidic conformers are described. Cross-reactive antibodies to the A. suis (1 → 6)-β-D-glucan could be detected in sera from a variety of species and in sera from specific pathogen free pigs. This cross-reactivity may arise from immunostimulation of organisms present in the surrounding environment that contain (1 → 6)-β-D-glucan, which may also explain the high incidence of false positive results in previous serological tests for A. suis. In addition, these (1 → 6)-β-D-glucan background antibodies may be protective against A. suis infection. The characterization herein of (1 → 6)-β-D-glucan is the foundation for the development of a serotyping system for A. suis. A cell surface antigen-typing system was devised for the swine pathogen Actinobacillus suis and used to examine the prevalence of different lipopolysaccharide (O) types in healthy and diseased pigs (slavic *et al.*, 2000). The strains examined in this study were isolated from a variety of locations in Canada and from Kansas. Lipopolysaccharide preparations of 151 isolates of *A. suis* were characterized by immunoblotting using polyclonal antisera generated to strains SO4 (O1/K1), H89-1173 (O2/K3), and VSB 3714, a rough strain. Approximately 54% (62 of 114) of *A. suis* isolates from diseased pigs, all (11 of 11) isolates from healthy pigs, and all (4 of 4) reference strains reacted with O1/K1 antiserum. More than 80% (18 of 22) of A. suis strains used for bacterin production and approximately 41% (47 of 114) of isolates from diseased pigs bound O2/K3 antiserum. One isolate appeared to be rough, and five were untypeable. O1/K1- and O2/K3-reactive strains were equally prevalent in Kansas, whereas O2/K3-reactive strains were more common in Québec and western Canada and O1/K1 strains were most common in Ontario. The fact that virtually all of the strains submitted for bacterin production were O2/K3-reactive strains is consistent with the notion that these strains may be more virulent than O1/K1 strains; alternatively, this may reflect geographic or other biases. Slavic *et al* (2000a) evaluated the pathogenicity of Actinobacillus suis serotypes O1/K1 (strain SO4), O1/K2 (strain C84), and O2/K2 (strain H91-0380) in specific-pathogen-free (SPF) piglets challenged by intraperitoneal inoculation with approximately 1 x 10(7) colony-forming units per mL. All 3 strains produced peritonitis, but differences were observed in the composite histopathologic scores ($P = 0.001$) and in their ability to spread ($P = 0.008$) at 7 h post challenge. The O2/K2 strain caused the most severe peritonitis and disseminated most widely to other tissues. Moderate lesions were seen with the O1/K2 strain while the O1/K1 strain caused mild lesions and remained largely localized to the peritoneum. In an attempt to explain the basis of observed differences, the serum sensitivity of 9 *A. suis* strains with different O and K types was assessed. Regardless of the O/K type, all of the isolates tested were serum resistant. Moreover, most *A. suis* isolates grew as well or better in complement-replete sera as they did in complement-depleted sera. These observations indicate that although 02 and K2 strains had a greater propensity to cause a disseminating septic inflammatory response in pigs, they were no more resistant to complement-mediated killing than O1 strains.

A cytotoxin in the RTX family, similar to the cycotoxin or haemolysin of *A.pleuropneumoniae* has been described but its role in pathogenesis is not clear. ApXIV toxins is not present. Genes responsible for encoding toxins have been characterized. Although *A. suis* is less pathogenic, it has a better capability to invade and persist in the blood stream than *A.pleuropneumoniae. A.suis* is able to resist bile and serum suggesting that it has additional virulence factors. A published report mentioning the binding of porcine transferrin (Tf) by at least one strain of *A. suis* suggested that *A. suis,* like other members of the Pasteurellaceae, can acquire Tf-bound iron by means of a siderophore-independent, receptor-mediated mechanism. The objective of the present study was to characterize the components involved in this process, if present. Growth assays, with seven strains, confirmed that *A. suis* can use porcine (but not human or bovine) Tf as an iron source for growth. In solid phase binding assays, total membranes derived from all strains exhibited strong binding of porcine Tf, but only if the membranes were from organisms grown under iron-restricted conditions. An affinity-isolation procedure allowed the isolation of putative Tf-binding polypeptides (approximately 100 and approximately 63 kDa) from comparable membranes from all strains. PCR approaches allowed the amplification, cloning and sequencing of A. suis tonB, exbB, exbD, tbpB and tbpA homologues. Reverse transcription (RT)-PCR, using RNA from organisms grown under iron-replete and iron-restricted conditions, revealed that tonB, exbB, exbD, tbpB and tbpA are transcribed as a single unit with expression being up-regulated in response to iron restriction. The calculated molecular masses of the predicted, mature TbpA (104.3 kDa) and TbpB (63.4 kDa) proteins suggest strongly that the affinity-isolated, approximately 100 and approximately 63 kDa Tf-binding polypeptides represent TbpA and TbpB, respectively. It is concluded that the acquisition of Tf-bound iron by *A. suis* involves mechanisms analogous to those found in other members of the Pasteurellaceae (Bahrami *et al.*, 2003).

As with other pathogens, the ability of *A. suis* to acquire iron within the host is crucial for virulence. Bahrami and Niven 2005) investigated the ability of seven strains of *A. suis* to acquire iron from haemoglobins. In growth assays, all strains could use porcine, bovine and human haemoglobins as iron sources for growth. Using solid phase binding assays, membranes derived from all strains, grown under iron-restricted conditions, were shown to bind all three haemoglobins. Competition binding assays indicated that these haemoglobins were bound by the same receptor and an affinity procedure allowed the isolation and identification of an iron-repressible, haemoglobin-binding polypeptide (approximately 105 kDa) from all strains. Nucleotide sequence analyses revealed that *A. suis* possesses a gene (hgbA) that encodes a homologue of the Actinobacillus pleuropneumoniae haemoglobin-binding protein, HgbA. hgbA, encoding a mature protein of 105 kDa, was shown to be preceded by a hugZ homologue; putative promoter sequences and a putative Fur box were located upstream of hugZ and RT-PCR revealed that hugZ and hgbA are co-transcribed and iron-repressible. It is concluded that the acquisition of haemoglobin-bound iron by *A. suis* involves a single-component receptor that is up-regulated in response to iron restriction (Bahrami and Niven 2005).

A study describes the application of a signature-tagged mutagenesis (STM) system to identify in vivo critical genes of *A. pleuropneumoniae* Fuller *et al.* 2000). Twenty pools representing over 800 *A. pleuropneumoniae* mutants were screened in a natural-host porcine infection model and presumptive attenuated mutants were selected. The identity of the disrupted gene in each mutant was determined using an inverse PCR approach to amplify DNA sequences adjacent to the transposon insertion, followed by sequencing of the PCR product and comparison to bacterial databases. *In vitro* and *in vivo* competitive indices were determined for each unique mutant, and a total of 20 unique, attenuating gene disruptions were identified including insertions into homologues of genes involved in biosynthesis, virulence determinants, regulation, translation and unknown functions. Three of the genes required for virulence of *A. pleuropneumoniae* in this study were also identified Seven of the STM-derived mutants were also evaluated for their potential as live vaccine strains and provided good protection against homologous challenge.

Diagnosis

The diagnostic protocols followed are similar to that of *A.pleuropneumoniae*. An ELISA kit is available in many western countries for diagnosis. Ojha *et al.* (2007) hypothesized that a mouse model of *A. suis* infection might be possible. To test this idea, the authors challenged CD1 mice with 3 strains of *A. suis* (2 porcine [SO4 and H91-0380] and 1 feline [96-2247]) by intranasal and intraperitoneal routes. They also evaluated the effects of coadministration of hemoglobin and immunosuppression by dexamethasone on the susceptibility of mice to *A. suis* infection. The feline and H91-0380 porcine strains induced clinical signs of acute disease and necrotizing pneumonia in mice similar to those seen in pigs. Although few bacteria were recovered, dissemination of A. suis was widespread. Generally, mice infected with the feline *A. suis* isolate had more severe clinical signs and higher bacterial titers than did mice infected with either of the porcine strains. Pretreatment of the mice with dexamethasone or addition of 2% porcine hemoglobin to the challenge inoculum appeared to hasten the onset of clinical signs by the porcine strains but had no significant effect on moribundity. These experiments demonstrate that mice can be infected with *A. suis* and subsequently develop pneumonia and bacteremia comparable to that seen in pigs, suggesting that mice may be used as a model for studying infection in swine. In swine gross lesions are visible in most of the internal organs. The necropsy findings are similar to *A.pleuropneumoniae* infection.

Treatment and Control

A.suis isolates are susceptible to most of the antibiotics. Penicillin is very effective. Use of oxytetracycline and streptomycin in feed is useful to limit the infection. Prompt treatment regime is required. The choice of antimicrobials is difficult because animal carry many strains at a given time. Most of the organisms are sensitive to Gentamicin and Ceftiofur. Autogenous bacterins are considered to be useful in controlling the infection.

Vaccines have been tested for control of the disease. Lapointe *et al.*((2001) assessed the kinetics of antibodies to *A. suis* in pigs from a herd showing clinical signs of *A. suis* infection and, evaluated the antibody response in gilts following vaccination with an autogenous vaccine. An enzyme-linked immunosorbent assay (ELISA) using a saline extract of boiled-formalinized whole cells of a field strain as the coating antigen was standardized. This ELISA was used as a tool for monitoring, in a comparative way, the variations in *A. suis* antibody levels. The herd selected for the serologic profile was negative for Actinobacillus pleuropneumoniae infection and showed clinical signs of *A. suis* infection in 16 to 19-week-old pigs. A cohort of 20 pigs was blood sampled at 5, 8, 12, and 16 weeks of age. The lowest level of serum antibodies was observed between weeks 8 and 12, this probably corresponding to a decrease in maternal immunity. A marked increase in the antibody response was seen at 16-week of age, at the approximate time of onset of *A. suis* clinical signs in the herd. The evaluation of serum antibody responses to an autogenous vaccine revealed that the humoral immunity of gilts further increased following vaccination although the level of antibodies was already high prior to vaccination. The magnitude of the response to vaccination was higher when the level of antibodies was low prior to the first injection. The ELISA test seems to detect antibodies against the O-chain LPS.

References

Aalbaek B., Ostergaard S., Buhl R., Jensen H.E., Christensen H. and Bisgaard M.2007. *Actinobacillus equuli* subsp. *equuli* associated with equine valvular endocarditis. APMIS. **115:** 1437-1442.

Ashhurst - Smith, C., Norton, R., Throrean, W. and Peel, M.M. 1998. *Actinobacillus equuli* septicaemia: an unusual zoonotic infection. J. Clin. Microbiol. **36:** 2789-2790.

Bahrami F., Ekins A. and Niven D.F.2003.Iron acquisition by *Actinobacillus suis*: identification and characterization of transferrin receptor proteins and encoding genes. Vet Microbiol. **94:** 79-92.

Bahrami, F., and Niven, D.F. 2005. Iron acquisition by *Actinobacillus suis*: Identification and characterization of a single - component haemoglobin receptor and encoding gene. Microb. Pathog. **39:** 45-51.

Belanger, M., Roiux, S., Foiry, B. and Jacques, M. 1992. Affinity for porcine respiratory tract mucus is found in some isolates of *Actinobacillus pleuropneumoniae*. Fed. Eur. Microbiol. Soc. Microbiol. Lett. **97:** 119-126.

Benaoudia F., Escande F. and Simonet M.1994.Infection due to *Actinobacillus lignieresii* after a horse bite. Eur. J. Clin. Microbiol. Infect. Dis. **13:** 439-440.

Berthoud H., Frey J., Sternberg S., Straub R. and Kuhnert P.2004.Antibodies to Aqx toxin of *Actinobacillus equuli* in horses and foals. Vet. Rec. **155:** 231-253.

Berthoud H., Frey J. and Kuhnert P.2002.Characterization of Aqx and its operon: the hemolytic RTX determinant of *Actinobacillus equuli*. Vet. Microbiol. **87:** 159-174.

Boltger, E.C., Jurs, A., Barrett, T., Washmuth, K., Metzger, S. And Bitter-Suermann, D. 1987. Qualitative and quantitative determination of enterobacterial common antigen (ECA) with monoclonal antibodies: Expression of ECA by 2 *Actinobacillus* species. J. Clin. Microbiol. **25:** 377-382.

Buettner F.F., Konze S.A., Maas A. and Gerlach G.F.2011Proteomic and immunoproteomic characterization of a DIVA subunit vaccine against *Actinobacillus pleuropneumoniae*. Proteome. Sci. **9**(1):23.

Carmalt J.L., Baptiste K.E. and Chirino-Trejo J.M. 1999. *Actinobacillus lignieresii* infection in two horses. J. Am. Vet. Med. Assoc. **215:** 826-828, 796.

Castagnetti, C., Rossi, M., Parmeggiani; F., Zanoni, R.G., Pirrone, A. and Marriella, J. 2008. Facial cellutitis due to *Actinobacillus equii* infection in a neonatal foal. Vet. Rec. **162:** 347-349.

Chiers, K., De Waele, T., Pasmans, F., Ducatelle, R. and Haesebrouck, F. 2010. Virulence factors of *Actinobacillus pleuropneumoniae* involved in colonization, persistence and induction of lesions in the porcine host. Vet. Res. **41:** 65-66.

Christensen, H. and Bisgaard, M. 2004. Revised detection of *Actinobacillus sensustricto* isolated from animals: A review with special emphasis on diagnosis. Vet. Microbiol. **99:** 13-30.

Christensen H., Bisgaard M., Angen O. and Olsen J.E.2002.Final classification of Bisgaard taxon 9 as Actinobacillus arthritidis sp. nov. and recognition of a novel genomospecies for equine strains of *Actinobacillus lignieresii*. Int. J. Syst. Evol. Microbiol. **52:** 1239-1246.

Costa, G., Oliveira, S., Torrison, J. & Dee, S. 2010. Evaluation of *Actinobacillus pleuropneumoniae* diagnostic tests using samples derived from experimentally infected pigs. Vet. Microbiol. 27. [http://www.ncbinlm.nih.gov/pubmed/20884132.]

Daignault D., Chouinard L., Møller K., Ahrens P., Messier S. and Higgins R.1999.Isolation of Actinobacillus suis from a cat's lung. Can. Vet. J. **40:** 52-53.

Dalai B., Zhou R., Wan Y., Kang M., Li L., Li T., Zhang S. and Chen H.2009.Histone-like protein H-NS regulates biofilm formation and virulence of Actinobacillus pleuropneumoniae. Microb Pathog. **46:** 128-134. Epub 2008 Dec 6.

Devenish, J., Brown, J.E. and Rosendal, S. 1992. Association of the RTX protein of *Actinobacillus pleuropneumoniae* with haemolytic, CAMP and neutrophil cytotoxic activities. Infect. Immun. **60:** 2139-2142.

Fenwick, B.W. 1990. Virulence attributes of the lipopolysacchanides of the HAP group organisms. Can. J. Vet. Res. **54:** 528-532.

Fuller T.E., Martin S., Teel J.F., Alaniz G.R., Kennedy M.J. and Lowery D.E. 2000. Identification of *Actinobacillus pleuropneumoniae* virulence genes using signature-tagged mutagenesis in a swine infection model. Microb. Pathog. **29:** 39-51.

Grasteau A., Tremblay Y.D., Labrie J., Jacques M.. 2011.Novel genes associated with biofilm formation of *Actinobacillus pleuropneumoniae*. Vet. Microbiol. 2011 Mar 30. [http://www.ncbi.nlm.nih.gov/pubmed/21530112].

Grondahl, G., Stemberg, S., Jensen-Waem, M. and Johannison, A. 2001. Opsonic capacity of foal serum for the two neonatal pathogens *Escherichia coli* and *Actinobacillus equuli*. Equine Vet. J. **33:** 670-675.

Holyoak, G.R., Smith, C.M., Boyette, R., Montelongo, M., Wray, J.H., Ayalew, S., Duggan, V.E. and Confer, A.W. 2007. Serum antibodies in mare and foals to *Actinobacillus equuli* whole cells, outer membrane proteins and AqX toxin. Vet. Immunol. Immunopathol. **118:** 310-316.

Hrièínová M., Holoda E., Mudroòová D. and Ondrašovièová S.2010.Multiplex PCR assay for detection of *Actinobacillus pleuropneumoniae*, Pasteurella multocida and *Haemophilus parasuis* in lungs of pigs from a slaughterhouse. Folia Microbiol. (Praha). **55:** 635-640. Epub 2011 Jan 21.

Huter V., Hensel A., Brand E. and Lubitz W.2000.Improved protection against lung colonization by *Actinobacillus pleuropneumoniae* ghosts: characterization of a genetically inactivated vaccine. J. Biotechnol. **83:** 161-172.

Inzana, T.J. 1991. Virulence properties of *Actinobacillus pleuropneumoniae*. Microbiol. Pathol. **11:** 305-316.

Ito H.2010.Development of a cps-based multiplex PCR for typing of *Actinobacillus pleuropneumoniae* serotypes 1, 2 and 5. J. Vet. Med. Sci. **72:** 653-655. Epub 2010 Jan 13.

Izano E.A., Sadovskaya I., Vinogradov E., Mulks M.H., Velliyagounder K., Ragunath C., Kher W.B., Ramasubbu N., Jabbouri S. and Perry M.B.2007.Poly-N-acetylglucosamine mediates biofilm formation and antibiotic resistance in *Actinobacillus pleuropneumoniae*. Microb Pathog. **43:** 1-9. Epub 2007 Mar 4.

Jeannotte M.E., Slaviæ D., Frey J., Kuhnert P. and MacInnes J.I.2000.Analysis of non-porcine isolates of *Actinobacillus suis*. Vet Microbiol. **85:** 83-93.

Jolie R.A., Mulks M.H. and Thacker B.J. 1994.Antigenic differences within *Actinobacillus pleuropneumoniae* serotype 1. Vet. Microbiol. **38:** 329-349.

Jolie R.A., Mulks M.H. and Thacker B.J.1995. Cross-protection experiments in pigs vaccinated with *Actinobacillus pleuropneumoniae* subtypes 1A and 1B. Ve.t Microbiol. **45:** 383-391.

Kaplan J.B., Velliyagounder K., Ragunath C., Rohde H., Mack D., Knobloch J.K. and Ramasubbu N.2004.Genes involved in the synthesis and degradation of matrix polysaccharide in Actinobacillus actinomycetemcomitans and *Actinobacillus pleuropneumoniae* biofilms. J. Bacteriol. **186:** 8213-8220.

Kim, J.M., Jung, D.I., Eom, Y.J., Park, S.M., Yoo, H.S., Jang, H.S., Jang, Y.S., Yang, M.S. and Kim, D.H. 2010. Surface displayed expression of a neutralizing epitope of ApxIIA exotoxin in Saccharomyces cerevisiae and oral administration of it for protective immune responses against challenge by *A.pleuropneumoniae*. Biosci. Biotechnol. Biochem. **74:** 1362-1367.

Kokotovic B., Angen Ø. And Bisgaard M.2011.Genetic diversity of *Actinobacillus lignieresii* isolates from different hosts. Acta. Vet. Scand. **53:** 6.

Kuhnert P., Berthoud H., Straub R. and Frey J. 2003a.Host cell specific activity of RTX toxins from haemolytic *Actinobacillus equuli* and *Actinobacillus suis*. Vet. Microbiol. **92:** 161-167.

Kuhnert, P., Berthound, H., Christensen, H., Bisgaard, M. and Frey, J. 2003. Phylogenetic relationship of equine *Actinobacillus* species and distribution of RTX toxin gene clusters. Vet. Res. **34:** 353-359.

Labrie J., Pelletier-Jacques G., Deslandes V., Ramjeet M., Auger E., Nash J.H. and Jacques M.2010.Effects of growth conditions on biofilm formation by *Actinobacillus pleuropneumoniae*. Vet. Res. **41:** 3. Epub 2009 Sep 10.

Lapointe L., D'Allaire S., . and Gottschalk M.2001.Serologic profile of a cohort of pigs and antibody response to an autogenous vaccine for *Actinobacillus suis*. Vet Res. **32:** 175-183.

Liao, Y., Deng, J., Zhang, A., Zhou, M., Hu, Y., Chen, H. and Jin, M. 2009. Immunoproteomic analysis of outer membrane proteins and extracellular proteins of *Actinobacillus pleuropneumoniae* JL 03 serotype 3. BMC Microbiol. **20:** 172-175.

Macinnes, J.I. and Smart, N.L. 1993. *Actinobacillus* and *Haemophilus*. In pathogenesis of Bacterial Infections in Animals. Ed. C.L. Gyles and C.O. Thoen pp. 188-200. Ames: Iowa State University Press.

MacInnes, J.L. and Desrosiers, R. 1999. Agents of the "Suis-ide diseases" of swine: *Actinobacillus suis, haemophilus parasuis* and *Streptococcus suis*. Can. J. Vet. Res. **63:** 83-89.

MacInnes, J.L., Gottaschalk, M., Lone, A.G., Metcalf, D.S., Ojha, S., Rosendal, T. Watson, S.B. and Friendship, R.M. 2008. Prevalence of *Actinobacillus pleuropneumoniae, Actinobacillus suis, Haemophilus parasuis, Pasteurella multocida* and *Streptococcus suis* in representative Ontario Swine herd. Can. J. Vet. Res. **72:** 242-248.

Matthews S., Dart A.J., Dowling B.A., Hodgson J.L. and Hodgson D.R.2001.Peritonitis associated with *Actinobacillus equuli* in horses: 51 cases. Aust. Vet. J. **79:** 536-539.

Moller, K., Nielsen, R., Andersen, L.V. and Kilian, M. 1992. Clonal analysis of the *Actinobacillus pleuropneumoniae* population in a geographically restricted area by multilocus enzyme delectroresis. J. Clin. Microbiol. **30:** 623-627.

Monteiro M.A, Slavic D., St Michael F., Brisson J.R., MacInnes J.I. and Perry M.B.2000.The .first description of a (1 – > 6)-beta-D-glucan in prokaryotes: (1 – > 6)-beta-D-glucan is a common component of actinobacillus suis and is the basis for a serotyping system. Carbohydr. Res. **329:** 121-130.

Nielsen, R. 1990. New diagnostic techniques: A review of the HAP group of bacteria. Can. J. Vet. Res. **54:** 568-572.

Ojha S., Hayes M.A., Turner P.V. and MacInnes J.I.2007.An experimental model of *Actinobacillus suis* infection in mice. Comp Med. **57:** 340-348.

Pusterla, N., Jones, M.E., Mohr, F.C., Higgins, J.F., Mapes, S., Jang, S.S., Samitz, E.M. and Byrne, B.A. 2008. Fatal pulmonary haemorrhages associated with RTX toxin producing *Actinobacillus equuli* subsp. *haemolyticus* infection in an adult horse. J. Vet. Diagn. Invest **20:** 118-121.

Ramos-Vara, J.A., Wu, C.C., Mitsui, I., Lin, T.L. and Miller, M.A. 2008. Metritis, valvular endocarditis and septicaemia by *Actinobacillus equuli* in a gilt in the United States. Vet. Pathol. **45:** 495-499.

Sanford, S.E., Josephson, K.A., Rehmtullah, A.J. and Tilker, A.M.E. 1990. *Actinobacillus suis* septicaemia in mature swine: Two outbreaks resembling erysipelas. Can. Vet. J. **31:** 443-447.

Schuchert J.A., Inzana T.J., Angen Ø. And Jessing S.*2004*. Detection and identification of *Actinobacillus pleuropneumoniae* serotypes 1, 2, and 8 by multiplex PCR. J Clin Microbiol. **42:** 4344-4348.

Shao, M., Wang, Y. Wang, C., Guo, Y., Peng, Y., Liu, J., Li, G., Liu, H. and Liu, S. 2010. Evaluation of multicomponent recombinant vaccines against *Actinobacillus pneumoniae* in mice. Acta Vet. Scand. **11:** 52-55.

Sheehan B.J., Bossé J.T., Beddek A.J., Rycroft A.N., Kroll J.S. and Langford P.R.2003.Identification of *Actinobacillus pleuropneumoniae* genes important for survival during infection in its natural host. Infect. Immun. **71:** 3960-3970.

Sidibe, M., Messier, S., Lariviere, S., Gottschalk, M. and Mittal, K.R. 1993. Detection of *Actinobacillus pleuropneuminae* in the porcine upper respiratory tract as a complement to serological tests. Can. J. Vet. Res. **57:** 204-208.

Slaviæ D., DeLay J., Hayes M.A. and MacInnes J.I. 2000a.Comparative pathogenicity of different *Actinobacillus suis* O/K serotypes. Can. J. Vet. Res. **64:** 81-87.

Slavic D., Toffner T.L., Monteiro M.A., Perry M.B. and MacInnes J.I.2000.Prevalence of O1/K1- and O2/K3-reactive *Actinobacillus suis* in healthy and diseased swine. J. Clin. Microbiol. **38:** 3759-3762.

Stemberg, S., 1998. Isolation of *Actinobacillus equuli* from the oral cavity of healthy horses and comparison of isolates by restriction enzyme digestion & pulse field gel electrophoresis. Vet. Microbiol. **59:** 147-156.

Tageldin M.H., el Sanousi S.M., Suliman T.A. and Fawi M.T.1988.Concurrent infection with Mycobacterium farcinogenes and *Actinobacillus lignièresi* in slaughtered cattle. J. Comp. Pathol. **99:** 431-437.

Thomas, E., Thomas, V. and Wilhelm, C. 2006. Antibacterial activity of Cefquinome against equine bacterial pathogens. Vet. Microbiol. **115:** 140-147.

Thompson A.B., Postey R.C., Snider T. and Pasma T.2010. *Actinobacillus equuli* as a primary pathogen in breeding sows and piglets. Can. Vet. J. **51:** 1223-1225.

Udez, F.A. and Kadis, S. 1992. Effect of *Actinobacillus pleuropneumonia* haemolysin on porcine neutrophil function. Infect. Immun. **60:** 1558-1567.

van den Bosch H. and Frey J.2003.Interference of outer membrane protein PalA with protective immunity against *Actinobacillus pleuropneumoniae* infections in vaccinated pigs. Vaccine. **21:** 3601-3607.

Varshney, J.P. and Uppal, P.K. 1993. Foal mortality in Thoroughbreds at an organized stud farm. Indian J. Vet. Med. **13:** 88.

Wang, C., Wang, Y., Shao, M., Si, W., Liu, H., Chang, Y., Peng, W., Kong, X. And Liu, S. 2009. Positive role for rApXIV VN in the immune protection of pigs against infection by *Actinobacillus pleuropneumoniae*. Vaccine **27:** 5816-5821.

Wilson R.J and McOrist S.2000.*Actinobacillus suis* infection in pigs in Australia. Aust Vet J. **78**(5): 317-319.

Xiao, G., Cao, S., Huang, X. and Wane, X. 2009. DNA microarray based identification and typing of *Actinobacillus pleuropneumoniae*. Can. J. Vet. Res. **73:** 1.

□□□

Chapter 11

Pseudomonas Infections

Dr. S.K. SRIVASTAVA
Former, Division of Bacteriology & Mycology
Indian Veterinary Research Institute, Izatnagar-243122
Bareilly (U.P.)

Pseudomonas infections

Pseudomonas is a gram-negative, aerobic or facultatively anaerobic short to medium sized rods. The organisms are free living, widely distributed in water and soil. The organisms are motile by means of polar flagella. Of many recognized species of *Pseudomonas*, only *P.aeruginosa* is of considerable veterinary importance. Its natural habitat is water, soil and decaying vegetation and it causes a wide variety of infections. *P.aeruginosa* also may be found on the skin and mucous membranes and in feces. The *Pseudomonas* species *Pseudomonas* stutzeri, *Pseudomonas fluorescens, Pseudomonas maltophilia* and *Pseudomonas* putida and other *Pseudomonas* are occasionally recovered from clinical specimens but they are rarely pathogenic in animals. The organism is aerobic but can grow anaerobically if nitrates and arginine is provided in the medium (Vasil 1986).

P. aeruginosa

Pseudomonas aeruginosa is member of the Gamma Proteobacteria class of Bacteria. It is a Gram-negative, aerobic rod belonging to the bacterial family Pseudomonadaceae. Since the revisionist taxonomy based on conserved macromolecules (e.g. 16S ribosomal RNA) the family includes only members of the genus *Pseudomonas* which are cleaved into eight groups. Pseudomonas aeruginosa is the type species of its group. which contain 12 other members. Much of our knowledge on pathogenic properties of this organism is drawn from studies of the human disease. The organism is ubiquitous in nature, found on skin and mucous membrane of healthy animals. It is physiologically a versatile organism and resists action of several antibacterial agents, hence, they are difficult to eliminate from the diseased host. Serotyping of organisms is based on recognition of the antigens exposed on the surface following one of the schemes available. Pyocin, a blue-green pigment produced by *P.aeruginosa,* typing is based on the sensitivity of the isolates to pyocins produced by a standard set of strains or by the activity of pyocin produced by the isolate against a set of indicator strains. Phage typing is based on the basis of the sensitivity of the isolate to a standard set of bacteriophages.

Pseudomonas aeruginosa is a common bacterium that can cause disease in animals, including humans. It is found in soil, water, skin flora, and most man-made environments throughout the world. It thrives not only in normal atmospheres but also in hypoxic atmospheres, and has, thus, colonized many natural and artificial environments. It uses a wide range of organic material for food; in animals, the versatility enables the organism to infect damaged tissues or people with reduced immunity. The symptoms of such infections are generalized inflammation and sepsis. If such colonization occur in critical body organs, such as the lungs, the urinary tract, and kidneys, the results can be fatal Because it thrives on most surfaces, this bacterium is also found on and in medical equipment, including catheters, causing cross-infections in hospitals and clinics. It is implicated in hot-tub rash. It is also able to decompose hydrocarbons and has been used to break down tar balls and oil from oil spills.

The G+C-rich *Pseudomonas aeruginosa* chromosome consists of a conserved core and a variable accessory part. The core genomes of *P. aeruginosa* strains are largely collinear, exhibit a low rate of sequence polymorphism, and contain few loci of high sequence diversity, the most notable ones being the pyoverdine locus, the flagellar regulon, *pilA*, and the O-antigen biosynthesis locus. Variable segments are scattered throughout the genome, of which about one-third are immediately adjacent to tRNA or tmRNA genes. The three known hot spots of genomic diversity are caused by the integration of genomic islands of the pKLC102/PAGI-2 family into $tRNA^{Lys}$ or $tRNA^{Gly}$ genes. The individual islands differ in their repertoire of metabolic genes, but share a set of syntenic genes that confer their horizontal spread to other clones and species. Colonization of atypical disease habitats predisposes to deletions, genome rearrangements, and accumulation of loss-of-function mutations in the *P. aeruginosa* chromosome. The *P. aeruginosa* population is characterized by a few dominant clones widespread in disease and environmental habitats. The genome is made up of clone-typical segments in core and accessory genome and of blocks in the core genome with unrestricted gene flow in the population.

It is commonly found in canine otitis externa and cystitis, the uteri of mares (specially those treated with antimicrobial drugs) and eyes of horses treated with topical steroids and antibiotic. It may also cause ulcerative keratitis in dogs and horse. It is an uncommon cause of bovine mastitis and septicaemia in immuno-compromised animals (Atherton & Pitt 1982). It is a causative agent of wound infection in all the species. It is commonly associated with bovine mastitis (Nam *et al.*, 2009). Outbreaks among more than 15 Israeli dairy sheep and goat herds presented clinical signs, including gangrenous infections. Characterization of the *P. aeruginosa* isolates revealed the presence of multiple environmental strains in the various farms, and it was hypothesized that the infected herds were temporarily immunocompromised. In spite of the variability of the isolates, (Leitner and Krifucks 2007).

It is an opportunist in weakened tissues (burns), wounds, debilitated patients, persons with malignancies and immunodeficiencies and young animals (Sabath 1980). Prolonged antibacterial agents given orally to calves may predispose to enteric infection by *P. aeruginosa.* The disease occurs sporadically in animals which are immunocompromised, however, in poultry outbreaks of septicaemia due to this organism have been recorded.

P. aeruginosa including other Pseudomonads are frequent contaminants in disease processes and isolation alone is not necessarily significant. However, repeated isolation is indicative of the involvement of the organism in the disease process.

The diseases caused by *P. aeruginosa* in different animal species are listed below;

All animals: Wound infections, abscess formation, ear, urinary and genital tract infections; diarrhoea.

Horse: Abortions; Corneal and guttural pouch infections

Cattle : Mastitis, abortion and genital infections

Dogs and Cats: Otitis externa, pneumonia, urinary tract infections, prostatitis, dermatitis, endocarditis.

Swine : Respiratory infections

Poultry: Septicaemia, keratitis, respiratory infections

Sheep: Pneumonia, mastitis, fleece rot

Chinchillas: Otitis media, pneumonia, septicaemia, enteritis, death.

Pathogenesis

Most *Pseudomonas* infections are both invasive and toxinogenic. The ultimate *Pseudomonas* infection may be seen as composed of three distinct stages: (1) bacterial attachment and colonization; (2) local invasion; (3) disseminated systemic disease. However, the disease process may stop at any stage. Particular bacterial determinants of virulence mediate each of these stages and are ultimately responsible for the characteristic syndromes that accompany thedisease.

Although colonization usually precedes infections by *Pseudomonas aeruginosa,* the exact source and mode of transmission of the pathogen are often unclear because of its ubiquitous presence in the environment. It is sometimes present as part of the normal flora of humans, although the prevalence of colonization of healthy individuals outside the hospital is relatively low (estimates range from 0 to 24 percent depending on the anatomical locale).

The pili of *Pseudomonas aeruginosa* will adhere to the epithelial cells of the upper respiratory tract and, by inference, to other epithelial cells as well. These adhesins appear to bind to specific galactose or mannose or sialic acid receptors on epithelial cells. Colonization of the respiratory tract by *Pseudomonas* requires pili adherence and may be aided by production of a protease enzyme that degrades fibronectin in order to expose the underlying pilus receptors on the epithelial cell surface. Tissue injury may also play a role in colonization of the respiratory tract, since *P. aeruginosa* will adhere to tracheal epithelial cells of mice infected with influenza virus but not to normal tracheal epithelium. This has been called opportunistic adherence, and it may be an important step in *Pseudomonas* keratitis and urinary tract infections, as well as infections of the respiratory tract.

The receptor on tracheal epithelial cells for *Pseudomonas* pili is probably sialic acid (N-acetylneuraminic acid). Mucoid strains, which produce an exopolysaccharide (alginate), have an additional or alternative adhesin which attaches to the tracheobronchial mucin (N-acetylglucosamine). Besides pili and the mucoid polysaccharide, there are possibly other cell surface adhesins utilized by *Pseudomonas* to colonize the respiratory epithelium or mucin. Also, it is possible that surface-bound exoenzyme S could serve as an adhesin for glycolipids on respiratory cells.

There are several extra cellular products that are involved in pathogenesis of the infection. *P.aeroginosa* produces an extra cellular slime (Knirel 1990), which is composed of cell wall polysaccharide, lipopolysaccharide and a glycolipoprotein (GLP). The biological activity of GLP resides in the glycolipid component of the molecule (Orr *et al.*, 1982). GLP possess mouse lethality, antipagocytic property and protective ability.

Mucoid strains produce a non-toxic hexopolysaccharide called acetylated alginate. This is of importance in strains causing cystic fibrosis in human beings. Chemically this is an heteropolymer of mannuronic and glucoronic acid and biologically possess antiphagocytic property. Alginate constitutes a surface layer of *P.aeruginosa* and renders the bacteria resistant to dehydration. This antigen is associated with the causation of cystic fibrosis in man. The alginate producing strains form biofilm which is composed of polysaccharide, protein and DNA. Biofilm forming mucoid strains show increased tolerance to phagocytosis and antibiotics. (Heiby *etal.*, 2010). Production of chromosomal â-lactamases, upregulated efflux pumps and mutation of bacteria also contribute to the survival of bacteria in biofilms. Bacteria in biofilm express less virulence factors and there is slow progression of disease. In cystic fibrous of lungs of patients, alginate interferes with complement mediated chemotaxis of neutorphils, as well as inhibit non-opsonic phagocytosis, scavenges hypochlorite and thereby resist against myeloperoxidase-driven bacterial killing and attaches bacteria to the tracheal epithelium (Gyles, 1993). Alginate allows bacteria to attach to each other during growth thus helps in the formation of microcolonies.

Lipopolysaccharide of *P.aeruginosa* is one of the virulence factor influencing the pathogenicity. It helps bacteria to protect against opsonization by compleme:.t in the absence of antibodies. A common protein antigen attached to the lipopolysaccharide in the cell wall has been reported. It's role in stimulating protective immunity has been identified. Patients with cystic fibrosis produce antibodies against all the three components of LPS. As a result patients show the presence of immune complexes which is enhanced in chronically infected patients. The amount of immune complexes is positively correlated to the amount of tumor necrosis factor-alpha in the sputum. The immune complexes also induce an oxidative burst response in polymorphonuclear cells (Kronborg, 1995).

Cell-surface polysaccharides play diverse roles in the bacterial *lifestyle*. They serve as a barrier between the cell wall and the environment, mediate host-pathogen interactions, and form structural components of biofilms. These polysaccharides are synthesized from nucleotide-activated precursors, and, in most cases, all the enzymes necessary for biosynthesis, assembly, and transport of the completed polymer are encoded by genes organized in dedicated clusters within the genome of the organism. Lipopolysaccharide is one of the most important cell-surface polysaccharides, as it plays a key structural role in outer membrane integrity, as well as being an important mediator of host-pathogen interactions. The genetics for the biosynthesis of the so-called A-band (homopolymeric) and B-band (heteropolymeric) O antigens have been clearly defined, and much progress has been made toward understanding the biochemical pathways of their biosynthesis. The exopolysaccharide alginate is a linear copolymer of β-1,4-linked D-mannuronic acid and L-glucuronic acid residues, and is responsible for the mucoid phenotype of late-stage cystic fibrosis disease. The *pel* and *psl* loci are two recently-discovered gene clusters, which also encode exopolysaccharides found to be important for biofilm formation. Rhamnolipid is a biosurfactant whose production is tightly regulated at the transcriptional level, but the precise role that it plays in disease is not well understood at present. Protein glycosylation, in particular of pilin and flagellin, is a recent focus of research by several groups, and it has been shown to be important for adhesion and invasion during bacterial infection.

A most toxic extra cellular product of *P.aeruginosa*, termed as Exotoxin A possessing diphtheria toxin like activity has been identified. This is one of the virulence factors of *P.aeruginosa* which is immunogenic *in vivo*. It cause inhibition of protein synthesis, causes tissue necrosis and contributes to lethality in severe infections. Pseudomonas exotoxin A (PE) is a highly toxic protein secreted by the opportunistic pathogen Pseudomonas aeruginosa. The modular structure and corresponding mechanism of action of PE make it amenable to extensive modifications that can redirect its potent cytotoxicity from disease to a therapeutic function. In combination with a variety of artificial targeting elements, such as receptor ligands and antibody fragments, PE becomes a selective agent for the elimination of specific cell populations The toxin catalyzes the transfer of adenosine diphosphate - ribosy/ moiety from nicotinamide adenine dinucleotide to elongation factor 2. the ribosylated elongation factor 2 is unable to mediate elongation of polypeptide chain and the protein synthesis ceases. This results in cytotoxicity to various cells and lethality for mice (Gyles 1993). The exotoxin has three structural domains; an amino terminal domain is responsible for cell surface binding whereas the second terminal causes translocation from endocytic vesicles to the cytoplasm whereas the C-terminal third domain possess the active site of the enzyme (Wick *et al.,* 1990). The immunosuppressive activity of exotoxin A may aid in long term residence of the bacteria in the lung of cystic fibrosis patients (Staugas *et al.,* 1992). In addition, an exoenzyme S is a second ADP transferase produced by *P.aeruginosa*. It preferentially ADP-ribosylate vimetin, a structural cell component and a number of low molecular weight, GTP binding membrane associated proteins of eukaryotic cells. The exoenzyme is immunogenic and antibodies against exoenzyme S protect against spread of infection. Baker *et al.* (1990) reported that exoenzyme S is an important adhesin that mediate binding of the bacteria to glycospingolipids. It's role in pathogenesis is unclear but strains lacking exoenzymes S are less virulent than the parent cells.

An exoenzyme U has been described by various workers possessing cytotoxic effect on epithelial cells and is lethal for mice. Mutation in the exoenzyme U genes renders the strain less toxic and of lower virulence (Allewelt *et al.*, 2000). It has been characterized as member of the phospholipase A family possessing phospholipase A2 activity. It requires eukaryotic specific modification or cofactor for its activity (Sato and Frank 2004). Besides Exoenzyme U, 3 different exoenzymes S, T and Y have been described. Exoenzyme S is responsible for dissemination of the pathogen from the original site of establishment in the host.

Zhuo *et al* (2010) studied the clinical significance of virulence genes exo U and exo S of type III secretion system (TTSS) of Pseudomonas aeruginosa (PA).One hundred and eighty-nine clinical isolates of PA were collected from five hospitals. The incidence of virulence genes exo U and exo S in PA were determined with PCR. Minimum inhibitory concentration of anti-bacterial drug for PA was determined with microdilution method. The clinical features and outcomes of 60 hospitalized patients colonized or infected with exo U+/ exo S- positive or exo U-/exo S+ positive PA isolated from sputum were analyzed retrospectively. Data were processed with chi-square test.Among the 189 PA isolates, 85.2% (161/189) harbored TTSS genes, including exo U-/exo S+ type (120 isolates), exo U+/exo S- type (31 isolates), exo U-/exo S- type (7 isolates), and exo U+/exo S+ type (3 isolates). 72.0% (72/100) isolates from sputum and 81.5% (44/54) isolates from blood belonged to exo U-/exo S+ genotype. Compared with those of TTSS-negative isolates, the antimicrobial resistance of TTSS-positive isolates to cefoperazone/sulbactam, ceftazidime, amikacin, and cefepime were lower (with $\div^2$ value respectively 10.1, 16.1, 9.3, 33.8, P values all below 0.01). The antimicrobial resistance to all examined drug between exo U-/exo S+ type and exo U+/exo S- type isolates was close (with $\div^2$ values from 0.08 to 2.04, P values all above 0.05). Patients detected with exo U+/exo S- positive PA isolated from sputum were significantly associated with PA infection, and they usually had history of tracheal intubation, ICU hospitalization, and combined use of drugs for anti-infection treatment. Patients detected with exo U-/exo S+ positive PA isolated from sputum were significantly associated with PA colonization, which had basic lung disease and better outcome than the former infection type. The TTSS exists in most clinical isolates of PA. Detection of exo U or exo S of PA isolated from sputum is helpful for the analysis of clinical features and outcome of patients.

P.aeruginosa produces 2 haemolytic factors, a phospholipase C and a detergent like glycolipid. The phospholipase C has effect on granulocytes and mast cells and the glycolipid induces release of histamine, serotonin and 12-hydroxyl eicosatetraenoic acid from platelets (Gyles 1993). Phospholipse C destroys a lecithin containing lipoprotein of alveolus and thus contributes to tissue destruction and atelectasis. This is an important virulence factor in causation of fleece rot in sheep.

P.aeruginosa also produces a 33kDa elastase, a zinc metalloprotease possessing weak elastolytic activity but has a strong proleotytic activity (Galloway 1991). It is an important invasin which causes destruction of cells. It is produced by many clinical isolates. It causes degradation of immunoglobulins, complement factors and alpha proteinase inhibitor. Elastase causes breakdown of elastin of lung tissues and blood vessels. Elastase appears to act together with the Las A protein which is another elastase. Damage elastin is initiated by LasA and the nicked elastin is then highly susceptible to attack by elastase and other proteases (Galloway 1991; Tamura *et al.*, 1992). Lecithinase produced by bacteria enhances invasiveness, destroys tissues and contribute to the inflammatory response.

P.aeruginosa produces either endogenous or exogenous infection which is usually an opportunistic infection. It contaminates areas of the body that posses reduced number of microflora, normally caused by antimicrobial therapy. The first phase of the infection which consists of establishment of the infection, is followed by the production of enzymes and toxic metabolites. The establishment of the infection is characterized by the adherence of the bacteria through exoenzyme S and *pili*. The *pili* mediated attachment is ordinarily protected by fibronectin. *Pili* can mediate attachment to buccal epithelial cells, damaged tracheal epithelial cells and mucous proteins. Pili are immunogenic in nature but antipilin antibodies provide protection from infection only partially. The organism expresses its binding to damaged epithelium through N-glycoproteins and haparam sulphate proteoglycans. Upregulation of epithelial N-glycasylation enhances the binding *in vitro* (Buci ro *et al.*, 2010). Following attachment of cells through the pili the exoenzyme S is released which interact with receptors to effect an irreversible attachment. The alginate also promotes the adherence through attachment to the tracheal epithelium. The adhered bacteria then undergo multiplication and form biofilm. The siderophores pyochelin and pyoverdin scavange the host iron by inducing iron - regulated membrane proteins for transportation of iron-siderophore complexes into the cell. Some secondary siderophores of lower affinity are also produced. These are pseudomonin, corrugatins, yersinia bactin and thioquinolobactins (Cornelis, 2010). Pseudononas acquire heme or iron from siderophores produced by other microbes (Xeno siderophores). This scavenging of iron by bacteria aids in the multiplication of cells. The bacterial toxic products are released which result in damage to the host tissue. These predominantly are Exotoxin A, elastase and protease.

The antiphagocytic LPS and slime also help in multiplication. The multiplication of cells, the toxin release and release of proteases result in tissue damage. Acute disease is due to the damage of tissues caused by the toxins whereas the chronic infection such as cystic fibrosis is due to the host immune response. The organisms produce tumor necrosis factor in cultured peripheral blood mononuclear leukocytes and also in lungs of cystic fibrosis patients which could contribute to the chronic inflammation (Staugas *et al.*, 1992). *P. aeruginosa* cause both local and generalized infection. Local lesions show inflammation and necrosis and may involve invasion of vascular walls and degenerative changes in epithelial and endothelial cells and leukocytes. In persistent infection, as seen in lung of human patients with cystic fibrosis, tissue damage is most probably caused by inflammation induced by immune complexes. This leads to the release of protease through complement activation and release of serotonin from thrombocytes.

The pathogenesis and the outcome of Pseudomonas aeruginosa ventilator-acquired pneumonia in man depend on the virulence factors displayed by the bacteria as well as the host response. Thus, quorum sensing, lipopolysaccharide, and type 3 secretion system have each individually been shown to be important virulence systems in laboratory reference strains. However, the relative contribution of these three factors to the *in vivo* pathogenicity of clinically relevant strains has never been studied. Le Berre *et al.* (2011) analyzed the virulence of 56 nonclonal Pseudomonas aeruginosa strains isolated from critically ill patients with ventilator-acquired pneumonia. To avoid the variation of human immune response, the authors used a murine model of pneumonia. The aim was to determine which virulence factor was the most important. Male adult BALB/c mice were used. *In vitro,* the phenotype of each strain was established as to the expression of quorum sensing-regulated factors (elastase and pyocyanin), type 3 secretion system exotoxin secretion (Exotoxin U, S and/or T, or "nonsecreting"), and lipopolysaccharide O-antigen serotype. Strain pathogenicity was evaluated in vivo in a mouse model of acute pneumonia through lung injury assessment by measuring alveolar-capillary barrier permeability to proteins, lung wet/dry weight ratio, and bacterial dissemination. Associations were then sought between virulence system phenotypes and levels of lung injury. In univariate analysis, elastase production, O11 serotype, and type 3 secretion system exotoxin secretion were associated with increased lung injury and exotoxin U was linked to an increase risk of bacteremia. In multivariate analysis, it was observed that type 3 secretion system exotoxin secretion and to a lesser degree elastase production were associated with increased lung injury. In conclusion In a murine model of pneumonia,it was suggested that type 3 secretion system and elastase are the most important virulence factors in clinically relevant *P. aeruginosa* strains. Respiratory isolates of *Pseudomonas aeruginosa* were collected from 58 critically-ill patients with ventilator-associated pneumonia. Expression of elastase and pyocyanin was assessed semi-quantitatively, while quorum-sensing activity was assessed by quantifying the levels of the autoinducers N-3-oxododecanoyl-L-homoserine lactone (C12-HSL) and N-butanoyl-L-homoserine lactone (C4-HSL). Correlations were sought between quorum-sensing activity and the expression of these two virulence factors, and all results were compared to those obtained with the laboratory reference strains PA103, a strain defective in quorum-sensing, and PAO1, a functional quorum-sensing strain. More than two-thirds of clinically pathogenic isolates had increased levels of elastase and/or pyocyanin, and high quorum-sensing activity, as assessed by autoinducer levels. However, a strong correlation between quorum-sensing activity and virulence factor production was revealed only for elastase and not for pyocyanin (C12-HSL/elastase, r = 0.7, p 2 x 10(-9); C4-HSL/elastase, r = 0.7, p 2 x 10(-9). These data suggest that the pathogenicity of P. aeruginosa isolates from critically-ill patients with ventilator-associated pneumonia is caused, at least in part, by an increase in elastase production regulated by quorum-sensing, while increased pyocyanin production in these isolates may be regulated predominantly by mechanisms other than quorum-sensing (Le Berre *et al.*2008).

Under certain circumstances the individuals of a bacterial population may find advantages in acting together and making "collective decisions". This phenomenon is better known as quorum sensing. When the concentration of signal molecules produced by the surrounding bacteria exceeds a certain threshold, the bacterial population acts as a single organism, collectively expressing virulence genes, biofilm forming genes, etc. Several mechanisms of quorum sensing are discussed, each with its distinct signal molecules and respective receptors. Some of these mechanisms are restricted to sensing intraspecies signalling, but interspecies and even interkingdom signalling have also been described. Several veterinary pathogens such as Staphylococcus aureus, Pseudomonas aeruginosa and Salmonella Typhimurium use quorum sensing as a means to optimize virulence gene expression and host colonization.

In Pseudomonas aeruginosa, cell-cell communication based on N-acyl-homoserine lactone (AHL) signal molecules (termed quorum sensing) is known to control the production of extracellular virulence factors. Hence, in pathogenic interactions with host organisms, the quorum-sensing (QS) machinery can confer a selective advantage on P. aeruginosa. However, as shown by transcriptomic and proteomic studies, many intracellular metabolic functions are also regulated by quorum sensing. Some of these serve to regenerate the AHL precursors methionine and S-adenosyl-methionine and to degrade adenosine via inosine and hypoxanthine. The fact that a significant percentage of clinical and environmental isolates of P. aeruginosa is defective for QS because of mutation in the major QS regulatory gene lasR, raises the question of whether the QS machinery can have a negative impact on the organism's fitness. In vitro, lasR mutants have a higher probability to escape lytic death in stationary phase under alkaline conditions than has the QS-proficient wild type. Similar selective forces might also operate in natural environments.

The pathogenesis of Pseudomonas infections is multifactorial and the production of many virulence factors is regulated by quorum sensing, a cell-to-cell communication mechanism. The two well defined QS systems in P. aeruginosa, the las and rhl systems, rely on N-acyl homoserine lactone signal molecules, also termed autoinducers. Karatuna and Yagci (2010) assessed the activity of QS-dependent virulence factors (including elastase, alkaline protease, pyocyanin and biofilm production) in respiratory isolates of P. aeruginosa and their relationship with antimicrobial susceptibility. Workers have identified sixteen isolates displaying impaired phenotypic activity; among them, eleven isolates were also defective in autoinducer production, and therefore considered QS-deficient. Six of the QS-deficient isolates failed to amplify one or more of the four QS regulatory genes (lasI, lasR, rhlI, rhlR) with PCR: one isolate was negative for rhlR, two isolates were negative for rhlI and rhlR and three isolates were negative for all four genes. The isolates that were negative for virulence factor production were generally less susceptible to the antimicrobials and statistically significant correlations were observed between the lack of elastase production and resistance to piperacillin and ceftazidime; between failure in alkaline protease production and resistance to tobramycin, piperacillin, piperacillin-tazobactam, cefepime, imipenem and ciprofloxacin; and between failure in pyocyanin production and resistance to amikacin, tobramycin, ceftazidime, ciprofloxacin and ofloxacin. The results obtained indicate that, despite the pivotal role of QS in the pathogenesis of P. aeruginosa respiratory infections, QS-deficient strains are still capable of causing infections and tend to be less susceptible to antimicrobials. Cotar et al (2010) investigated by real-time RT-qPCR the influence of probiotic culture soluble factors on the QS genes expression in 30 Ps. aeruginosa strains isolated from patients hospitalized in the National Institute for Cardiovascular Infections, Bucharest. The results of the real time RT-qPCR have shown that in all Ps. aeruginosa strains grown in the presence of probiotic culture sterile filtrates, the level of QS genes expression was reduced comparatively with those from control cultures. In conclusion, these results proved that the inhibition of virulence factors regulation mechanisms by soluble molecules secreted by probiotics could represent an interesting way pathogenicity and virulence attenuation in Ps. aeruginosa nosocomial strains.

Two quorum-sensing systems (las and rhl) regulate virulence gene expression in Pseudomonas aeruginosa. The las system consists of a transcriptional activator, LasR, and LasI, which directs the synthesis of the autoinducer N-(3-oxododecanoyl) homoserine lactone (PAI-1). Induction of lasB (encoding elastase) and other virulence genes requires LasR and PAI-1. The rhl system consists of a putative transcriptional activator, RhlR, and RhlI, which directs the synthesis of N-butyryl homoserine lactone (PAI-2). Rhamnolipid production in P. aeruginosa has been reported to require both the rhl system and rhlAB (encoding a rhamnosyltransferase). Pearson *et al.* (1997) reported the generation of a delta lasI mutant and both delta lasI delta rhlI and delta lasR rhlR::Tn501 double mutants of strain PAO1. Rhamnolipid production and elastolysis were reduced in the delta lasI single mutant and abolished in the double-mutant strains. rhlAB mRNA was not detected in these strains at mid-logarithmic phase but was abundant in the parental strain. Further RNA analysis of the wild-type strain revealed that rhlAB is organized as an operon. The rhlAB transcriptional start was mapped, and putative sigma 54 and sigma 70 promoters were identified upstream. To define components required for rhlAB expression, we developed a bioassay in Escherichia coli and demonstrated that PAI-2 and RhlR are required and sufficient for expression of rhlA. To characterize the putative interaction between PAI-2 and RhlR, we demonstrated that [3H]PAI-2 binds to E. coli cells expressing RhlR and not to those expressing LasR. Finally, the specificity of the las and rhl systems was examined in E. coli bioassays. The las system was capable of mildly activating rhlA, and similarly, the rhl system partly activated lasB. However; these effects were much less than the activation of rhlA by the rhl system and lasB by the las system. The results presented here further characterize the roles of the rhl and las quorum-sensing systems in virulence gene expression. The impact of quorum sensing (QS) in in vivo models of infection has been widely investigated, but there are no descriptions for ischemic wound infection. To explore the role of QS in Pseudomonas aeruginosa in the establishment of ischemic wound infection, Nakagami et al (2011) challenged a pressure ulcer model in rats with the PAO-1, PAO-1 derivatives ÄlasIÄrhlI and ÄlasRÄrhlR strains, which cannot induce the virulence factor under QS control, thus the reduced tissue destruction was expended in these mutant strains. However unexpectedly, on postwounding day 3, the inflammatory responses in the three groups were similarly severe and the numbers of bacteria in tissue samples did not differ among the three strains. Biofilm formation was immature in QS-deficient strains, defined by the absence of dense bacterial aggregates and extracellular polymeric substance, which was confirmed by scanning electron microscopy. The Pseudomonas aeruginosa QS signal, acylated homoserine lactone, was only quantified from wound samples in the PAO-1 group. The swimming and twitching motilities were significantly enhanced in the ÄlasRÄrhlR group compared with the PAO-1 group in vitro. A significantly larger wound area was correlated with the bacterial motility. The inflammation in the early phase of bacterial challenge to wounds with immature biofilm formation in the QS-deficient strains indicated that the role of QS was more crucial for the chronic phase than for the acute phase of infection. The present findings indicate a difference in the importance of QS in ischemic wound infections compared with other infection models.

Current literature suggests that pockets with reduced oxygen tension exist in the CF airway mucus. However, virulence features of this opportunistic pathogen under such conditions are largely unknown. Cell-free supernatant of the standard laboratory P. aeruginosa strain PAO1 obtained from anaerobic culture, but not aerobic culture, failed to kill A549 human airway epithelial cells (Lee *et al.*, 2011). Further investigation revealed that this reduced cytotoxicity upon anaerobiosis was due to the suppressed secretion of elastase, a virulence factor controlled by *P. aeruginosa* quorum sensing. Both a lacZ-reporter fusion assay and quantitative RT-PCR analysis demonstrated that transcription of the elastase-encoding lasB gene was substantially decreased during anaerobic growth compared with aerobic growth. Moreover, transcription of other genes controlled by the LasI/R QS system, such as rhlR, vqsR, mvfR, and rsaL, was also repressed under the same anaerobic growth conditions. Importantly, synthesis of 3-oxo-C12 HSL (PAI-1), an autoinducer molecule that mediates induction of the LasI/R QS system, was >22-fold decreased during anaerobic growth while C4-HSL (PAI-2), which mediates RhlI/R QS, was non-detectable under the same growth conditions. Transcription of the lasB gene was restored by exogenous supplementation with autoinducers, with PAI-2 more effective than PAI-1 or PQS at restoring transcription of the lasB gene. Together, these results suggest that anaerobiosis deprives *P. aeruginosa* of the ability to regulate its virulence via QS and this misregulation attenuates the pathogenic potential of this important pathogen.

Biofilm of *Pseudomonas aeruginosa* can cause chronic opportunistic infections. These kinds of infections are a serious problem for medical care in industrialized societies, especially for immunocompromised patients and the elderly. They often cannot be treated effectively with traditional antibiotic therapy. Biofilms seem to protect these bacteria from adverse environmental factors. *Pseudomonas aeruginosa* can cause nosocomial infections and is considered a model organism for the study of antibiotic-resistant bacteria. Researchers consider it important to learn more about the molecular mechanisms that cause the switch from planktonic growth to a biofilm phenotype and about the role of interbacterial communication in treatment-resistant bacteria such as *Pseudomonas aeruginosa*. This should contribute to better clinical management of chronically infected patients, and should lead to the development of new drugs.

Many Gram-negative bacteria possess a type III secretion system (TTSS (paragraph sign)) that can activate the NLRC4 inflammasome, process caspase-1 and lead to secretion of mature IL-1beta. This is dependent on the presence of intracellular flagellin. Reports have suggested that this activation is independent of extracellular K(+) and not accompanied by leakage of K(+) from the cell, in contrast to activation of the NLRP3 inflammasome. However, non-flagellated strains of Pseudomonas aeruginosa are able to activate NLRC4, suggesting that formation of a pore in the cell membrane by the TTSS apparatus may be sufficient for inflammasome activation. Thus, Arlehamn et al (2010) set out to determine if extracellular K(+) influenced *P. aeruginosa* inflammasome activation. It was found that raising extracellular K(+) prevented TTSS NLRC4 activation by the non-flagellated P. aeruginosa strain PA103DeltaUDeltaT at concentrations above 90 mm, higher than those reported to inhibit NLRP3 activation. Infection was accompanied by efflux of K(+) from a minority of cells as determined using the K(+)-sensitive fluorophore PBFI, but no formation of a leaky pore. We obtained exactly the same results following infection with Salmonella typhimurium, previously described as independent of extracellular K(+). The inhibitory effect of raised extracellular K(+) on NLRC4 activation thus reflects a requirement for a decrease in intracellular K(+) for this inflammasome component as well as that described for NLRP3. IL-1β is produced from inactive pro-IL-1β by activation of caspase-1 brought about by a multi-subunit protein platform called the inflammasome. Many bacteria can trigger inflammasome activity through flagellin activation of the host protein NLRC4. However, strains of the common human pathogen Pseudomonas aeruginosa lacking flagellin can still activate the inflammasome. We set out to identify what non-flagellin components could produce this activation. Using mass spectroscopy, Arlehamn and Evans (2011) identified an inflammasome-activating factor from *P. aeruginosa* as pilin, the major component of the type IV bacterial pilus. Purified pilin introduced into mouse macrophages by liposomal delivery activated caspase-1 and led to secretion of mature IL-1β, as did recombinant pilin purified from Escherichia coli. This was dependent on caspase-1 but not on the host inflammasome proteins NLRC4, NLRP3 or ASC. Mutants of *P. aeruginosa* strain PA103 lacking pilin did not activate the inflammasome following infection of macrophages with live bacteria. Type III secretion remained intact in the absence of pili, showing this was not due to a lack of effector delivery. These observations show pilin is a novel activator of the inflammasome in addition to flagellin and the recently described PrgJ protein family, the basal body rod component of the type III apparatus. This could influence the pathogenesis of the infection caused by Pseudomonas.

Dermatitis in sheep is caused due to wetness. This is followed by the leakage of plasma onto the skin surface from damaged follicles. The bacteria multiply at this site which causes discolouration of fleece, mainly green colour due to the production of pyocyanin. The phospholipase C is produced which exacerbates the dermatitis and influence the inflammatory cascade that draws neutrophils and lymphocytes into the skin.

Specific immune response doesn't seem to play much of a role in pathogenesis.

Laboratory Diagnosis

P.aeruginosa grows well on most of the ordinary bacteriology media including nutrient agar. Rich growth is attained on blood agar. Colonies are large, translucent, spreading gray usually with a zone of haemolysis. The colonies emit characteristic grape like odour. Colonies also have bluish-metallic sheen. The organism does not grow anaerobically. It forms a blue green chloroform soluble pigment pyocyanin. Another pigment produced is fluorescein or pyoverdin (Yellowish green) which is not chloroform soluble. Occasionally a dark red pigment may be observed. This is termed as pyorubin. Additionally a brown black pigment (Pyomelanin) may be produced. Fluorescein fluoresces under ultraviolet light. Medium size gram-negative rods are seen in smears. They cannot be distinguished morphologically from members of the family Enterobacteriaceae. All strains are oxidase positive which differentiate them from enterobacteria. The organisms are motile, liquefy gelatin, uses citrate, is indole negative and reduce nitrate. The oxidation/ fermentation (O/F) test is positive for oxidation. Definitive identification is based on biochemical tests. The study by Stehling et al (2010) had as objective to evaluate the genotypic diversity and biological characteristics, such as hemolysin, protease, elastase of 56 clinical strains of Pseudomonas aeruginosa isolated from 13 cystic fibrosis (CF) patients attending at the School Hospital of Campinas State University (UNICAMP), Brazil. Genotypic diversity has been determined by Ribotyping (RT) and the pattern of the enterobacterial repetitive intergenic consensus PCR (ERIC-PCR) of each strain. The production of elastase was significantly different only among mucoid and nonmucoid isolates. Joint results obtained by (RT) and ERIC-PCR methods were able to discriminate all strains isolated from both the same and different patients.

Additionally, we observed four strain clusters with low diversity. The most infective strains were located in just two clusters. These results suggest that either there is a strong selection towards a specific genotype or that specific isolates could be responsible for the initial and subsequent colonization processes.

Strains can also be typed by bacteriophage and pyocins. In recent years nucleic acid fingerprinting has largely replaced the other typing schemes. The method is expensive and time consuming. A rapid polymerase chain reaction (PCR) to identify strains from cases of cystic fibrosis has been described (Anuj *et al.*, 2010) Williams *et al.*, (2010) reported a diagnostic PCR for the detection of cases of cystic fibrosis in Australia.

Current procedures for the detection of Pseudomonas aeruginosa require sophisticated equipment, skilled technicians, and a great deal of time. Immunochromatography assays (ICA) are simple and rapid diagnostic procedures that can be performed and interpreted on the spot or at the bedside without a machine. Wang *et al.* (2011) developed a rapid, 1-step immunochromatographic test strip that is well suited to the on-site detection of P. aeruginosa with high sensitivity and specificity. In brief, a monoclonal antibody targeting the outer membrane protein F (OprF) of P. aeruginosa, 3C3B5, was conjugated to colloidal gold and used as a detection antibody. An OprF polyclonal antibody was developed as the capture antibody. Eighty-three clinical samples were examined for P. aeruginosa by rapid 1-step ICA and compared with Multiplex-polymerase chain reaction (M-PCR). Results: The detection limit of this method is 5 × 10(5) CFU/ml for P. aeruginosa and 10 ng/ml for the OprF protein. The immunochromatographic strip test demonstrated a slightly lower sensitivity (84.8%), but a similar specificity (100%), to multi-PCR, which is an accurate method for the detection of *P. aeruginosa* in the laboratory. We observed no cross-reactivity with non-*P. aeruginosa* bacterial microbes. The detection of P. aeruginosa by the ICA strip can be completed within 5-10 min and is at least 10-fold faster than M-PCR. Conclusions: The ICA test strip developed in this study has proved to be a rapid, simple, effective and economical method for the detection of P. aeruginosa infection in clinical samples.

Agarwal *et al.* (2002) studied 38 children with CF attending the Paediatric Chest Clinic at the All India Institute of Medical Sciences, New Delhi, India during October 2000-January 2001 who were regularly followed up at the clinic. Patients were divided into 2 groups, Group 1 included all patients chronically infected with *P. aeruginosa* and Group 2 included patients who were infrequently colonized with this organism. Different colony morphological types of *P. aeruginosa* on culture media were identified. They were characterized by phenotypic methods using antibiograms and genotypic methods using enterobacterial repetitive intergenic consensus (ERIC) polymerase chain reaction and PCR-ribotyping.Fourteen of the 38 patients were colonized at least once with *P. aeruginosa*. Eight patients belonged to Group 1 and 42 isolates were obtained from these patients. Group 2 had 6 patients and 9 isolates were obtained from them. All patients in Group 1 harboured different colony morphotypes (Types 1-6) while all 6 patients in Group 2 showed a single type of colony morphology (Type 1). The isolates from Group 1 patients showed higher antimicrobial resistance as compared to Group 2 patients. Molecular typing of the isolates revealed 10 ERIC-PCR patterns and 2 PCR-ribotyping patterns among Group 1 and 2 ERIC-PCR and 1 PCR-ribotyping pattern among patients of Group 2.The frequency of different morphotypes of *P. aeruginosa* and antibiotic resistance was higher among Group 1 patients. On molecular typing, more than one genotype was isolated from Group 1 patients while only one genotype was isolated from patients in Group 2. We conclude that at a given time, chronically infected patients can be colonized by phenotypically and genotypically distinct strains of P. aeruginosa which has an implication in the management of these patients.

In one study, the suitability of two repetitive-element-based PCR (rep-PCR) assays, enterobacterial repetitive intergenic consensus (ERIC)-PCR and BOX-PCR, to rapidly characterize *Pseudomonas aeruginosa* strains isolated from patients with cystic fibrosis (CF) was examined. ERIC-PCR utilizes paired sequence-specific primers and BOX-PCR a single primer that target highly conserved repetitive elements in the *P. aeruginosa* genome were examined (Syrmis et al2004). Using these rep-PCR assays, 163 P. aeruginosa isolates cultured from sputa collected from 50 patients attending an adult CF clinic and 50 children attending a paediatric CF clinic were typed. The results of the rep-PCR assays were compared to the results of PFGE. All three assays revealed the presence of six major clonal groups shared by multiple patients attending either of the CF clinics, with the dominant clonal group infecting 38% of all patients. This dominant clonal group was not related to the dominant clonal group detected in Sydney or Melbourne (pulsotype 1), nor was it related to the dominant groups detected in the UK. In all, PFGE and rep-PCR identified 58 distinct clonal groups, with only three of these shared between the two clinics. The results of this study showed that both ERIC-PCR and BOX-PCR are rapid, highly discriminatory and reproducible assays that proved to be powerful surveillance screening tools for the typing of clinical *P. aeruginosa* isolates recovered from patients with CF.

Pseudomonas aeruginosa is associated with infectious endometritis in horses. Although infectious endometritis is often considered a venereal infection, there is relatively limited genotypic-based evidence to support this mode of transmission. The study by Kidd et al (2011) sought to determine the relatedness between genital *P. aeruginosa* isolates collected from a limited geographical region using molecular strain typing. Enterobacterial repetitive intergenic consensus PCR typing was performed on 93 isolates collected between 2005 and 2009 from 2058 thoroughbred horses (including 18 stallions) at 66 studs. While *P. aeruginosa* was not detected in the stallions, 53/93 (57%) mares harbouring *P. aeruginosa* had clonally related strains, which included a single dominant genotype detected in 42 (45%) mares from 13 different studs. These novel findings suggest that most equine genital *P. aeruginosa* infections in this region may have been acquired from mechanisms other than direct horse to horse transmission. Instead, other potential acquisition pathways, as well as strain specific adaptation to the equine genital tract, should be investigated.

Two molecular-typing strategies were used in an attempt to determine the genomic relationship(s), if any, of the *P. aeruginosa* strains isolated from the various herds and to verify whether the same strain was responsible for each outbreak. Thirty-six isolates from the mastitis outbreaks were tested and compared to fourteen clinical isolates from Cork University Hospital. With one exception, all outbreak-linked strains produced identical patterns when ribotyped with ClaI and PvuII enzymes. Eight of the clinical isolates gave the same ClaI ribotype pattern as the mastitis-causing strains. However, PvuII proved more discriminatory, with only the outbreak isolates producing identical patterns. Similar results were obtained with RW3A-primed DNA amplification fingerprinting, with all outbreak isolates except one displaying the same fingerprint array. The clinical strains produced several fingerprint patterns, all of which were different from those of the mastitis-causing isolates. Fine-resolution DNA fingerprinting with a fluorescence-labelled RW3A primer also identified a number of low-molecular-weight polymorphisms that would have remained undetected by conventional methods (Daly *et al.*, 1999).

Treatment and Control

Treatment involves the use of antimicrobial agents. Antimicrobial susceptibility testing should be done to select the most suitable drug. *P.aeruginosa* is usually susceptible to gentamicin, tobramycin, amikacin, carbenicillin, ciprofloxacin and ticarcillin clavulanic acid. Resistance may develop to a single drug thus a combination of a β-lactam agent with an aminoglycoside may be preferred for serious infections. Some strains readily develop resistance of antibiotics because of low metabolic activity, particularly in cystic fibrosis patients and formation of biofilms (Heiby *et al.*, 2010). For such strains a combination of colistin-tobramycin is most effective for treatment of patients with cystic fibrosis (Herrman *et al.*, 2010). Polymyxin is highly effective in urinary tract infections. In the canine urinary tract tetracycline achieves the concentration sufficient to kill most isolates. In otic infections, enrofloxacin, neomycin, polymyxin, chloramphenicol and gentamicin are effective. Control of the infection requires minimum exposure to the organism using sanitary precautions. Effective disinfectants should be used in animal premises.

Pseudomonas aeruginosa is notorious for its resistance to antibiotics and is, therefore, a particularly dangerous and dreaded pathogen. The bacterium is naturally resistant to many antibiotics due to the permeabiliity barrier afforded by its Gram-negative outer membrane. Also, its tendency to colonize surfaces in a biofilm form makes the cells impervious to therapeutic concentrations antibiotics. Since its natural habitat is the soil, living in association with the bacilli, actinomycetes and molds, it has developed resistance to a variety of their naturally-occuring antibiotics. Moreover, *Pseudomonas* maintains antibiotic resistance plasmids, both R-factors and RTFs, and it is able to transfer these genes by means of the bacterial mechanisms of horizontal gene transfer (HGT), mainly transduction and conjugation.

Background Multidrug resistance has become a quandary in the treatment of bacterial infections. The effect of resistance mutations and the fitness cost on the pathogenicity of *Pseudomonas aeruginosa* is not well established (Abdelraouf *et al.*, 2011). The objective of this study was to examine the impact of multidrug resistance on the fitness and virulence of *P. aeruginosa*. Methods Fourteen *P aeruginosa* strains with various resistance mechanisms were used. In vitro growth of these isolates was investigated in full-strength and 0.25-strength Mueller-Hinton broth (MHB). Exponential growth rates were estimated from serial bacterial burden over 24 h. In vitro growth of two multidrug-resistant strains (PAO1ÄmexRÄoprD and PA9019) was studied when each was grown in co-culture with wild-type strain PAO1. *In vivo* growth was compared between PAO1 and PAO1ÄmexRÄopD using a murine pneumonia model; virulence over 10 days was studied in six isolates. Results Significant reduction in growth rate was observed in selected mutants (P<0.01). PAO1 out-competed PAO1ÄmexRÄoprD and PA9019 in vitro, and in vivo growth of PAO1 was faster than PAO1ÄmexRÄoprD. Compared with PAO1, PAO1ÄmexR and PAO1ÄoprD showed a slight reduction in mortality rate; significantly lower mortality was seen in PAO1ÄmexRÄoprD (P<0.01). However, virulence of PA9019 was not significantly different from that of PAO1. Conclusions Specific resistance mutations were associated with fitness cost in *P. aeruginosa*, and accumulation of such mutations was associated with a reduction in virulence.

Only a few antibiotics are effective against *Pseudomonas aeruginosa*, including fluoroquinolones, gentamicin and imipenem, and even these antibiotics are not effective against all strains. The futility of treating *Pseudomonas* infections with antibiotics is most dramatically illustrated in cystic fibrosis patients, virtually all of whom eventually become infected with a strain that is so resistant that it cannot be treated.

Treatment of cystic fibrosis (CF) patients chronically infected with *P. aeruginosa* with the macrolide antibiotic azithromycin (AZM) has been demonstrated to improve the clinical outcome. Several studies indicate that AZM may accomplish its beneficial action in CF patients by impeding QS, thereby reducing the pathogenicity of *P. aeruginosa*. Skindersoe *et al.* (2008) investigated whether QS inhibition is a common feature of antibiotics. The workers present the results of a screening of 12 antibiotics for their QS-inhibitory activities using a previously described QS inhibitor selector 1 strain. Three of the antibiotics tested, AZM, ceftazidime (CFT), and ciprofloxacin (CPR), were very active in the assay and were further examined for their effects on QS-regulated virulence factor production in *P. aeruginosa*. The effects of the three antibiotics administered at subinhibitory concentrations were investigated by use of DNA microarrays. Consistent results from the virulence factor assays, reverse transcription-PCR, and the DNA microarrays support the finding that AZM, CFT, and CPR decrease the expression of a range of QS-regulated virulence factors. The data suggest that the underlying mechanism may be mediated by changes in membrane permeability, thereby influencing the flux of N-3-oxo-dodecanoyl-L-homoserine lactone.

A total of 39 non-duplicate isolates of carbapenem-resistant *Pseudomonas aeruginosa* and Acinetobacter species isolated from blood and endotracheal secretions were tested for metallo-β-lactamase (MBL) production by modified-EDTA disc synergy and double disc synergy tests. The prevalence of MBLs was 33.33% by both the above tests. All patients with MBL-positive isolates were multidrug resistant and had multiple risk factors like > 8 days hospital stay, catheterization, IV lines, previous antibiotic use, etc. These were risk factors for imipenem resistance also. The overall mortality in MBL-positive patients was 46.15% (De *et al.* 2010). A study was designed to investigate the molecular epidemiological characteristics of multidrug-resistant outbreak-related *Pseudomonas aeruginosa* isolates collected in a university hospital in northern Greece. Of 29 nonreplicate *P. aeruginosa* isolates resistant to carbapenems and ceftazidime, 14 were positive for metallo-beta-lactamase production. PCR analyses with primers specific for bla(VIM) and bla(IMP) revealed that 13 isolates carried a novel bla (VIM-2) gene variant, designated bla (VIM-17), and only 1 isolate carried bla (VIM-2), a gene predominant among P. aeruginosa strains in Greek hospitals (Siarkou *et al.* 2009). Pulsed-field gel electrophoresis of XbaI-digested genomic DNAs showed a close genetic relationship for 12 of 13 bla (VIM-17)-carrying outbreak-related isolates, which were of the O11 serotype; the clonally unrelated isolate carrying bla(VIM-17) was of the O12 serotype. PCR mapping strategies for the detection of class 1 integrons and sequencing approaches revealed the presence of integrons containing one bla(VIM) cassette flanked by two aacA29 cassettes. These integrons were similar but not identical to In59 (GenBank accession number AF263519) initially described in France. All isolates carrying bla(VIM-17), regardless of their genetic profile, had an identical integron, named In59.3, indicating that although the hospital outbreak was mainly due to clonal dissemination, the horizontal transmission of the bla(VIM-17)-containing integron among *P. aeruginosa* isolates should also have occurred. An outbreak-related isolate and a control strain, both of which carried the bla(VIM-2) gene but which were clonally distinct, had an identical integron, named In59.2, which differed only at the level of the bla(VIM) gene from In59.3 integrons, suggesting a common ancestry. The spread of the bla(VIM-17)-containing integron in clonally unrelated *P. aeruginosa* isolates without any evidence of plasmid carriage is probably associated with a transposon.

The first controlled clinical trial of a therapeutic bacteriophage preparation showed efficacy and safety in chronic otitis because of chemo-resistant *P. aeruginosa* (Wright *et al.* 2009). Further, in an evaluation of a bacteriophage treatment for infection, ten dogs were included with chronic *Pseudomonas aeruginosa* otitis. Each received, directly into the auditory canal of one ear, a single dose of a topical preparation containing approximately 1 × 10(5) plaque forming units (PFU) of each of 6 bacteriophage strains, active against *P. aeruginosa*. At the time of bacteriophage administration and 48 h later each dog's core temperature was taken, its ear was assigned a clinical score (higher=worse condition) and aural swabs were taken for bacteriophage and *P. aeruginosa* counts. Forty eight hours after treatment the clinical score and *P. aeruginosa* count of all ears had fallen (mean score fall: 30.1%, range 7.7-56.3%, $p<0.0001$; mean count fall: 67%, range 29.4-96.8%, $p<0.001$). The bacteriophage counts had risen from the administered dose (mean rise: 99.1-fold, range 2.8-433.3-fold). No treatment related inflammation or other adverse events were detected during the trial period. This is the first report of a veterinary clinical trial of a bacteriophage treatment of infection. The results show that administration of this topical bacteriophage mixture leads to lysis of *P. aeruginosa* in the ear without apparent toxicity and that it has potential to be a convenient and effective treatment for *P. aeruginosa* otitis in dogs (Hawkins *et al.* 2010). Knezevic *et al.* (2011) reported that all phages were significantly stable at pH 5-9, and phages δ and 001A even at pH 3. Most of the examined carbohydrates and exopolysaccharides of the original host efficiently inactivated phage ä, while phages ó-1 and J-1 were inactivated considerably only by the amino acid alanine. Silver-nitrate efficiently inactivated all the phages, while Siphoviridae were more resistant to povidone-iodine. Serum of non-immunized rats had no influence on phage inactivation and adsorption. Only phage δ showed ability to effectively inhibit The examined *in vitro* bacterial growth and biofilm formation. Conclusions: environmental parameters can significantly influence the adsorption and viability of *P. aeruginosa* specific phages. The phage δ is a good candidate for The study biocontrol of *P. aeruginosa.* Significance and Impact of the Study: provides important data on *P. aeruginosa* specific phage adsorption, inactivation and in vitro lytic efficacy.

The spread of *P. aeruginosa* can best be controlled by observing proper isolation procedures, aseptic technique, and careful cleaning and monitoring of respirators, catheters, and other instruments. Topical therapy of burn wounds with antibacterial agents such as silver sulfadiazine, coupled with surgical debridement, dramatically reduces the incidence of *P. aeruginosa* sepsis in burn patients.

Vaccines against *P.aeruginosa* infection in animals and human have been tried. Because there are several immunotypes of *P.aeruginosa,* it is difficult to ensure protection against all using a single vaccine. Humoral antibody against lipopolysaccharide and exotoxin A provide protective immunity (Cryz *etal.,* 1987).

A formalin killed culture of *P.aeruginosa* isolated from an outbreak of disease has been reported to be effective in protecting mink. Killed vaccines have been used in human burn patients, however, the immunity is short lived and there is no specific immunity to re-infection. *Pseudomonas aeruginosa* is most often associated with sporadic clinical mastitis

Characterization of the *P. aeruginosa* isolates revealed the presence of multiple environmental strains in the various farms, and it was hypothesized that the infected herds were temporarily immunocompromised. In spite of the variability of the isolates, because of the economic impact on the small-ruminant farms, leitner and Krifucks (2007) decided to search for common antigens that might induce an immune response that would protect the animals from the various P. aeruginosa strains present in the herds. Responses to selected isolates, representative of various animals and farms, were further studied in mouse models for capability to induce antibodies and to protect from homologous and heterologous challenge after immunization with an experimental primary vaccine. 1-D-SDS-PAGE tests revealed two patterns of protein bands among the various *P. aeruginosa* isolates, whereas the immunoblot and ELISA tests of sera of mice immunized with either MA-58, GE-61 monovalent, or (MA-58 + GE-61) bivalent bacterial vaccine preparations revealed two subgroups with low mutual cross-reactivity. Immunization with a vaccine prepared from either of the subgroups protected mice only from the homologues but not from the heterologues, whereas the bivalent vaccine protected mice from both subgroups.

References

Abdelraouf K., Kabbara S., Ledesma K.R., Poole K. and Tam VH. 2011.Effect of multidrug resistance-conferring mutations on the fitness and virulence of *Pseudomonas aeruginosa*. J. Antimicrob. Chemother. **66:** 1311-1317. Epub 2011 Mar 17.

Agarwal G., Kapil A., Kabra S.K., Chandra R., Das B. and Diwedi S.N. 2002.Phenotypic & genotypic variants of *Pseudomonas aeruginosa* isolated from children with cystic fibrosis in India. Indian J. Med. Res. **116:** 73-81.

Allewelt, M., Coleman, F.T., Grout, M., Priebe, G.P. and Pier, G.B. 2000. Acquisition of expression of the *Pseudomonas aeruginosa* ExoU cytotoxin leads to increased bacterial virulence in a murine model of acute pneumonia and systemic spread. Infect. Immun. **68:** 3998-4004.

Anuj, S.N., Whiley, D.M., Kidd, T.J., Ramsay, K.A., Bell, S.C., Syrmis, M.W. Grimwood, K., Wain Wright, C.E., Nlissen, M.D. and Sloots, T.P. 2010. Rapid SNP- based identification of clonal *Pseudomonas aeruginosa*. Isolates from patients with cystic fibrosis using real time PCR and high resolution multicurve analysis. Clin. Microbiol. Infect. **1111:** 1469-1591.

Arlehamn C.S., Evans T.J. 2011.*Pseudomonas aeruginosa* pilin activates the inflammasome. Cell. Microbiol. **13:** 388-401. doi: 10.1111/j.1462-5822.2010.01541.x. Epub 2010 Nov 3.

Arlehamn C.S., Pétrilli V., Gross O., Tschopp J. and Evans T.J.2010.The role of potassium in inflammasome activation by bacteria. J. Biol. Chem. **285:** 10508-18. Epub 2010 Jan 22.

Atherton, J.G. and Pitt, L.T. 1982. Types of *Pseudomonas aeruginosa* isolated from horses. Equine Vet. J. **14:** 329-332.

Baker, N.R., Minor, V., Deal, C., Shahrabadi, M.S., Simpson, D.A. and Woods, D.E. 1992. *Pseudomonas aeruginosa* exoenzyme S is an adhesin. Infect. Immun. **60:** 2859-2863.

Bucior, I., Mostov, K. and Engel, J.N. 2010. *Pseudomonas aeruginosa* – mediated damage requires distinct receptors at the apical and basolateral surfaces of the polarized epithelium. Infect. Immun. **78:** 939-953.

Cornelis, P. 2010. Iron uptake and metabolism in *pseudomonas*. Appl. Microbiol. Biotechnol. **86:** 1637-1645.

Cotar A.I., Chifiriuc M.C., Dinu S., Pelinescu D., Banu O. and Lazăr V.2010.Quantitative real-time PCR study of the influence of probiotic culture soluble fraction on the expression of *Pseudomonas aeruginosa* quorum sensing genes. Roum. Arch. Microbiol. Immunol. **69:** 213-223.

Cryz, S.J. Furer, E., Sadoff, J.C. and Germanair, R. 1987. A polyvalent *Pseudomonas aeruginosa* O polysaccharide – Toxin A conjugate vaccine. Antibiot. Chemother. **39:** 249-255.

Daly M., Power E., Björkroth J., Sheehan P., O'Connell A., Colgan M., Korkeala H. and Fanning S 1999. Molecular analysis of *Pseudomonas aeruginosa*: epidemiological investigation of mastitis outbreaks in Irish dairy herds. Appl. Environ. Microbiol. **65:** 2723-2729.

De A.S., Kumar S.H. and Baveja S.M.2010.Prevalence of metallo-β-lactamase producing *Pseudomonas aeruginosa* and Acinetobacter species in intensive care areas in a tertiary care hospital. Indian J. Crit. Care Med. **14:** 217-219.

Galloway, D.R. 1991. *Pseudomonas aeruginosa* elastase and elastolysis revisited: recent developments. Mol. Microbiol. **5:** 2315-2321.

Gyles, C.L. 1993. Pseudomonas and Moraxella. In pathogenesis of Bacterial infection in animals. Pp. 248-261. Ames, Iowa State University Press.

Heiby, N., Ciofu, O. and Bjarnsholt, T. 2010. *Pseudomonas aeruginosa* biofilms in cystic fibrosis. Future Microbiol. **5:** 1663-1674.

Hawkins C., Harper D., Burch D., Anggård E. and Soothill J.2010.Topical treatment of *Pseudomonas aeruginosa* otitis of dogs with a bacteriophage mixture: a before/after clinical trial. Vet Microbiol. **146:** 309-313. Epub 2010 May 12.

Herrmann, G., Yang, L., Wu, H., Song, Z., Wang, H., Haiby, N., Ulrich, M., Molin, S., Riethmuller, J. and Doring, G. 2010. Colistin- tobramycin combinations are superior to monotherapy concerning the killing of biofilm *Pseudomonas aeruginosa*. J. Infect. Dis. **202:** 1585-1592.

Karatuna O. and Yagci A. 2010..Analysis of quorum sensing-dependent virulence factor production and its relationship with antimicrobial susceptibility in *Pseudomonas aeruginosa* respiratory isolates. Clin. Microbiol. Infect. **16:** 1770-1775. doi: 10.1111/j.1469-0691.2010.03177.x.

Kidd T.J., Gibson J.S., Moss S., Greer R.M., Cobbold R.N., Wright J.D., Ramsay K.A., Grimwood K. and Bell S.C.2011.Clonal complex *Pseudomonas aeruginosa* in horses. Vet. Microbiol. **149:** 508-512. Epub 2010 Dec 1.

Knezevic P., Obreht D., Curcin S., Petrusic M., Aleksic V., Kostanjsek R. and Petrovic O. 2011.Phages of *Pseudomonas aeruginosa*: response to environmental factors and in vitro ability to inhibit bacterial growth and biofilm formation. J. Appl. Microbiol. 2011 May 7. doi: 10.1111/j.1365-2672.2011.05043.x. [http://www.ncbi.nlm.nih.gov/pubmed/21554503]

Knirel, Y. A. 1990. Polysaccharide antigens of *Pseudomonas aeruginosa*. Rev. Microbiol. **17:** 273-304.

Kronborg, G. 1995. Lipopolysaccharide (LPS), LPS-immune complexes and cytokines as inducers of pulmonary inflammation in patients with cystic fibrosis and chronic *Pseudomonas aeruginosa* lung infection. APIMS suppl. **50:** 1-30.

Lee K.M., Yoon M.Y., Park Y., Lee J.H. and Yoon S.S. 2011.Anaerobiosis-induced Loss of Cytotoxicity is Due to Inactivation of Quorum Sensing in *Pseudomonas aeruginosa*. Infect. Immun. 2011 May 9. [http://www.ncbi.nlm.nih.gov/pubmed/21555402]

Le Berre R., Nguyen S., Nowak E., Kipnis E., Pierre M., Ader F., Courcol R., Guery B.P. and Faure K. 2008. Quorum-sensing activity and related virulence factor expression in clinically pathogenic isolates of *Pseudomonas aeruginosa*. Clin. Microbiol. Infect. **14:** 337-343. Epub 2008 Jan 7.

Le Berre R., Nguyen S., Nowak E., Kipnis E., Pierre M., Quenee L., Ader F., Lancel S., Courcol R., Guery B.P. and Faure K; 2011. Relative contribution of three main virulence factors in *Pseudomonas aeruginosa pneumonia*. Crit. Care Med. 2011 May 12. [http://www.ncbi.nlm.nih.gov/pubmed/21572326]

Leitner G. and Krifucks O.2007.*Pseudomonas aeruginosa* mastitis outbreaks in sheep and goat flocks: antibody production and vaccination in a mouse model. **119:** 198-203. Epub 2007 Jun 2.

Nakagami G., Morohoshi T., Ikeda T., Ohta Y., Sagara H., Huang L., Nagase T., Sugama J. and Sanada H.2011.Contribution of quorum sensing to the virulence of *Pseudomonas aeruginosa* in pressure ulcer infection in rats. Wound Repair Regen. **19:** 214-222. doi: 10.1111/j.1524-475X.2010.00653.x.

Nam H.M., Lim S.K., Kang H.M., Kim J.M., Moon J.S., Jang K.C., Kim J.M., Joo Y.S. and Jung S.C.2009.Prevalence and antimicrobial susceptibility of gram-negative bacteria isolated from bovine mastitis between 2003 and 2008 in Korea. J. Dairy Sci. **92:** 2020-2026.

Orr, T., Koepp, L.H. and Bartell, P.F. 1982. Carbohydrate mediation of the glycolipoprotein of *Pseudomonas aeruginosa*. J. Gen. Microbiol. **128:** 2631-2638.

Pearson J.P., Pesci E.C. and Iglewski B.H.1997.Roles of *Pseudomonas aeruginosa* las and rhl quorum-sensing systems in control of elastase and rhamnolipid biosynthesis genes. J. Bacteriol. **179:** 5756-5767.

Sabath, L.D. 1980. *Pseudomonas aeruginosa*: The organism, Disease it causes and their treatment. Bern, Switz. Hans Huber.

Sato, H. and Frank, D.W. 2004. ExoU is a potent intracellular phospholipase. Mol. Microbiol. **53:** 1279-1290.

Siarkou V.I., Vitti D., Protonotariou E., Ikonomidis A. and Sofianou D.2009.Molecular epidemiology of outbreak-related *Pseudomonas aeruginosa* strains carrying the novel variant blaVIM-17 metallo-beta-lactamase gene. Antimicrob. Agents Chemother. **53:** 1325-1330. Epub 2009 Jan 21.

Skindersoe M.E., Alhede M., Phipps R., Yang L., Jensen P.O., Rasmussen T.B., Bjarnsholt T., Tolker-Nielsen T., Høiby N. and Givskov M..2008.Effects of antibiotics on quorum sensing in *Pseudomonas aeruginosa*. Antimicrob. Agents Chemother. **52:** 3648-3663. Epub 2008 Jul 21.

Staugas, R.E., Harvey, D.P., Ferrante, A., Nandoskar, M. and Allison, A.C. 1992. Induction of tumor necrosis factor (TNF) and interleukin – 1 (IL – 1) by *Pseudomonas aeruginosa* and exotoxin A induced suppression of lymphoproliferation and TNF, lymphotoxin, gamma interferon and IL-1 production in human leukocytes. Infect. Immun. **60:** 3162-3168.

Stehling E.G., Leite D.S. and Silveira W.D.2010.Molecular typing and biological characteristics of *Pseudomonas aeruginosa* isolated from cystic fibrosis patients in Brazil. Braz J Infect Dis. **14:** 462-467.

Syrmis M.W., O'Carroll M.R., Sloots T.P., Coulter C., Wainwright C.E., Bell S.C. and Nissen M.D. 2004.Rapid genotyping of *Pseudomonas aeruginosa* isolates harboured by adult and paediatric patients with cystic fibrosis using repetitive-element-based PCR assays. J. Med. Microbiol. **53:** 1089-1096.

Tamura, Y., Suzuki, S. and Sawada, T. 1992. Role of elastase as a virulence factor in experimental *Pseudomonas aeruginosa* infection in mice. Microb. Pathog. **12:** 237-244.

Vasil, M.L. 1986. *Pseudomonas aeruginosa:* biology, mechanism of virulence, epidemiology. J. Pediatr. **108:** 800-805.

Wang Y., Dou H., Chen K., Zhang H. and Hu C.2011.Development of a colloidal gold-based immunochromatographic test strip for the rapid, on-site detection of *Pseudomonas aeruginosa* in clinical samples. Scand. J. Infect. Dis. **43:** 329-338. Epub 2011 Feb 2.

Wick, M.J., Frank, D.W., Storey, D.G. and Igleoski, B.H. 1990. Structure, function and regulation of *Pseudomonas aeruginosa* exotoxin A. Ann. Rev. Microbiol. **44:** 335-363.

Williams, H.L., Turnbull, L., Thomas, S.J., Murphy, A., Stinear, T., Armstrong, D.S. and Whitchurch, C.B. 2010. A diagnostic PCR assay for the detection of an Australian epidemic strain of *Pseudomonas aeruginosa*. Ann. Clin. Microbiol. Antimicrob. **16:** 9-18.

Wright A., Hawkins C.H., Anggård E.E. and Harper D.R.2009.A controlled clinical trial of a therapeutic bacteriophage preparation in chronic otitis due to antibiotic-resistant *Pseudomonas aeruginosa*; a preliminary report of efficacy. Clin. Otolaryngol. **34:** 349-357.

Zhuo C., Wang L.X., Xiao S.N., Li H.Y., Qiu G.X. and Zhong N.S.. 2010. [Clinical significance of virulence-related genes of type III secretion system of *Pseudomonas aeruginosa*]. Zhonghua. Shao. Shang. Za. Zhi.**26:** 354-359. [Article in Chinese].

□□□

Chapter 12

Yersinia Infections

Dr. S.K. SRIVASTAVA
Former, Division of Bacteriology & Mycology
Indian Veterinary Research Institute, Izatnagar-243122
Bareilly (U.P.)

Yersinia infections

Yersinae are bipolar gram negative rods that are facultatively anaerobic, oxidase negative and fermentative. The organism belong to genus Enterobacteriaceae and has 10 species of which only yersinia pestis, Yersinia pseudotuberculosis and yersinia enterocolitica are pathogenic to man and animals. Even though the 3 species use different routes to infect host and provoke disease of different intensity, they share common tropism for the lymphoid tissue and they resist the initial immune response of host. *Yersinia rucheri* is a fish pathogen. All species except *Y.pestis* are motile at 22-30°C and their optimum temperature for growth is 25-28°C. Other non-pathogenic species are *Yersinia frederiksenii, Yersinia intermedia, Yersinia kristenii, Yersinia pereovieri, Yersinia mollaretti, Yersinia rodhei* and *Yersinia aldovae*. These can be differentiated on biochemical tests (Bercovier and Mollareet 1984). *Y.pseudotuberculosis* attacks many birds and rodents but occasionally domestic animals and primates. The habitat of *Y.pseudotuberculosis* and *Y.pestis* is the intestine of domestic and wild animals and birds. Plague, caused by *Y.pestis* is a rodent based zoonosis. The zoonotic aspects of other species is uncertain. *Y.rohdei* has been recovered from feces of dogs and humans. *Y.pseudotuberculosis* is classified into 10 serovars and *Y.enterocolitica* into 57 serotypes and 5 biotypes. *Y.pseudotuberculosis* serovars I, II & III contain strains that are pathogenic for both farm animals and humans. *Y.entercolitica* serotype 09 is antigenically very similar to Brucella spp. and infection with this serotype is a cause of false positive reaction to Brucella agglutination and complement fixation tests. Strong molecular evidence supports the fact that *Y. pestis* recently diverged from *Y. pseudotuberculosis* and is therefore closely related. *Y. enterocolitica* has evolved into a more heterogeneous group, classified into 6 biogroups including biotype 1B, associated with human infection. Biotype 1B includes the most virulent serotype O8, primarily isolated in North America.

Yersinia pestis

It is an important disease of rats and human but of minor significance for animals. It has been reported rarely in dogs, cats, camels, elephants, buffaloes, deer and some other animals. Cats usually acquire the infection from eating dead rodents. Characteristics of the disease are high fever, lethargy, swelling and abscessation of lymph nodes. *Y.pestis* is an intracellular pathogen. Urban or domestic plague is characterized by transmission of the pathogen from rats to human and from rats to rats. A flea, *Xenopsiella cheopis,* is involved in transmission of pathogen from rats to rats and rats to human beings. The organisms ingested by the flea multiply in the gut. When the flea bites, the blood containing the organisms is regurgitated into the bite wound. Domestic animals including cats and dogs may become infected during the outbreak. Sylvatic plague occurs in wild rodents other than rats. At least 38 species of wild rodents including marmots and squirrels have been found to be susceptible. Sylvatic plague may lead to epidemics of bubonic plaque and rarely pneumonic plaque. The prevalence of antibodies against Yersinia pestis in domestic carnivores (dogs and cats), in plague areas in the State of Ceará, was analyzed to establish the importance of monitoring these animals within the routine practice of the plague control program(Aragao et al.2009). Over the decade 1997-2006, 146,732 serum samples were examined (95,883 from dogs and 50,849 from cats), of which 2,629 (2,234 from dogs and 395 from cats) proved to be positive. The prevalence among dogs (85%) was higher than among cats (15%) throughout the decade and in all places, except in Ibiapina in 1998. Following natural infection both cats and dogs develop antibodies to plague which can be measured for several months after infection. Besides being helpful in the diagnosis of plague in domestic carnivores, the antibody titer has important implications in outbreak investigation and surveillance programs. The authors reported the first serological survey for plague in domestic carnivores conducted in California between 1979 and 1991 in five different settings or programs. A total of 4115 dogs and 466 cats were tested for plague antibody by the passive hemagglutination test (Chomel et al.1994). 86 dogs (2.09%) and 15 cats (3.22%) had plague antibody titers > or = 1:16. The percentage of positive dogs and cats were respectively 3.96% and 0% on reservations, 3.27% and 1.39% on military bases, 0.74% and 1.25% in Los Angeles County and 0% and 4.61% in veterinary clinics, but 41.38% and 41.2% from outbreak investigations. Titers ranged from 1:16 to 1:4096 in dogs and cats, but were low in dogs and cats in the Los Angeles County survey and on the military bases.

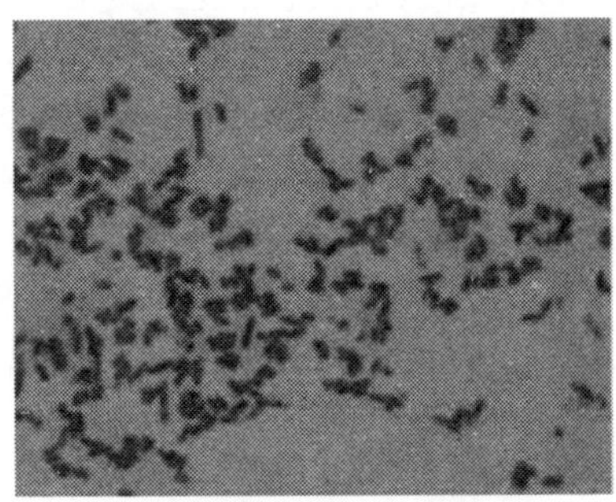

Y. pestis gram stained

Bubonic plague progresses rapidly to a life-threatening septicemia, but septicemia without a prior bubonic phase (primary septicemic plague), may also result from direct injection of plague bacilli into a blood vessel during the flea bloodmeal. Other less common clinical presentations that can follow flea-borne transmission include pestis minor (a benign form of bubonic plague) and carbuncular plague with or without palpable buboes . These rare forms of plague have not been attributed to atypical strains of *Y. pestis.* However, atypical strains have been isolated from around the world and it remains unclear whether these isolates produce one or another form of plague. Typical *Y. pestis* strains form red colonies (pigmented or Pgm$^+$) after growth at =34°C on media containing Congo red, but white colonies (Pgm$^-$) may be isolated at a frequency of 10^{-4}. Most spontaneous Pgm$^-$ mutants result from the deletion of a 102-kb chromosomal region termed the *pgm* locus. This locus includes the haemin storage operon (*hmsHFRS*) which is essential for the pigmentation phenotype and for the production of a biofilm in the flea gut that can block normal blood feeding; the blockage of the flea's digestive tract is considered to be an important process for flea-borne transmission. The *pgm* locus also contains the Yersinia high-pathogenicity island (HPI), which carries among other genes the *irp1-irp2-ybtU-ybtT-ybtE,* the *ybtP-ybtQ-ybtX-ybtS* and the *psn* loci that encode the yersiniabactin (Ybt) siderophore-based iron acquisition and transport system. The *irp* genes encode the high molecular weight proteins (HMWP) 1 and 2 which act in concert with YbtU, YbtE, YbtS and probably YbtT to synthesize the Ybt siderophore . Ybt is secreted, acquires iron from transferrin and lactoferrin in host tissues, then is transported back into *Y. pestis* by the TonB-dependent outer membrane receptor Psn and the inner membrane ABC-transporter YbtP-YbtQ. A critical role of the Ybt system in bubonic plague is indicated by the fact that Ybt$^-$ *Y. pestis* strains are essentially avirulent by the subcutaneous inoculation route that mimics the flea bite, although these strains retain complete or nearly complete virulence when inoculated intravenously. Presumably, Ybt is required to provide sufficient iron at the peripheral injection site, in the draining lymphatic system, and/or in the lymph nodes, suggesting that Ybt would be an essential virulence factor for flea-borne bubonic plague.

Despite the importance of the Hms and Ybt system for flea-borne transmission and for disease in bubonic plague models, respectively, the *pgm* locus is subject to complete or partial loss at relatively high frequency by genomic rearrangements; and $Pgm^- Ybt^-$ and Pgm^-Ybt^+ strains from natural plague foci have been described. Furthermore, human cases of plague have been associated with non-pigmented strains.

Pathogenesis

Y.pestis produces a highly invasive disease in humans and animals. This is owing to the possession of several virulence factors by the causative organism. The Fraction 1 antigen is a glycoprotein associated with the capsule of *Y.pestis* and produced during growth at 37ºC. There is molecular heterogeneity but has a single immunogenic specificity. The gene fra which encodes production of F1 is carried on a 60 MDa plasmid. It is antiphagocytic and protective (Gyles, 1993). Besides, V and W antigens have been identified. V is a 38 kDa protein whereas W is a 145 kDa lipoprotein. It is present in all 3 pathogenic species. It is a virulence marker encoded by a 42- to 48- MDa virulence plasmid. These antigens promote resistance to intracellular killing but have no resistance against phagocytosis. The production of VW antigen is Ca++ dependant. It is more likely that low calcium ion concentration mimics as yet unknown *in vivo* one. A plasmid (pCAD) is associated with calcium dependence in *Y.pestis*. Important products encoded by genes residing on these plasmids include YopS (Yersinia outer membrane protein) Yad A (Yersinia adherence protein); Ler V (low calcium response virulence) and YpKA (Yersinia protein kinase). V antigen is also protective in mice (Gyles 1993). Antigen W is a complex of Ler V and the heat shock protein Gro EL. Transcription of calcium responsive proteins is also temperature regulated. At 26ºC transcription of YopS, LerV and YpkA is repressed while at 37ºC transmission is de-repressed.

The three human pathogenic *Yersinia* species harbor the 70-kb low calcium response plasmid that encodes essential virulence factors including the type III secretion system and the adherence protein YadA (not functional in *Y. pestis*). LcrV is a secreted, multifunctional protein that is central to the activity of the type III secretion system apparatus. LcrV affects effector secretion by binding the negative regulator LcrG and in conjunction with YopB and YopD, is essential for the translocation of effectors into eukaryotic cells. LcrV is highly immunogenic, inducing a protective immune response, and is therefore a component of most plague vaccines. It is highly conserved among the *Yersiniae*, although some protein polymorphism has been described which is especially evident in *Y. enterocolitica* strains. As a result of this polymorphism, there are two distinct types of LcrV, LcrV-YenO8, derived from *Y. enterocolitica* serotype

O8 and LcrV-Yps, which includes LcrV from *Y. pestis, Y. pseudotuberculosis* and other *Y. enterocolitica* serotypes. While the two LcrV types differ at a number of amino acids across the protein, the most notable difference lies in a hypervariable region between aa 225 and 232 that includes a 9 aa insertion in the LcrV-YenO8 group. One exception is the O8 strain *Y. enterocolitica* 8081, which synthesizes an LcrV protein that is more like LcrV-Yps across aa 225–232. Monospecific antisera against the two types of LcrV used in passive immunization studies, protected mice against challenge with strains expressing the homologous LcrV, but not strains expressing LcrV from the other group. In addition, LcrV contributes to pathogenicity via TLR2-mediated IL-10 induction: LcrV-YenO8 of *Y. enterocolitica* causes TNF-ásuppression in macrophages in a CD14 and TLR2-dependant manner by inducing IL-10. However, the TLR2-LcrV interaction seems to play less of a role in *Y. pestis* and *Y. pseudotuberculosis* pathogenicity. Administration of TNF-á and INF-ã can promote survival after *Y. pestis* challenge.

A plasmid mediated 63 kDa peptidoglycan hydrolase called Pesticin is produced by *Y.pestis* when grown at 30⁰C. The role pesticin play as a virulence factor is not known. The 10 kb plasmid pPCPI carry virulence genes besides the pesticin gene eg. genes for coagulase, fibrinolysin and C3 degradative activity. Coagulase is active at 25⁰C but not at 37⁰C and promotes blood clotting in the flea. On the contrary fibrinolysin dissolves clot and is more active at 37⁰C than at 35⁰C (Butter 1983). Transcription of gene, pla which resides on a plasmid pPCPI is higher at 37⁰C but is not calcium dependent. What role pla plays in the pathogenesis of *Y.pestis* is not known.

Other virulence factors involve a protein toxin and lipopolysaccharide (LPS). The protein is composed of 2 proteins, a 240 kDa toxin A and toxin B (120 kDa). The toxin is lethal for mice by causing blockage of beta-adrenergic nerves and inhibiting the action of epinephrine. The toxin is coded by a plasmid pMT1. This also carries a gene encoding for a capsular structure F1. The F1 gene is transcribed at 37⁰C but not at 26⁰C and is not calcium dependant. F1 is related to virulence. LPS is responsible for inducing fever, vascular collapse and disseminated intravascular coagulation, resulting in focal necrosis and death.

Yops (Yersinia outer membrane protein, a misnomer – they are not outer membrane proteins) are secreted by all virulent yersiniae. There are at least 11 Yops. They are responsible for depolymerization of actin and disruption of signal transduction resulting in inhibition of phagocytosis and the oxidative burst. The Yop proteins are secreted by a specific secretion system, called type III. After secretion they are immediately internalized into the cytosole of target eukaryotic cells. Three *Y.pestis* adhesions facilitate Yop delivery to eukaryotic cells (Felek *et al.,* 2010).

A fibrillar structure composed of a protein produced at pH 6.0 serve as adhesion for *Y.pestis* for entry into phagocytic cells in order to deliver Yops. Transient survival with in phagocytic cells is due to GsrA, a protein induced following phagocytosis. YadA is an adhesion protein present on many yersiniae. The YadA gene is located on 70 kb virulence plasmid. It is also a classical serum resistance factor as it inhibits the classical complement activation (Tahir and Skumik 2001).

Y.pestis colonies bind hemoglobin or congo red. This phenotype is known as HmS (Hemin storage). This phenotype is related to blockage of transfer of the microbes in the flea. This property of binding of pigment is associated with virulence in *Y.pestis* as strains lacking the property of binding pigment are markedly reduced in virulence. Virulence is restored to binding deficient mutants when iron is supplied exogenously. Using various techniques such as PCR, the low calcium response - congo red positive clones can be isolated for use in the development of growth models of virulent *Y.pestis* in food (Bhaduri *et al.,* 2010).

Shaw *et al* (2008) identified a homolog of the Salmonella enterica serovar Typhimurium lipoprotein (lpp) gene in Yersinia species and prepared lpp gene deletion mutants of *Y. pseudotuberculosis* YPIII, Y. pestis KIM/D27 (pigmentation locus minus), and Y. pestis CO92 with reduced virulence. Mice injected via the intraperitoneal route with 5 x 10(7) CFU of the Deltalpp KIM/D27 mutant survived a month, even though this would have constituted a lethal dose for the parental KIM/D27 strain. Subsequently, these Deltalpp KIM/D27-injected mice were solidly protected against an intranasally administered, highly virulent Y. pestis CO92 strain when it was given as five 50% lethal doses (LD(50)). In a parallel study with the pneumonic plague mouse model, after 72 h postinfection, the lungs of animals infected with wild-type (WT) *Y. pestis* CO92 and given a subinhibitory dose of levofloxacin had acute inflammation, edema, and masses of bacteria, while the lung tissue appeared essentially normal in mice inoculated with the Deltalpp mutant of CO92 and given the same dose of levofloxacin. Importantly, while WT *Y. pestis* CO92 could be detected in the bloodstreams and spleens of infected mice at 72 h postinfection, the Deltalpp mutant of CO92 could not be detected in those organs. Furthermore, the levels of cytokines/chemokines detected in the sera were significantly lower in animals infected with the Deltalpp mutant than in those infected with WT CO92. Additionally, the Deltalpp mutant was more rapidly killed by macrophages than was the WT CO92 strain. These data provided evidence that the Deltalpp mutants of *Yersiniae* were significantly attenuated and could be useful tools in the development of new vaccines.

A siderophore-dependent iron transport system of the pathogenic *Yersiniae* plays a role in the pathogenesis of these organisms. The structure of the yersiniabactin (Ybt) siderophore produced by *Yersinia enterocolitica* has been elucidated. Perry *et al.* (1999) reports the purification of Ybt from Yersinia pestis and demonstrates that it has the same structure as Ybt from Y. enterocolitica. Purified Ybt had a formation constant for Fe3+ of approximately 4x10(-36). Addition of purified Ybt from *Y. pestis* enhanced iron uptake by a siderophore-negative (irp2) strain of *Y. pestis*. Maximal expression of the Ybt outer-membrane receptor, Psn, in this strain was dependent upon exogenously supplied Ybt. Regulation of Psn expression by Ybt occurred at the transcriptional level. *Y. pestis* DNA was used to construct irp2 and psn mutations in Yersinia pseudotuberculosis. The irp2 mutant strain no longer synthesized Ybt and the psn mutant strain could not use exogenously supplied Ybt. As in *Y. pestis,* Ybt was required for maximal expression of Psn. Regulation by Ybt occurred at the transcriptional level. In contrast to *Y. pestis,* in which a psn mutation does not repress synthesis of Ybt siderophore or expression of the iron-regulated HMWP1 and HMWP2 proteins, the same mutation in *Y. pseudotuberculosis* partially repressed these products.

Iron acquisition from the host is an important step in the pathogenic process. While *Yersinia pestis* has multiple iron transporters, the Ybt siderophore-dependent system plays a major role in iron acquisition in vitro and in vivo. In one study, it was determined whether the Ybt system is required for the use of iron bound by transferrin and lactoferrin and examined the importance of the Ybt system for virulence in mouse models of bubonic and pneumonic plague (Fetherston *et al.* 2010). *Y. pestis* mutants unable to either transport Ybt or synthesize the siderophore were both essentially avirulent via subcutaneous injection (bubonic plague model). Surprisingly, via intranasal instillation (pneumonic plague model), the authors saw a difference in the virulence of Ybt biosynthetic and transport mutants. Ybt biosynthetic mutants displayed an approximately 24-fold-higher 50% lethal dose (LD_{50}) than transport mutants. In contrast, under iron-restricted conditions in vitro, a Ybt transport mutant had a more severe growth defect than the Ybt biosynthetic mutant. Finally, a Delta pgm mutant had a greater loss of virulence than the Ybt biosynthetic mutant, indicating that the 102-kb pgm locus encodes a virulence factor, in addition to Ybt, that plays a role in the pathogenesis of pneumonic plague.

Y. pestis mutants lacking the Ybt siderophore-based iron transport system are avirulent when inoculated intradermally but fully virulent when inoculated intravenously in mice. Presumably, Ybt is required to provide sufficient iron at the peripheral injection site, suggesting that Ybt would be an essential virulence factor for flea-borne plague. Sebbane (2010) showed that a *Y. pestis* strain lacking the Ybt system causes fatal plague at low incidence when transmitted by fleas. Bacteriology and histology analyses revealed that a Ybt-negative strain caused only primary septicemic plague and atypical bubonic plague instead of the typical bubonic form of disease. The results provide new evidence that primary septicemic plague is a distinct clinical entity and suggest that unusual forms of plague may be caused by atypical *Y. pestis* strains. Yersiniabactin (Ybt) is a siderophore-dependent iron uptake system encoded on a pathogenicity island that is widespread among pathogenic bacteria including the *Yersiniae*. While biosynthesis of the siderophore has been elucidated, the secretion mechanism and a few components of the uptake/utilization pathway are unidentified. ybt genes are transcriptionally repressed by Fur but activated by YbtA, likely in combination with the siderophore itself. The Ybt system is essential for the ability of *Yersinia pestis* to cause bubonic plague and important in pneumonic plague as well. However, the ability to cause fatal septicemic plague is independent of Ybt (Perry and Fetherston 2011). All identified genes required for the regulation, synthesis, and transport of Ybt, except for *ybtD*, are carried within a high-pathogenicity island (HPI) that has been spread among enteric pathogens but is essentially identical in the pathogenic yersiniae. In *Y. pestis*, the ~36-kb HPI is located within the 102-kb *pgm* locus; the entire *pgm* locus undergoes spontaneous deletion *in vitro* at a frequency of about 10^{-5}. The Ybt system produces a siderophore composed of one salicylate, one thiazoline, and two thiazolidine rings via a nonribosomal peptide/polyketide synthesis mechanism involving high-molecular-weight protein 1 (HMWP1), HMWP2, YbtD, YbtT, YbtE, YbtU, and YbtS. The formation constant of this siderophore with ferric iron is 4×10^{36}, and the crystal structure of the ferric complex has been solved.

Iron from the Ybt-Fe complex is transported into the cell via the TonB-dependent outer membrane (OM) receptor Psn (which is also required for sensitivity to the bacteriocin pesticin) and an ABC transporter consisting of two inner membrane (IM), fused-function permease/ATP-binding proteins, YbtP and YbtQ. A mutation in any of these three genes prevents Ybt-dependent uptake of iron but does not prevent Ybt secretion. YbtX is encoded in an apparent four-gene operon (*ybtPQXS*) and is a predicted IM protein which resembles an exporter, with 12 predicted transmembrane domains . It has weak homology to *Escherichia coli* EntS and *Bordetella* AlcS, exporters for enterobactin and alcaligin, respectively, but stronger similarities to RhtX and FptX, which import rhizobactin and pyochelin in *Sinorhizobium meliloti* and *Pseudomonas aeruginosa*, respectively. A mutation in *ybtX* does not cause a significant defect in either Ybt synthesis or the ability to use Ybt as an iron source. Thus, the role of YbtX, if any, in the Ybt system remains an enigma.In addition to typical Fur-Fe repression, maximal activation of the Ybt biosynthetic and transport operons requires an AraC-like positive regulator, YbtA, and its cognate siderophore, Ybt. Similar mechanisms activate diverse siderophore systems in a number of bacteria.

With in a few hours of bite of the flea the organism are carried to the regional lymph nodes where multiplication occurs. Once inside the host adherence and invasion allow bacteria to be taken up by non phagocytic cells in the mucosa of ileum and colon. After this the bacteria are phagocytosed by the neutrophils and macrophages. In the macrophages the organisms survive and multiply but not inside neutrophils (Straley 1991). Some protection against phagocytosis is provided by the protein- complex capsule. The VW antigens and outer membrane protein (YopS) are responsible for antiphagocytic property and subsequently the survival inside the cells. The intracellular environment of the phagocytes (37ºC low Ca++) results in induction of lcr operon and in production of surface proteins, which also resist killing. Straley (1991) has speculated that the role of lcr is to protect the organism when extracellular. The role of the highly mouse toxic murine toxin in plague is unknown but it is also probably an antiphagocytic factor. Once inside the tissues and lymph nodes, bacteria and dead phagocytes results in formation of abscesses, and focal necrosis.

Bacterial multiplication elicits haemorrhagic inflammatory lesions, followed by local lymph node involvement ("bubo"). The infection commonly become septicaemic and if untreated terminates fatally. This form is called bubonic plague.

Pneumonia also develops in some patients characterized by dyspnea, fever and presence of organisms in the sputum under epidemic conditions. This form is nearly always fatal.

Among domestic animals cats acquire clinical infection. Signs include lymphadenitis, fever, depression, anorexia, sneezing, coughing and occasionally central nervous system involvement. Human may acquire the infection from infected cats through cuts, bites, scratches and airborne routes.

Diagnosis

Exudates, edematous tissues, lymph nodes, blood from the abscess should be sent to a specialized laboratory for demonstration of the pathogen. Utmost hygienic precautions are required to handle the material. A mask and gloves should be used when handling the infected animal. Direct smears are examined following immuno-fluorescent, "bipolar (Wayson's) and Gram staining. The organisms can also be isolated from blood and tissues and inoculated on blood agar. Identification is confirmed by immuno-fluorescence or bacteriophage susceptibility. Animal inoculation involves use of mice or guinea pigs. The laboratory animals die with in 3 to 8 days when injected subcutaneously with the *Y.pestis* culture.

Serological tests such as haemagglutination, haemagglutination-inhibition, enzyme linked immunosorbant assay are useful for retrospective diagnosis of clinical cases.

For humans, a real time polymerase chain reaction has been described for diagnosis of bubonic plague (Richm *et al.*, 2010).

Treatment and Control

If plague is suspected in cats it must be euthanized, if not, must be kept under strict isolation with great exercise to prevent infection. When handling such cats, mask gown and gloves must be used. Abscesses (buboes) should be lanced and drained. Streptomycin, doxycline, gentamycin or chloramphenicol are effective for treatment. Levofloxacin was tested for primary pneumonic plague treatment in a nonhuman primate model mimicking human disease.Twenty-four African Green monkeys (AGMs, Chlorocebus aethiops) were challenged via head-only aerosol inhalation with 3-145 (mean = 65) 50% lethal (LD(50)) doses of *Y. pestis* strain CO92. Telemetered body temperature >39°C initiated intravenous infusions to seven 5% dextrose controls or 17 levofloxacin treated animals. Levofloxacin was administered as a "humanized" dose regimen of alternating 8 mg/kg and 2 mg/kg 30-min infusions every 24-h, continuing until animal death or 20 total infusions, followed by 14 days of observation. Fever appeared at 53-165 h and radiographs found multilobar pneumonia in all exposed animals. All control animals died of severe pneumonic plague within five days of aerosol exposure. All 16 animals infused with levofloxacin for 10 days survived. Levofloxacin treatment abolished bacteremia within 24 h in animals with confirmed pre-infusion bacteremia, and reduced tachypnea and leukocytosis but not fever during the first 2 days of infusions. Levofloxacin cures established pneumonic plague when treatment is initiated after the onset of fever in the lethal aerosol-challenged AGM nonhuman primate model, and can be considered for treatment of other forms of plague. Levofloxacin may also be considered for primary presumptive-use, multi-agent antibiotic in bioterrorism events prior to identification of the pathogen (Layton *et al.* 2011).

Live attenuated and killed whole cell vaccines against disease caused by *Yersinia pestis* have been available for man since the early part of the last century. Although these vaccines indicate the feasibility of protecting against disease, they have a number of shortcomings. The live attenuated vaccine is highly reactogenic and is not licensed for use in humans. The killed whole cell vaccine, also reactogenic, provides poor protection against pneumonic plague and immunisation requires multiple doses of the vaccine. Against this background, a range of candidate vaccines, including rationally attenuated mutants, subunit vaccines and naked DNA vaccines have been described. Of these, an injected subunit vaccine is likely to offer the best near-term solution to the provision of a vaccine that protects against both bubonic and pneumonic plague.

For man, formalin killed vaccine has been used since a long time. Live vaccines have also been used but side effects are common. Moreover, variability in the efficacy of vaccine from batch to batch has been observed. The antibacterial immunity is short lived, hence, revaccination is recommended every 6 months. Cell mediated immunity is more important than the humoral immunity for protecting the individuals against the disease. Tests for delayed type hypersensitivity to pestin have been developed (Wake and Morgan, 1986). Cynomolgus macaques, immunised at the 80μg dose level with an rF1+rV vaccine (two doses, three weeks apart), were fully protected against pneumonic plague following inhalational exposure to a clinical isolate of Yersinia pestis (strain CO92) at week 8 of the schedule (Williamson *et al.* 2011). At this time, all the immunised animals had developed specific IgG titres to rF1 and rV with geometric mean titres of 96.83±20.93μg/ml and 78.59±12.07μg/ml, respectively, for the 40μg dose group; by comparison, the 80μg dose group had developed titres of 114.4±22.1 and 90.8±15.8μg/ml to rF1 and rV, respectively, by week 8. For all the immunised animals, sera drawn at week 8 competed with the neutralising and protective Mab7.3 for binding to rV antigen in a competitive ELISA, indicating that a functional antibody response to rV had been induced. All but one of the group immunised at the lower 40ìg dose-level were protected against infection; the single animal which succumbed had significantly reduced antibody responses to both the rF1 and rV antigens. Although a functional titre to rV antigen was detected for this animal, this was insufficient for protection, indicating that there may have been a deficiency in the functional titre to rF1 and underlining the need for immunity to both vaccine antigens to achieve protective efficacy against plague. This demonstrated to protect cynomolgus macaques, immunised in the clinical regimen, against pneumonic plague.

A fully recombinant sub-unit vaccine comprising the protein antigens rF1 + rV has been demonstrated to protect immunized guinea pigs against exposure to 10(5) colony-forming units (CFU) of virulent *Yersinia pestis* (Jones *et al.* 2003). Additionally, IgG purified from rF1 + rV-immunized guinea pig serum, protected the mouse by passive immunization against challenge with *Y. pestis* whereas IgG purified from the serum of guinea pigs immunized with a licensed killed whole cell (KWC) vaccine for plague, protected less well. Guinea pigs immunized with the licensed killed whole cell vaccine developed an IgG titre for fraction 1 (F1) but not for V antigen. The differential in protection conferred on the mouse by passive immunization with guinea pig IgG, was abrogated by the use of IgG purified from guinea pigs immunised with killed whole cell vaccine supplemented with V antigen. These findings indicate that the reduced efficacy of the licensed killed whole cell vaccine formulation previously observed in the mouse can be attributed to lack of the V antigen. Cross-protection of the mouse with guinea pig IgG suggests that the recognition of neutralising epitopes in the F1 and V proteins is conserved between these two species.

A fusion recombinant protein vaccine comprising of Fraction 1 capsular antigen and V antigen has been developed against plague. *In vitro* model suggested it to be a useful preparation for vaccination of humans (Goodin *et al.*, 2010). The recombinant vaccines expressing 2 important antigen of *Y.pestis*; the fraction 1 capsular antigen (F1) and the low calcium response virulent antigen (V) either in combination or as a fusion protein has been tested. These have been expressed in plants and proved to be effective vaccines (Alvarez and Cardineau 2010). For vaccine development Ler V virulence protein has also been targeted. The vaccine elicits humoral and cellular immunity and induce protection in mouse model (Do *et al.*, 2010). The chemokine, lymphotactin (LTN), was tested as a molecular adjuvant using bicistronic DNA vaccines encoding the protective Yersinia capsular (F1) antigen and virulence antigen (V-Ag) as a F1-V fusion protein (Yamanaka *et al* 2010). The LTN-encoding F1-V or V-Ag vaccines were given by the intranasal (i.n.) or intramuscular (i.m.) routes, and although serum IgG and mucosal IgA antibodies (Abs) were induced, F1-Ag boosts were required for robust anti-F1-Ag Abs. Optimal efficacy against pneumonic plague was obtained in mice i.m.-, not i.n.-immunized with these DNA vaccines. These vaccines stimulated elevated Ag-specific Ab-forming cells and mixed Th cell responses, with Th17 cells markedly enhanced by i.m. immunization. These results show that LTN can be used as a molecular adjuvant to enhance protective immunity against plague.

No vaccine is available for animals. Experimentally, a vaccine for animals comprising of F1 capsular protein and the LcrV type III secretion component of *Y.pestis* has been reported (Bhattacharya *et al.*, 2010).

For long term elimination of the infection rodent control is essential.

Yersinia pseudotuberculosis and *Yersinia enterocolitica*

Yersinia pseudotuberculosis is basically pathogen of man and animals. It is very closely related to *Y.pestis*. The morphological features of both the species are indistinguishable from *Y.pestis*. The organisms *Y.pseudotuberculosis* share several antigens with *Y.pestis* as well as susceptibility to phages. *Yersinia pseudotuberculosis* is a parasite of wild rodents, rabbits and birds and persist in the environment. Both the organisms occurs world wide. Cases commonly tend to occur in cold months. The species *Y.pseudotuberculosis* was previously included with the family Pasteurellaceae but was transferred to Enterobacteriaceae because of their oxidase negative reaction and their relatedness to *E.coli*.

Y.pseudotuberculosis is a common inhabitant of the intestine in a wide variety of domestic and wild mammals and birds. The organisms are acquired through the ingestion of the organisms. There are differences in the host specificity of different serotypes and strains. Rodents and birds may be the major reservoirs of serotypes I and II, which infect deer and goats, whereas sheep may be the maintenance host for serotype III. Following ingestion, the organisms are sometimes contained by the mesenteric lymph nodes but may progress further to cause septicaemia characterized by the formation of miliary nodules in the organs.

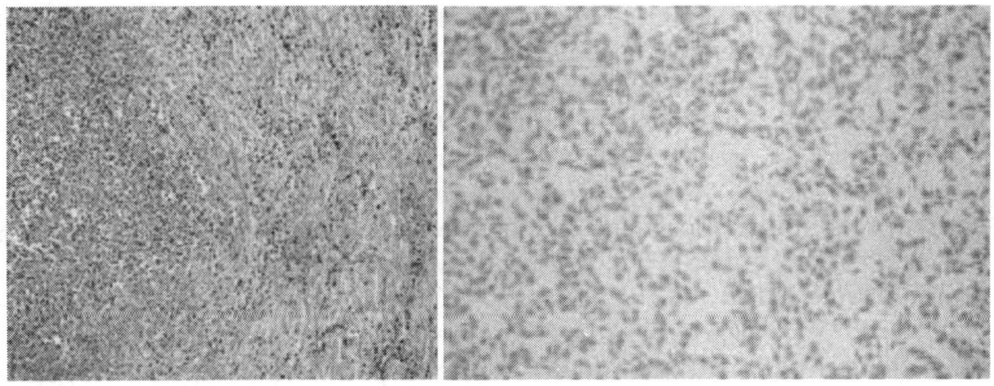

Y. enterocolitica gram stained

Y.pseudotuberculosis may also cause sporadic abortion in cattle and sheep, occasionally caprine mastitis and orchitis in rams. It is also associated with sporadic cases of abscessation and lymphangitis in ruminants. Tonsils of 457 fattening pigs from Estonia (n = 151), Latvia (n = 109), and the Leningrad Region of Russia (n = 197) were collected between 2004 and 2007 to study the prevalence of enteropathogenic *Yersinia* in slaughter pigs Martinez *et al.* 2009). Yersinia enterocolitica and *Yersinia pseudotuberculosis* were isolated by selective and cold enrichment. Pathogenic *Y. enterocolitica* and *Y. pseudotuberculosis* were identified by PCR targeting the chromosomal genes ail and inv, respectively. The presence of the virulence plasmid was confirmed by PCR targeting the virF gene of *Y. enterocolitica* and *Y. pseudotuberculosis*.

The prevalence of ail-positive *Y. enterocolitica* was 89% in Estonia, 64% in Latvia, and 34% in Russia, with 81% of ail-positive samples being virF-positive. A statistically significant ($p < 0.05$) difference between Estonian and Latvian pigs and between pigs from Latvia and the Leningrad Region of Russia was observed when assuming randomized sampling. Y. enterocolitica bioserotype 4/O:3 was the only pathogenic type found. The prevalence of inv and virF-positive *Y. pseudotuberculosis* was higher in Russia (7%) than in Latvia (5%) and Estonia (1%), with a statistically significant difference between pigs from Estonia and the Leningrad Region of Russia when assuming both randomized sampling and clustering at farms. All *Y. pseudotuberculosis* isolates were bioserotype 2/O:3. A total of eight pigs (2%), one pig from Latvia and seven pigs from the Leningrad Region of Russia, carried both pathogenic *Y. enterocolitica* and *Y. pseudotuberculosis* in the tonsils. Cold enrichment was found to be a more efficient method compared to selective enrichment to isolate both species. Pigs seem to be an important reservoir of human enteropathogenic *Y. enterocolitica* 4/O:3 and *Y. pseudotuberculosis* 2/O:3 in these countries.

The prevalence of *Yersinia enterocolitica* and *Yersinia pseudotuberculosis* was determined in slaughter pigs from 47 farms in Latvia(Terentieva and Berzins 2010). Tonsils from 404 pigs representing farms from four geographical areas (Kurzeme, Latgale, Vidzeme, and Zemgale) were collected at slaughter in 2007 and 2008. The prevalences of *Y. enterocolitica* and *Y. pseudotuberculosis* were 35 and 3%, respectively. All *Y. enterocolitica* isolates belonged to bioserotype 4/O:3. *Y. enterocolitica* was recovered from 35 of 47 pig farms, and Y. pseudotuberculosis was found on 6 farms. The prevalence of Yersinia was highest in Latgale (90%) followed by Kurzeme (39%), Zemgale (33%), and Vidzeme (21%). *Y. enterocolitica* 4/O:3 was sensitive to amoxicillin-clavulanic acid, aztreonam, cefotaxime, ceftriaxone, chloramphenicol, ciprofloxacin, nalidixic acid, trimethoprim, and trimethoprim-sulfamethoxazole and resistant to ampicillin, cephalothin, erythromycin, streptomycin, sulfamethoxazole, and tetracycline. *Y. pseudotuberculosis* exhibited resistance to erythromycin and sulfamethoxazole but not to the other antimicrobial agents tested.

Yersinia enterocolitica 4/O:3 is commonly isolated from fattening pigs in Finland, but its prevalence in sows is relatively unknown. During the study the workers determined the prevalence of yadA-positive *Y. enterocolitica* in sows and fattening pigs with polymerase chain reaction (PCR) and culture methods (Korte *et al.* 2004). The strains were characterized with pulsed-field gel electrophoresis (PFGE) using NotI DNA-restriction enzyme. Pathogenic *Y. enterocolitica* was detected in only 14% of sow tonsils compared with 56% of tonsils of fattening pigs. The prevalence varied between seven slaughterhouses from 0% to 30% in sows and from 30% to 87% in fattening pigs. A total of 37 NotI profiles were obtained from 148 *Y. enterocolitica* 4/O:3 strains isolated from 134 tonsil samples: eight profiles were obtained from 26 sow strains and 34 from 122 fattening pig strains. Two types predominated in both sows and fattening pigs. The prevalence of yadA-positive *Y. enterocolitica* in fattening pigs increased from 1995 versus 1999; the mean prevalence in five slaughter houses for the 2 years was 33% and 64%, respectively. Seven NotI profiles, including the two common types, were found both years. In conclusion, pathogenic *Y. enterocolitica* was detected at a significantly lower rate in sows than in fattening pigs. Moreover, the prevalence of this pathogen in fattening pigs was significantly higher in 1999 than in 1995. Some *Y. enterocolitica* 4/O:3 strains persisting among slaughter swine were demonstrated to be very stable genetically. This study shows that fattening pigs are an important reservoir of different genotypes of *Y. enterocolitica* 4/O:3 strains.

Subclinical mastitis with a raised somatic cell count was diagnosed in a cow in her fifth lactation (Sampimon et al.2005). It was caused by *Yersinia pseudotuberculosis,* which can also infect humans. This is the first time that *Yersinia pseudotuberculosis* has been isolated from a mastitis sample in The Netherlands. Despite treatment with antibiotics in the dry period, *Yersinia pseudotuberculosis* was still present in the same quarter in the subsequent lactation. The somatic cell count was still high and milk production was much lower than in previous lactation. The pathogen did not spread to other quarters of the same cow or to herd mates on the farm over a 1-year period. *Y. pseudotuberculosis* was isolated from mastitis cases in nine dairy cows in Israel (Shwimmer *et al.* 2007). Six cases occurred on one farm (three instances of two cows, 2 months apart) and three cases on one farm each. Seven cows suffered from clinical and two from subclinical mastitis.

Pigs are assumed to be the main reservoir of pathogenic *Y. enterocolitica* because pig is so far the only animal species from which pathogenic strains have frequently been isolated. Fredricksson *et al.* (2007) conducted a study to know the frequency of ail-positive *Y. enterocolitica* in pigs slaughtered at a Swiss abattoir. In total, 212 pig tonsils were screened by real-time PCR and culture methods. The prevalence rate of ail-positive *Y. enterocolitica* in pigs at slaughter was 88% and 34% with PCR and culture methods, respectively. The 148 ail-positive isolates from the 72 culture-positive tonsils were bio-and serotyped. The most common bioserotype was 4/O:3 found in 96% (69/72) of the culture-positive samples. However, pig was also shown to be a reservoir for ail-positive *Y. enterocolitica* belonging to bioserotypes 2/O:5,27 and 2/O:9, which were detected in 8% (6/72) and 1% (1/72) of the culture-positive samples, respectively. Using PFGE with NotI, only a limited number of different patterns was found. In all, 6 genotypes were obtained when 86 isolates of bioserotype 4/O:3 from 69 samples were characterised and two genotypes (N1 and N4) dominated. The biotype 4 differs clearly from biotype 2 with PFGE. Antimicrobial resistance testing of 77 ail-positive *Y. enterocolitica* isolates from 72 samples studied with disc-diffusion revealed that all strains were sensitive to cefotaxime, chloramphenicol, ciprofloxacin and tetracycline, which are antimicrobial agents used for treatment of human disease. The isolates of bioserotype 2/O: 5, 27 differed from the isolates of bioserotypes 2/O: 9 and 4/O: 3 in resistance to ampicillin and amoxicillin/clavulanic acid.

Y.enterocolitica is represented by six biovars (1A, 1B2-5). Biovar 1A is generally regarded as non-virulent as they lack pYv plasmid and major chromosal genes (Bhagat and Virdi, 2010). Based on selected genes of virulence, *Y.enterocolitica* serotypes can be differentiated as different genotypes and bioserotypes eg. Yst B gene is a marker for biotype 1a (Kot *et al.,* 2010).

Y.enterocolitica biotype 5, serotype O:2, 3 is commonly associated with enterocolitis in sheep and goats of less than one year of age. It also causes abortion in sheep. Diarrheal disease has been reported in several species including dogs, chinchillas, hares, deer and cattle. The organisms are carried in the tonsils of healthy pigs in Europe and North America. Carriage is associated with microscopic inflammation in the tonsil crypts. The prevalence of *Y.enterocolitica* bioserotype 2 / 0:9 and 2/0:5 is high in English pigs than other European countries where biotype 4/0:3 predominate (Ortiz-Martinez *et al.,* 2010). Invasion of the intestinal epithelium is followed by inflammation in the mucosa and the formation of microabscesses in the lamina propria and mesenteric lymph nodes. There is loss of fluid and function due to ulcers and disruption of intestinal mucosa. There is villous atrophy that may lead to malabsorption and diarrhoea. Gross lesions are usually absent in the intestine. Some sheep may have thickening of mucosa of the small intestine with enlargement of cecum and colon.

Pathogenesis

Both, *Y.pseudotuberculosis* and *Y.enterocolitica* exhibit several virulence factors which are responsible for cellular damage and signs seen in the disease. V and W antigens are produced by both the species. V is responsible for virulence and W is associated with V antigen (Butler 1983). The Lcr V gene encodes the V antigen (Yop 41) of *Y.enterocolitica.* The gene vwa+ is located on a 42 to 48 MDa virulence plasmid. The V antigen is a protein whereas the W antigen is a lipoprotein. VW antigens promote resistance to intracellular killing, thus the organisms are disseminated. After oral ingestion, the bacteria move to the small intestine and invade the intestinal epithelium via interactions with the specialized M cells overlying the Peyer's patches. This interaction is mediated by the *inv* and *ails* genes. Once established, they colonize the underlying lymph tissues. Occasionally, *Y. enterocolitica* but not *Y. pseudotuberculosis* may spread to the spleen and liver, causing systemic disease.

Some strains of *Y.enterocolitica* produce a heat stable enterotoxin at 25^{0}C *in vitro*. This is antigenically related to heat stable enterotoxin (STa) of *Escherichia coli*. The enterotoxin a 30 amino acid long structure causes diarrhoea through activation of guanylate cyclase in intestinal epithelial cells. In vivo the toxin is not produced hence it role as a virulence factor is doubtful. It is postulated that loss of function of absorptive epithelium as a result of the invasion may account for diarrhoea.

Yersiniae possess a single gene inv or ail that encodes Invasins, a protein comprising of 957 amino acid whose C-terminal portion mediates invasion. This protein binds to the specific eukaryotic cells through a integrin receptors. The binding of invasions through these receptors results in internalization of the protein.

Mutants of *Y.enterocolitica* lacking inv poorly invade cells in culture. Both the species invades across the intestinal epithelium. The infection is usually contained at this level but *Y.pseudotuberculosis* often cause septicaemia and induces abscess for formation in liver, spleen and other organs. Barrier dysfunction due to *Y.enterocolitica* infection is due to circumscribed epithelial TJ protein changes and necrotic cell loss as a consequence of which leak flux diarrhoea and antigen - uptake provoking extra intestinal arthritis may be triggered (Hering *et al.*, 2010).

The enteropathogenic species share three adhesins: invasin, YadA and Ail. Invasin is the first adhesin required for enteric infection; it binds to â(1) integrins on microfold cells in the distal ileum, leading to the ingestion of the bacteria and allows them to cross the intestinal epithelium. YadA is the major adhesin in host tissues. It is a multifunctional protein, conferring adherence to cells and extracellular matrix components, serum and phagocytosis resistance, and the ability to autoagglutinate. Ail has a minor role in adhesion and serum resistance. *Y. pestis* lacks both invasin and YadA, but expresses several other adhesins. These include the pH 6 antigen and autotransporter adhesins. Also the plasminogen activator of *Y. pestis* can mediate adherence to host cells (Leo and Skurnik 2011). Although the adhesins of the pathogenic yersiniae have been studied extensively, their exact roles in the biology of infection remain elusive.

PCR-based assays were developed for the detection of plasmid- and chromosome-borne virulence genes in *Yersinia enterocolitica* and *Yersinia pseudotuberculosis*, to investigate the distribution of these genes in isolates from various sources (Thoerner *et al.*, 2003). The results of PCR genotyping, based on 5 virulence-associated genes of 140 strains of *Y. enterocolitica,* were compared to phenotypic tests, such as biotyping and serotyping, and to virulence plasmid-associated properties such as calcium-dependent growth at 37 degrees C and Congo red uptake. The specificity of the PCR results was validated by hybridization. Genotyping data correlated well with biotype data, and most biotypes resulted in (nearly) homogeneous genotypes for the chromosomal virulence genes (ystA, ystB, and ail); however, plasmid-borne genes (yadA and virF) were detected with variable efficiency, due to heterogeneity within the bacterial population for the presence of the virulence plasmid. Of the virulence genes, only ystB was present in biotype 1A; however, within this biotype, pathogenic and apathogenic isolates could not be distinguished based on the detection of virulence genes. Forty *Y. pseudotuberculosis* isolates were tested by PCR for the presence of inv, yadA, and lcrF. All isolates were inv positive, and 88% of the isolates contained the virulence plasmid genes yadA and lcrF. In conclusion, this study shows that genotyping of *Yersinia* spp., based on both chromosome- and plasmid-borne virulence genes, is feasible and informative and can provide a rapid and reliable genotypic characterization of field isolates. Zheng et al (2008) investigated the distribution of virulence genes in clinical isolates of pathogenic *Yersinia enterocolitica.* Two thousand six hundred stool samples were collected from 2600 patients with diarrhea, and were tested using the culture method and real-time PCR. Then, all isolates of pathogenic *Y. enterocolitica* cultured from the culture method were examined for virulence genes (inv, ail, ystA, ystB, ystC, yadA, virF) by PCR and for the presence of plasmid by four phenotypic tests. As a result, 160 pathogenic strains were successfully detected by the culture method, including bio/serotype 1A/unknown (4), 1B/unknown (8), 2/O:9 (39), 2/unknown (7), 3/O:3 (22), 3/unknown (6), 4/O:3 (55), 4/unknown (10) and 5/unknown (9). The positive rate of virulence genes tested in 160 isolates was inv (100%), ail (94%), ystA (93%), ystB (7.5%), ystC (5%), yadA (89%) and virF (82%) while the phenotypic test included autoagglutination (87%), binding of crystal violet (89%), calcium-dependent growth (74%) and Congo red absorption (78%), respectively. Finally, it was found that not all pathogenic *Y. enterocolitica* necessarily carry all traditional virulence genes in both chromosomes and plasmids to cause illness. Perhaps, some of them, lacking some traditional virulence genes, contain other unknown virulence markers that interact with each other and play an important role in the diverse pathogenesis of pathogenic *Y. enterocolitica.*

Molecular typing and virulence markers were used to evaluate the genetic profiles and virulence potential of 106 *Yersinia enterocolitica* strains (Falcao *et al.* 2006). Of these strains, 71 were bio-serotype 4/O : 3, isolated from human and animal clinical material, and 35 were of biotype 1A or 2 and of diverse serotypes, isolated from food in Brazil between 1968 and 2000. Drug resistance was also investigated. All the strains were resistant to three or more drugs. The isolates showed a virulence-related phenotype in the aesculin, pyrazinamidase and salicin tests, except for the food isolates, only two of which were positive for these tests. For the other phenotypic virulence determinants (autoagglutination, Ca(++) dependence and Congo red absorption), the strains showed a diverse behavior. The inv, ail and ystA genes were detected in all human and animal strains, while all the food isolates were positive for inv, and 3 % of them positive for ail and ystA. The presence of virF was variable in the three groups of strains. The strains were better discriminated by PFGE than by enterobacterial repetitive intergenic consensus PCR (ERIC-PCR). A higher genomic similarity was observed among the 4/O : 3 strains, isolated from human and animal isolates, than among the food strains, with the exception of two food strains possessing the virulence genes and grouped close to the 4/O : 3 strains by ERIC-PCR. Unusually, the results revealed the virulence potential of a bio-serotype 1A/O : 10 strain, suggesting that food contaminated with *Y. enterocolitica* biotype 1A may cause infection. This also suggests that ERIC-PCR may be used as a tool to reveal clues about the virulence potential of *Y. enterocolitica* strains. Furthermore, the results also support the hypothesis that animals may act as reservoirs of Y. enterocolitica for human infections in Brazil, an epidemiological aspect that has not been investigated in this country, confirming data from other parts of the world.

The 150 *Y. enterocolitica* strains isolated from humans and from pigs belonged to biotypes 4 (68.7%), 1A (18.7%) and 2 (4%), or were biochemically untypeable (8.6%) (Kot et al.2010). Biotype 4 was comprised of *Y. enterocolitica* strains representing serotype O:3, within biotype 1A the strains either belonged to serotypes O:5 and O:6 or were untypeable, and biotype 2 was represented by the strains of serotype O:9. The strains which were biochemically untypeable belonged to serotypes O:5, O:6 and O:3. Among the strains tested there also were those of an unidentified biotype and serotype. Nearly all the strains of biotype 1A represented genotype ystB+myfA+, and few belonged to genotype ystB+. The presence of the ystB gene in the strains of biotype 1A and only occasional occurrence of the gene in the other biotypes makes ystB a distinguishing marker of biotype 1A. The strains of genotype ystA+ail+myfA+yadA+ predominated in biotype 4 (serotype O:3). The strains of biotype 2 (serotype O:9) represented genotype ystA+ail+myfA+, and the plasmid yadA gene was detected in some of them. Within the group of biochemically untypeable strains ystB- and myfA-specific PCR products were mainly obtained. The genotypes determined for the tested biotypes and serotypes of Y. enterocolitica, based upon the selected genes of virulence, can be applied as distinguishing markers and indicators of the potential virulence of *Y. enterocolitica* strains, excluding bioserotyping.

Another protein a 17 kDa outer membrane protein, Ail mediates attachment of cells followed by invasion is present in *Y.enterocolitica* (Miller *et al.*, 1988). Loss of Ail results in a decrease in invasion of tissue culture and decrease in mice virulence. *Y.enterocolitica* plasmid pYV also encodes a protein that mediates adhesion (Paerregaard 1992). YadA is also responsible for pYV encoded adhesion. YadA, however, also mediates binding to one or more constituents present in intestinal mucus. Such binding decreases penetration to ileal brush border membrane vesicles. YadA is encoded by the Yad gene located in the 70 Kb virulence plasmid of *Yersinia enterocolitica* and *Y.pseudotuberculosis*. It is hydrophobic and expressed at 37^{0}C. It is also a serum resistance factor as it inhibits the classical complement pathway (Eltahir and Skurnik, 2001). Adhesion of *Y. enterocolitica* was quantitatively studied by methods that measured binding to cultured epithelial cells, mucosal constituents immobilized on polystyrene, intestinal tissue, and nonbiological solid surfaces(Paerregaard 1992). The chromosomal inv and ail gene products have been shown by others to be independently able to mediate adhesion to and invasion of cultured epithelial cells. However, the *Yersinia virulence* plasmid, pYV, also encodes for at least one product that may mediate adhesion. It was shown that pYV carrying *Y. enterocolitica* strains adhered more efficiently than their isogenic pYV cured derivatives to rabbit and human ileal intestinal tissue and to rabbit ileal brush border membrane vesicles (BBVs). Using *Y. enterocolitica* mutants that were defective for production of the pYV encoded outer membrane protein, YadA, and *Escherichia coli* strains carrying the cloned yadA gene it was verified that YadA was responsible for the pYV encoded adhesion. The YadA promoted adhesion was found likely to be non-specific and, at least in part, mediated by hydrophobic interaction. YadA, however, also mediated binding to one or more constituents present in intestinal mucus. Such binding led to decreased ability to penetrate a layer of mucus in vitro and subsequent decreased ability to adhere to BBVs. Based upon these results, it remains uncertain whether *Y. enterocolitica* is able to benefit from the YadA mediated adhesion in the intestinal millieu. In vivo results have suggested that expression of YadA confers on *Y. enterocolitica* an increased ability to colonize the intestine, but no definitive conclusions have been reached so far. A large number of antigens were identified in *Y. enterocolitica* by means of crossed immunoelectrophoresis (XIE).

Yersinae harbour Yop genes as virulence determinants. The gene is organized in several operons scattered around a plasmid (VWa+). Yops are expressed at 37^{0}C *in vitro* in *Y.enterocolitica* and *Y.pseudotuberculosis* but not in *Y.pestis,* in which they are expressed only *in vivo.* They are regulated by a 20 Kb region of the plasmid called the calcium region or low calcium response (lcr) region.

The lcr region is conserved in both the species (Gyles 1993). YopN, which is part of the lcr E locus of *Y.pseudotuberculosis* encodes a surface exposed outer membrane protein of 33 kDa that work as a sensor along with calcium send a signal to inhibit transcription of Yop genes (Forsberg *et al.,* 1990).

At least 10 Yops have been described for *Y.enterocolitica.* Yad A is responsible for rendering *Y.enterocolitica* to complement mediated killing. Besides, YopS inhibit complement deposition on the bacteria thereby providing resistance to phagocytosis.

Laboratory Diagnosis

Diagnosis involves isolation of the agent from feces or lymph nodes aspirates. The organisms are shed by animals in the feces thus isolation alone is not of much value. The organisms grow well on blood agar and MacConkey agar at room temperature. If the number of organisms is suspected to be small, "cold enrichment" method is followed. In this procedure the incubation of a 10% mixture of inoculum in a minimal medium for several weeks at 4^{0}C is followed.

An ISO 10273 certified method for detecting pathogenic Yersinia using cultural techniques has been described by Fondrenez *et al.* (2010) from slaughtered pig tonsils. 900 tonsil swabs were taken from pigs at one slaughterhouse in Brittany, France. The swabs were vortexed in 10 ml PSB broth, then 1 ml was added to 9 ml ITC broth. The media were incubated for 48 h at 25°C. The PSB enrichment broth was streaked on CIN plates and the ITC enrichment broth on SSDC plates. In addition to the ISO 10273 method, we also streaked ITC enrichment broth on CIN plates. The plates were incubated for 24h at 30°C, and we then streaked a maximum of four typical colonies per plate onto a plate containing chromogenic medium (YeCM), for the isolation of pathogenic *Y. enterocolitica* isolates. In parallel, biochemical assays were carried out to confirm the identification of the isolates as *Yersinia* and to determine biotype. After passage on a YeCM plate and biochemical tests, 380 strains were confirmed to be pathogenic *Y. enterocolitica.* Finally, with the ISO 10273 method, 9.1% (CI(95%) [5.8-12.4]) of tonsil swabs and 60% (CI(95%) [45.4-74.6]) of the batches were positive. With the ITC-CIN method, 14.0% (CI95% [10.7-17.3]) of the tonsil swabs and 68.9% (CI(95%) [54.3-83.5]) of the batches were positive. Identification as pathogenic *Y. enterocolitica* was confirmed for 97.0% of the typical colonies obtained on the chromogenic medium, YeCM. The most prevalent biotype was biotype 4

(80.5% of the isolates), followed by biotype 3. This study demonstrates that the ITC-CIN method, followed by streaking on YeCM, may be an effective approach to the isolation of pathogenic *Y. enterocolitica* from tonsil swabs and the recovery of positive samples. This method is less time-consuming than the ISO 10273 method and reduces the number of biochemical tests required for the confirmation of *Yersinia* identification, through the use of YeCM.

Both the organisms are motile at 22-25⁰C. The organisms are gram-negative, non-spore forming, facultatively anaerobic rods or coccobacilli. Final species identification rests on biochemical characterization of isolates. The serotyping is also essential since, in case of *Y.pseudotuberculosis,* more than 90% of infections in human and animals are caused by O-group 1 strains. Guaranteed differentiation of typical strains is provided only by PCR-analysis using appropriate primers (Arseneva *et al.,* 2010). A multiplex PCR assay was developed for the detection and differentiation of the *Yersinia enterocolitica* and *Yersinia pseudotuberculosis* isolates in both pure bacterial cultures and pig tonsils (Kot *et al.,* 2007). The assay was based on the amplification of the ail, inv, yadA, and ystB genes. The PCR products, corresponding to the ail gene and the plasmid-borne yadA gene or only one product corresponding to the ail gene, were detected in *Y. enterocolitica* 4 biotype isolates. All of the *Y. pseudotuberculosis* isolates (n=6) tested gave a positive PCR reaction for the inv gene. For all tested *Y. enterocolitica* 1A biotype isolates (n=31), one product corresponding to the ystB gene was observed. The multiplex PCR assay was used to detect *Y. enterocolitica* and *Y. pseudotuberculosis* strains in pig tonsil samples obtained from 80 slaughtered pigs from three different herds. The presence of at least one of the specific PCR amplification products of ail-, ystB-, yadA-, and inv-specific sequences was observed in 11 samples (13.75%). These results of the multiplex PCR assay were compared with the results of conventional, microbiological testing. *Y. enterocolitica* isolates were cultured from only 3 (3.75%) of the 80 pig tonsils examined. The multiplex PCR assay was shown to be an efficient tool for differentiation between the pYV plasmid-bearing Y. enterocolitica isolates, the plasmidless *Y. enterocolitica* isolates, the *Y. enterocolitica* biotype 1A isolates, and the *Y. pseudotuberculosis* isolates with and without the pYV plasmid in naturally contaminated pig tonsils. This indicates that this assay is useful to control food processing and track the source of contamination.

Based on differences within the yopT-coding region of *Yersinia.* enterocolitica, *Y. pseudotuberculosis* and *Y. pestis,* a rapid and sensitive one-step polymerase chain reaction assay with high specificity for pathogenic *Y. enterocolitica* was developed (Arnold *et al.* 2003). By this method pathogenic isolates of *Y. enterocolitica* can be easily identified and discriminated from other members of this genus. The entire coding sequence of the yopT effector gene of *Y. pseudotuberculosis* Y36 was determined. Horisaka *et al.* (2004) developed a loop-mediated isothermal amplification method able to detect *Yersinia pseudotuberculosis* strains in 30 min by using six primers designed by targeting the inv gene. This method is more sensitive than PCR and might be a useful tool for detecting and identifying Y. pseudotuberculosis. A real time multiplex PCR assay for detection of *Yersinia pestis* and *Y.pseudotuberculosis* using a set of four primers has been described. The assay was found to be sensitive and specific (Matero *et al.,* 2009). Various target genes have been tested. Presently ail is the primary target gene for nucleic acid detection of pathogenic *Y.enterocolitica* (Huang *et al.,* 2010).

Treatment and Control

Tetracycline, trimethoprin- sulfonamides, aminoglycosides and chloramphenicol are antimicrobics of choice. Sulfonamides-trimethoprim is not found to be effective in cattle.

Pig strains of *Y.enterocolitica* have been found to be sensitive to amoxicillin, cefotaxime, chloramphenicol, ciprofloxacin, trimethoprim-sulfamethaxozole and resistant to ampicillin, cephalothin, erythromycin, streptomycin and tetracycline (Terentieva and Berzins, 2010).

There is no conventional vaccine for the control of disease. The only vaccine currently available in zoos is Pseudovac (a mixture of killed strains of various serotypes), but its efficacy is not well established. It was shown that Pseudovac does not protect guinea pigs against a severe *Y. pseudotuberculosis* infection. Quintard *et al.* (2010) evaluated the possibility of using a live attenuated *Y. pseudotuberculosis* strain (IP32680) as an oral vaccine against animal *pseudotuberculosis.* It was reported that IP32680 is avirulent for guinea pigs and induces a strong IgG response against various serotypes of *Y. pseudotuberculosis.* One and two oral inoculations of IP32680 provided 50% and 83% protection, respectively against a severe infection with a highly pathogenic strain. The avirulent *Y. pseudotuberculosis* IP32680 is therefore much more protective than Pseudovac and may represent a valuable oral vaccine against *pseudotuberculosis* in zoo animals. The use of live recombinant attenuated Salmonella vaccines (RASV) synthesizing *Yersinia* proteins is a promising approach for controlling infection by *Yersinia* species. Branger et al.(2009) constructed attenuated Salmonella strains which synthesize a truncated form of LcrV, LcrV196 and evaluated the immune response and protective efficacy elicited by these strains in mice against two other major species of *Yersinia: Yersinia pseudotuberculosis* and *Yersinia enterocolitica.* Surprisingly, it was found that the RASV strain alone was sufficient to afford nearly full protection against challenge with *Y. pseudotuberculosis,* indicating the likelihood that Salmonella produces immunogenic cross-protective antigens. In contrast, lcrV196 expression was required for protection against challenge with *Y. enterocolitica* strain 8081, but was not sufficient to achieve significant protection against challenge with *Y. enterocolitica* strain WA, which expressed a divergent form of lcrV. The plasmid encoded V antigen (Vag) of pathogenic *Yersinia* spp. is a major virulence factor as well as a protective immunogen. Recently, two main types of Vag, represented by either Yersinia enterocolitica 0:8 or *Yersinia pseudotuberculosis*, have been identified and it has been suggested, that antibodies generated against one type are unable to protect against *Yersinia* spp. carrying the other type. By using a recombinant Vag (rVagHis) of the *Y. enterocolitica* 0:8 type Schmidt et al(1999) have shown, that actively immunized mice were completely protected against challenge with both, *Y. enterocolitica* 0:8 and *Y. pseudotuberculosis* serotype III. In addition, passive protection was possible with polyclonal rabbit anti-rVagHisIgG. However, while a single antibody dose (200 microgramg) was sufficient to protect against challenge with *Y. enterocolitica* 0:8, repetitive injections at intervals of 2 to 3 days were needed to protect against challenge with *Y. pseudotuberculosis* III. The apparent difference in protection correlated with a rapid disappearance of anti-rVagHisIgG from the circulation by days 3 to 4. The data therefore indicate, that expression of distinct types of Vag by Yersinia spp. does not necessarily exclude immunoprotection in mice immunized with the other type of Vag. It rather appears, that differences in immunoprotection between *Yersinia* species relate to the amount of cross-protective antibody. Finally, as revealed by the lack of complement-mediated killing and the lack of immunostaining of Yersiniae with anti-rVagHisantibodies, evidence is provided to indicate that immunoprotection does not occur via opsonisation or complement lysis.

There is no specific control but the maintenance of good nutrition is believed to be an important factor in avoiding clinical disease.

References

Alvarez, M.L. and Cardineau, G.A. 2010. Prevention of bubonic and pneumonic plague using plant derived vaccines. Biotechnol. Adv. **28:** 184-196.

Arnold T., Hensel A., Hagen R., Aleksic S., Neubauer H. and Scholz H.C.2001.A highly specific one-step PCR - assay for the rapid discrimination of enteropathogenic *Yersinia enterocolitica* from pathogenic *Yersinia pseudotuberculosis* and *Yersinia pestis*. Syst. Appl. Microbiol. **24:** 285-289.

Arseneva, T.E., Lebedeva, S.A., Trukhacher, A.L., Vasileva, E.A., Ivanova, V.S. and Bozko, N.V. 2010. [comparison of efficacy of tests for differentiation of typical and atypical strains of *Yersinia pestis* and *Yersinia pseudotuberculosis*] Zh. microbiol. Epidemiol. Immunobiol. July-Aug. **4:** 75-81.

Aragão A.I., Pinheiro K.M., Seoane A.C., Tavares C. and Almeida A.M.2009. [Prevalence of antibodies against *Yersinia pestis* in domestic carnivores, in plague foci in the State of Ceará]. Rev Soc Bras Med Trop. **42:** 711-715 [Article in Portuguese].

Bercovier, H. and Mollaret, H.M. 1984. Genus XIV. Yersinia Van Log hem 1944. In Bergey's Manuel of systematic bacteriology. Vol. 1 Ed. N.R. Krieg and J.G. Holtz, pp. 498-506. Baltimore; Williams and Wilkins.

Bhaduri, S., Chaney- Pope K. and Smith, J.F. 2010. A procedure for monitoring the presence of the virulent plasmid (pYV) in *Yersinia pestis* under culture conditions. Food borne Pathog. Dis. [http://www.ncbi.nlm.nih.gov/pubmed/ 21034234].

Bhagat, N. and Virdi, J.S. 2010. The enigma of *Yersinia enterocolitica* biovar 1A. Crit. Rev. Microbiol. [http://www.ncbi.nlm.nih.gov/pubmed/20883083].

Bhattacharya, D., Mecsas, J. and Hu L.T. 2010. Development of a vaccinia virus based reservoir – targeted vaccine against *Yersinia pestis*. Vaccine. **28:** 7683-7689.

Branger C.G., Torres-Escobar A., Sun W., Perry R., Fetherston J., Roland K.L. and Curtiss R. 2009.Oral vaccination with LcrV from Yersinia pestis KIM delivered by live attenuated Salmonella enterica serovar Typhimurium elicits a protective immune response against challenge with *Yersinia pseudotuberculosis* and *Yersinia enterocolitica*.Vaccine. **27:** 5363-5370. Epub 2009 Jul 9.

Butter, T. 1983. Plague and other *Yersinia* infection. New York: Plenum Press.

Chomel B.B., Jay M.T., Smith C.R., Kass P.H., Ryan C.P. and Barrett L.R.1994.Serological surveillance of plague in dogs and cats, California, 1979-1991. Comp. Immunol. Microbiol. Infect. Dis. **17:** 111-123.

DoY., Koh, H., Park, C.G., Dudziak, D., Seo, P., Mehandru, S., Choi, J.H., Cheong, C., Park, S., Perlin, D.S., Powell, B.S. and Steinman, R.M. 2010. Targetting of Ler V virulence protein from *Yersinia pestis* to dendritic cells protect mice against pneumonic plague. Eur. J. Immunol. **40:** 2791-2796.

El-Tahir, Y. and Skumik, M. 2010. Yad A, the multifaceted Yersinia adhesion. Int. J. Microbiol. **291:** 209-218.

Falcão J.P., Falcão D.P., Pitondo-Silva A., Malaspina A.C. and Brocchi M.2006.Molecular typing and virulence markers of *Yersinia enterocolitica* strains from human, animal and food origins isolated between 1968 and 2000 in Brazil. J. Med. Microbiol. **55** (Pt 11): 1539-48.

Felek, S., Tsang, T.M. and Krukonis, E.S. 2010. Three *Yersinia pestis* adhesions facilitate Yop delivery to eukaryotic cells and contribute to plague virulence. Infect. Immun. **78:** 4134-4150.

Fetherston J.D., Kirillina O., Bobrov A.G., Paulley J.T. and Perry R.D.2010.The yersiniabactin transport system is critical for the pathogenesis of bubonic and pneumonic plague. Infect Immun. **78:** 2045-2052. Epub 2010 Feb 16

Fondrevez, M., Labbe, A., Hourad, E., Fravalo, P., Madec, F. and Denis, M. 2010. A simplified method for detecting pathogenic *Yersinia enterocolitica* in slaughtered pig tonsils. J. Microbiol. Methods. **83:** 244-249.

Forsberg, A., Viitawn, A.M., Skurnika, M., Wolf-Watz, H. and Straley, S.C. 1990. The surface located Yop N protein is involved in calcium transduction in *Yersinia pseudotuberculosis*. Mol. Microbiol. **5:** 997-986.

Fredriksson-Ahomaa M., Stolle A. and Stephan R.2007.Prevalence of pathogenic *Yersinia enterocolitica* in pigs slaughtered at a Swiss abattoir. Int. J. Food Microbiol. **119:** 207-212. Epub 2007 Aug 6.

Goodin, J.L., Powell, B.S., Enama, J.T., Raab, R.W., McKown, R.L., Coffman, G.L. and Andrews, G.P. 2010. Purification and characterization of a recombinant Yersinia pestis VF-1 Reversed fusion protein for use as a new subunit vaccine against plague. Protein Expr. Purif. [http://www.ncbi.nlm.nih.gov/pubmed/21055471].

Gyles, C.L. 1993. Yersinia. In pathogenesis of bacterial infections in animals. Ed. C.L. Gyles and C.O. Thoen. Pp. 226-235. Ames: IOWA State University press.

Hering, N.A., Richter, J.F., Krug, S.M., Gunzel, D., Fromm, A., Bohn, E., Rosenthal, R., Bucker, R. Fromm, M., Troegar, H. and Schulzke, J.D. 2010. *Yersinia enterocolitica* induces epithelial barrier dysfaction through regional tight junction changes in colorie HT-29/B6 cell monolayer Lab. Invest. [http://www.ncbi.nlm.nih.gov/pubmed/20956974].

Horisaka T., Fujita K., Iwata T., Nakadai A., Okatani A.T., Horikita T., Taniguchi T., Honda E., Yokomizo Y. and Hayashidani H.2004.Sensitive and specific detection of *Yersinia pseudotuberculosis* by loop-mediated isothermal amplification. J. Clin. Microbiol. **42:** 5349-5352.

Huang, Y., Wang, X., Cut, Z., Yang, Y., Xiao, Y., Tang, L., Kan, B., Xu, J. And Jing, H. 2010. Possible use of ail and fox A polymorphisms for detecting pathogenic *Yersinia enterocolitica*. BMC Microbiol. **10:** 211.

Jones S.M., Griffin K.F., Hodgson I. and Williamson E.D.2003.Protective efficacy of a fully recombinant plague vaccine in the guinea pig. Vaccine. **21**(25-26): 3912-8.

Korte T., Fredriksson-Ahomaa M., Niskanen T. and Korkeala H.2004.Low prevalence of yadA-positive *Yersinia enterocolitica* in sows. Foodborne Pathog. Dis. **1:** 45-52.

Kot, B., Piechota, M. and Jakubczak, A. 2010. Analysis of occurrence of virulence genes among *Yersinia enterocolitica* isolates belonging to different biotypes and serotypes. Pol. J. Vet. Sci. **13:** 13-19.

Kot B., Trafny E.A. and Jakubczak A.2007.Application of multiplex PCR for monitoring colonization of pig tonsils by *Yersinia enterocolitica*, including biotype 1A, and *Yersinia pseudotuberculosis*. J. Food Prot. **70:** 1110-1115.

Layton R.C., Mega W., McDonald J.D., Brasel T.L., Barr E.B., Gigliotti A.P. and Koster F.2011Levofloxacin cures experimental pneumonic plague in African green monkeys. PLoS Negl Trop Dis. **5:** e959.

Leo JC, Skurnik M.2011Adhesins of human pathogens from the genus yersinia. Adv Exp Med Biol. 2011; **715:** 1-15.

Martínez P.O., Fredriksson-Ahomaa M., Sokolova Y., Roasto M., Berzins A. and Korkeala H.2009.Prevalence of enteropathogenic *Yersinia* in Estonian, Latvian, and Russian (Leningrad region) pigs. Foodborne Pathog. Dis. **6:** 719-724.

Matero, P., Pasanen, T., Laukkanen, R., Tissari, P., Tarkka, E., Vaara, M. and Skurmik, M. 2009. Real time multiplex PCR assay for detection of *Yersinia pestis* and *Yersinia pseudotuberculosis*. APMIS. **117:** 34-44.

Miller, V.L., Finlay, B.B. and Falkow, S. 1988. Factors essential for the penetration of mammalian cells by *Yersinia*. Curr. Top. Microbiol. Immunol. **138:** 15-39.

Ortiz Martinez, P., Nylona, S., Drake, I., Fredriksson-Ahomaa, M., Korkeala, H. and Corry, J.E. 2010. Wide variety of bioserotypes of enteropathogenic *yersinia* in tonsils of English pigs at slaughter. Int. J. Food. Microbiol. **139:** 64-69.

Paerregaard A.1992. Interactions between *Yersinia enterocolitica* and the host with special reference to virulence plasmid encoded adhesion and humoral immunity. Dan Med Bull. **39:** 155-172.

Paerregaard, A. 2010. Interactions between *Yersinia enterocolitica* and the host with special reference to virulence plasmid encoded adhesion and humoral immunity. Don Med. Bull. **39:** 155-172.

Perry R.D. and Fetherston J.D.2011.*Yersiniabactin* iron uptake: Mechanisms and role in Yersinia pestis pathogenesis. Microbes Infect. 2011 May 12. [http://www.ncbi.nlm.nih.gov/pubmed/21609780].

Perry R.D., Balbo P.B., Jones H.A., Fetherston J.D. and DeMoll E.1999.Yersiniabactin from *Yersinia pestis*: biochemical characterization of the siderophore and its role in iron transport and regulation. Microbiology. **145**(Pt 5): 1181-1190.

Quintard B., Petit T., Ruvoen N., Carniel E. and Demeure C.E.2010.Efficacy of an oral live vaccine for veterinary use against *pseudotuberculosis*. Comp. Immunol. Microbiol. Infect. Dis. **33:** e59-65. Epub 2010 Jan 19.

Riehm, J.M., Rahalison, L., Scholz, H.C., Thoma, B., Pfeffer, M., Razanakoto, L.M., Al Dahouk, S., Newbauer, H. and Tomaso, H. 2010. Detection of *Yersinia pestis* using real time PCR in patients with suspected bubonic plague. Mol. Cell. Probes. [http://www.ncbi.nlm.nih.gov/pubmed/20933595].

Sampimon, O.C., Sol, J., Koene M.G., Van der Schaaf A. and Kock R.A.2005.[Mastitis caused by *Yersinia pseudotuberculosis* in a cow].Tijdschr. Diergeneestd. **30:** 307-308.

Sebbane F., Jarrett C., Gardner D., Long D. and Hinnebusch B.J.2010.Role of the Yersinia pestis *yersiniabactin* iron acquisition system in the incidence of flea-borne plague. PLoS One. **5:** e14379.

Schmidt A., Schaffelhofer S., Müller K., Röllinghoff M. and Beuscher H.U.1999Analysis of the *Yersinia enterocolitica* 0:8 V antigen for cross protectivity. Microb. Pathog. **26:** 221-233.

Sha J., Agar S.L., Baze W.B., Olano J.P., Fadl A.A., Erova T.E., Wang S., Foltz S.M., Suarez G., Motin V.L., Chauhan S., Klimpel G.R., Peterson J.W.. and Chopra A.K.2008.Braun lipoprotein (Lpp) contributes to virulence of yersiniae: potential role of Lpp in inducing bubonic and pneumonic plague. Infect. Immun. **76:** 1390-1409. Epub 2008 Jan 28.

Shwimmer A., Freed M., Blum S., Khatib N., Weissblit L., Friedman S. and Elad D.2007.Mastitis caused by *Yersinia pseudotuberculosis* in Israeli dairy cattle and public health implications. Zoonoses Public Health. **54:** 353-357.

Straley, S.C. 1991. The low - Ca + response virulence regulon of human pathogenic *yersinae*. Microb. Pathog. **10:** 87-91.

Terentieva, M. and Berzins, A. 2010. Prevalence and antimicrobial resistance of *Yersinia enterocolitica* and *Yersinia pseudotuberculosis* in slaughter pigs in Latvia. J. Food Prot. **73:** 1335-1338.

Thoerner P., Bin Kingombe C.I., Bögli-Stuber K., Bissig-Choisat B., Wassenaar T.M., Frey J. and Jemmi T.2003.PCR detection of virulence genes in *Yersinia enterocolitica* and *Yersinia pseudotuberculosis* and investigation of virulence gene distribution. Appl. Environ. Microbiol. **69:** 1810-1816.

Wake, A. and Moyan, H.R. 1986. Host parasite relationships and the *Yersinia* model. New York: Springer - Verlag.

Williamson E.D., Packer P.J., Waters E.L., Simpson A.J., Dyer D., Hartings J., Twenhafel N. and Pitt M.L.2011.Recombinant (F1+V) vaccine protects cynomolgus macaques against pneumonic plague. Vaccine. 2011 May 2. [http://www.ncbi.nlm.nih.gov/pubmed/21570437]

Yamanaka H., Hoyt T., Yang X., Bowen R., Golden S., Crist K., Becker T., Maddaloni M. and Pascual D.W.2010.A parenteral DNA vaccine protects against pneumonic plague. Vaccine. **28:** 3219-3230. Epub 2010 Mar 1.

Zheng H., Sun Y., Mao Z. and Jiang B..2008. Investigation of virulence genes in clinical isolates of *Yersinia enterocolitica*. FEMS Immunol. Med. Microbiol. **53:** 368-374. Epub 2008 Jun 28.

□□□

Chapter 13

Mycobacterium Avium Subsp. Paratuberculosis

Dr. S.K. SRIVASTAVA
Former, Division of Bacteriology & Mycology
Indian Veterinary Research Institute, Izatnagar-243122
Bareilly (U.P.)

Mycobacterium avium subsp. paratuberculosis

M.avium subsp. paratuberculosis (*M.paratuberculosis*) is the causative agent of a transmissible chronic wasting disease involving intestine of ruminants called paratuberculosis (Chiodini *et al.*, 1984). It is a rod shaped bacillus, acid-fast, non-spore forming and strictly aerobe. It does not stain by gram method because of the rich mycolic acid content of the cell wall. Extracts of broth cultures of *M.paratuberculosis* contain the protein derivative called johnin which is responsible for eliciting delayed type hypersensitivity reaction in skin of affected animals. Two genotypically and microbiologically distinct strains of *M.paratuberculosis* exist- S and C MAP strains that primarily infect sheep and cattle, respectively (Janagama *et al.*, 2010). *M.paratuberculosis* like organisms have been isolated from humans with crohn's disease (regional ileitis), a disease remarkably similar to johne's disease.

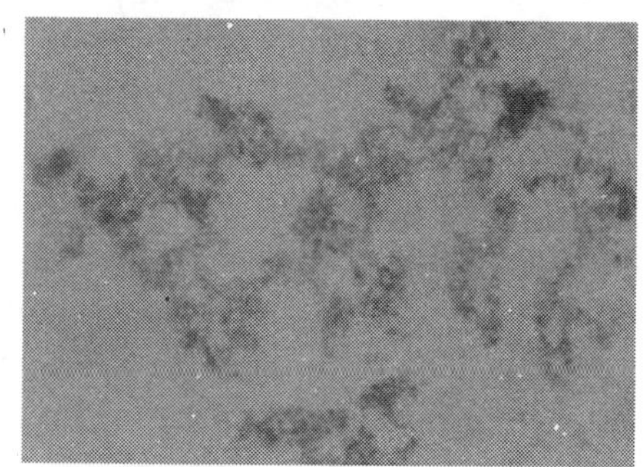

M.paratuberculosis gram stained

Iron-acquiring substances exochelins and mycobactin (a complex lipid) may be responsible for intracellular growth. Exochelins are protein in nature responsible for removing ferric iron from ferritin. Mycobactin in the cell membrane of the organisms perform the function of transferring iron from the exochelin to the bacterium. M.paratuberculosis depend on mycobactin for its growth. This property is shared with other mycobacteria eg. M.avium. Most *M.paratuberculosis* strains are stimulated by pyruvate.

On the basis of cultural phenotypes and IS 1311 PCR-REA, strains have been genotyped as "Cattle type", "Sheep type" and "Bison type". Recently a new Indian Bison type has been reported as a strain causing disease in India (Sohal *et al.*, 2000). Genotype diversity among Indian animal strains has been reported on the basis of IS900 and IS 1311 PCR-REA. Majority was "Indian Bison type" and remaining cattle type (Singh *et al.*, 2010).

The disease affects cattle, sheep, goats and other wild and domestic ruminants. It is present worldwide however, exact incidence of the disease is difficult to assess. It may be sufficiently prevalent in some herds to constitute a real problem. In some herds the prevalence is increasing. It is most common in cattle followed by sheep and goats. Sheep are easily infected experimentally and excrete large number of organisms but may recover spontaneously. Pigs mixed with infected cattle may develop enlargement of the lymph nodes suggestive of tuberculosis and from which the causative agent can be isolated. The salvage value of clinically affected animals is usually negligible because of severe emaciation.

Paratuberculosis of camels, locally called Silag in the Arab world, is a serious and invariably fatal disease in the Arabian camel. Six camels were used in this study. Five camels with clinical paratuberculosis were used to study the pathology of the disease and confirm its aetiology. The sixth camel was clinically healthy and used as a control. The camels were examined clinically and bled for haematological and blood chemistry analysis. They were then humanely killed with a high intravenous dose of thiopental sodium (10 mg/kg) for pathological studies as well as obtaining tissues for microbiological and molecular studies. The clinical signs of the disease were emaciation, diarrhoea, alopecia, wry neck and pale mucous membranes. Laboratory diagnosis showed reduced haemoglobin concentration, low haematocrit and high activity of the serum enzyme alanine aminotransferase. Serum creatinine concentration was normal. These results indicated the infected camels were anaemic and the function of their livers was affected. Postmortem examination showed thickened and corrugated intestinal mucosa, enlarged granulomatous mesenteric lymph nodes, miliary and diffuse granulomas in the liver (in four camels), generalized lymph node granulomas (in one camel), splenic granuloma (in one camel) and mediastinal lymph node granuloma (in two camels). Histopathological examination showed diffuse infiltration of macrophages in all organs showing lesions. Ziehl-Neelsen staining of tissue scraping and tissue sections showed masses of acid fast bacilli, except for the spleen. Infection with *Mycobacterium avium* subsp. paratuberculosis was confirmed by PCR by targeting the IS900 gene (Alharbi *et al.*, 2011).

A distinguishing characteristic of johne's disease is that infection occurs in animals at a very early age usually under 30 days of age and clinical disease does not occur until 3-5 years of age. However, on extreme circumstances the disease can occur at 12-18 months of age in calves kept under contaminated environment. Stress, including parturition, transportation and nutritional deficiencies may influence the development of clinical disease.

In cattle, clinical signs commonly appear at 2-6 years of age. Emaciation with submandibular oedema are commonly observed. The submandibular oedema disappears as the diarrhoea develops. A fall in milk yield is observed before the diarrhoea. In the feces there is absence of blood, epithelial debris and mucus. Diarrhoea may be marked or intermittent with the tendency to improve in late pregnancy which reappears after the parturition. The course of disease varies from a few weeks to months but severe dehydration, emaciation and weakness is common. In sheep and goats the disease is manifested principally by emaciation, with shedding of wool in sheep. There is loss of weight in both species with soft and pasty feces.

Calves experimentally infected via Payer's patches show colonization of M.paratuberculosis in ileocecal lymph nodes and ileocecal junction were consistently observed. Flow cytometry revealed the presence of interferon gamma and interleukin locally and systematically (Plattner et al., 2010). Clinical disease occurs mostly under conditions of domestication or captivity especially in association with stress factors such as parturition, crowding, shipment or faulty dietary regimes.

Pathogenesis

Infection with M.paratuberculosis occurs primarily in young animals through the fecal-oral route. The organisms, interacts with M cells in intestine through payer's patches. Studies have shown that M.paratuberculosis enters the intestinal mucosa through enterocytes with absence of M cells. It was also shown to interact with epithelial cells by an alpha (5) beta (1) integrin-in dependent pathway (Bermudez et al., 2010). Transplacental and transuterine routes have also been suggested. In utero infection of cattle may retard the success of the disease control programme if postnatal transmission is controlled (Whittington and Windsor 2009). After an incubation period of 1-5 years animals develop a general weakness, rough hair coat, chronic weight loss and intermittent diarrhoea. After a few months, severe diarrhoea, emaciation, ventral oedema, debility and death occurs. After the oral ingestion the organisms localizes in the mucosa of the small intestine, its associated lymph nodes and to a lesser extent in the tonsils and suprapharyngeal lymph nodes. Bacteria primarily multiply in the terminal part of the small intestine and large intestine. The organism has been isolated from the udder and reproductive tract of both male and female cattle. Disseminated paratuberculosis of both kidneys of cows have been reported. The animal may resist the infection at the first stage and the shedder stage does not develop or shed intermittently. The ileum and colon are usually involved and the infection may extend up to rectum in advanced cases. The mucous membrane become corrugated and thickened because of epithelioid and giant cells both of which contain many cells. The organisms are phagocytozed by macrophages which in turn proliferate in large number in large intestinal particularly in ileo-cecal region, and infiltrate the intestinal submucosa. Ingested microbes limit production of superoxides and discourage fusion of lysosomes with phagosomes and multiply in macrophages. This results in decreased absorption, chronic diarrhoea and resulting malabsorption. The penetration of epithelial cells is through the M cells (Momotani et al., 1988). If the infection progresses there is an immune mediated granulomatous reaction in the submucosa with the accumulation of large number of macrophaes and lymphocytes. The mortality is caused in large part by this mal absorption of amino acids and loss of protein in the intestine (protein losing enteropathy). The migration of macrophages and lymphocytes is mediated by cytokines such as IL-12 and gamma - interferon. These are aided by T-helper cells secreting cytokines associated with a cell mediated immune response. These infected macrophages do not respond well to these cytokines signal, subsequently they accumulate in the submucosa and later sloughed off. A study has shown that T helper cell activity is hindered in animals with clinical disease. It has also been shown that general cellular responses in infected cattle are depressed as compared to normal cattle (Kruger and Snider 1992) which suggest a predominance of type-2 activity. A suppressed helper cell activity does not properly activate mono-nuclear phagocytes which lead to bacterial proliferation. This may result in energy at the later stage of the disease. Studies have suggested role of gamma/delta T lymphocytes in immuno-pathogenesis of *M.paratuberculosis* infection. These cells are toxic to specific $CD4^+$ TH1 lymphocytes. This toxicity is regulated by CD8+ T lymphocytes. No serological or cellular immunity test will identify all the infected animals. The lymphocytes proliferation test is positive because their circulating lymphocytes are sanitized. Interleukin 10 (IL-10) activity is lowered as animals reach terminal stage of the disease. IL-10 can suppress Th-1 type and enhance Th-2 type cytokine production. The IL-10 production increase soon after exposure of animals to *M.paratuberculosis* suggesting that IL-10 production may play a role in disease outcome (de Silva *et al.,* 2010).

The intracellular *M.paratuberculosis* acquires iron for growth with the excretion of exochelins which remove iron from macrophage ferritin. There is evidence that iron-availability dictates the distribution of *M.paratuberculosis* with most iron available with in macrophages of nodules in the ileocecal area.

Release of IL-12 by affected macrophages initiates the imflammatory and immune response. The responses are initiated by the recruitment of specific CD4+ TH1 cells and subsequent release of cytokines leading to the attraction of macrophages to the site of interaction of M.paratuberculosis and macrophages. Gamma-interferon activates macrophages to tackle effectively the ingested mycobacteria although gamma interferon released by lymphocytes is a poor activator of *M.paratuberculosis* infected macrophages.

The interaction between these cells results in formation of a slowly progressing granulomations reaction. The granulomatous response and cellular infiltrate, which is within the lamina propria ultimately leads to sloughing of the mucosal epithelium and release of infected macrophages and mycobacteria into the human. However the extent of infiltration is not always related to the severity of the disease.

The key features of host immunity to *M. avium* subsp. paratuberculosis infection include an appropriate early proinflammatory and cytotoxic response (Th1-like) that eventually gives way to a predominant antibody-based response (Th2-like). Clinical disease symptoms often appear subsequent to waning of the Th1-like immune response. Understanding why this shift in the immune response occurs and the underlying molecular mechanisms involved is critical to future control measures and diagnosis. Previous studies have suggested that M. avium subsp. paratuberculosis may suppress gene expression in peripheral blood mononuclear cells (PBMCs) from infected cows, despite a continued inflammatory reaction at sites of infection. In the present study, we tested the hypothesis that exposure to *M. avium* subsp. *paratuberculosis* suppresses a proinflammatory gene expression pattern in PBMCs from infected cows. Cossens et al.(2004) examined expression of genes encoding interleukin-1alpha (IL-1alpha), IL-2, IL-4, IL-5, IL-6, IL-8, IL-10, IL-12p35, IL-16, and IL-18, as well as genes encoding γ interferon (IFN-γ), transforming growth factor beta (TGF-β), and tumor necrosis factor alpha (TNF-α), in PBMCs, intestinal lesions, and mesenteric lymph nodes of cattle naturally infected with *M. avium* subsp. *paratuberculosis*. Cytokine gene expression in these cells and tissues was compared to expression in similar cells and tissues from control uninfected cattle. Our comprehensive results demonstrate that for most cytokine genes, including the genes encoding IFN-gamma, TGF-β,

TNF-α, IL-α, IL-4, IL-6, IL-8, and IL-12p35, differential expression in PBMCs from infected and control cattle did not require stimulation with *M. avium* subsp. *paratuberculosis*. In fact, stimulation with *M. avium* subsp. paratuberculosis tended to reduce the differential expression observed in infected and uninfected cows for genes encoding IFN-γ, IL-α, and IL-6. Only IL-10 gene expression was consistently enhanced by *M. avium* subsp. *paratuberculosis* stimulation of PBMCs from subclinically infected cattle. In ileal tissues from *M. avium* subsp. paratuberculosis-infected cattle, expression of the genes encoding IFN-γ, TGF-β, IL-5, and IL-8 was greater than the expression in comparable tissues from control uninfected cattle, while expression of the gene encoding IL-16 was lower in tissues from infected cattle than in control tissues. Mesenteric lymph nodes draining sites of *M. avium* subsp. *paratuberculosis* infection expressed higher levels of IL-α, IL-8, IL-2, and IL-10 mRNA than similar tissues from control uninfected cattle expressed. In contrast, the genes encoding TGF-β and IL-16 were expressed at lower levels in lymph nodes from infected cattle than in tissues from uninfected cattle. Taken together, our results suggest that cells or other mechanisms capable of limiting proinflammatory responses to *M. avium* subsp. *paratuberculosis* develop in infected cattle and that a likely place for development and expansion of these cell populations is the mesenteric lymph nodes draining sites of infection.

Although the presence or absence of intestinal lesions cannot be used as a definitive indicator of *M. avium* subsp. *paratuberculosis* infection, most infected cattle exhibit significant changes to intestinal mucosa, with the focus of pathology surrounding the ileal cecal junction. Typical pathology of *M. avium* subsp. *paratuberculosis* infection includes inflammation, thickening of the lumenal wall, and hyperplasia in draining lymph nodes. To further understand the pathology of Johne's disease, we compared the gene expression profiles of ileal tissues from Johne's disease-positive (n = 6), and Johne's disease-negative (n = 5) Holstein cattle. Gene expression profiles were compared with a bovine total leukocyte (BOTL-3) cDNA microarray. Genes that were expressed at significantly higher levels (>1.5-fold; $P < 0.05$) in tissues from Johne's disease-infected animals relative to noninfected animals included those encoding tumor necrosis factor receptor-associated protein 1 (TRAF1), interleukin-1alpha (IL-1alpha), MCP-2, N-cadherin, and beta1 integrin (CD29). Dramatic upregulation of IL-1alpha (21.5-fold) and TRAF1 (27.5-fold) gene expression in tissues of Johne's disease-positive cows relative to tissues from control cows was confirmed by quantitative real-time PCR. Western blot analysis confirmed that IL-1alpha and TRAF1 mRNA levels resulted in increased protein expression in tissues of Johne's disease-positive cattle relative to tissues from control cattle. High levels of IL-1alpha can produce symptoms similar to those found in clinical Johne's disease. Taken together, the data presented in this report suggest that many outward symptoms of Johne's disease may be due to IL-1alpha toxicity. In addition, enhanced levels of TRAF1 could result in cells within the lesions of Johne's disease-positive cattle that are highly resistant to TNF-alpha-induced signaling(Aho *et al.*, 2003).

A theme among many pathogenic mycobacterial species affecting both humans and animals is a prolonged asymptomatic or latent period that can last years to decades. The mechanisms that favor progression to active disease are not well understood. Pathogen containment is often associated with an effective cell-mediated or T-helper 1 immune profile. With certain pathogenic mycobacteria, such as *Mycobacterium avium* subspecies *paratuberculosis*, a shift to active clinical disease is associated with loss of T-helper 1 immunity and development of an ineffective humoral or T-helper 2 immune response. Recently γδ T cells have been shown to play a role early in mycobacterial infections and have been hypothesized to influence disease outcome (Plattner and Hostetter 2011).

Extra intestinal localization indicates a hematogenous phase of the disease. There is a direct correlation between the degree of dissemination and the number of *M.tuberculosis* in feces. Infected blood monocytes have been demonstrated which may help in dissemination of the bacteria to other sites. The post primary dissemination of lesions is more widespread in adult animals than in calves. A recombinant heparin binding haemagglutinin from M.paratuberculosis has been reported (Sechi *et al.*, 2006). This protein was found to be immunogenic with cross reactivity observed with M.bovis. Report has suggested that this could be associated with virulence of M.paratuberculosis.

The lesion and host responses are manifestation of cellular immunity. Problems such as decreased milk production and increased calving intervals may be due to generalized immunosuppression observed in infected animals. There is also development of sensitization to johnin and to mammalian and avian tuberculin. The sensitivity usually develops in the preclinical stage but disappears in most cases by the time clinical sign are evident.

Laboratory Diagnosis

Sample collection and their microscopic examination are carried out. From cattle samples (intestinal or lymph nodes) ileocecal areas are collected and obtained for necropsy and stained by Ziehl-Neelson method. From live animals mucosal scraping from the rectum are collected. On average, the rectal smear will only detect about 25% of infected animals. Rectal pinch examination is useful than fecal examination. From sheep and goats lymph nodes from ileocecal areas are examined. Sheep may also express the organism in blood during the late phase of the infection (Bower *et al.,* 2010). On staining the organisms appear as short pinkish red rods occurring in bunches. Other acid fast staining bacteria will be singly located or quite large in size. Bovine feces contain several saprophytic bacteria that can be mistaken for Johne's bacilli. Masses of intra and extra cellular organisms are demonstrated in typical granulomatous lesions.

For isolation fecal samples or tissues are examined. The samples are first decontaminated with hexadecyl pyridinium chloride and placed in Herrold egg yolk medium containing mycobactin – J. Because some strains are inhibited by sodium pyruvate, egg yolk medium with or without pyruvate are used for isolation. Nicotinic acid, nicotinamide and α – and β- NAD enhances the growth of *M.paratuberculosis* (Greenstein *et al.,* 2010). Time taken to develop visible colonies is about 8 weeks. Identification is based on cultural (including growth rate and mycobactin dependency), morphologic and staining characteristics and seroagglutination.

Detection of MAP from milk and dairy products has been reported from countries on the European continent, Argentina, the UK and Australia. In one study three different methods (quantitative real time PCR, combined phage IS900 PCR and conventional cultivation) were used to detect the presence of MAP in bulk tank milk (BTM) and cheese originating from sheep, goat and mixed milks from farms and products in Cyprus (Botsaris et al.2010). During the first survey the presence of MAP was detected in 63 (28.6%) of cows' BTM samples by quantitative real time PCR. A second survey of BTM used a new combined phage IS900 PCR assay, and in this case MAP was detected in 50 (22.2%) samples showing a good level of agreement by both methods. None of the herds tested were known to be affected by Johne's disease and the presence of viable MAP was confirmed by conventional culture in only two cases of cows BTM. This suggests that either rapid method used is more sensitive than the conventional culture when testing raw milk samples for MAP. The two isolates recovered from BTM were identified by IS1311 PCR REA as cattle and sheep strains, respectively. In contrast when cheese samples were tested, MAP DNA was detected by quantitative real time PCR in seven (25.0%) samples (n=28). However no viable MAP was detected when either the combined phage IS900 PCR or conventional culture methods were used.

Grant *et al.* (2000) tested the potential use of a novel immunomagnetic PCR (IMS-PCR) technique as a rapid method to screen milk samples for the presence of *Mycobacterium avium* subsp. *paratuberculosis* (*M. ptb*). Immunomagnetic separation (IMS) for *M. ptb*, developed at Queen's University, Belfast, was applied to milk samples prior to IS900 PCR in order to selectively concentrate any *M. ptb* cells present and, at the same time, separate the cells from constituents of milk likely to inhibit subsequent PCR. This increased the sensitivity of IS900 PCR. IMS-PCR sensitivity could be further increased by initial centrifugation (2500 g for 20 min) of larger volumes of milk (10 and 50 ml), and resuspension of the sediment into a 1 ml volume appropriate for IMS treatment. Following IMS, template DNA for IS900 PCR was obtained by heating the bead-cell suspension in a thermal cycler at 100 degrees C for 15 min. It was estimated that the IMS-PCR assay could detect approximately 10(3)CFU of M. ptb per 50 ml of milk (equivalent to 20 CFU/ml), whereas the minimum detection limit of direct IS900 PCR was estimated at 10(5)CFU of *M. ptb* per 50 ml (equivalent to 2000 CFU/ml). A blind trial was carried out in which a total of 40 spiked (10(6)CFU M. ptb) and unspiked, raw and laboratory-pasteurized milk samples were independently tested by IMS-PCR and conventional IS900 PCR. IMS-PCR correctly identified 97. 5% of milk samples (sensitivity 100%, specificity 95%), including spiked milk samples before and after laboratory-pasteurization. One false positive result was obtained which may have resulted from carryover between samples during the IMS procedure. Conventional IS900 PCR correctly identified only 72.5% of the same 40 milk samples (sensitivity 23%, specificity 100%). IMS-PCR was also shown to be capable of detecting natural *M. ptb* infection in raw sheep's milk, and raw and commercially pasteurized cows' milk.

A polymerase chain reaction (PCR)-based assay was developed for detection of insertion sequence 900 (IS900) of Mycobacterium avium subsp. paratuberculosis in raw milk (Pillai and Jayarao 2002). This IS900 PCR assay included DNA extraction and PCR assay using commercially available kits. The DNA extraction and PCR assay were optimized to detect the IS900 sequence directly from raw milk. The IS900 PCR assay was evaluated by inoculating raw bulk milk and Middlebrook's 7H9 broth with 0 to 10(8) cfu/ml of each of four American Type Culture Collection strains of M. paratuberculosis. Under experimental conditions, both milk culture on Herrold's egg yolk medium slants, and IS900 PCR could detect 10 to 100 cfu/ml of M. paratuberculosis. Detection of M. paratuberculosis by IS900 PCR was consistent (24/24 PCR assays) when about 100 cfu/ml were present, whereas detection was variable (12/24 PCR assays) at concentrations as low as 10 cfu/ml. Based on the findings of the experimental study, IS900 PCR was further evaluated with pooled quarter milk samples from 211 cows from five herds with known history of Johne's disease. Out of 211 animals examined, nine (4%) and 69 (33%) were positive for *M. paratuberculosis* by milk culture and IS900 PCR from milk, respectively. A total of 20 bulk tank milk sample aliquots (one sample, four aliquots from each herd) were also examined, of which 10 (50%) were positive for *M. paratuberculosis* by IS900 PCR. By contrast, only one out of 20 (5%) bulk tank milk sample aliquots was positive by culture. The IS900 PCR amplified product of 229-bp obtained on testing of quarter milk and bulk tank milk samples was confirmed to be the IS900 of *M. paratuberculosis* by DNA sequence analysis. The results of this study suggest that M. paratuberculosis can be detected directly from quarter milk and bulk tank milk by IS900 PCR. Shankar et al.(2010) evaluated commercially available unpasteurized and pasteurized milk and its products for the presence of viable MAP or MAP DNA from an area of northern India with a population of 150 million people. 43 samples (16 unpasteurized, 27 pasteurized) purchased in Mathura, Agra, or New Delhi, for the presence of MAP by culture or by PCR for IS900 MAP DN were stdied. A. Positives results were confirmed as MAP by restriction endonuclease analysis and/or DNA sequencing.Colonies appeared in 1.5-20 months post-inoculation. Of the unpasteurized samples, 44% (7/16) were MAP culture-positive and 6% (1/16) were positive for IS900 MAP DNA. Of the pasteurized samples, 67% (18/27) were MAP culture-positive and 33% (9/27) were IS900-positive. Subsequently, 100% (25/25) of the cultured colonies were IS900 and IS1311 MAP DNA-positive.This is the first report from a developing country of MAP cultured from both pasteurized and unpasteurized milk and milk products. With the increasing concern that MAP may be zoonotic, these findings have major implications for healthcare in India. The decreased sensitivity in detecting MAP DNA by PCR directly from milk should be ascribed to employing only one set of PCR primers.

A study was conducted to evaluate sensitivity, specificity, and predictive value of IS900-PCR assay for detection of *Mycobacterium avium* subspecies *paratuberculosis* in pooled quarter milk and bulk tank milk (Jayarao et al 2004). Feces, blood and pooled quarter milk from 1493 lactating cattle on 29 herds were analyzed. Bulk tank milk (n = 29 bulk tanks) samples were also examined. Culture analysis revealed that 10.9%, 2.8%, and 20.6% of fecal, pooled quarter milk samples and bulk tanks were positive for *M. avium* subsp. *paratuberculosis,* respectively. While 13.5% and 27.5% of pooled quarter milk samples and bulk tanks were positive by IS900 PCR assay, respectively. Moderate to high antibody titers for *M. avium* subsp. *paratuberculosis* were detected in 223 of 1493 (14.4%) cows. Cows positive on fecal culture were taken as true positives relative to which the IS900 PCR assay was evaluated. The sensitivity and predictive value of KELA, pooled quarter milk culture, and IS900 PCR assay increased with lactation age. While the specificity of the tests decreased with increase in lactation age. Overall, the IS900 PCR assay using pooled quarter milk samples had a sensitivity, specificity and predictive value of 0.87, 0.95 and 0.71, respectively. The IS900 PCR assay using bulk tank milk had poor sensitivity (0.21), specificity (0.5) and predictive value (0.6). Pooled quarter milk culture analysis had a very low sensitivity (0.17).

The kinetics ELISA had lower sensitivity (0.59), specificity (0.90) and predictive value (0.43) as compared to the IS900 PCR assay using pooled quarter milk samples. Results from our study suggest that IS900 PCR assay using bulk tank milk may not be useful for screening herds with M. avium subsp. paratuberculosis infected animals. In conclusion, use of IS900 PCR assay for cows in 2(nd) lactation and higher, using aseptically collected pooled quarter milk samples, can be a useful tool for screening and monitoring lactating cattle in herds with *M. avium* subsp. *paratuberculosis* infection.

Numerous reports have described diagnostic methods based on the polymerase chain reaction (PCR) used to detect Mycobacterium avium subsp. paratuberculosis, the causative agent of Johne's disease. The result of conventional PCR tests has been only qualitative, either positive or negative; it does not present any quantitative information about the number of the agents in the specimen. A quantitative PCR method (IS900 TaqMan) was developed to measure the number of *M. paratuberculosis* organisms present in field and clinical samples. The sensitivity of IS900 TaqMan was 1 colony-forming unit (CFU) for *M. paratuberculosis* ATCC 19698. The specificity of the method was determined by testing 14 mycobacterial species (*M. abscessus, M. asiaticum, M. avium* subsp. *avium, M. bovis, M. fortuitum* subsp. *fortuitum, M. intracellulare, M. kansasii, M. marinum, M. phlei, M. scrofulaceum, M. simiae, M. smegmatis, M. terrae,* and *M. ulcerans*) and 9 nonmycobacterial species (*Borrelia burgdorferi, Chlamydia psittaci, Ehrlichia canis, E. equi, E. risticii, Escherichia coli, E. coli* O157:H7, *Streptococcus equi,* and *S. zooepidemicus*). Even at high cell numbers (10(5) CFU/reaction), most of the organisms tested negative for the IS900 insertion element except *M. marinum* and *M. scrofulaceum* (Kim *et al.*, 2002). This finding for *M. scrofulaceum* was consistent with previous reports that several *M. scrofulaceum*-like isolates were positive for IS900. Those isolates had 71-79% homology with M. a. paratuberculosis in the region of IS900. When used in conjunction with the new liquid medium-based ESP culture system II for bovine clinical fecal samples, IS900 TaqMan confirmed that the ESP II-positive samples contained 10(5)-10(6) CFU/ml of M. a. paratuberculosis. All of the 222 ESP II-positive and acid-fast bacilli-positive samples tested in this study were positive by IS900 TaqMan. IS900 TaqMan was also useful in the study of growth characteristics of 3 groups of *M. paratuberculosis* strains in bovine fecal samples from 3 shedding levels (heavy, medium, and low) based on cell numbers measured by Herrold egg yolk (HEY) agar culture. When cultured in ESP medium, *M. paratuberculosis* reached 10(5)-10(6) CFU/ml within 2 weeks for heavy shedders, 3-4 weeks for medium, and 6-8 weeks for low shedders. No significant growth was observed after up to 5 weeks of incubation for some of low shedders. No or extremely slow growth characteristic of low shedders might be a possible explanation for frequent false-negative results by HEY. The detection time was dependent on the inoculum size and the growth rate of *M. paratuberculosis*. Generation times were inversely proportional to the shedding level: 1-2 days for medium and heavy shedders and >4 days for low shedders. IS900 TaqMan could be a useful tool for determining viable cell counts by measuring changes in cell numbers over the incubation period.

Stabel and Banantine (2005) describe the development of a nested PCR assay that uses a unique element (ISMap02) for Mycobacterium avium subsp. paratuberculosis that is present at six copies within the genome. In addition, the sensitivity of the assay with this element was compared to the sensitivity of detection of the IS900 element in both conventional and real-time PCR assays. The specificity of the ISMap02 element was evaluated by PCR of the DNA extracted from isolates of *M. avium* subsp. *paratuberculosis* and *M. avium* subsp. avium, as well as DNA from *M. fortuitum, M. scofulaceum, M. phlei, M. smegmatis,* and *M. gordonae*. Only *M. avium* subsp. *paratuberculosis* DNA was detectable after amplification with the ISMap02 primers. The sensitivity of detection for the ISMap02 element in either a conventional or a real-time PCR format was less than 100 fg DNA or 10(2) CFU/ml in serial titration curves with pure bacteria. These results were comparable to those obtained for the IS900 element. Experimental spiking of a negative fecal sample followed by M. avium subsp. paratuberculosis DNA extraction resulted in detection thresholds of 10(2) CFU/g for the IS900 element and 10(3) CFU/g for the ISMap02 element by using a real-time PCR format, but this sensitivity dropped 10-fold for both elements in a conventional PCR format. Analyses of fecal samples obtained from naturally infected animals demonstrated a sensitivity for the detection of *M. avium* subsp. *paratuberculosis* DNA by use of the ISMap02 element similar to that achieved by use of the IS900 element when it was used in a conventional PCR format. The real-time PCR format improved the levels of detection of both elements, but not to a significant degree. In conclusion, the ISMap02 element provides a very sensitive and specific alternative as a diagnostic reagent for use in PCR assays for the detection of paratuberculosis.

A polymerase chain reaction for amplification of insertion sequence IS 900, a M.paratuberculosis specific sequence of DNA, has been described for rapid identification of the organisms in the bovine feces, tissues and blood monocytes. Use of monocytes is more sensitive than feces. A real time PCR assay targeting Mptb52.16 sequence has been used for quantification of low level of cells in raw and pasteurized milk. The target Mptb52.16 is promising with regard to the detection of viable cells (Dzieciol *et al.*, 2010) Chui et al. (2010) developed an immunocapture - polymerase chain reactions assay using

IgY to detect M. paratuberculosis in bovine feces. Real time Quantitative PCR is as effective as cultural method for detection of infection using fecal samples from affected animals (Aly *et al.*, 2010). The recent completion of the M. avium subsp. paratuberculosis genome sequence has provided some alternative genes that may be useful for diagnostic tests. Although the majority of the specific genes that have been identified thus far have been present at a single copy within the genome, one element has been found to be present at six copies. This element has been named ISMap02 and has no readily identifiable function at this time. However, due to its multiplicity within the genome, it may be useful as a target gene for diagnostic assays. The current study is an evaluation of the sensitivity and specificity of the newly identified ISMap02 element in both conventional and real-time PCR tests for the detection of M. avium subsp. paratuberculosis in bovine fecal samples in comparison to the sensitivity and specificity of the IS900 element target.

Immunodiagnosis

Immunodiagnositic procedures help in diagnosis of johne's disease. Several serological tests are performed for detection of antibodies. Simultaneously delayed type hypersensitivity test (Johne's testing) is also performed to confirm the disease. During the early stages of infection the host response is primarily cell mediated, with little to no humoral immunity noted. A reciprocal shift in host immunity is generally noted during the clinical stage of infection, with reduced cell-mediated immunity and strong humoral responses. Therefore, serologic tools such as enzyme-linked immunosorbent assay and agar gel immunodiffusion are more useful during the clinical stages of disease, when the titers of antibodies to M. avium subsp. paratuberculosis are measurable. A single diagnostic tool for use in the early stages of disease has not yet been identified, but the gamma interferon test has shown promise for the early detection of infection in cattle and sheep

Serological test used complement fixation test (CFT), the agar gel diffusion test (AGID) and the enzyme linked immunosorbant assay. The later 2 tests are more specific and the first one which detect about 75% false positive reactors. The diagnostic efficacy of CFT is reduced when applied to subclinical conditions, hence can't be used for detection of cases. False positive results with CFT in infected herds are due to cross-reaction with other bacteria. ELISA detects shedders before the AGID which become positive only after large numbers of *M. paratuberculosis* are shed in the feces. ELISA detects less number of positive cases than direct culture examination or PCR (Clark *et al.*, 2008). AGID is considered to be the most appropriate test for the diagnosis of clinical disease. It is rapid, inexpensive and accurate and results are available with in 48 hrs. Various form of ELISA tests are available. A lipoarabinomannan ELISA is considered superior to both CFT and AGID. An ELISA using ethanol extracted antigen from M.paratuberculosis has been described to have a better specificity than the commercial ELISA. Sera absorbed with Mycobacterium phlei to inhibit the cross-reactivity are suggested for this test (Scott *et al.*, 2010).

For performing johnin testing, 2 types of tests are available, an intradermal (ID) test and an intravenous (IV) johnin test. The ID is performed by intradermal injection of the johnin preferably on the cervical region of the animal followed by examination for swelling 48 to 72 hrs. later. This test may result in as high as 75% false positive reactors. It is due to sensitization by saprophytic mycobacteria including Mycobacterium avium.

The IV johnin testing is more specific. Following administration of johnin intravenously the animal develop fever of 1.5^{0}F or higher after 5-8 hours. This test detects 80% of the cases showing clinical signs but not asymptomatic shedder. A systemic reaction including anorexia, depression, dyspnea, erection of hair coat and severe scouring may accompany the temperature rise.

An in vitro lymphocyte stimulation test can be performed to detect the development of delayed hypersensitivity in animals. Peripheral blood lymphocytes are collected and exposed to johnin. Lymphocytes from exposed animals in which delayed hypersensitivity has developed will respond to the johnin by proliferating which is measured by the addition of a radio-labeled nucleic acid precursor (Thymidine). This test increase the specificity of the detection but animals test positive at a stage when clinical signs are visible, Lymphocytes stimulation assay has been reported to be a useful test in assessing the disease status in sheep (de Silva *et al.*, 2010b).

Treatment and Control

M.paratuberculosis is quite resistant to chemotherapeutic agents in vitro so that prospects for an effective treatment are rather bleak. Isoniazid has a minor degree of activity against the organism but does not cure the clinical cases. Clofazimine is effective to some degree in sheep and cattle. The new macrolide, clarithromycin are effective in vitro but it is too expensive to use clinically.

For achieving control following step are under taken:

- Animals showing signs of disease should be immediately isolated and maintained in an isolation barn.
- Fecal culture examination should be carried out at every 6 months on all the animals of 2 years old or more. Animals found positive should be segregated.

- Continue surveillance until there have been four consecutive negative fecal cultures of all animals 2 years of age or more. Animal less than 2 years also have been found to shed the organisms for control programme. This criteria must also be kept in mind (Weber *et al.*, 2010)
- Purchase of only the johnin-negative animals or from johnin-negative herd is carried out.
- For artificial insemination purpose use of semen from paratuberculosis free bulls is advisable. Breeding bulls with infected semen are a source of paratuberculosis infection through natural mating (Khol *et al.*, 2010). Bull calves born in infected herd can be source of infection when later used for natural mating or artificial insemination since subclinically infected bulls released the microbes in the semen (Ayele *et al.*, 2004).

For effective control, correct detection of cases of paratuberculosis is of utmost importance. The lack of accurate tests and the long incubation period of the disease combine to make the control impossible. In the usual plan for containing the disease without eradicating it, the separation of the infected resistant animal from the early developing clinical carriers is of paramount importance.

Besides the above described methods for control of the disease a number of hygienic precautions can be taken to limit the spread of infection. Supply of clean drinking water, fencing of marshes and ponds and closing up of contaminated pastures for 2-3 years are useful measures or else frequent ploughing of pasture to break dung pats facilitates killing of the bacteria by exposing the pathogens to sun and drying. Calves should be kept separately and fed colostrum to develop passive immunity.

Settled dust samples were collected on a commercial dairy farm in the Netherlands with a high prevalence of *Mycobacterium avium* subspecies *paratuberculosis* (MAP) (barn A) and on a Dutch experimental cattle farm (barn B) stocked with cattle confirmed to be MAP shedders (Eisenberg et al.2011). Barns were sampled while animals were present, after both barns were destocked and cleaned by cold high-pressure cleaning, and after being kept empty for two weeks (barn A) or after additional disinfection (barn B). MAP DNA was detected by IS900 real-time PCR and viable MAP were detected by liquid culture. MAP DNA was detected in 78 per cent of samples from barn A and 86 per cent of samples from barn B collected while animals were still present. Viable MAP was detected in six of nine samples from barn A and in three of seven samples from barn B. After cold high pressure cleaning, viable MAP could be detected in only two samples from each barn. After leaving barn A empty for two weeks, and following additional disinfection of barn B, no viable MAP could be detected in any settled dust sample.

Vaccine provides protection against clinical disease and reduces the prevalence. Vallee's vaccine of live *M.paratuberculosis* organisms in a paraffin oil pumice stone vehicle or the Sigurdsson vaccine containing killed cells are the commonly used vaccines. Sigurdsson vaccine is effective in controlling disease in sheep. Vaccines which contain killed whole bacterial cells have superior immunizing power in cattle as compared to vaccines prepared from fractionated cells. In cattle vaccination is carried out only in calves less than 1 month of age. Revaccination is not carried out. Vaccinated animals become positive to johnin and tuberculin testing. The reaction is less to mammalian tuberculin than avian tuberculin. Studies have shown that both humoral and cellular immunity develops in animals following vaccination. In a study it has been found that a single dose of a lipid based live cell vaccine generate CMI but more than elicited by killed vaccine. All immunization regimes tended to decrease the proportion of CD4 (+) T cells but increase the proportions of gamma delta TCR (+) T cells and CD25 (+) cells. The CD8(+): gamma delta TCR (+) T cell ratio represent a reduced regulatory capacity among T cells which increased following vaccination with either killed or live vaccine (Gillan *et al.*, 2010). In order to develop an effective third generation vaccine, a multi-antigen virally vectored vaccine secreting 2 antigen and 2 cell surface antigens of M.paratuberculosis has been developed. The full length expression of a 95kDa fusion protein was observed. The vaccine proved to be highly immunogenic and protective in mice without showing any side effects (Bull *et al.*, 2007).

Glycolipids are presented to T cells by human group 1 CD1 proteins, but are not used as subunit vaccines yet. Experimental immunizations with pure mycobacterial glucose monomycolate (GMM) and keyhole limpet haemocyanin (KLH) in cattle, a species which, unlike mice, expresses group 1 CD1, showed that GMM was equally efficient as KLH in generating T cell responses in blood, but not in the draining lymph node. Also, KLH induced strong antibody responses whereas GMM did not. These data suggest that non-overlapping T cell populations are targeted and demonstrate the potential of glycolipids as a special class of subunit vaccine candidates.Strong anti glycolipid IgG responses can occur in humans and animals, but contrary to anti protein responses and anti glycoprotein responses, the exact mechanism of induction is unknown. Nguyen *et al.* (2011) have previously shown that experimental immunization with the glycolipid glucose monomycolate (GMM) causes the development of specific T cell responses, but not of anti GMM antibodies. However, cattle naturally infected with Mycobacterium avium ssp. paratuberculosis produce high levels of anti GMM IgG. In the present study, The authors tested whether vaccination with GMM conjugated to a protein mimics natural infection in its capacity to induce the production of antibodies against GMM. Cattle were immunized (n=5 per group) with GMM conjugated to a protein, or GMM and protein non-conjugated and administered at contralateral locations, or carrier only. Although immunization with the GMM-protein conjugate vaccine and the non-conjugated vaccine induced protein specific antibody responses, GMM specific antibodies were not detected in either of the groups. In conclusion, the generation of isotype-switched anti lipid antibodies appears to require more than providing peptide epitopes for T helper cells to support glycolipid specific B cells in antibody production.

A DNA vaccine expressing 2 mycobacterial antigens has been tested for protection against paratuberculosis in lambs. Strong protective immune response against *M.paratuberculosis* was observed suggesting that this approach may be useful in vaccinating the animals against paratuberculosis (Sechi *et al.,* 2006).

References

Aho A.D., McNulty A.M. and Coussens P.M.2003.Enhanced expression of interleukin-1alpha and tumor necrosis factor receptor-associated protein 1 in ileal tissues of cattle infected with *Mycobacterium avium* subsp. *paratuberculosis*. Infect. Immun. **71:** 6479-6486.

Alharbi K.B., Al-Swailem A., Al-Dubaib M.A., Al-Yamani E., Al-Naeem A., Shehata M., Hashad M.E., Albusadah K.A. and Mahmoud O.M.2011.Pathology and molecular diagnosis of paratuberculosis of camels. Trop/ Anim/ Health Prod. 2011 Jun 4. [http://www.ncbi.nlm.nih.gov/pubmed/21643659].

Aly, S.S., Mangold, B.L., Whitlock, R.H., Sweeney, R.W., Anderson, R.J., Jiang, J., Schukken, Y.H., Hoving, E. and Gardner, I.A. 2010. Correlation between Harrold egg yolk medium culture and real time quantitative polymerase chain reaction results of *Mycobacterium avium* subsp. *paratuberculosis* in pooled fecal and environmental samples. J. Vet. Diag. Invest. **22:** 677-683.

Ayele, W.Y., Bartos, M., Svastova, P. and Pavlik, I. 2004. Distribution of *Mycobacterium avium* subsp. *paratuberculosis* in organs of naturally infected bull calves and breeding bulls. Vet. Microbiol. **103:** 209-217.

Bermudez, L.E., Petrofsky, M., Sommer, S. and Barletta, R.G. 2010. Payer's patches deficient mice demonstrate that *Mycobacterium avium* subsp. *paratuberculosis* translocates across the mucosal barrier via both M cells and enterocytes but has inefficient dissemination. Infect. Immun. **78:** 3570-3577.

Botsaris G., Slana I., Liapi M. and Dodd C. Economides C, Rees C, Pavlik I.2010.Rapid detection methods for viable *Mycobacterium avium* subspecies *paratuberculosis* in milk and cheese. Int. J. Food Microbiol. 141 Suppl 1: S87-S90. Epub 2010 Mar 16

Bower, K.L., Begg, D.J. and Whittington, R.J. 2010. Culture of *Mycobacterium avium* subsp. *paratuberculosis* from blood are extra intestinal tissues in experimentally infected tissues. Vet. Microbiol. [http://www.ncbi.nlm.nih. gov/pubmed/206095333].

Bull, T.J., Gilbert, S.C., Sridhar, S., Linedale, R., Dierkes, N., Sidi Boumedine, K. and Hermon, Taylor, J. 2007. A novel multi-antigen virally vectored vaccine against *Mycobacterium avium* subsp. *paratuberculosis*. PLoS one **2:** 1229.

Chiodini, R.J., Van Kruiningen, H.J. and Merkal, R.S. 1984. Ruminant paratuberculosis (Johne's disease): the current status and future prospects, Cornell Vet. **74:** 218-62.

Chui, L.W., King, R. and Sim. J. 2010. Development of an immuno capture polymerase chain reaction assay using IgY to detect *Mycobacterium avium* subsp. *paratuberculosis*. Can. J. Vet. Res. **74:** 102-7.

Clark, D.L., Jr., Koziczkowski, J.J., Radcliff, R.P., Carlson, R.A. and Ellingson, J.L. 2008. Detection of *Mycobacterium avium* subsp. *paratuberculosis* comparing fecal culture versus serum enzyme linked immunosorbant assay and direct fecal polymerase chain reaction. J. Dairy Sci. **91:** 2620-7.

Cytokine gene expression in peripheral blood mononuclear cells and tissues of cattle infected with *Mycobacterium avium* subsp. *paratuberculosis*: evidence for an inherent proinflammatory gene expression pattern. Infect Immun. **72:** 1409-1422.

de Silva, K., Begg, D. and Whittington, R. 2010a. The interleukin 10 response in ovine Johne's disease. Vet. Immunol. Immunopathol. [http://www.ncbi.nlm. nih.gov/pubmed/20817276].

de Silva, K., Begg, D., Carter, N., Taylor, D., Di Fiore, L. and Whittington, R. 2010b. The early lymphocyte proliferation response in sheep exposed to *Mycobacterium avium* subsp. *paratuberculosis* compared to infection status. Immunobiology. **215:** 12-25.

Dzieciol, M., Volgger, P., Khol, J., Baumgartner, W., Wagner, M. And Hein, I. 2010. A novel real time PCR assay for specific detection and quantification of *Mycobacterium avium* subsp. *paratuberculosis* in milk with the inherent possibility of differentiation between viable and dead cells. BMC Res. Notes **3:** 251.

Mycobacterium avium subspecies paratuberculosis in bioaerosols after depopulation and cleaning of two cattle barns. Vet Rec. **168:** 587. Epub 2011 May 24.

Gillan, S., Huges, A.D., O'Brien, R. and Griffin, J.F. 2010. Ovine immuno parameters following immunization against *Mycobacterium avium* subsp. *paratuberculosis* using a lipid-base live cell vaccine. Vet. Immunol. Immunopathol. **137:** 109-119.

Grant I.R., Pope C.M., O'Riordan L.M., Ball H.J. and Rowe M.T. 2000.Improved detection of *Mycobacterium avium* subsp. *paratuberculosis* In milk by immunomagnetic PCR. Vet Microbiol. **77:** 369-378.

Greenstein, R.J., Su, L. and Brown, S.T. 2010. Growth of *M.avium* subsp. *paratuberculosis* in culture is enhanced by Nicotinic Acid, Nicotinamide and alpha and beta nicotinamide adenine dinucleotide. Dig. Dis. Sci. 29. [http://www.ncbi.nlm.nih.gov/pubmed/20585983].

Janagama, H.K., Kumar, S., Bannantine, J.P. Kugadas, A., Jagtap, P., Higgins, L., Witthuhn, B. and Sreevatsan, S. 2010. Iron sparing response of *Mycobacterium avium* subsp. *paratuberculosis* is strain dependent. BMC Microbiol. **10:** 268-271.

Jayarao B.M., Pillai S.R., Wolfgang D.R., Griswold D.R., Rossiter C.A., Tewari D., Burns C.M. and Hutchinson L.J.2004. Evaluation of IS900-PCR assay for detection of *Mycobacterium avium* subspecies *paratuberculosis* infection in cattle using quarter milk and bulk tank milk samples. Foodborne Pathog. Dis. **1:** 17-26.

Khol, J.L., Kratik, P., Slana, I., Beram, V., Aurich, C., Baumgartner, W. and Pavlik, I. 2010. Consecutive excretion of *Mycobacterium avium* subsp. *paratuberculosis* in semen of a breeding bull compared to the distribution in feces, tissue and blood by IS900 and F57 quantitative real time PCR and culture examinations. J.Vet. Med. Sci. **72:** 1283-1288.

Kim S.G., Shin S.J., Jacobson R.H., Miller L.J., Harpending P.R., Stehman S.M., Rossiter C.A. and Lein D.A. 2002.Development and application of quantitative polymerase chain reaction assay based on the ABI 7700 system (TaqMan) for detection and quantification of *Mycobacterium avium* subsp. *paratuberculosis*. J. Vet. Diagn. Invest. **14:** 126-131

Kruger, J.M. and Snider, T.G. 1992. Measurement of lymphoblast proliferative capacity of stimulated blood mononuclear cells from cattle with chronic paratuberculosis. Am. J. Vet. Res. **53:** 392-395.

Momotani, E., Whipple, D.L., Thierman, A.B. and Cheville, N.F. 1988. Role of M cells and macrophages in the entrance of *Mycobacterium paratuberculosis* into domes of ileal Payers' Patches in calves. Vet. Pathol. **25:** 131-137.

Nguyen T.K., Wieland W., Santema W., Hoeboer J., van Eden W., Rutten V., Koets A. and Van Rhijn I.2011.Immune response of cattle immunized with a conjugate of the glycolipid glucose monomycolate and protein. Vet. Immunol. Immunopathol. 2011 May 13. [http://www.ncbi.nlm.nih.gov/pubmed/21640388].

Pillai S.R. and Jayarao B.M.2002.Application of IS900 PCR for detection of *Mycobacterium avium* subsp. *paratuberculosis* directly from raw milk. J. Dairy Sci. **85:** 1052-1057.

Plattner, B.L., Chiang, Y.W., Roth, J.A., Platt, R., Huffman, E., Zylstra, J. and Hostetter, J.M. 2010. Direct inoculation of *M.avium* subsp. *paratuberculosis* into ileocecal payer patches results in colonization of the intestine in a calf model. Vet. Pathol. [http://www.ncbi.nlm.nih.gov./ pubmed/20930105].

Plattner B.L. and Hostetter J.M.2011.Comparative gamma delta T cell immunology: a focus on mycobacterial disease in cattle. Vet. Med. Int. 214384. Epub 2011 May 16.

Scott. M.C., Bannantine, J.P., Kaneko, Y., Branscum, A.J., Whitlock, R.H., Mori, Y., Speerc, A. and Eda, S. 2010. Absorbed EVELISA: A diagnostic test with improved specificity for Johne's disease in cattle. Food borne Pathog. Dis. **7:** 1291-1296.

Sechi, L.A., Ahmad, N., Felis, G.E., Dupre, I., Cannas, S., Fadda, G., Bua, A. and Zanetti, S. 2006. Immunogenicity and cytoadherence of recombinant heparin binding haemagglutinin (HBHA) of *Mycobacterium avium* subsp. *paratuberculosis*: functional promiscuity or a role in virulence vaccine. **24:** 236-243.

Sechi, L.A., Mara, L., Cappai, P., Frothingam, R., Ortu, S., Leoni, A., Ahmad, N. and Zanetti, S. 2006. Immunization with DNA vaccines encoding different mycobacterial antigens elicit a Th1 type immune response in lambs and protects against *Mycobacterium avium* subsp. *paratuberculosis* infection. Vaccine **24:** 229-235.

Shankar H., Singh S.V., Singh P.K., Singh A.V., Sohal J.S. and Greenstein R.J.2010 Presence, characterization, and genotype profiles of *Mycobacterium avium* subspecies *paratuberculosis* from unpasteurized individual and pooled milk, commercial pasteurized milk, and milk products in India by culture, PCR, and PCR-REA methods. Int. J. Infect. Dis. **14:** e121-6. Epub 2009 Jul 2.

Singh, A.V., Singh, S.V., Singh, P.K. and Sohal, J.S. 2010. Genotype diversity in Indian isolates of *Mycobacterium avium* subsp. *paratuberculosis* recovered from domestic and wild ruminants from different agro-climatic regions. Comp. Immunol. Microbiol. Infect. Dis. [http://www.ncbi.nlm.nih.gov/pubmed/20832117].

Sohal, J.S., Singh, S.V., Singh, P.K. and Singh, A.V. 2010. On the evolution of "Indian Bison type" strains of *Mycobacterium avium* subsp. *paratuberculosis*. Microbiol. Res. **165:** 163-171.

Stabel J.R. and Bannantine J.P. 2005.Development of a nested PCR method targeting a unique multicopy element, ISMap02, for detection of *Mycobacterium avium* subsp. *paratuberculosis* in fecal samples. J. Clin. Microbiol. **43:** 4744-4750.

Weber, M.F., Kogut, J., deBree, J., van Schaik, G. and Nielen, M. 2010. Age at which dairy cattle become *Mycobacterium avium* subsp. *paratuberculosis* fecal culture positive. Prev. Vet. Med. **97:** 29-36.

Whittington, R.J. and Windsor, P.A. 2009. In utero infection of cattle with *Mycobacterium avium* subsp. *paratuberculosis*: A critical review and meta analysis. Vet. J. **179:** 60-69.

□□□

Chapter 14

Dichelobactor nodosus

Dr. S.K. SRIVASTAVA
Former, Division of Bacteriology & Mycology
Indian Veterinary Research Institute, Izatnagar-243122
Bareilly (U.P.)

Dichelobactor nodosus

Dichelobactor nodosus is the causative agent of infectious foot rot in sheep. The disease is of world wide occurrence including India (Hussain *et al.,* 2009). Rather *et al.* (2011) determined the prevalence, economic impact of virulent footrot in central Kashmir, India, along with isolation and molecular characterization of *Dichelobacter nodosus* (*D. nodosus*) where so far no such work has been carried out. Over all 12.54% prevalence of footrot was recorded in central Kashmir with highest (15.84%) in district Srinagar, and least (10.89%) in district Budgam, while it was 13.28% in district Ganderbal. Overall economic impact of footrot was estimated to the tune of Rs 15.82 million annually to the sheep farming in central Kashmir. Out of 370 samples collected from footrot lesions of naturally infected sheep, 200 (54.05%) detected *D. nodosus* positive by polymerase chain reaction (PCR). Out of these, 132 (66.00%) samples carried serogroup B of *D. nodosus,* five (2.50%) serogroup E, one (0.50%) serogroup I, while, 53 (26.50%) had mixed infection of serogroups B and E, four (2.00%) of serogroups B and I, two (1.00%) of serogroups B and G and the remaining three (1.50%) samples harboured the mixed infection of serogroups B, E and I. Serogroup G was detected for the first time in India. Over all serogroup B was most frequent (97.0%) followed by E (30.5%), while serogoups I (4.0%) and G (1.0%) were least prevalent. A total of 265 D.nodosus strains were isolated out of which 194 (73.20%) were typed as serogroup B, 61 (23.01%) as serogroup E, eight (3.01%) as serogroup I and remaining two (0.75%) belonged to serogroup G. Out of 265 D. nodosus isolates, 164 (61.88%) possessed intA (integrase) gene, thus were considered as virulent strains. Serogroup wise intA gene was found in 121(62.37%) isolates of serogroup B, 36 (59.01%) of E, two (100%) of G and five (62.50%) of I. Out of 20 randomly selected isolates subjected to gelatin gel test, 16 isolates with intA gene produced thermostable protease while four isolates without intA gene revealed the production of thermolabile protease. This indicated a good co-relation between presence of intA gene and gelatin gel test in determination of the D. nodosus virulence.

The first cases of footrot in Bhutan were reported in sheep in 1990 at the National Sheep Breeding Centre (NSBC), which supplies breeding animals to village sheep flocks throughout Bhutan. Despite the presence of footrot at the Centre the distribution of apparently disease-free sheep continued. Cases of footrot were reported in village flocks soon after the disease was diagnosed at NSBC. A national survey was designed to establish the distribution and prevalence of footrot in Bhutan. This detected footrot in 19/94 village sheep flocks surveyed. The 19 affected flocks were distributed among nine different administrative districts whereas the villages selected were in 13 of a total of 16 sheep growing districts. The highest within-flock prevalences were among the seven flocks sampled in Bumthang district (mean 20.4%). The prevalence of the disease within flocks was generally much lower in other affected districts and in three districts a single affected animal was identified in the sample of 14 sheep examined in each village. Nationally, footrot prevalence was estimated to be 3.1% (95% CI 2.16-4.04%). There was a positive association between the receipt of animals from NSBC and the presence of footrot. The prevalence of the disease was higher in flocks with a migratory system of management than in those using a sedentary system. The relative risk of there being footrot in a migratory flock was nine-times higher than in a non-migratory flock. Only one strain of Dichelobacter nodosus (serogroup B) was identified among the 234 isolates obtained from the 19 affected flocks.

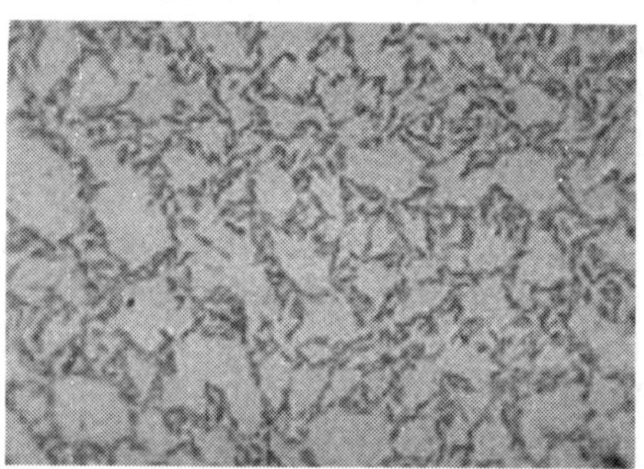

Dichelobacter nodosus

It is a debilitating disease of sheep resulting in lameness and production losses. The causative organism is a large gram-negative, non-motile anaerobic rod. *Fusobacterium necrophorum* and *Archanobacterium pyogenes* are common secondary invaders and *Treponema penotha* is a non-pathogenic species which is frequently isolated from lesions. The organism is often heavily fimbriated with several hundred fimbriae arranged in a polar distribution. These help the organisms to mediate to adherence of cells to host surfaces. The bacteria can survive in soil, bedding etc. for no longer than several days under optimal conditions of high humidity and temperature over 1^{0}C but it can survive in infected feet for considerable period. Bovine isolates are avirulent for sheep. At least nine serogroup (A-1) have been characterized with different serotypes identified within these groups. The current Australian antigenic classification system, based on variation in the fimbriae, classifies *D. nodosus* into at least 10 serogroups (A-I and M) and 18 serotypes. The serogrouping is based on slide agglutination test and polymerase chain reaction methods. Several strains can infect a single hoof at a time. Based on the extent of conservation of pilin amino acid sequence outside the major N-terminal region, serogroup A-H have been divided into 2 distinct categories, an A set (6 serogroups and A B set (2 serogroups). The degree of amino acid conservation within the sets corresponds to the degree of serological cross-reaction and cross protection (Elleman 1988). Different typing schemes have been suggested. The Australian schemes divided the strains into 10 serogroup whereas a British scheme identifies 17 and a U.S. scheme identifies 21 strains. Pilin engender high specific immunity to infection. Wani *et al.* (2007) investigated the serological diversity of *D. nodosus* in this region of Kashmir, India. Exudates of footrot lesions were collected from 24 naturally infected sheep and 42 goats located in the Kashmir valley. Of these 66 samples, 24 yielded evidence of *D. nodosus* by PCR using 16SrDNA specific primers. Multiplex PCR using serogroup specific primers revealed the presence of serogroup B in all the samples except two, which showed the presence of serogroup E D. nodosus.

Caqatay and Hickford (2005) aimed to isolate, identify, and characterize as many *D. nodosus* strains as possible from NZ farms by using polymerase chain reaction (PCR)-based technology. Understanding the virulence of this bacterium and showing extensive genomic variation in the fimbrial subunit gene (fimA) in different *D. nodosus* strains was very important to produce serogroup specific and effective vaccine for NZ. More than 100 footrot samples were collected from four different farming regions in NZ. Thousands of primary plates were cultured anaerobically and examined with Gram-staining in order to detect single colonies of *D. nodosus*. Approximately 500 plates that had potential *D. nodosus* colonies were subcultured several times to eliminate contaminating colonies until single colonies were obtained. Variable and a part of the conserved regions of the fimbrial subunit gene (fimA) were amplified directly from bacterial DNA extracted from footrot lesions and also from cultured NZ *D. nodosus* isolates, using the polymerase chain reaction. Different fimA amplimers were analyzed by DNA sequencing. On the basis of DNA sequence analysis, 16 new *D. nodosus* isolates belonging to eight different serogroups were identified from NZ. These new *D. nodosus* fimA sequences from NZ were different to previously reported strains and strains used in a commercial vaccine. The antigenic diversity of *D. nodosus* is due to variations in the DNA sequence of its fimbrial subunit gene (fimA) and provides the basis for classification of the organism into at least 10 major serogroups (A-I and M), the distribution of which varies with different geographical locations.

There are a number of strains of *B.nodosus* with varying virulence and they have been subdivided into benign, intermediate and virulent strains which conform with the type of disease observed. The level of virulence of each strain depends on its keratolytic capacity. The most virulent strains possess the capacity to produce a heat stable protease with a single isoenzyme pattern. Recently, it has been shown that only the virulent strains carry a polymorphic proline-glycine repeat gene suggesting that it could be an epidemiological marker for future studies (Calvo Bado *et al.*, 2010).

Foot rot is an economically important disease of sheep, cattle, goats and deer. Based on clinical observations and comparison with diseases known to affect domestic ungulates, it was hypothesized these wild ungulates were affected by foot rot associated with infection with *Dichelobacter nodosus*. *Dichelobacter nodosus* has been shown to be the essential pathogen for initiation and establishment of foot rot. Because these bacteria could not be cultivated from affected ibex, Belloy *et al.* (2007) developed a nested polymerase chain reaction that allowed detection of *D. nodosus* without culture. Using this assay, the authors were able to diagnose *D. nodosus* infections of ibex, mouflon, and domestic sheep in natural outbreaks. From these results it was concluded that *D. nodosus* plays an etiological role in foot rot not only in domestic but also in wild Caprinae.

Following exposure to continuous rain of stratum corneum the inter digital space is colonized by various pathogens including *D.nodosus* and *F.necrophorum*. The organism invade the germinal layer of the epidermis of the inter-digital skin leading to destruction and lameness. This results in acute interdigital dermatitis. Eventually it is so severe that hoof may separate. Other bacteria also act synergistically and enhance the lesions. *F.necrophorum* is invariably present in the lesions. Other bacterial species usually involved is *P.asaccharolytica*. The severely inflamed inter digital lesions are characterized by superficial ulceration, necrosis, fissuring and hyperkeratosis. Sole ulcers, interdigital fibroma and hoof overgrowth may also occur (Egerton *et al.*, 1989).

Pathogenesis

Prolonged wet conditions leads to exposure of interdigital skin causing local dermatitis by *F.necrophorum* at the skin which may be complicated by

D.nodosus leading to the development of foot rot. The interdigital dermatitis, may resolve soon but involvement of *D.nodosus* leads to the chronic infection. The hyperkeratosis is induced by the primary infection which facilitates infection by *D.nodosus.* Pili present on these bacteria probably mediate the adherence on epidermal matrix of hoof surface. Based on pilus antigen at least 10 serologically distinct groups of *D.nodosus* have been identified. Research that has used a classical molecular genetics approach has led to major advances in our understanding of the role of the key virulence factors of *D. nodosus* in the disease process. *D. nodosus* strains produce polar type IV fimbriae and extracellular serine proteases. Mutagenesis of the fimbrial subunit gene fimA and the pilT gene, which is required for fimbrial retraction, and subsequent testing of these mutants in sheep virulence trials has shown that type IV fimbriae-mediated twitching motility is essential for virulence. The extracellular protease genes aprV2, aprV5 and bprV have also been mutated. Analysis of these mutants has shown that ArpV5 is the major extracellular protease and that AprV2 is the thermostable protease that is responsible for the extracellular elastase activity. Structural analysis of AprV2 has revealed that it contains several novel loops, one of which appears to act as an exosite that may modulate substrate accessibility. Finally, virulence experiments in sheep have shown that the AprV2 protease is required for virulence.These pilin are small in size (16-18 kDa) with 32 amino acids are highly hydrophobic. These pilin are type 4 pili because they possess a common N-methyl phenylalanine as a modified terminal residue. This also produces a keratinolytic protease which digests interdigital skin and horn matrix. These extracellular protease are likely serine protease that require divalent cations for activity. This subtilisin like serine protease comprise of proteases AprV2, AprV5 and BprV which is produced by virulent strains whereas strains causing benign foot rot produce AprB2, AprB5 and BprB. Recently the proteases have been crystallized and a the proteases contain one molecule in the asymmetric unit with a solvent content ranging from 36 to 40% (Wong *et al.,* 2010). The proteases from virulence strains are more thermostable than from benign strains. There is considerable variation in the virulence among strains and the lesions produced vary accordingly. Serine protease are produced by both virulent and a virulent strains. Subtle differences in proteases is important for virulence. *D.nodosus* posses 2 chromosomal regions that have a genotype association with virulence (Billington *et al.,* 1996). The non-pathogenic strains causes benign foot rot or non-progressive foot rot. An intermediate stage has also been described which is characterized by less severe disease than virulent foot rot. A polynucleotide phosphorylase has been identified as a putative virulence factor in *D.nodosus* strains. This activity is lower in virulent strains. This activity is virulence repressor in benign strains (Palanisamy *et al.,* 2010). Host genetic factors are increasingly recognized as determining the outcome of infection (Skerman 1989). Affected animals show in the beginning lameness due to the inflammation.

The fimbriae of *D. nodosus* are classified as type IV because of their highly conserved amino-terminal region, polar location, association with twitching motility, and the presence of an N-methylphenylalanine residue as the N-terminal amino acid. *D. nodosus* fimbriae are highly immunogenic, with agglutination reactions involving the fimbrial antigens providing the basis of the classification of *D. nodosus* into nine major serogroups designated A to I. Vaccination of sheep with whole cells of *D. nodosus* or with purified fimbriae protects against the disease, although this protection is serogroup specific. Multivalent recombinant fimbrial vaccines have been prepared by overexpression of each of the nine fimbrial subunit genes in *Pseudomonas aeruginosa* . However, antigenic competition has limited the application of these vaccines so that the most effective strategies are based on univalent and divalent formulations.

The *fimA* genes encoding the major fimbrial subunit from each of the nine major serogroups have been sequenced, which has allowed the division of *D. nodosus* isolates into two major classes based on the genetic organisation of the fimbrial gene region. In class I strains (serogroups A, B, C, E, F, G, and I), the *fimA* gene is followed by *fimB*, which encodes a potential 29.5-kDa membrane protein of unknown function but which is postulated to play a role in the export of fimbrial subunits to the cell surface . Strains of serogroups D and H belong to class II and have three additional genes downstream of *fimA*, namely, *fimC*, *fimD*, and *fimZ*. The *fimD* gene is postulated to be a functional homologue of *fimB*, *fimC* has sequence similarity to *traX* from the F plasmid, and *fimZ* may represent a redundant fimbrial subunit.

Cagaty and Hickford (2008) revealed that these fimbriae are glycosylated. This was demonstrated in several ways: by the detection of carbohydrate on fimbrial protein using periodic acid Schiff reagent (PAS) staining of SDS-PAGE gels and by demonstrating enzymatic deglycosylation and by analysis of the amino acid sequences derived from the *fimA* gene, whereby the gene from isolates of *D. nodosus* that appeared to be glycosylated had potential glycosylation sites both inside and outside of the variable region of fimA. The results would also explain the observation that the calculated molecular weight of *fimA* from some *D. nodosus* serotypes does not correlate with the apparent size determined from electrophoretic mobility.

To examine the role of the fimbriae in virulence, allelic exchange was used to insertionally inactivate the *fimA* gene, which encodes the fimbrial subunit protein, from the virulent type G D. nodosus strain VCS1703A. Detailed analysis of two independently derived *fimA* mutants revealed that they no longer produced the fimbrial subunit protein or intact fimbriae and did not exhibit twitching motility. In addition, these mutants were no longer capable of undergoing natural transformation and did not secrete wild-type levels of extracellular proteases. These effects were not due to polar effects on the downstream *fimB* gene because insertionally inactivated *fimB* mutants were not defective in any of these phenotypic tests. Virulence testing of the mutants in a sheep pen trial conducted under controlled environmental conditions showed that the *fimA* mutants were avirulent, providing evidence that the fimA gene is an essential *D. nodosus* virulence gene (Kennan *et al.* 2001).

Mutation of either the pilT or pilU gene eliminated the ability to carry out twitching motility. However, the pilT mutants displayed decreased adhesion to epithelial cells and reduced protease secretion, whereas the pilU mutants had wild-type levels of extracellular protease secretion and adherence. These data provided evidence that PilT is required for the type IV fimbria-dependent protease secretion pathway in *D. nodosus*. It was postulated that sufficient fimbrial retraction must occur in the pilU mutants to allow protease secretion, but not twitching motility, to take place. Although no cell movement was detected in a pilU mutant of *D. nodosus*, aberrant motion was detected in an equivalent mutant of Pseudomonas aeruginosa. These observations explain how in *D. nodosus* protease secretion can occur in a pilU mutant but not in a pilT mutant. In addition, virulence studies with sheep showed that both the pilT and pilU mutants were avirulent, providing evidence that mutation of the type IV fimbrial system affects virulence by eliminating twitching motility, not by altering cell adherence or protease secretion.

Parker *et al.* (2006) identified a two-component signal transduction system (PilR/S) and an alternative sigma factor (sigma 54) that were shown by insertional inactivation to be required for the regulation of fimbrial biogenesis in *D. nodosus*. Western blots showed that in both pilR and rpoN mutants, fimbrial subunit production was significantly reduced by a process that was shown to occur at a PilR- and sigma 54-dependent promoter. The mutants lacked surface fimbriae, which were shown to be required for the adherence of D. nodosus cells to tissue culture monolayers. The reduction in fimbrial subunit production in these mutants also resulted in a concomitant loss of the ability to secrete extracellular proteases. A maltose binding protein-PilR fusion protein was purified and was shown to bind specifically to a region located 234 to 594 bp upstream of the fimA transcriptional start point. To determine additional targets of PilR and sigma 54, genome-wide transcriptional profiling was performed using a whole-genome oligonucleotide microarray. The results indicated that PilR and sigma 54 regulated genes other than *fimA*; these genes appear to encode surface-exposed proteins whose role in virulence is unknown. In conclusion, this study represents a significant advancement in our understanding of how the ability of *D. nodosus* to cause ovine footrot is regulated, as it has been shown that the biogenesis of type IV fimbriae in *D. nodosus* is regulated by a sigma 54-dependent PilR/S system that also indirectly controls protease secretion.

Both claws of one foot is involved and often all the foot is involved. At the advanced stage there is distinctive, foul smelling exudates in small amount.

Foot rot caused by *D.nodosus* in goats is manifested by severe inter digital dermatitis with some separation of skin-horn junction at the axial surface but rarely involving foot as in sheep. In cattle, also there is lameness due to severe inter digital dermatitis. The fissuring and hyperkeratosis of the inter digital skin with pitting and erosion at the skin-horn junction is visible.

Diagnosis

The disease can be diagnosed by the demonstration of the organisms in the gram-stained smears collected from typical lesions. Deep smearing is required. The rods of *D.nodosus* are straight or slightly curved gram-negative rods and vary from 0.6 to 1.2 μm in length. The organism is non-sporing and non-encapsulated. When stained with Loffler's methylene blue, one, two or more red staining granules can be seen at either end or along the rod.

Cultural examination of the organism requires the procedures involving anaerobic techniques. An anaerobic plastic chamber with glove box is preferred. Anaerobic media used are cooked meat media and thioglycollate broth. Special oxygen free media are used for conducting biochemical tests. Dichelobacter nodosus is confirmed by culture and polymerase chain reaction (PCR) using species-specific 16S ribosomal RNA primers. When cultured, the organism appeared as flat colourless colonies having a fine granulated structure with irregular margins, and showing characteristic Gram-negative rods with swollen ends. Detection by PCR from cultured bacteria resulted in amplification of a 783 base pairs (bp) product.

Use of elastase test, gelatin gel test and electophoretic zymogram are carried out to determine virulence of the *D.nodosus* strains (Liu and Yong 1993). Southern blot analysis has shown a remarkable correlation between the virulence and IntA gene.

An antigen extracted from Dichelobacter nodosus with potassium thiocyanate (KSCN) is currently used in enzyme-linked immunosorbent assay (ELISA) for serological diagnosis of ovine footrot, but the test lacks specificity in mature sheep (Whittington *et al.*, 1997). Other antigens were therefore evaluated for use in this test. Structural components of the cell envelope of *D. nodosus* including outer membrane, cytoplasmic membrane, lipopolysaccharide and pilus and extracellular proteases were purified from cultured *D. nodosus* while recombinant membrane proteins, protease and pilus antigens were also evaluated. Many antigenic components of *D. nodosus* participated in reactions in ELISA that were not specific for infection with *D. nodosus* and apart from pilus, none of the antigens resulted in improved specificity of the ELISA. Using a positive-negative cut-off to yield sensitivity of 70%, ELISA using pili from cultured *D. nodosus* serogroup A had a specificity of 98.3% compared with 89.7% for the ELISA with KSCN-extract as antigen ($P < 0.001$). Recombinant pili morphogenetically expressed in *Pseudomonas aeruginosa* were unsuitable for use in ELISA due to copurification of *Pseudomonas antigens* to which apparently healthy sheep directed antibodies.

The humoral response of goats to *D. nodosus* antigens and the possibility of a serological diagnosis of footrot in goats have not been studied. With the aim of evaluating a diagnostic ELISA test, Ghimire *et al.* (2002) investigated the primary immune response of goats to experimental and natural infection, the memory response in recovered animals, and the transfer and persistence of colostral antibodies in kids. Footrot stimulated the goat's immune system and, as in sheep, under-running lesions were the primary stimulus for production of anti-*D. nodosus* antibodies. The immune response could be detected in ELISA using either fimbrial or outer membrane protein (KSCN) antigens of *D. nodosus*. Antibody titres resulting from infection declined quickly after recovery and reached pre-infection levels within 3-4 months. Previously affected animals, however, mounted a memory response when injected with purified *D. nodosus* antigens. Antibody levels attained after anamnestic challenge were correlated with the maximum levels attained during infection, and were therefore indicative of the infection status. Anti-*D. nodosus* antibodies were also transferred to kids via colostrum, but these antibodies did not persist and therefore were unlikely to interfere with the diagnostic ELISA after 3 months of age. Though these ELISA tests were highly specific, their sensitivity was rather low. Therefore, they are only suitable for a herd diagnosis of footrot in goats and are dependent on the development of advanced under-running infections in a proportion of affected goats.

A PCR is used for detection of IntA gene to identify the virulent strains (Cheetham *et al.*, 2006). The differentiation of ovine foot rot strains of *D.nodosus* is also possible through Gene probes. The probes also differentiate between virulent and benign isolates. Additionally PCR can also be used for differentiation of isolates and diagnosis of disease (Rood *et al.*, 1996; Hussain *et al.*, 2009).

Treatment and Control

Topical bactericidal agents after trimming of under run hoof surface is adequate. Very sharp instruments including a knife and hoof secateurs are required. Local application include 10% tincture of chloramphenicol, oxytetracycline (5% tincture), Cetyltrimethyl ammonium bromide (10% solution), copper sulfate (10% solution) and dichlorophen (10% solution) is preferred. Foot bathing is a more practical approach to topical treatment. Copper sulfate, formalin and zinc sulfate is used for foot bathing. Systemic use of penicillin, tetracyclines, tylosin, erythromycin and streptomycin is of value when accompanied with other measures such as culling, segregating affected sheep, use of dry pastures and vaccination. From observational studies, farmers who use parenteral antibacterials to promptly treat all sheep with footrot (FR) or interdigital dermatitis (ID) have a prevalence of lameness of < 2% compared with a prevalence of 9% lameness reported by farmers who treat lame sheep by trimming affected feet. Wassink et al.(2010.) tested the hypothesis that prompt treatment of sheep lame with naturally developing FR or ID with parenteral and topical antibacterials reduces the prevalence and incidence of lameness with these conditions compared with less frequent treatment with trimming of hoof horn and applying topical antibacterials.A further hypothesis was that reduction of ID and FR would improve productivity. A lowland sheep flock with 700 ewes was used to test these hypotheses in an 18-month within farm clinical trial with four groups of ewes: two interventions and two control. The duration and severity of lameness was used to categorise sheep into three weighted scores of lameness (WLS): never lame (WLS0), mildly lame/lame for < 6 days (WLS1) and severely or chronically lame (WLS2). The intervention reduced the prevalence of lameness due to FR and ID in ewes and lambs and the incidence of lameness in ewes. The WLS was also significantly lower in sheep in the intervention groups. Ewes with a higher WLS were subsequently significantly more likely to have a body condition score < 2.5 and to have lame lambs. Significantly more ewes lambed and successfully reared more lambs that were ready for slaughter at a younger age in the intervention versus control groups. There was an increase in the gross margin of Pound630/100 ewes mated in the intervention group, including the cost of treatment of Pound150/100 ewes mated. We conclude that prompt parenteral and topical antibacterial treatment of sheep lame with ID and FR reduced the prevalence and incidence of these infectious conditions and led to improved health, welfare and productivity.

The agar dilution method was used to determine the inhibitory activity of 25 antimicrobial agents against 69 strains of *Dichelobacter nodosus* and 108 strains of the genus Fusobacterium, all of which were isolated from 90 clinical cases of ovine footrot between October 1998 and November 2000

(Jimenez *et al.*, 2004). In the case of the micro-organisms belonging to the genus Fusobacterium, the six beta-lactams studied (benzyl penicillin, ampicillin, cloxacillin, cefadroxil, cefuroxime and cephalexine) proved to be, in general, the most effective antimicrobial agents. Chloramphenicol, clindamycin and doxycycline were also quite active against *Fusobacterium* spp. With regard to the 69 strains of *D. nodosus* tested, the levels of resistance remained low.

An outbreak of virulent footrot was investigated in a flock of 605 Merino cross-bred sheep in Bhutan (Gurung *et al.*, 2006). Conventional control methods in the preceding eight years had reduced its prevalence from 36-79% in different components of the flock to about 15% overall. Only one serogroup (B) of *Dichelobacter nodosus* was identified among 40 isolates cultured from affected sheep. A vaccine prepared from this strain was used in a pilot trial to compare the response of 14 treated and 14 untreated sheep. All affected, vaccinated animals in this trial healed quickly and were protected against re-infection while additional cases developed among untreated sheep during a period favourable for the spread of footrot. The serogroup B vaccine was administered to the whole flock for two successive years. No other footrot treatment was given during these or subsequent years. The whole flock was examined three times, foot by foot, for two years and twice yearly for another two years. When vaccination began there were 88 affected sheep in the flock, an affected sheep being defined as an animal with a foot-score of 2 or greater in one or more feet. There were neither affected sheep in the flock 30 days after the first dose of vaccine nor were any identified in later inspections. Virulent footrot, originating from the farm under investigation, persisted in neighbouring village flocks during this period. It was concluded that whole flock specific *D. nodosus* vaccination made a major contribution to the elimination of all clinical signs of footrot from the flock of 605 sheep where the condition had previously persisted for 10 years.

Commercial multivalent footrot vaccines containing nine fimbrial serogroups (A through I) of *D. nodosus* produce relatively low and short term antibody responses due to antigenic competition, in contrast to higher and longer responses provided by monovalent or bivalent vaccines. The latter were important components of successful eradication programs for endemic footrot caused by either one or two serogroups of *D. nodosus* in Nepal, Bhutan, and several flocks in Australia (Dhungyel and Whittington 2009). However, the presence of up to six serogroups in some Australian flocks and the use of an annual bivalent vaccination regime to progressively eradicate serogroups would require a long term program. In this study a sequential vaccination trial testing different time intervals between different bivalent vaccinations was carried out. Intervals of 12, 9, 6, 3 and 0 months were tested. The 1st vaccination was with recombinant fimbrial antigens for serogroups A and B while the 2nd vaccination was with D and E. There were no significant differences between the antibody responses for time intervals of 3, 6, 9 and 12 months whereas there was a reduced response when sheep were vaccinated with two bivalent vaccines (four antigens) concurrently, indicating antigenic competition. Therefore an inter-vaccination interval of 3 months can be applied between two different bivalent vaccines without detrimental impact on the humoral immune responses to the various fimbrial antigens of *D. nodosus*. These results could have wider applications in vaccination against diseases caused by multivalent or multistrain microbes.

A recent study has suggested that both parenteral antibacterials treatment and trimming hoof is useful for treatment of foot rot and interdigital dermatitis (Wassnik *et al.*, 2010). However, the parenteral treatment was more effective. The pilus antigens are the major host-protective immunogens and confer longer immunity against homologous strain. Protection is chiefly humoral but high concentration of antibodies is required for adequate diffusion into the epidermis.

The immunoglobulins can be passively transferred from ewes to lambs through colostrum. An alum adjuvanted vaccine is useful. Oil is also used as an adjuvant. Local reactions with adjuvanted vaccines are quite common. A recent study has shown that administration of melatonin increases the immune response in sheep to vaccination (Regodon *et al.*, 2009). In milk goat and sheep vaccination can result in a significant drop in milk production. Current vaccine consists of 8-10 strains of common strains of *D.nodosus*. Protective vaccine response to several distinct serogroups can be readily measured by serogroup specific, K-agglutinating antibody titers. The antigenic competition in multivalent vaccines is a problem which can be tackled by modulating the vaccine at suitable inter-vaccination intervals (Dhungyel and Whittington 2009). Recombinant pilus antigen has been tested as vaccine with useful results. In order to find out a putative immunogen of *D.nodosus* for vaccine production, Myers *et al.* (2007) sequenced gene from the organism and identified 8 immunogenic proteins which could be used for producing third generation vaccines.

Vaccination targeted at up to two specific serogroups can eliminate those serogroups from infected flocks, but requires identification of serogroups present in infected flocks. Serogroups can be identified using slide agglutination or polymerase chain reaction (PCR) methods. The objectives of the work of Hill *et al.* (2010) was to use stochastic simulation modeling to estimate the efficacy of sampling strategies encompassing 5-40 sheep per flock and 2-4 colonies per sheep, and to compare efficacies based on slide agglutination or multiplex PCR test results. Foot swabs collected from sheep in 12 flocks were used as the basis for a sampling strategy simulation model. None of the evaluated sampling strategies identified the two most common serogroups in the flock, or all serogroups present in the flock, in 95% of iterations. However, a simulated sample of 22 sheep/flock and 2 colonies/ sheep resulted in a simulated vaccine that protected 95% of the sheep that could be protected by a single bivalent vaccine, while a sample of 24 sheep/ flock and 2 colonies/sheep resulted in a series of simulated bivalent vaccines that protected 95% of diseased infected sheep. The difference in outcome was due to the distribution and frequency of serogroups within certain flocks where some serogroups were uncommon and others dominant. A sampling strategy (>40 sheep/flock, 4 colonies/sheep) that will identify the two most common serogroups in a flock 95% of the time may not be cost effective. Evaluating efficacy based on the expected effect on the flock may be more useful than one which seeks to determine the most common serogroups. These findings are broadly applicable to diseases where more than one strain or type of pathogen may be present and must be represented in a vaccine.

The identification of *Dichelobacter nodosus* present in a flock is a prerequisite to specific (autogenous) vaccination. Current methods of identification of the serogroup present in a population requires that the organisms be isolated, identified visually in mixed culture on streak plates, subcultured to purify and subjected to antigenic analysis. This process takes at least 3 to 4 weeks. One study describes the development of a simple and rapid serogroup specific PCR test for *D. nodosus* (Dhungyel *et al.*, 2002). A common forward primer was designed from the conserved amino-terminal region of the fimbrial gene (fimA) and 9 (A-I) serogroup specific reverse primers were designed from the carboxy-terminal regions of fimA of the different serogroups. To verify the specificity within *D. nodosus*, each specific primer pair was tested in PCR against 18 serogroups/serotypes (prototypes) and found to be specific for all the serotypes within the homologous serogroups. Eighty four other bacterial strains, either commonly occurring in sheep or found in the environment of sheep, and including organisms related taxonomically to *D. nodosus*, were used to check the specificity of these assays. They were found to be specific for *D. nodosus* as none of the 84 bacterial stains reacted. These primers detected 1 pg of purified chromosomal DNA, or 50-100 cells of *D. nodosus* in crude lysates. Sensitivity was markedly improved when an immuno-magnetic capture was employed. Single tube multiplex PCRs were tested with different combinations of common forward primer and groups of 3, 4 or 5 reverse primers chosen so that amplicon size for each reaction product was different. These were able to amplify DNA of isolates from all the relevant serogroups included in the reactions. These tests were evaluated with samples taken directly from lesions of footrot, either directly or preceded by DNA purification, immuno-magnetic capture, enrichment broth culture and culture on hoof agar media. Of these methods only PCR on mixed colonies from 4-day-old cultures on 4% hoof agar media yielded results of practical value.

For the past 20 years footrot vaccines have evolved from simple bacterins to highly specific recombinant DNA (rDNA) fimbrial vaccines (O'Meara *et al.* 1993). The development of these vaccines has left a trail of discoveries, challenges and solutions; these processes continue as we move closer to understanding the requirements of a footrot vaccine. The initial whole cell vaccines were unsuccessful due to the short duration of immunity and incorporation of limited serotypes. A multistrain vaccine eliminated the problem of serotype inclusion, although the duration of immunity in many cases is still inadequate. The proteases of *Dichelobacter nodosus* appear to be cross protective; however, little is known of their ability to protect sheep against footrot. The major protective immunogen is the bacterial fimbriae, which also forms the basis for the K-agglutination serotyping system. *K-agglutinin* titre correlates directly with resistance to challenge. The protective fimbrial epitope is conformationally dependent, suggesting little advantage in the development of synthetic peptide vaccines. To enhance the efficiency of vaccine production *D. nodosus* fimbrial genes were eventually cloned and successfully expressed in *P. aeruginosa*. Monovalent vaccines based on recombinant fimbriae are omnipotent, inducing high levels of agglutinins and long lasting immunity. In multivalent vaccines, on the other hand, incorporation of each additional serogroup into the vaccine results in reduced efficacy both in terms of reduced *K-agglutinin* titres and reduced protection following challenge. The least effective are multivalent formulations representing all major serogroups. In addition, considerable genetic variation has been observed in the ability of sheep to respond optimally to each serogroup in a multivalent vaccine. Results show that the limitation of the sheep to mount an effective immune response, rather than the quality or quantity of the immunogen, limits the efficacy of current footrot vaccines. Melatonin has been shown to exert immunomodulatory properties with broad application in veterinary medicine. Regodon *et al.* (2009) investigated the effect of exogenous melatonin in the improvement of the immune response to administration of an immune-preparation of two stumps of A1 and C strains of *Dichelobacter nodosus* in sheep. Subcutaneous administration of melatonin enhanced plasma levels of melatonin from days 42 to 120. Administration of melatonin to vaccinated animals enhanced both the titer of antibodies and serum IgG levels to A1 and C strains of *D. nodosus* compared to vaccinated animals not treated with melatonin. These results suggest that melatonin increased the immune response to vaccination and open new perspectives in the design of prophylactic strategies.

Myers *et al.* (2007) sequenced its 1.4-Mb genome, the smallest known genome of an anaerobe. It differs markedly from small genomes of intracellular bacteria, retaining greater biosynthetic capabilities and lacking any evidence of extensive ongoing genome reduction. Comparative genomic microarray studies and bioinformatic analysis suggested that, despite its small size, almost 20% of the genome is derived from lateral gene transfer. Most of these regions seem to be associated with virulence. Metabolic reconstruction indicated unsuspected capabilities, including carbohydrate utilization, electron transfer and several aerobic pathways. Global transcriptional profiling and bioinformatic analysis enabled the prediction of virulence factors and cell surface proteins. Screening of these proteins against ovine antisera identified eight immunogenic proteins that are candidate antigens for a cross-protective vaccine.

References

Belloy L., Giacometti M., Boujon P. and Waldvogel A. 2007.Detection of Dichelobacter nodosus in wild ungulates (Capra ibex ibex and Ovis aries musimon) and domestic sheep suffering from foot rot using a two-step polymerase chain reaction. J. Wildl. Dis. **43:** 82-88.

Billington, S.J., Johnston, J.L. and Rood, J.I. 1996. Virulence regions and virulence factors of the ovine foot rot pathogen, *Dichelobacter nodosus*. FEMS Microbiol. Lett. **145:** 147-156.

Cagatay T.I. and Hickford J.G. 2008.Glycosylation of type-IV fimbriae of *Dichelobacter nodosus*. Vet Microbiol. **126:** 160-167. Epub 2007 Jun 17.

Calvo-Bado, L.A., Green, L.E., Medley, G.F., Ul-Hassan, A., Grogono-Thomas, R., Buller, N., Kaler, J., Russell, C.L., Kennan, R.M., Rood, J.I. and Wellington, E.M. 2010. Detection and diversity of a putative novel heterogenous polymorphic proline-glycine repeat (Pgr) protein in the foot rot pathogen *Dichelobacter nodosus*. Vet. Microbiol. [http://www.ncbi.nlm.nih.gov/pubmed/ 20655152].

Cagatay I.T. and Hickford J.G.2005.Update on ovine footrot in New Zealand: isolation, identification, and characterization of *Dichelobacter nodosus* strains [corrected]. Vet. Microbiol. **111:** 171-180. Epub 2005 Nov 8.

Cheetham, B.F., Tanzing, L.R., Sutherland, M., Dreitt, J., Green, G., McFarlane, J., Bailey, G.D., Seaman, J.T., and Katz, M.E. 2006. Improved diagnosis of virulent ovine foot using the int A gene. Vet. Microbiol. **116:** 166-174.

Dhungyel O.P., Whittington R.J. and Egerton J.R.2002.Serogroup specific single and multiplex PCR with pre-enrichment culture and immuno-magnetic bead capture for identifying strains of *D. nodosus* in sheep with footrot prior to vaccination. Mol. Cell Probes. **16:** 285-296.

Dhungyel, O.P. and Whittington, R.J. 2009. Modulation of intervaccination interval to avoid antigenic competition in multivalent foot rot (*Dichelobacter nodosus*) vaccine in sheep. Vaccine **28:** 470-473.

Egerton, J.R. Yong, W.K. and Reffkin, G.g. (eds) 1989. Foot rot and foot abscess of ruminants. Boca Raton, Fla: CRC Press.

Elleman, T.C. 1988. Pilin of *Bacteroides nodosus*: Molecular basis of serotypic variation and relationships to other bacterial pilin. Microbiol. Rev. **52:** 233-247.

Ghimire S.C., Whittington R.J., Dhungyel O.P., Joshi H.D. and Egerton J.R 2002.Diagnosis of footrot in goats: application of ELISA tests for response to antigens of *Dichelobacter nodosus*. Vet. Microbiol. **87:** 237-251.

Gurung R.B., Dhungyel O.P., Tshering P. and Egerton J.R 2006.The use of an autogenous *Dichelobacter nodosus* vaccine to eliminate clinical signs of virulent footrot in a sheep flock in Bhutan. Vet J. **172:** 356-363. Epub 2005 Jul 12.

Hill A.E., Dhungyel O.P. and Whittington R.J.2010.Diagnostic sampling strategies for virulent ovine footrot: simulating detection of *Dichelobacter nodosus* serogroups for bivalent vaccine formulation. Prev. Vet. Med. **95:** 127-136. Epub 2010 Mar 19.

Hussain, I., Wani, S.A., Qureshi, S.D. and Farooq, S. 2009. Serological diversity and virulence determination of *Dichelobacter nodosus* from foot rot in India. Mol. Cell. Probes. **23:** 112-114.

Jiménez R., Píriz S., Mateos E. and Vadillo S. 2004.Minimum inhibitory concentrations for 25 selected antimicrobial agents against *Dichelobacter nodosus* and *Fusobacterium* strains isolated from footrot in sheep of Portugal and Spain. J. Vet. Med. B Infect. Dis. Vet. Public. Health. **51:** 245-248.

Kennan R.M., Dhungyel O.P., Whittington R.J., Egerton J.R. and Rood J.I. 2001.The type IV fimbrial subunit gene (fimA) of *Dichelobacter nodosus* is essential for virulence, protease secretion, and natural competence. J. Bacteriol. **183:** 4451-4458.

Liu, D. and Yong, W.K. 1993. Use of elastase test, gelatine gel test and electrophoretic zymogram to determine virulence of *Dichelobacter nodosus* isolated from ovine foot rot. Res. Vet. Sci. **55:** 124-129.

Mattick, J.S., Anderson, B.J., Cox, P.T., Dalrymple, B.P., Bills, M.M., Hobbs, M. and Egerton, J.R. 1991. Gene sequences and comparison of the fimbrial subunits representative of *Bacteroides nodosus* serotype A to I class I and class II strains. Mol. Microbiol. **5:** 561-573.

Myers G.S., Parker D., Al-Hasani K., Kennan R.M., Seemann T., Ren Q., Badger J.H., Selengut J.D., Deboy R.T., Tettelin H., Boyce J.D., McCarl V.P., Han X., Nelson W.C., Madupu R., Mohamoud Y., Holley T., Fedorova N., Khouri H., Bottomley S.P., Whittington R.J., Adler B., Songer J.G. and Rood J.I., Paulsen I.T. 2007.Genome sequence and identification of candidate vaccine antigens from the animal pathogen *Dichelobacter nodosus*. Nat Biotechnol. **25:** 569-575. Epub 2007 Apr 29.

O'Meara T.J., Egerton J.R. and Raadsma HW.1993.Recombinant vaccines against ovine footrot. Immunol. Cell Biol. **71**(Pt 5): 473-488.

Palanisamy, S.K., Fletcher, C., Tanjung, L., Katz, M.E. and Cheetham, B.F. 2010. Deletion of C-twitching motility, a virulence characteristics of the anaerobic bacterial pathogen *Dichelobacter nodosus*. FEMS Microbiol. Lett. **302:** 39-45.

Parker D., Kennan RM., Myers G.S., Paulsen I.T., Songer J.G., and Rood J.I. 2006. Regulation of type IV fimbrial biogenesis in *Dichelobacter nodosus*. J. Bacteriol. **188:** 4801-4811.

Rather M.A., Wani S.A., Hussain I., Bhat M.A., Kabli Z.A. and Magray S.N. 2011. Determination of prevalence and economic impact of ovine footrot in central Kashmir India with isolation and molecular characterization of *Dichelobacter nodosus*. Anaerobe. **17:** 73-77. Epub 2011 Mar 21.

Regodon, S., Ramos, A., Morgado, S. Tarazona, R., Martin-Palomino, P., Rosado, J.A. and Miguez Mdel, P. 2009. Melatonin enhances the immune response to vaccination against A1 and C strains of *Dichelobacter nodosus*. Vaccine **27:** 1566-1570.

Rood, J.I., Howarth, P.A., Haring, V., Billington, S.J., Yong, W.K., Liu, D., Palmer, M.A., Pitman, D.R., Links, I., Stewart, D.J. and Vaughan, J.A. 1996. Comparison of gene probe and conventional methods for the differentiation of ovine foot isolates of *Dichelobacter nodosus*. Vet. Microbiol. **52:** 127-141.

Skerman, T.M. 1989. Isolation and identification of *Dichelobacter nodosus*. In Foot rot and Foot Absecess of ruminants. Ed. J.R. Egerton, W.K. Yong and G.G. Riffkin. Boca Raton, Fla: CRC Press.

Wani S.A., Samanta I. and Kawoosa S. 2007.Isolation and characterization of *Dichelobacter nodosus* from ovine and caprine footrot in Kashmir, India. Res. Vet .Sci. **83:** 141-144. Epub 2007 Jan 23.

Wassnik, G.J., King, E.M., Grogono-Thomas, R., Brown, J.C., Moore, L.J. and Green, L.E. 2010. A within farm clinical trial to compare 2 treatments (parenteral antibacterial hoof trimming) for sheep lameness with foot rot. Prev. Vet. Med. **96:** 93-103.

Whittington R.J., Saunders V.F. and Moses E.K. 1997. Antigens for serological diagnosis of ovine footrot. Vet. Microbiol. **54:** 255-274.

Wong, W., Kannan, R.M., Rosado, C.J., Rood, J.I., Whisstock, J.C., Poster, C.J. 2010. Acta. Crystallogr. Sect. F. Struct. Biol. Cryst. Commun. **66:** 289-293.

Chapter 15

Helicobacter

Dr. S.K. SRIVASTAVA
Former, Division of Bacteriology & Mycology
Indian Veterinary Research Institute, Izatnagar-243122
Bareilly (U.P.)

Helicobacter

Helicobacter is a spiral organism commonly prevalent in gastric environment of man and animals. It was previously classified in the genus Campylobacter. Since the discovery of *Helicobacter pylori* from gastric tissues of man in 1982, it has been isolated from stomach of ferrets, non-human primates, dogs, cats, cheetals and laboratory animals. Since 1989, the strains have been grouped into its own genus. These bacteria are gram-negative motile and curved to spiral shaped. The organisms are microaerophilic. The type species *H.pylori* is commonly prevalent in stomach of 20% to 95% of human beings throughout the world. Helicobacter is highly adaptive; can live in a single host for years. The organism is responsible for causing persistent gastritis mainly in the antrum of stomach leading to peptic ulcer in humans. Gastric adenocarcinoma has been epidemiologically associated with this organism. Helicobacter spp. are also carried in the stomach or intestine of animals without causing apparent disease. They live beneath the mucous coating where the pH may reach 7.4. *H.pylori* infection has been associated with patients with chronic renal failure receiving dialysis (Sugimoto & Yamoaka 2011). The table enlists several species of *Helicobacter* isolated from human and animals. At least 20 species have been identified. The 16 S rRNA analysis has been useful for identifying and studying similar gastric bacteria in a variety of animal species. *Helicobacter pylori* strains exhibit a high degree of genomic heterogeneity due in part to nucleotide substitutions among strains. However, *H.pylori,* lacks an SOS mutagenesis pathway and the large number of nucleotides substitutions are probably due to replication fidelity deficiencies or mismatch repair defects.

Table : Some of the commonly isolated Helicobacter species and their hosts

Species	Hosts	Primary site of isolation
H.pylori	Human, macaque, cat	Stomach
H.mustelae	Ferret, mink	Stomach
H.felis	Cat, Dog	Stomach
H.heilmanii	Dog, Cat, human, monkey	Stomach
H.suis	Swine	Stomach
H.rappini	Sheep, dog, human, mice	Intestine*
H.canis	Dog, human	Intestine, liver of dog
H.hepaticus	Mice	Intestine, liver
H.rodentium	Mice	Intestine
H.muridarum	Mice, rat	Intestine, stomach of mice
H.bilis	Research mice	Intestine
H.cinaedii	Human, hamster	Intestine
H.fenneliae	Human	Intestine
H.pullorum	Chicken, human	Intestine
H.pameteusis	Bird, swine	Intestine

* Also from liver of sheep.

Non-pyloric *Helicobacter* spp. encompasses two groups, gastric and enterohepatic, showing different organ specificity. Some species such as *H.hepaticus, H.mustelae* and probably *H.bilis* exhibit carcinogenic potential in animals. Gastric helicobacters such as *H.suis, H.felis, H.bizzozeroni* and *H.salomonis* cause chronic gastritis and peptic ulcer in humans and lymphoma compared to *H.pylori*. Enterohepatic species such as *H.hepaticus, H.bilis* and *H.ganmani* cause hepatobiliary disease.

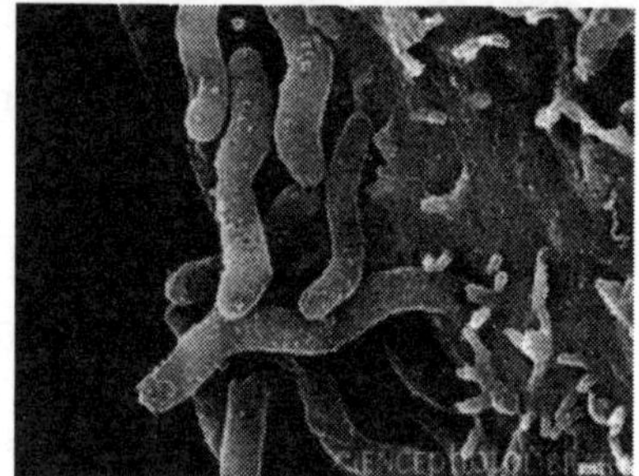

Helicobacter pylori scanning microscopic picture

H.rappini, is entwined with periplasmic fibres that cover the entire surface of the organism. The periplasmic fibres in *H.felis* are sparsly distributed and visible singly or in groups of two, three or four. *H.heilmanni* is very tightly coiled devoid of periplasmic fibres. All *Helicobacter* species have sheathed flagella except *H.pullorum* and *H.rodentium.*

There have been some doubts on the pathogenic significance of Helicobacter in dogs and cats. However, evidence suggests that they can cause gastritis and some serous implications. Besides, vomiting, regurgitation, abdominal pain, fever, diarrhoea, anorexia, weight loss and debilitated condition can be caused. These conditions are due to colonization of bacteria gastric tissues and induction inflammatory response which increase the level of oxygen species. The type strain, *H.pylori,* has evolved adaptive mechanisms to minimize oxidative damage by utilizing its enzymes, superoxide dismutase and catalase. The type of helicobacter traditionally found in the stomach of cats, namely *H.felis* and *H.heilmanni* have been referred as gastric *Helicobacter* whereas commonly found in intestine, are referred as enteric Helicobacter (Lecoindre *et al.,* 2000). *H.cinaedi* from feces of dogs and a cat has been recently isolated. *H.fenneliae* has also been identified in the feces of dogs and macaques. Similarly *H.canis* also has been isolated from feces of normal and diarrheic dogs. It has also been isolated from liver of a puppy diagnosed as having an active multifocal hepatitis. *H.equorum* sp. Nov. has been isolated from horse feces. The organism is urease negative (Moyaert *et al.,* 2007). *H.cynogastricus* a new species, was reported by Van den Bukk *et al.,* (2006) from canine gastric mucosa. A study was carried out primarily, to determine the existence of Helicobacter spp. in the oral secretions of stray cats as one of the possible routes of transmission and secondly, to evaluate the accordance between oral and gastric colonization of Helicobacter spp. in these cats(Shojaee et al2010). Forty-three adult stray cats were thus studied for the presence of Helicobacter species by quantitative rapid urease test (RUT), cytology and PCR. Helicobacter spp. were found in the oral secretions and gastric biopsies of 93% and 67.5% of the stray cats, respectively. There was not, however, any agreement observed between Helicobacter colonization at these two locations, at neither genus nor species level. These findings suggest that the oral cavity is routinely exposed to transient forms of bacteria and may temporarily harbor *Helicobacter* spp. Thus, oral cavity as a source of *Helicobacter* spp. may act as a reservoir for transmission and may not necessarily reflect the colonization status of the gastric mucosa.

Ulceration in the non-glandular part of the stomach of pigs has been reported in several countries. It is a disease of complex etiology in which multiple factors are involved including dietary and stress conditions such as small particle sizes of feed, interruption of feed intake and the presence of highly fermentable carbohydrates. Its etiology also seems to be associated with various infectious diseases such as porcine reproductive respiratory syndrome (PRRS), post-weaning multisystemic wasting syndrome (PMWS) and porcine dermatitis nephrophathy syndrome (PDNS). Ulcers of the non-glandular part of the stomach have been associated with *Helicobacter* (*H.*) *suis,* but the exact role of *H. suis* in porcine gastric pathology is a subject of considerable debate. Indeed, several authors did not find this association while it has been recently reported that gastric ulcers of the non-glandular part of the stomach were induced in pigs experimentally infected with *H. suis* . In any case, it was demonstrated that *H. suis* causes gastritis in experimentally and naturally infected pigs. *H. suis* is the main *Helicobacter* species colonizing the stomachs of pigs and is the most prevalent gastric non-*H. pylori Helicobacter* species in humans. There are strong indications that pigs may be a source of *H. suis* infection in humans, while animals may be occasionally infected with *H. pylori*; Krakowka et al. [1995] demonstrated the occurrence of gastric ulcers in gnotobiotic piglets experimentally infected with *H. pylori*. Our study was conducted to evaluate the presence of *Helicobacter* spp., *H. suis* and *H. pylori* by PCR in swine affected by gastric ulcers. Moreover, the presence of *Helicobacter* spp. was investigated in feces and saliva samples in order to assess the feasibility of an *in vivo* detection method.

Using 16 S rRNA sequencing *H.suis* have been identified. A higher incidence of *H.suis* in swine with gastric ulcers located in parsoesophagea has been identified. In pigs *H.suis* normally colonize the mucus layer and gastric pits of the antral and body mucosa. Helicobacter (H.) heilmannii" type 1 is the most prevalent gastric non-H. pylori Helicobacter species in humans suffering from gastric disease. It has been shown to be identical to H. suis, a bacterium which is mainly associated with pigs. To obtain better insights into the long-term pathogenesis of infections with this micro-organism, experimental infections were carried out in different rodent models.Mongolian gerbils and mice of two strains (BALB/c and C57BL/6) were infected with H. suis and sacrificed at 3 weeks, 9 weeks and 8 months after infection. Gastric tissue samples were collected for PCR analysis, histological and ultrastructural examination. In gerbils, bacteria mainly colonized the antrum and a narrow zone in the fundus near the forestomach/stomach transition zone. In both mice strains, bacteria colonized the entire glandular stomach. Colonization with H. suis was associated with necrosis of parietal cells in all three animal strains. From 9 weeks after infection onwards, an increased proliferation rate of mucosal epithelial cells was detected in the stomach regions colonized with H. suis. Most gerbils showed a marked lymphocytic infiltration in the antrum and in the forestomach/stomach transition zone, becoming more pronounced in the course of time. At 8 months post infection, severe destruction of the normal antral architecture at the inflamed sites and development of mucosa-associated lymphoid tissue (MALT) lymphoma-like lesions were observed in some gerbils. In mice, the inflammatory response was less pronounced than in gerbils, consisting mainly of mononuclear cell infiltration and being most severe in the fundus (Flahou *et al.* 2010). It is concluded that H. suis causes death of parietal cells, epithelial cell hyperproliferation and severe inflammation in mice and Mongolian gerbil models of human gastric disease. Moreover, MALT lymphoma-like lesions were induced in *H. suis*-infected Mongolian gerbils. Therefore, the possible involvement of this micro-organism in human gastric disease should not be neglected.

The aim of one study was to evaluate the presence of Helicobacter spp. in swine affected by gastric ulceration (Casagrande et al.2010). Stomachs from 400 regularly slaughtered swine were subjected to gross pathological examination to evaluate the presence of gastric ulcers. Sixty-five samples collected from ulcerated pars esophagea and 15 samples from non-ulcerated pyloric portions were submitted to histopathological and molecular analyses, to detect *Helicobacter* spp., *H. suis* and *H. pylori* by PCR. Feces and saliva swabs were also collected from 25 animals in order to detect in vivo the presence of *Helicobacter* spp.. Gastric ulcers were detected in 373 cases (93%). The presence of ulcers in association with inflammatory processes was further confirmed by histological examination. Forty-nine percent (32/65) of the ulcerated esophageal portions as well as 53% (8/15) of the non-ulcerated pyloric portions were positive for Helicobacter spp. by PCR. The Helicobacter spp. positive samples were also positive for *H. suis*, while *H. pylori* was not detected. These results were confirmed by restriction enzyme analysis. With regard to feces and saliva samples, 15/25 (60%) and 16/25 (64%) were positive for *Helicobacter* spp. PCR, respectively but all were negative in H. suis and H. pylori specific PCR.

In order to obtain better insight into the genes involved in pathogenicity and in the specific adaptation to the gastric environment of *H. suis*, a genome analysis was performed of two *H. suis* strains isolated from the gastric mucosa of swine(Vermoote et al.2011). Homologs of the vast majority of genes shown to be important for gastric colonization of the human pathogen *H. pylori* were detected in the *H. suis* genome. *H. suis* encodes several putative outer membrane proteins, of which two similar to the *H. pylori* adhesins HpaA and HorB. *H. suis* harbours an almost complete comB type IV secretion system and members of the type IV secretion system 3, but lacks most of the genes present in the cag pathogenicity island of *H. pylori*. Homologs of genes encoding the *H. pylori* neutrophil-activating protein and γ-glutamyl transpeptidase were identified in *H. suis*. *H. suis* also possesses several other presumptive virulence-associated genes, including homologs for mviN, the *H. pylori* flavodoxin gene, and a homolog of the *H. pylori* vacuolating cytotoxin A gene. It was concluded that although genes coding for some important virulence factors in *H. pylori*, such as the cytotoxin-associated protein (CagA), are not detected in the *H. suis* genome, homologs of other genes associated with colonization and virulence of *H. pylori* and other bacteria are present.

The experimental evidence that long-term colonization of Helicobacter pylori results in the development of gastric cancer in Mongolian gerbils has been reported only by two Japanese groups to date. Zheng *et al.* (2004) carried out a study aimed to investigate the carcinogenicity of *H. pylori* infection in a Mongolian gerbil model. Thirty-six Mongolian gerbils (inner Mongolian origin) were divided into two groups (male to female ratio, 1:1) and orally inoculated with a standard *H. pylori* strain (ATCC43504) or *H. pylori* 161 (isolated from a Chinese patient with gastric adenocarcinoma), respectively, once a week for 5 weeks. Another 10 control gerbils were given phosphate-buffered saline. The animals were killed 8, 20, 28 and 84 weeks after inoculation for bacterial and histological examination. Seven inoculated gerbils died at the week 42. Overall, H. pylori colonization was detected in 24 (83%) of the 29 available inoculated gerbils. The gastric lesions were aggravated gradually over time. At week 84, moderate to severe gastritis, characterized by diffuse infiltration of mononuclear cells and formation of multiple lymphoid follicles in mucosa and submucosa, and even the lymphoepithelial lesions, were observed. Epithelial hyperplasia were dominant in almost all gerbils. Four (24%) of the 17 animals had hyperplastic polyps. Intestinal metaplasia were rarely seen (in three gerbils). Well-differentiated gastric adenocarcinomas developed in three (18%) of the 17 gerbils after 84 weeks. Of the three gerbils, one female gerbil was infected with *H. pylori* 161 and the others (one male and one female) were infected with ATCC43504.

The present study reconfirms that *H. pylori* infection alone can induce gastric adenocarcinoma in Mongolian gerbils and suggests that different species of gerbil and both standard and clinically isolated *H. pylori* strains can be used for investigating the carcinogenesis of H. pylori. This is the first report of the development of gastric cancer in female gerbils, which highlights the importance of using both sexes to investigate the pathogenesis of *H. pylori* and whether host susceptibility is influenced by sex.

Flexispira rappini, isolated for the first time from humans with diarrohoea and also from feces of a young asymptomatic dog, has been cultured from aborted ovine fetuses. The organism can cross the placenta in pregnant sheep, cause acute hepatic necrosis in sheep fetuses and induce abortion. This organism was later designated as *Helicobacter rappini.*

Since, the original observation of helicobacters in mice in the 1990s, it is now known that helicobacter spp. are prevalent in many rodent colonies throughout the world, persisting in the intestine for the life of the animal. *H.bilis, H.hepaticus* and *H.rodentium* have been most frequently isolated.

Pathogenesis

Transmission of helicobacters is via the fecal oral or oral routes. There is a controversy that some non-culturable cocoid *Helicobacter* are present in the environment which may be transmitted to the host to cause the disease. The organisms occur in the gastric mucus layer and variety of animals and their capacity to breakdown urea with the production of ammonia and carbon dioxide with the consequent raising of the pH contributes to their survival. Urease is produced by *Helicobacter* spp. which locally raises the pH from less than 2 to a more biocompatible range of 6-7. The ecological niche of intestinal *helicobacter* is the crypts of the colon and cecum and in some cases it colonizes the bile canaliculi of the liver.

The virulence factors of *Helicobacter* include adhesion, flagella, cytotoxin, urease, acid inhibitory protein, mucinase, catalase, superoxide dismutase, vacuolating cytotoxin (VacA) and Cytotoxin associated gene (Cag A).

A number of other putative virulence factors for Helicobacter pylori have been identified including cagA, vacA and iceA (Graham and Yamaoka 2000). The criteria for a true virulence factor includes meeting the tests of biologically plausibility with the associations being both experimentally and epidemiologically consistent. Although disease-specific associations have been hypothesized/claimed, there are now sufficient data to conclusively state that none of these putative virulence factors have disease specificity. CagA has been claimed to be associated with increased mucosal IL-8 and inflammation, increased density of *H. pylori* in the antrum, duodenal ulcer (DU), gastric cancer, and protection against Barrett's cancer. Only the increase in IL-8/ inflammation is direct and substantiated. Different *H. pylori* strains with functional cag pathogenicity islands do not vary in virulance as it has been shown that mucosal IL-8 levels are proportional to the number of cagA + H. pylori independent of the disease from which the *H. pylori* were obtained. It is now known that the density of either cagA + and cagA-*H. pylori* in the antrum of patients with *H. pylori* gastritis is the same. In contrast, the mean density of *H. pylori* in the antrum in DU is greater than in the antrum of patients with H. pylori gastritis. Of interest, the density of *H. pylori* is higher in the corpus of patients with *H. pylori* gastritis than those with DU, suggesting that acid secretion plays a critical role in these phenomena. The presence of a functional cag pathogenicity island increases inflammation and it is likely that any factor that results in an increase in inflammation also increases the risk of a symptomatic outcome. Nevertheless, the presence of a functional cag pathogenicity island has no predictive value for the presence, or the future development of a clinically significant outcome. The hypothesis that iceA has disease specificity has not been confirmed and there is currently no known biological or epidemiological evidence for a role for iceA as a virulence factor in *H. pylori*-related disease. The claim that vacA genotyping might prove clinically useful, e.g. to predict presentation such as duodenal ulcer, has been proven wrong. Analysis of the worldwide data show that vacA genotype s1 is actually a surrogate for the cag pathogenicity island. There is now evidence to suggest that virulence is a host-dependent factor. The pattern of gastritis has withstood the test of time for its relation to different *H. pylori*-related diseases (e.g. antral predominant gastritis with duodenal ulcer disease). The primary factors responsible for the different patterns of gastritis in response to an *H. pylori* infection are environmental (e.g. diet), with the H. pylori strain playing a lesser role. Future studies should work to eliminate potential bias before claiming disease associations. Controls must exclude regional or geographic associations related to the common strain circulation and not to the outcome.

Although the cag pathogenicity island, especially the cagA gene, has been linked with adenocarcinoma, few data concerning *H. pylori* pathogenic factors involved in low-grade gastric MALT lymphoma are available. The goal of one study was to analyze the prevalence of and correlation between genes coding for seven *H. pylori* virulence factors (cagA, cagE, vacA, iceA, babA, hopQ, and oipA) and two novel adhesins (sabA and hopZ) by comparing a collection of 43 *H. pylori* strains isolated from patients with low-grade gastric MALT lymphoma to 39 strains isolated from age-matched patients with gastritis only Lehours *et al.*, 2004). These results show that taken individually, none of the nine genes tested can be considered associated with MALT strains and allows one to conclude that MALT pathogenesis is not linked with more proinflammatory *H. pylori* strains. The study demonstrated that in patients infected with strains harboring the iceA1 allele, sabA functional status, and hopZ "off" status, the odds of developing a MALT lymphoma were 10 times higher. However, the low prevalence of such strains (10 of 43 MALT strains) renders this triple association a low-sensitivity marker for MALT strains. These data confirmed that *H. pylori* virulence factors are correlated with one another. If the involvement of *H. pylori* in MALT lymphoma is well established, the pathomechanism by which gastric lymphoma occurs remains to be identified.

Urease and flagella are necessary to colonize Helicobacter spp. in the gastric mucus. Phenotypic expression of gamma-glutamyl transpeptidase by *H.pylori* strains has been correlated with colonization of the bacteria in mice (Chevalier *et al.*, 1999). Cytotoxins and urease and certain proteins are required to induce chronic inflammation. Vac A protein is toxic to human cells. Besides a cytotoxin associated protein is important for causing peptic ulcer by *H.pylori*. It has MW of 120-140 kDa (Perez - Perez *et al.*, 1999). These virulence factors which are present persistently in the gastric environment probably initiate sustained production of a series of inflammatory cytokines.

Breakdown of urea as a result of production of urease by Helicobacter releases ammonia which causes tissue irritation. The presence of these urease producing bacteria in stomach and liver may damage cells adjacent to the colonizing bacterial cells. Vacuolating cytotoxin (Vac A) is an important factor in induction of gastric ulcer as well as chronic atrophic gastritis, a precancerous gastric lesion. Gastric erosion may be caused by *H.pylori* exotoxin. A soluble cytotoxin exists in *H.hepatica* directly affecting the murine hepatic cell live.

In order to live in the gastric environment, it has developed a repertoire of acid resistance mechanisms that can be classified into time-independent, acute, and chronic responses. Time-independent acid resistance depends on the structure of the organism's inner and outer membrane proteins that have a high isoelectric point, thereby reducing their proton permeability. Acute acid resistance depends on the constitutive synthesis of a neutral pH optimum urease that is an oligomeric Ni(2+)-containing heterodimer of UreA and UreB subunits. Gastric juice urea is able to rapidly access intrabacterial urease when the periplasmic pH falls below approximately 6.2 owing to pH-gating of a urea channel, UreI. This results in the formation of NH3, which then neutralizes the bacterial periplasm to provide a pH of approximately 6.2 and an inner membrane potential of -101 mV, giving a proton motive force of approximately -200 mV. UreI is a six-transmembrane segment protein, with homology to the amiS genes of the amidase gene cluster and to UreI of *Helicobacter hepaticus* and *Streptococcus salivarius*. Expression of these UreI proteins in Xenopus oocytes has shown that UreI of *H. pylori* and *H. hepaticus* can transport urea only at acidic pH, whereas that of *S. salivarius* is open at both neutral and acidic pH. Site-directed mutagenesis and chimeric analysis have identified amino acids implicated in maintaining the closed state of the channel at neutral pH and other amino acids that play a structural role in channel function. Deletion of ureI abolishes the ability of the organism to survive in acid and also to colonize the mouse or gerbil stomach. However, if acid secretion is inhibited in gerbils, the deletion mutants do colonize but are eradicated when acid secretion is allowed to return, showing that UreI is essential for gastric survival and that the habitat of *H. pylori* at the gastric surface must fall to pH 3.5 or below. The chronic response is from increased Ni(2+) insertion into the apo-enzyme, which results in a threefold increase in urease, which is also dependent on expression of UreI. This allows the organism to live in either gastric fundus or gastric antrum depending on the level of acidity at the gastric surface. There are other effects of acid on transcript stability that may alter levels of protein synthesis in acid. Incubation of the organism at acidic pH also results in regulation of expression of a variety of genes, such as some outer membrane proteins, that constitutes an acid tolerance response. Understanding of these acid resistance and tolerance responses should provide novel eradication therapies for this carcinogenic gastric pathogen (Sach *et al.*, 2003).

In dogs, various *Helicobacter* spp. localize within the surface mucus, the lumen of gastric glands and inside parietal cells. They also colonize small intestine of dogs. In the cecum and colon, high concentration of *H.billis, H.cinaedi* and *H.canis* are localized with in the mucus and crypts (Recordati *et al.*, 2009). Helicobacter spp. are normally present in the feces of cats as detected by PCR (Shen *et al.*, 2001). Coinfection with Campylobacter is normally observed.

H.felis and *H.heil*mannii when inoculated in dogs in high number, induction of lymphoreticular hyperplasia was observed. In pet dogs and cats, helicobacters was associated with reduction of mucus of surface epithelia possibly due to the presence of mucinase. Abnormal findings in stomach are vacuolation, enlarged cell size and nuclear degeneration. The presence of large number of *H.pylori* in the gastric mucosa of commercially reared cats was associated with lymphofollicular gastritis, characterized by lymphoid aggregates and diffuses inflammation in the deep mucosa and lamina propria.

H.mustelae is located on the surface of mucosa of stomach but not in crypts. In the distal antrum, inflammation occupied the full thickness of the mucosa in humans. In *H.hepaticus* infected mice liver lesions are observed characterized by inflammation and necrosis involving hepatic parenchyma, the portal triad and small intralobular hepatic virnles. *H.canis* has also been observed in dog liver with multifocal hepatitis. *H.hepaticus* and *H.bilis* infection are associated with inflammatory bowel disease in immunodeficient mice and only in frequently in *H.hepaticus* infected immunocompetent mice.

Lipopolysaccharide (LPS) is considered as an important virulence factor of *H.pylori* and contributes to disease persistence and severity. It also helps bacteria to adhere on cells (Chang *et al.*, 2011). The O specific chain of LPS mimics Lewis blood group antigen in structure which is present in the gastric mucosa. The expression of Lewis antigens on the bacterial surface may camouflage the bacterium and aid survival of bacterium. LPS mediate the binding of the bacterium to laminin and interferes with gastric cell receptor thereby contributing to the loss of mucosal integrity (Moran 1996).

Helicobacter LPS exhibits reduced endotoxic potency and this may account for the escape mechanism from the host immunosurveillance exerted by this bacterium. Despite its low immunological activity, LPS promotes production of an array of proinflammatory cytokines such as interleukin (IL)

& IL-1 and tumor necrosis factor from epithelial cells and macrophages (Pece *et al.*, 1997). *Helicobacter pylori* exhibit adhesion to gastric mucosa through a protein HpaA. Non-gastric helicobacters do not show this protein (Evans *et al.*, 1995). The adhesion proteins are present on outer membrane protein of bacterial cells (Evans and Evans 2000) namely BabA protein which recognize Leb antigen of gastric mucosa. The SabA adhesin bind to sialyated antigens. Other OMP are Alp AB or HopZ which bind to gastric epithelial cells (Odenbreit 2005).

The 128 kDa CagA protein has been established as a useful marker of H. pylori strains associated with more severe forms of disease(Stephens *et al.*, 1996). A mouse monoclonal antibody raised against the CagA protein has been produced and characterised as belonging to the IgG1 subtype. It identified the protein in all clinical isolates (10/10) from this laboratory and in two NCTC reference strains (NCTC 11637 and NCTC 11961). No cross-reacting proteins were detected in H. pylori L2, a well characterised strain known not to contain the cagA gene, or in four *Helicobacter* sp. from non-human sources (H. canis, H. mustelidae, *H. muridarum* and H. acinonyx). The monoclonal antibody was used to develop an antigen capture ELISA system for detecting the presence of antibodies to the CagA protein in human serum samples.

Laboratory Diagnosis

Isolation and identification or demonstration of helical bacteria from samples from patients with gastritis is suggestive of *Helicobacter*. The organisms can be isolated routinely from the gastric tissues of infected animals and man. It is more difficult to isolate *H.felis* from dogs and cats and also *H.heilmanni*. They do not form distinct colonies but rather bacterial growth consisting of a very fine spreading film. The organisms are not routinely cultured from gastric juices or feces. The medium of choice is the selective antibiotic media. It consists of Brucella agar with 10% horse blood and vancomycin (10mg/lit), polymyxin B (2500μ/lit) and Trimethoprim (5 mg/lit). Incubation for up to a week may be required for appreciable growth. Use of 0.45μ or 0.65μ filter to selectively filter feces helps minimize contamination from other enteric organisms during primary culture or selective agar. Fresh media are recommended for optimal growth. The organisms grow best under microaerophilic condition (5% Co_2, 90% N_2, 5% H_2).

Scrapings of the gastric mucosa can be directly examined under phase contrast microscope for demonstration of helicobacters. The organisms are motile and helical-shaped. The organisms can also be seen in smears and stained sections of gastric biopsies. The objective of one study was to improve the visual localization of urease activity of Helicobacter pylori-like organisms (HPLO) on swine gastric mucosa by in vitro optimization of the urea concentration and pH indicator of a urease test reagent (McIntosh et al 2010). Five 21-day-old conventional pigs were infected orally with HPLO (3 pigs) or Brucella broth alone (2 pigs). At 17 d after infection the pigs were euthanized and their stomachs excised and tested for HPLO by a modified urease test formulation sprayed onto the gastric mucosa, as well as confirmatory culture and isolation of HPLO from urease-positive sites. This study showed improved detection of HPLO in porcine gastric mucosa with the use of a modified urease test formulation containing 5% urea and the pH indicator bromocresol purple compared with the use of a conventional formulation of 2% urea and phenol red. This test can readily be applied to achieve a presumptive diagnosis of HPLO in cases of gastritis or gastric esophageal ulceration in pigs.

Bacterial urease hydrolyzes urea, resulting in ammonia production and a subsequent rise in the microenvironmental pH. This increase in pH is indirectly detected by a urease test reagent that contains urea and a pH indicator. The customary reagent formulation for the detection of cultured urease-producing organisms is 2% urea (w/v) and the indicator phenol red, which changes from yellow-orange to pink-red at a pH of 6.8 to 8.2. However, this indicator is problematic for use on *Helicobacter*-infected gastric mucosa because modest color changes cannot, in confidence, be distinguished from the normal color of the gastric mucosa.For presumptive diagnosis of the helicobacters urease activity of the bacteria can be performed. The urease activity is visible in gastric tissues between 15 minutes to 3 hours. The helicobacters are oxidase positive and do not ferment carbohydrates, and with the exception of *H.felis,* are catalase positive. *Helicobacter heilmanni,* the most common species in dogs and cats, do not grow on artificial media. *H.felis* is difficult to isolate. *H.bellis, H.canis* and *H.cinaedi* from dogs and cats have been identified using whole cell protein profile, phenotypic tests, PCR-RFLP of gyrB and phylogenetic study of partial groEL and 16sRNA sequence (Rossi *et al.,* 2008).

Gastric brushing cytology can be performed during gastric endoscopy before obtaining gastric biopsies. Cells and mucus that adhere to the brush are applied to a glass slide, air dried, Giemsa stained and observed under microscope (100X).

An ELISA is used to determine the antibody response in animals and man following infection. The antigen used for ELISA is glycin extracted antigen or whole cell sonicate of the bacteria. An increase in *H.pylori* specific IgG and IgA in gastric secretions is suggestive of the infection. These antibodies are not protective. Recombinant antigens have also been used (Kendall *et al.,* 2004). Antigen consisting of a 128 kDa CagA protein, a virulence marker of *H.pylori,* can also be used for conducting ELISA. An enzyme immune assay for detection of *H.pylori* is in use to detect antigen in feces. The test is better than conducting histology and rapid urease test (Forne *et al.*, 2000). A rapid stool antigen test using monoclonal antibody to catalase for detection of *H.pylori* infection has been developed and found useful (Shimoyama *et al.*, 2011). The stool antigen test has been reported to be the most sensitive and specific and cost effective detection method for *H.pylori* in stool (Gisbert and Pajares 2001).

Polymerase chain reaction is useful for detection of Helicobacter in the stool or drinking water. Ge *et al.* (2001) described a fluorogenic PCR based assay for quantitative detection of *H.hepaticus* in mouse ceca and feces using ABI prism 7700 sequence detection system using a primer generated from the *H.hepaticus* Cdt B gene (encoding subunit B of the *H.hepaticus* cytolethal distending toxin). The test was found to possess high sensitivity and specificity. *H.pylori* PCR is used for detection of the organism in feces and saliva. PCR can also be used for detection of virulence factors such as cytotoxin associated genes and vacuolating Cytotoxin gene (VacA) in feces and saliva (Kabir 2004). Appino et al.(2006)evaluated by PCR the presence of Helicobacter spp. in gastric mucus from the fundic region of the stomach and investigated its role in oesophagogastric ulcers in swine bred and regularly slaughtered in Piedmont (Northern Italy). Stomachs from 595 regularly slaughtered swine were subjected to gross pathological examination in order to evaluate the presence of gastric ulcers (revealed in 75 cases, 12.6%). Histopathological examination was performed to better characterise erosions and ulcers. DNA extracted from gastric mucus collected from all the ulcer-affected and from 25 normal stomachs was submitted to PCR using Helicobacter spp. 16S rRNA gene target primers. Sixty-three percent (47/75) of the affected stomachs was positive as well as 24% (6/25) of the non-affected ones. Sequence analysis from 5 positive samples showed 99% homology with Helicobacter candidatus suis 16S ribosomal RNA gene.

Treatment and Control

For dogs and cats, metronidazole with amoxicillin or metronidazole with tetracycline given for 2-3 weeks is effective. Amoxicillin with omeprazole, (proton pump inhibitor) to inhibit gastric acid secretion is used. Ranitidine is also used to reduce gastric acid. Khosnegah et al.(2011) assessed the efficacy and safety of a 14-day quadruple Helicobacter species therapy in cats with naturally acquired infection. Thirteen asymptomatic adult stray cats with Helicobacter species infection (identified by analysis of gastric biopsies using polymerase chain reaction and Helicobacter-specific primers) received omeprazole 0.7mg/kg q 8h plus amoxicillin 20mg/kg q 12h, metronidazole 20mg/kg q 12h and clarithromycin 7.5mg/kg q 12h, for 14 days. Second molecular analysis of gastric biopsies revealed persistence of Helicobacter species DNA in four cats that were negative on quantitative urease testing, cytology and histopathology. Our results suggest that antibiotic regimens that are effective against *Helicobacter pylori* in people cannot eradicate Helicobacter species in cats with naturally acquired infection, although transient suppression may occur.Studies in ferrets indicate that the triple therapy consisting of amoxicillin, metronidazole and bismuth subsalicylate 3 times a week for 3 to 4 weeks has successfully eradicated *H.mustelae* from ferrets.

Helicobacter pylori, the major cause of gastric cancer, have mechanisms that allow colonization of the inhospitable gastric mucosa, including enzymes such as superoxide dismutase (SOD) which protect against reactive oxygen species (Every et al.2011). As SOD is essential for *in vivo* colonization, it was theorized that it might constitute a viable vaccine target. *H. pylori* SOD was expressed in *E. coli* and a purified recombinant protein used to vaccinate mice, prior to live *H. pylori* challenge. Partial protective immunity was induced, similar to that commonly observed with other antigens tested previously. This suggests SOD may have utility in a combination vaccine comprising several protective antigens.

It is well documented that the enzymatic active site of *Helicobacter pylori* urease is present in the beta-subunit. An important sequence of 135 amino acids of the beta-subunit was determined from the structure of *H. pylori* urease and by a homology-based study of the urease of other bacteria and plants (Fujii *et al.*, 2004). The sequence (UreB) was expressed in *Escherichia coli* as a recombinant fusion protein with glutathione-S-transferase (GST). Seventeen monoclonal antibodies, UA-1-17, were produced using the UreB-GST as the immunogen. The obtained monoclonal antibodies showed a high specificity to UreB, and some of the MAbs cross-reacted with Jack bean urease. About 70% of the established MAbs displayed an inhibitory effect on the enzymatic activity of the urease. Among them, UA-15 MAb could reduce the activity by 53% and it immunologically binds to the bacterium infecting the human stomach mucosa. The antiserum induced by immunization with a recombinant UreB-GST into rabbits displayed a specific binding to mucosal surfaces of the human stomach infected with the pathogen *H. pylori*. Moreover, the antiserum suppressed the enzymatic activity of *H. pylori* urease, while the purified H. pylori urease could not induce such an antiserum.

Yang *et al.* (2005) prepared the live recombinant vaccine of attenuated Salmonella typhimurium SL3261 expressing *Helicobacter pylori* (*H. pylori*) B subunit (UreB) and determined whether it could be used as an oral vaccine against *H. pylori* infection. Using genomic DNA of *H. pylori* Sydney strain (SSI) as template, the *H. pylori* UreB gene fragment was amplified by PCR and subcloned into the expression vector pTC01. The recombinant plasmid pTC01-UreB was then transferred into LB5000 to obtain modified forms, and further conversed into the attenuated Salmonella typhimurium SL3261 to obtain recombinant SL3261/pCT01-UreB as an oral immunization reagent, which was then used to orally immunize Balb/c mice twice at a three-week interval. Twelve weeks later, anti-UreB IgA antibodies in intestinal fluid and IgG antibodies in sera were determined by ELISA. The relating data in control groups (including body weight, gastric inflammation, etc.) were also collected. The sequencing analysis showed that the UreB gene fragment amplified by PCR was consistent with the sequence of the *H. pylori* UreB gene. The restriction enzyme digestion revealed that the correct pTC01-UreB was obtained. SDS-PAGE and Western blot showed that a 61KD protein was expressed in SL3261/pTC01-UreB, which could be recognized by anti-*H. pylori* UreB antiserum and was absent in the control containing only Salmonella typhimurium SL3261 strain. The multiple oral immunization with SL3261/pTC01-UreB could significantly induce *H. pylori* specific mucosal IgA response as well as serum IgG responses. IFN-gamma and IL-10 levels were significantly increased in SL3261/pTC01-UreB group, and no obvious side effect and change in gastric inflammation were observed.The attenuated vaccine of Salmonella typhimurium expressing *H. pylori* UreB can be used as an oral vaccine against *H. pylori* infection.

Xu *et al.* (2007) constructed a recombinant live attenuated Salmonella typhimurium DNA vaccine encoding *H. pylori* ureB gene and mouse IL-2 gene and to detect its immunogenicity in vitro and *in vivo*. *H. pylori* ureB and mouse IL-2 gene fragments were amplified by polymerase chain reaction (PCR) and cloned into pUCmT vector. DNA sequence of the amplified ureB and IL-2 genes was assayed, then cloned into the eukaryotic expression vector pIRES through enzyme digestion and ligation reactions resulting in pIRES-ureB and pIRES-ureB-IL-2. The recombinant plasmids were used to transform competent *E. coli* DH5alpha, and the positive clones were screened by PCR and restriction enzyme digestion. Then, the recombinant pIRES-ureB and pIRES-ureB-IL-2 were used to transform LB5000 and the recombinant plasmids extracted from LB5000 were finally introduced into the final host SL7207. After that, recombinant strains were grown in vitro repeatedly. In order to detect the immunogenicity of the vaccine in vitro, pIRES-ureB and pIRES-ureB-IL-2 were transfected to COS-7 cells using Lipofectamine 2000, the immunogenicity of expressed UreB and IL-2 proteins was assayed with SDS-PAGE and Western blot. C57BL/6 mice were orally immunized with 1 x 10(8) recombinant attenuated Salmonella typhimurium DNA vaccine. Four weeks after vaccination, mice were challenged with 1 x 10(7) CFU of live *H. pylori* SS1. Mice were sacrificed and the stomach was isolated for examination of H pylori 4 wk post-challenge.The 1700 base pair ureB gene fragment amplified from the genomic DNA was consistent with the sequence of *H. pylori* ureB by sequence analysis. The amplified 510 base pair fragment was consistent with the sequence of mouse IL-2 in gene bank. It was confirmed by PCR and restriction enzyme digestion that H pylori ureB and mouse IL-2 genes were inserted into the eukaryotic expression vector pIRES. The experiments in vitro showed that stable recombinant live attenuated Salmonella typhimurium DNA vaccine carrying ureB and IL-2 genes was successfully constructed and the specific strips of UreB and IL-2 expressed by recombinant plasmids were detected through Western blot. Study *in vivo* showed that the positive rate of rapid urease test of the immunized group including ureB and ureB-IL-2 was 37.5% and 12.5% respectively, and was significantly lower than that (100%) in the control group (P<0.01). it is concluded that recombinant attenuated Salmonella typhimurium DNA vaccine expressing UreB protein and IL-2 protein with immunogenicity can be constructed. It can protect mice against *H. pylori* infection, which may help the development of a human-use *H. pylori* DNA vaccine.

HpaA is a *Helicobacter pylori*-specific lipoprotein that has been shown to be an effective protective antigen for mucosal vaccination against *H. pylori* infection in mice. However, detergents are needed for the purification of full-length HpaA (HpaA(full)), which might confer toxicity, thus making HpaA(full) unsuitable for use in a human vaccine. We here describe a recombinantly produced truncated version of HpaA (HpaA(trunc)), which is easily purified without the use of detergents. Evaluation in the murine *H. pylori* infection model showed that sublingual immunization with HpaA(trunc) was equally immunogenic and protective as immunization with HpaA(full). Immunization with a combination of HpaA(trunc) and recombinant UreB protein induced strong immune responses to both antigens and importantly had a strong synergistic effect on protection, associated with synergistically increased expression of IL-17 in the stomach. Notably, sublingual immunization with HpaA(trunc) and UreB was superior to corresponding intragastric immunization with regard to the level of protection induced. In conclusion, HpaA(trunc) is a promising, readily produced, non-toxic recombinant antigen for inclusion in a mucosal vaccine against *H. pylori* infection, which may preferably be given sublingually together with UreB.

HpaA is a *Helicobacter pylori*-specific lipoprotein that has been shown to be an effective protective antigen for mucosal vaccination against H. pylori infection in mice. However, detergents are needed for the purification of full-length HpaA (HpaA(full)), which might confer toxicity, thus making HpaA(full) unsuitable for use in a human vaccine. Flach *et al.* (2011) here describe a recombinantly produced truncated version of HpaA (HpaA(trunc)), which is easily purified without the use of detergents. Evaluation in the murine

H. pylori infection model showed that sublingual immunization with HpaA(trunc) was equally immunogenic and protective as immunization with HpaA(full). Immunization with a combination of HpaA(trunc) and recombinant UreB protein induced strong immune responses to both antigens and importantly had a strong synergistic effect on protection, associated with synergistically increased expression of IL-17 in the stomach. Notably, sublingual immunization with HpaA(trunc) and UreB was superior to corresponding intragastric immunization with regard to the level of protection induced. In conclusion, HpaA(trunc) is a promising, readily produced, non-toxic recombinant antigen for inclusion in a mucosal vaccine against *H. pylori* infection, which may preferably be given sublingually together with UreB.

References

Appino S., Guarda F., Pregel P., Amedeo S., Cutufia M.A., Bellonio G. and Ponzetto A.2010.Detection of *Helicobacter* candidatus suis by PCR in oesophagogastric ulcers of swine in Italy. Acta. Vet. Hung. **54:** 517-524.

Casagrande Proietti P., Bietta A., Brachelente C., Lepri E., Davidson I. and Franciosini M.P.2010.Detection of *Helicobacter* spp. in gastric, fecal and saliva samples from swine affected by gastric ulceration. J. Vet. Sci. **11:** 221-225.

Chang, P.C., Wang, C.J., Yon, C.K. and Kao, M.C. 2011. Effects of a HP0859 (rfa D) knockout mutation on lipopolysaccharide structure of *Helicobacter pylori* 26695 and the bacterial adhesion on AGS cells. Biochem. Biophys. Res. Commun. 20 [http://www.ncbi.nlm.nih.gov/pubmed/21256827].

Chevalier, C., Thiberge, J.M., Ferrero, R.L. and Labigne, A. 1999. Essential role of *Helicobacter pylori* gamma glutamyl transpeptidase for the colonization of the gastric mucosa of mice. Mol. Microbiol. **31:** 1359-1372.

Evans, D.G., Lampert, H.C., Nakano, H., Eaton, K.A., Burnens, A.P., Bronsdon, M.A. and Evans, D.J. Jr. 1995. Genetic evidence for host specificity in the adhesion-encoding genes hna A of *Helicobacter acinomyx*, hna A of *Helicobacter nemestrinae* and hpa A of *H.pylori*. Gene. **163:** 97-102.

Evans, D.J. Jr. and Evans, D.G. 2000. *Helicobacter pylori* adhesions: review and perspectives. Helicobacter **5:** 183-195.

Every A.L., Stent A., Moloney M.B., Ng G.Z., Skene C.D., Edwards S.J. and Sutton P. 2011.Evaluation of superoxide dismutase from *Helicobacter pylori* as a protective vaccine antigen. Vaccine. **29:** 1514-1518. Epub 2010 Dec 18.

Flach C.F., Svensson N., Blomquist M., Ekman A., Raghavan S. and Holmgren J.2011.A truncated form of HpaA is a promising antigen for use in a vaccine against *Helicobacter pylori*. Vaccine. **29:** 1235-1241. Epub 2010 Dec 13.

Forne, M., Dorminguez, J., Fernandez-Banares, F., Lite, J., Esteve, M., Gali, N., Espinos, J.C., Quintana, S. and Viver, J.M. 2000. Accuracy of an enzyme immunoassay for the detection of *Helicobacter pylori* in stool specimens in the diagnosis of infection and post-treatment check-up. Am. J. Gastroenterol. **95:** 2200-2205.

Fujii R., Morihara F., Fukushima K., Oku T., Hifumi E. and Uda T.2004.Recombinant antigen from Helicobacter pylori urease as vaccine against *H. pylori*-associated disease. Biotechnol. Bioeng. **86:** 737-746.

Ge Z., White, D.A., Whary, M.T. and Fox. J.G. 2001. Fluorogenic PCR-based quantitative detection of a murine pathogen, *Helicobacter hepaticus*. J. Clin. Microbiol. **39:** 2598-2602.

Gisbert, J.P. and Pajares, J.M. 2001. Diagnosis of *Helicobacter pylori* infection by stool antigen determination: a systematic review. Am. J. Gastroenterol. **96:** 2829-2838.

Kabir, S. 2004. Detection of *Helicobacter pylori* DNA in feces and saliva by polymerase chain reaction: a review. Helicobacter **9:** 115-123.

Graham D.Y. and Yamaoka Y. 2000.Disease-specific *Helicobacter pylori* virulence factors: the unfulfilled promise. *Helicobacter*. 5 Suppl **1:** S3-9; discussion S27-31.

Kendall, L.V., Feng, S., Hodzic, E., Freet, K. and Barthold, S.W. 2004. Use of the P167 recombinant antigen for serodiagnosis of *Helicobacter bilis*. Comp. Med. **54:** 44-48.

Khoshnegah J., Jamshidi S., Mohammadi M. and Sasani F.2011The efficacy and safety of long-term *Helicobacter* species quadruple therapy in asymptomatic cats with naturally acquired infection. J. Feline Med. Surg. **13:** 88-93. Epub 2010 Dec 8.

Krakowka S., Eaton K.A. and Rings D.M.1995. Occurrence of gastric ulcers in gnotobiotic piglets colonized by *Helicobacter pylori*. Infect Immun. **63:** 2352-2355.

Lecoindre, P., Chevallier, M., Peyrol, S., Boude, J., Ferrero, R.L., Labigne, A. 2000. Gastric *Helicobacters* in cats. J. Faline Med. Surg. **2:** 19-27.

Lehours P., Ménard A., Dupouy S., Bergey B., Richy F., Zerbib F., Ruskoné-Fourmestraux A., Delchier J.C. and Mégraud F.2004.Evaluation of the association of nine *Helicobacter pylori* virulence factors with strains involved in low-grade gastric mucosa-associated lymphoid tissue lymphoma. Infect Immun. **72:** 880-888.

McIntosh K.A., Krakowka S., Ringler S.S. and Ellis J.A.2010.In situ detection of urease-positive *Helicobacter pylori*-like organisms on swine gastric mucosa. Can. J. Vet. Res. **74:** 237-240.

Moran, A.P. 1996. The role of lipopolysaccharide in *Helicobacter pylori* pathogenesis. Aliment. Pharmocol. Ther. Suppl. **1:** 39-50.

Moyaert, H., Decostere, A., Vandamme, P., Debruyne, L., Mast, J., Baele, M., Cedent, Ducatelle, R. and Haesebroack, F. 2007. *Helicobacter equorum* sp. nov., a urease negative Helicobacter species isolated from horse feces. Int. J. Syst. Evol. Microbiol. **57:** 213-218.

Odenbriet, S. 2005. Adherence properties of *Helicobacter pylori*: impact on pathogenesis and adaptation to the host. Int. J. Med. Microbiol. **295:** 317-324.

Pece, S., Guiliani, G., DiLeo, A., Fumarola, D., Antonaci, S. and Jirillo, E. 1997. Role of lipopolysaccharide and related cytokines in *Helicobacter pylori* infection. Recenti. Prog. Med. **88:** 237-241.

Perez-Perez, G.I., Peck, R.M., Legath, A.J., Heine, P.R. and Gaff, L.B. 1999. The role of cag A status in gastric and extragastric complication of *Helicobacter pylori*. J. Physiol. Pharmacol. **50:** 833-845.

Recordeti, C., Ganldi, V., Craven, M., Sala, L., Luini, M., Lanzoni, A., Rishniw, M., Simpson, K.W. and Scanziani, E. 2009. Spatial distribution of *Helicobacter* spp. in the gastrointestinal tract of dogs. Helicobacter **14:** 180-191.

Rossi, M., Hanninen, M.L., Revez, J., Hannula, M., and Zanoni, R.G. 2008. Occurrence and species level diagnostic of *Campylobacter* spp., enteric *Helicobacter* spp. and *Anaerobiospirillum* spp. in healthy and diarrheic dogs and cats. Vet. Microbiol. **129:** 304-314.

Sachs G. Weeks DL, Melchers K, Scott DR2003The gastric biology of *Helicobacter pylori*. Annu. Rev. Physiol. **65:** 349-369.

Shen, Z., Feng, Y., Dewhirst, F.E. and Fox, J.G. 2001. Confection of enteric Helicobacter spp. and *Campylobacter* spp. in cats. J.. Clin.. Microbiol. **39:** 2166-2172.

Shimoyama, T., Sawaya, M., Ishiguro, A., Hanabata, N., Yoshimura, T. and Fukuda, S. 2011. Applicability of a rapid stool antigen test using monoclonal antibody to catalase for the management of *Helicobacter pylori* infection. J. Gastroenterol. 25 [http://www.ncbi.nlm.nih.gov/ pubmed/21264478].

Shojaee Tabrizi A., Jamshidi Sh., Oghalaei A., Zahraei Salehi T., Bayati Eshkaftaki A. and Mohammadi M.2010.Identification of *Helicobacter* spp. in oral secretions vs. gastric mucosa of stray cats. Vet. Microbiol. **140:** 142-146. Epub 2009 Aug 8.

Smet A., Duchateau L., Chiers K. and Ducatelle R.. 2010.Helicobacter suis causes severe gastric pathology in mouse and mongolian gerbil models of human gastric disease. PLoS One. **5:** e14083.

Stephens JC, Larkins A, James RF, Rathbone BJ.1996. Production of a monoclonal antibody against the 128 kDa (CagA) protein of *Helicobacter pylori*.J Immunol Methods. **190:** 163-169.

Sugimoto, M. and Yamaoka, A. 2011. Review of *Helicobacter pylori* infection and chronic renal failure. Ther. Apher. Dial. **15:** 1-9.

Vanden Bulck, K., Decostere, A., Baele, M., Vandamme, P., Mast, J., Ducatelle, R. and Haesebrouck, F. 2006. *Helicobacter cynogastricus* sp. nov. isolated from the canine gastric mucosa. Int. J. Syst. Evol. Microbiol. **56:** 1559-1564.

Vermoote M., Vandekerckhove T.T., Flahou B., Pasmans F., Smet A., De Groote D., Van Criekinge W., Ducatelle R. and Haesebrouck F. 2011.Genome sequence of *Helicobacter suis* supports its role in gastric pathology. Vet. Res. **42:** 51.

Xu C., Li Z.S., Du Y.Q., Gong Y.F., Yang H., Sun B. and Jin J.2007.Construction of recombinant attenuated Salmonella typhimurium DNA vaccine expressing H pylori ureB and IL-2. World J. Gastroenterol. **13:** 939-944.

Yang X.L., Liu W.C., Yang W.W., Zhong D., Liu Y.H., Zhang J.D., Jiang J.H. and Li S.S.2005.Oral immunization of mice with vaccine of attenuated Salmonella typhimurium expressing *Helicobacter pylori* urease B subunit. Biomed. Environ. Sci. **18:** 411-418.

Zheng Q., Chen X.Y., Shi Y. and Xiao SD.2004.Development of gastric adenocarcinoma in Mongolian gerbils after long-term infection with *Helicobacter pylori*. J Gastroenterol Hepatol. Oct; **19**(10): 1192-1198.

□□□

Chapter 16

Erysipelothrix rhusiopathiae

Dr. S.K. SRIVASTAVA
Former, Division of Bacteriology & Mycology
Indian Veterinary Research Institute, Izatnagar-243122
Bareilly (U.P.)

Erysipelothrix rhusiopathiae

Erysipelothrix rhusiopathiae is the causative agent of erysipelas in turkey and swine. It also causes disease in poultry, ducks, emus and sheep. The causative agent is a thin, gram-positive bacilli which may take the form of filaments. It is non-motile, alpha-haemolytic and catalase negative. It is a fermentative facultatively anaerobic bacteria that grow in the range of 15-45^{0}C. Erysipelothrix has 2 species, *E.rhusiopathiae* and *E.tonsillarum,* of them the former is of importance. *E.tonsillarum* has been recovered from water and tonsils of normal swine and not considered pathogenic. The 2 species can be differentiated on the basis of deoxyribonucleaic acid (DNA) homology and biochemically.

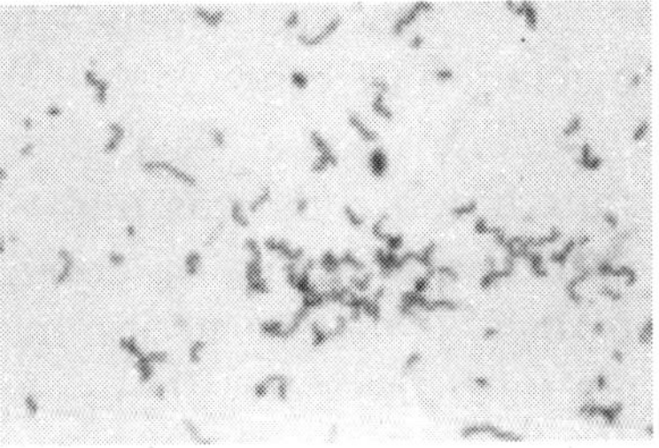

E.rhuseopathiae gram stained

The E. rhusiopathiae genome (1,787,941 bp) is one of the smallest genomes in the phylum Firmicutes. Phylogenetic analyses based on the 16S rRNA gene and 31 universal protein families suggest that E. rhusiopathiae is phylogenetically close to Mollicutes, which comprises Mycoplasma species (Ogawa *et al.*2011). Genome analyses show that the overall features of the E. rhusiopathiae genome are similar to those of other Gram-positive bacteria; it possesses a complete set of peptidoglycan biosynthesis genes, two-component regulatory systems, and various cell wall-associated virulence factors, including a capsule and adhesins. However, it lacks many orthologous genes for the biosynthesis of wall teichoic acids (WTA) and lipoteichoic acids (LTA) and the dltABCD operon, which is responsible for d-alanine incorporation into WTA and LTA, suggesting that the organism has an atypical cell wall. In addition, like Mollicutes, its genome shows a complete loss of fatty acid biosynthesis pathways and lacks the genes for the biosynthesis of many amino acids, cofactors, and vitamins, indicating reductive genome evolution. The genome encodes nine antioxidant factors and nine phospholipases, which facilitate intracellular survival in phagocytes. Thus, the E. rhusiopathiae genome represents evolutionary traits of both Firmicutes and Mollicutes and provides new insights into its evolutionary adaptations for intracellular survival.

Infectious cases with clinical symptoms in cats have not been reported. E. rhusiopathiae was recovered from a 4-month Russian blue breed cat with a very poor body condition score of 1 (BCS: 1/5). The isolate was typed as serotype 2b. Mice experimentally infected with the clinical isolate of E. rhusiopathiae through subcutaneous or intraperitoneal routes survived, and the organism was recovered from the spleen and synovial and pericardial fluids(Lee *et al.*2011). Cats experimentally inoculated with the isolate either orally or subcutaneously survived but commonly exhibited depression and emaciation together with localized erythemal lesion of the skin accompanied by purulent ocular discharge. On hematological analysis, the number of total white blood cells was high compared with that in normal cats. Histological examination revealed congestion and moderate inflammation with focal necrosis. This observation may provide insight on *E. rhusiopathiae* infection in cats with the possible epidemiological significance and implications as a potential source of infection to other animals and humans.

As this bacterium has been isolated from the poultry red mite (Dermanyssus gallinae), this parasite has been suggested as a possible means of transmission of *E. rhusiopathiae* on and between poultry farms. To further elucidate the capacity of the mite as a reservoir, Ericksson *et al*. (2010) analysed and compared 56 bacterial isolates from laying hens and nine isolates from mites by pulsed-field gel electrophoresis (PFGE), using the restriction enzyme SmaI. The isolates originated from one outbreak in a laying hen flock housed in an indoor litter-based aviary system. Except for two isolates, a homogeneous banding pattern was obtained from all isolates analysed, suggesting that a single strain was the cause of the outbreak. Another finding was that isolates from individual hens could exhibit slightly different PFGE patterns. Mites collected from the same house at the end of the production period of the following flock were negative for the presence of *E. rhusiopathiae*. An increasing number of erysipelas outbreaks as well as escalating problems with D. gallinae are expected in other European countries related to the forthcoming changes in housing systems for laying hens.

Erysipelothrix rhusiopathiae is found on the mucous membrane of normal swine. It is also found in fresh water and saltwater fish and crustacea. The organisms lives and multiplies during the warm months in alkaline soil throughout the world. The organism can be isolated from the environment of clinically affected pigs (Bender *et al.*, 2010). The organisms have been recovered from a wide variety of wild and domestic animals including mammals, birds, reptiles, amphibians and fish. It is reported that 30-50% of pigs carry the bacterium in their tonsils and other lymphoid tissues. Turkeys carry the organisms in their cecal tonsils, liver and other organs. It can survive in feces for several months. Carrier pigs are primarily the reservoir of the organism and may transmit the infection to the susceptible population through direct contact and fomites (Wood 1992). The mode of infection is mainly by ingestion. Fish meals may be the source of infection.

E.rhusiopathiae is divided into 23 serotypes and the non-typeable strains are designated N. strains of serotype 1 are subdivided into Ia & Ib. Serotype Ia, Ib and 2 predominantly cause disease in swine, however, some Ia strains are avirulent (Takahashi *et al.*, 1987a, b). Seven serovars (3, 7, 1G, 20, 22, 23 and 31) of *E.rhusiopathiae* have been placed in the species *E.tonsillarum* based on DNA-DNA hybridization studies.

The disease in pigs is found throughout the world. Economic losses are due to death of the animals and devaluation of pig carcasses due to arthritis. There is considerable variation in the case with which the disease can be produced. Many factors such as age, health and intercurrent disease, exposure to erysipelas and heredity govern the case of both natural and artificial transmission. Smooth strains can cause the disease successfully but rough strains are non-pathogenic. Pigs of all ages are susceptible. Piglets from an immune sow may get sufficient antibodies in the colostrums to give them immunity for some weeks. Specimens from 70 carcasses with lesions suspect for swine erysipelas were collected at an abattoir in Iowa from October 2007 to February 2009. Erysipelothrix spp. were isolated from 59 of 70 carcasses (84.3%). Abattoir inspectors classified lesions as acute, subacute, or chronic; 8 of 8 (100%) were acute cases, 31 of 32 (96.9%) were subacute cases, and 20 of 30 (66.6%) were chronic cases that were isolation positive (Bender *et al.*2011). The following serotypes were identified: 1a (40.7%; 24/59), 2 (49.2%; 29/59), 7 (1/59), 10 (1/59), 11 (1/59), and untypeable (5.1%; 3/59). Serotypes 1a and 2 were identified in pigs with acute, subacute, or chronic clinical manifestations, whereas serotypes 7, 10, and 11 were only present in chronic cases. Fifty-seven of the 59 isolates were determined to belong to *E. rhusiopathiae*, and 2 of 59 of the isolates were determined to be *E. tonsillarum* by multiplex real-time polymerase chain reaction. Surface protective antigen (spa) A was detected in all *E. rhusiopathiae* isolates but not in *E. tonsillarum* serotypes 7 and 10. The results of the present study indicate that *E. rhusiopathiae* serotypes 1a and 2 continue to be commonly isolated from condemned pig carcasses and that spaA is the exclusive spa type in U.S. abattoir isolates. Interestingly, *E. tonsillarum*, thought to be avirulent for swine, was isolated from systemic sites from 3.4% of the carcasses that were negative for *E. rhusiopathiae*, indicating the potential importance of this genotype in erysipelas pathogenesis.

The disease occurs in several forms in swine; acute septicaemia, urticarial or diamond skin lesions, vegetative endocarditis and arthritis (Wood 1992). These symptoms may occur alone or in combinations. In pigs acute septicaemic form is most common, so is the case with turkeys. In sheep, it causes polyarthritis. Rheumatoid arthritis is associated with dogs. *E.rhusiopathiae* causes a zoonotic problem. In human, erysipeloid is a cutaneous infection that frequently occurs in veterinarians, fish handlers, and meat processing workers (Gyles 1993).

In turkeys, the disease is usually evident by the sudden death of birds in the flock. Cutaneous lesions, particularly those affecting the snood may be evident. During a chronic course birds may develop vegetative endocarditis or arthritis and become gradually emaciated. Diarrhoea are sometime observed, Erysipelas is not a very common infection in cattle. Organisms have been isolated from tonsils of healthy animals. Very rarely cases of septicaemia with abscesses in liver and lungs are observed at post mortem. Non-suppurative arthritis is associated with *E.rhusiopathiae* infection in calves manifested by lameness, recumbency and emaciation. In sheep, pneumonia due to *E.rhusiopathiaei* has been recorded with sudden death. Generalized infections are rare. Other manifestations recorded in sheep are valvular endocarditis, cutaneous infections, septicaemia and polyarthritis.

Pathogenesis

If the disease is caused by a fully virulent form of bacteria in a highly susceptible host, invasion of the blood stream occurs as a first sign of pathogenesis. This is likely to lead to acute septicaemia. Coagulase activity is a possible virulence factor and concurrent viral infection such as hog cholera may increase susceptibility of the host. Carrier animals are important source of infection. Localization of the pathogen is commonly seen in skins joints and heart valve with subsequent bacteremic episodes. Selective adherence of some strains of *E.rhusiopathiae* to heart valve may be a factor in the pathogenesis of endocarditis (Takahashi *et al.,* 1987a). The bacterial structure required for adherence is heat labile and trypsin sensitive.

Three avirulent insertional mutants of Erysipelothrix rhusiopathiae were obtained by the technique of transposon mutagenesis with the self-conjugative transposon Tn916 (Shimoji *et al.,* 1994). The interactions between murine polymorphonuclear leukocytes and parent and mutant strains were studied in vitro. In the presence of normal serum, the virulent parent strain was resistant to phagocytosis, whereas the avirulent mutant strains were efficiently phagocytosed. In the presence of immune serum, the parent and the mutant strains were both efficiently phagocytosed. Electron microscopic examination of the parent strain demonstrated the presence of a structure resembling a capsule which was absent on the mutant strains, suggesting that a capsule may be involved in virulence. This was confirmed in studies in which an avirulent mutant strain reverted to virulence following acquisition of a capsule when the transposon was lost by spontaneous excision. These results strongly suggest that virulence of *E. rhusiopathiae* is associated, at least in part, with resistance to phagocytosis by polymorphonuclear leukocytes and that this antiphagocytic ability of the bacterium results from its possession of a capsule.

To investigate the role of hyaluronidase in the pathogenicity of Erysipelothrix rhusiopathiae, transposon Tn916 was transferred from *Enterococcus faecalis* CG110 to a virulent strain of *E. rhusiopathiae,* and hyaluronidase-deficient mutants were isolated (Shimoji *et al*2002). A virulence assay in the mice showed that of the seven hyaluronidase-deficient mutants tested, six mutants were avirulent, but that one mutant, designated AST121, was as virulent as its parental strain. Western immunoblotting with a monoclonal antibody specific to the capsule, a major virulence factor of the organism, revealed that all of the avirulent mutants had lost the capsular antigen, whereas the mutant AST121 did not. These results suggest that the lack of virulence of the six hyaluronidase-negative mutants could be due to a loss of the capsule and that hyaluronidase does not contribute to the lethality of E. rhusiopathiae infection in mice.

RspB is a surface adhesin of Erysipelothrix rhusiopathiae. A recombinant form of the collagen-binding region of this protein, RspB((31-348)), has been overexpressed in *Escherichia coli* in native and selenomethionine-derivative forms and purified using affinity and gel-permeation chromatography (Devi *et al*.2010). Thin plate-like crystals were obtained by the hanging-drop vapour-diffusion method using the same condition for both forms. The native crystals diffracted to a resolution of 2.5 A using an in-house X-ray source, while the selenomethionine-derivative crystals diffracted to a resolution of 2.2 A using synchrotron radiation. The crystals belonged to the monoclinic space group P2(1), with unit-cell parameters a = 46.19, b = 66.65, c = 101.72 A, beta = 94.11 degrees.

Shimoji *et al.* (2003) found two adhesive surface proteins of *E. rhusiopathiae* and determined the nucleotide sequences of the genes, which were colocalized and designated rspA and rspB. The two genes were present in all of the serovars of *E. rhusiopathiae* strains examined. The deduced RspA and RspB proteins contain the C-terminal anchoring motif, LPXTG, which is preceded by repeats of consensus amino acid sequences. The consensus sequences are composed of 78 to 92 amino acids and repeat 16 and 3 times in RspA and RspB, respectively. Adhesive surface proteins of other gram-positive bacteria, including Listeria monocytogenes adhesin-like protein, Streptococcus pyogenes protein F2 and F2-like protein, Streptococcus dysgalactiae FnBB, and Staphylococcus aureus Cna, share the same consensus repeats. Furthermore, the N-terminal regions of RspA and RspB showed characteristics of the collagen-binding domain that was described for Cna. RspA and RspB were expressed in *Escherichia coli* as histidine-tagged fusion proteins and purified. The recombinant proteins showed a high degree of capacity to bind to polystyrene and inhibited the binding of *E. rhusiopathiae* onto the abiotic surface in a dose dependent manner. In a solid-phase binding assay, both of the recombinant proteins bound to fibronectin, type I and IV collagens, indicating broad spectrum of their binding ability. It was suggested that both RspA and RspB were exposed on the cell surface of *E. rhusiopathiae,* as were the bacterial cells agglutinated by the anti-RspA immunoglobulin G (IgG) and anti-RspB IgG. RspA and RspB were present both in surface-antigen extracts and the culture supernatants of *E. rhusiopathiae* Fujisawa-SmR (serovar 1a) and SE-9 (serovar 2). The recombinant RspA, but not RspB, elicited protection in mice against experimental challenge. These results suggest that RspA and RspB participate in initiation of biofilm formation through their binding abilities to abiotic and biotic surfaces.

The organisms enter the host through ingestion and reaches small intestine where they adhere to the epithelium. Subsequently they penetrate the intestine and become hematogenous leading to bacteremia. Vascular damage, arthritis, endocarditis and skin lesion are due to localization of the organisms in different tissues. Bacteremia also leads to vascular damage and thrombosis and pyrexia. In joints there is proliferation of synovial villi and thickening of joint capsule. Discospondylitis also occurs in association with chronic polyarthritis. Amyloidosis may also occur in pigs.

The early lesions in septicaemic disease are dominated by vascular disturbances (Wood 1984). In the acute form there is swelling of the endothelium of caprillaries and venules and hyaline thrombosis which progresses to fibrinous thrombosis.

Haemolysis and ischemic necrosis may also develop. Involvement of joints, heart valve and arteries is visible in subacute and chronic form. Lesions of arthritis are produced as a primary manifestation of the disease which is later enhanced by immunological mechanisms to persistent antigen at the size. The slowly progressive course and morphological changes observed are similar to human rheumatoid arthritis (Schulz *et al.*, 1980).

The organisms do not secrete any toxin which could be incriminated with the disease but the enzyme neuraminidae has been suggested to play a role in the virulence as there is some correlation between the amount of neuraminidase produced and the virulence of the strains (Muller 1980). The enzyme removes the N-acetyl neuraminic acid from a number of substrates and enhances the bacterial cell penetration. Removal of N-acetyl neuraminic acid from mucin, fibrinogen and erythrocytes results in a reduction in protection afforded by mucin, formation of fibrin like structure in blood vessels, increased viscocity of blood and haemolysis. Effects attributable to the removal of N-acetyl neuraminic acid from heart cells and immunoglobin G (IgG) are disturbance in control of calcium exchange in the heart and deposition of IgG in the kidneys (Gyles 1993). Hyaluronidase is another virulence factor, though its role is controversial. The presence of heat labile capsule supports antiphagocytic property (Wang *et al.*, 2010). Infected animals produce anti neuraminidase antibodies capable of neutralizing the enzymes suggesting a role of this enzyme in the pathogenesis. Furthermore, these antibodies are proven to be protective in mice.

Similarly active immunization of mice with neuraminidase also confers protection.Makino *et al.*(2000) isolated the spaA gene encoding the surface protective antigen A, SpaA, of Erysipelothrix rhusiopathiae, and found that the N-terminal region of SpaA was responsible for protective immunity against erysipelas and that the C-terminal region contained eight repeat units consisting of 20 amino acids comprising the binding domain on the Erysipelothrix cell surface. In this study, using recombinant SpaA proteins, the authors showed that the repeat region bound to the cell surfaces of various Gram-positive bacterial cells, SpaA was a membrane-associated protein, this association depended on the interaction with choline residues in teichoic acid, and SpaA bound to lipoteichoic acid (LTA) of Bacillus subtilis and Staphylococcus aureus. These results showed that LTA was required for the surface association of SpaA in E. rhusiopathiae and that such an association might be common among Gram-positive bacterial cells. It is suggested that an LTA-SpaA complex might have an important role in the E. rhusiopathiae infection process.

Diagnosis

Clinical specimen are collected from appropriate sites according to the signs visible and subjected to the examination. Blood cultures collected during the bacteremic phase helps in the diagnosis. Necropsy specimen include liver, spleen, kidney, heart and synovial tissues. In chronic cases specimen from joints or heart valves may be subjected to the examination.

The organisms are gram positive bacilli which may be observed in the clinical samples from acute, sub acute or chronic cases.

For bacteriological culture, blood agar are streaked with the specimen and incubated at 37°C in 10% CO_2 tension. Colonies are often non-haemolytic and pin point after 24 hrs. of incubation. At 48 hrs. a greenish haemolysis may be seen. Selective media containing various aminoglycosides and vancomycin may be used to isolate *Erysipelothrix* from contaminated tissues. Other selective media contain Sod. azide (0.001%). Enrichment broth culturing technique is superior than direct plating for isolates on *E. rhusiopathiae* from pig samples (Bender *et al.*, 2009).

The objective of the current study was to compare the diagnostic performance of a direct isolation method for *Erysipelothrix* spp. with a broth-based enrichment technique (Bender *et al.*, 2009). Samples were obtained from three sources: 1) experimentally inoculated pigs, 2) porcine tissue samples submitted to the Iowa State University Veterinary Diagnostic Laboratory (Ames, IA), and 3) tissues from condemned carcasses at an abattoir. Culture plates from direct isolation and broth-based technique were evaluated for growth at 24 and 48 hr. Results indicated that the broth enrichment method was markedly more sensitive for the isolation of Erysipelothrix spp. Interestingly, in several samples, a Gram-positive bacterium with almost identical growth characteristics to Erysipelothrix spp. was detected and identified as a Vagococcus sp. through 16S ribosomal RNA gene sequencing. The results of this study indicate that the broth-based enrichment method should be used for the isolation of *Erysipelothrix* spp. from clinical samples with a history suggestive of erysipelas and that Vagococcus spp. is potentially an important differential diagnosis.

Erysipelothrix is catalase and oxidase negative and non-motile. An acid reaction is visible in triple sugar iron agar slants. H_2S production is also apparent. Various other biochemical reactions can be performed to identify the bacteria. Erysipelothrix rhusiopathiae can be differentiated from *E.tonsillarum* on the basis of the ability of the former to ferment saccharose while the latter does not.

Opriessnig *et al* (2010) developed an immunohistochemical (IHC) assay for rapid detection of *Erysipelothrix rhusiopathiae*. Serotypes 1a, 1b, and 2 are most frequently associated with clinical disease in pigs. Antiserum against serotypes 1a, 1b, and 2 was produced in rabbits, pooled, and applied to formalin-fixed, paraffin-embedded tissue sections of pigs (lungs, heart, spleen, and skin). The results obtained with the IHC assay were compared with direct culture on tissue samples from experimentally inoculated pigs either treated (n = 6) with antibiotics or untreated (n = 8) as well as on samples from field cases (n = 170) submitted to the Veterinary Diagnostic Laboratory at Iowa State University. The agreement between direct culture and IHC staining was found to be substantial. The results of the present study indicate that the IHC assay is highly sensitive and specific in detecting *E. rhusiopathiae* antigen in formalin-fixed, paraffin-embedded tissues. Results indicated that the IHC is particularly useful in cases in which pigs had been treated with antibiotics prior to submission and in which direct cultures of organs were negative. In addition, the IHC was found to be useful for detection of *E. rhusiopathiae* antigen in skin lesions, which are often culture negative.

In meat inspection, it is very important to distinguish *E. rhusiopathiae* from other bacteria showing similar clinical signs of disease or similar bacterial characteristics. To distinguish *E. rhusiopathiae* from Erysipelothrix tonsillarum, 2 polymerase chain reaction (PCR) systems were combined (Yamazaki 2006). The primer sets ERY-1F and ERY-2R were designed to amplify 2210 base pairs (bp) of nucleotide sequence specific for *E. rhusiopathiae* chromosomal DNA, and the primer sets MO101 and ERS-1R were designed to amplify 719 bp of nucleotide sequence including a highly conserved region of genus Erysipelothrix 16S rRNA. Two fragments were amplified when *E. rhusiopathiae* was used as the PCR template using the primer sets, whereas a single fragment was amplified when *E. tonsillarum* was used as the template. No fragments were amplified when nucleic acid from other bacteria that cause clinical signs similar to swine erysipelas were used as the template. Moreover, 5 specimens collected from postinspected swine carcasses were diagnosed as E. rhusiopathiae using the PCR described in this study, in agreement with results of microbiological tests for the genus Erysipelothrix, whereas negative samples were negative both in conventional bacterial tests and by PCR. The detection limit of multiplex PCR ranged from 10(2) to 10(4) colony forming units per reaction tube for positive samples.

One hundred and fifty-one Erysipelothrix spp. isolates from diseased and carrier swine from Brazil were identified by PCR, submitted to serotyping and analyzed by amplified fragment length polymorphism with a single enzyme (AFLP)(Coutinho *et al.*, 2011). Reference strains from Australia and the United Kingdom were also examined. The 151 strains were classified into

18 different serotypes (1a, 1b, 2a, 2b, 4, 5, 6, 7, 8, 10, 11, 12, 15, 17, 19, 21, 24 and 25), being serotype 2b the most frequent (39.7%). By associating serotyping and PCR results, it was possible to identify 146 strains as *E. rhusiopathiae* and five strains as *E. tonsillarum*. Despite the fact that for this genus AFLP did not cluster all isolates according to serotype, origin, disease or isolation data, the execution of the technique was easy and fast, demonstrating high discriminatory power. The results produced by the AFLP analysis of *Erysipelothrix* spp. could also support its use as a discriminatory tool for E. rhusiopathiae and *E. tonsillarum* species.

Shen *et al.*(2010) developed spa multiplex real-time and conventional PCR assays to detect and differentiate between spaA, spaB and spaC genes within *Erysipelothrix* spp. For evaluation of the assays, 28 *Erysipelothrix* spp. reference strains, 25 tissues from pigs inoculated with reference strains of serotypes 1, 2, 5, 10 or 18, and 15 diagnostic samples were used. SpaA was found to be present in *Erysipelothrix* rhusiopathiae serotypes 1a, 1b, 2, 5, 9, 12, 15, 16, 17, 23 and N; spaB was detected in *E. rhusiopathiae* serotypes 4, 6, 8, 11, 19 and 21 and spaC was detected in E. sp. strain 2 serotype 18. Spa-related genes were not detected in *E. tonsillarum* strains (serotypes 3, 7, 10, 14, 20, 22, 24, 25, 26) or E. sp. strain 1 (serotype 13). With the spa multiplex real-time PCR assay, it was also possible to further differentiate spaB into spaB1 (serotypes 4, 6, 8, 19 and 21) and spaB2 (serotype 11). Overall, spaA was detected in seven experimental tissue samples and six diagnostic tissue samples, and spaC in two experimental tissue samples. The detection limits were determined to be five colony-forming units (CFU) per reaction for the spa CFU per reaction for the multiplex real-time PCR assay and 4000 conventional PCR assay.Both spa PCR assays were specific and reproducible in the identification of spa types in *Erysipelothrix* spp.The described spa PCR assays may be useful tools for investigating Spa prevalence among strains isolated from field tissues and to determine the role of the Spa proteins in vaccine protection and pathogenesis.

Quantitative real-time polymerase chain reaction (qPCR) assays were developed and validated in combination with enrichment culture for the detection and discrimination of *Erysipelothrix* rhusiopathiae and other *Erysipelothrix* species from tissue samplesTo *et al.*, 2009). The targets for SYBR green qPCR assays were the 16S ribosomal RNA gene for *Erysipelothrix* species and a gene involved in capsular formation for *E. rhusiopathiae*. The specificity of the assays was assessed with Erysipelothrix species and other related bacterial species. The limit of detection was found to be 5 colony-forming units per reaction. Amplification of DNA extracted from spleen and joint samples spiked with increasing quantities of *Erysipelothrix* cells was shown to be equally sensitive to DNA extracted from a pure bacterial culture. The assays were evaluated with 88 tissue samples from 3 experimentally infected pigs and 50 mice and with 36 tissue samples from 3 naturally infected pigs and 11 noninfected pigs. Results were compared with those of direct qPCR and conventional culture. The qPCR after enrichment increased the diagnostic sensitivity over that of culture and qPCR, thereby significantly reducing the total time taken for the detection of *E. rhusiopathiae* and other *Erysipelothrix* species.

Treatment and Control

Penicillin is the antibiotic of choice for pigs and turkeys. Tetracycline and tylosin are other antibiotics, however, resistance to oxytetracycline and some macrolides has been reported. In turkeys injectable erythromycin is a recommended alternative. Many strains are resistant to erythromycin, lincomycin, ofloxacin and enrofloxacin (Chuma *et al.,* 2010).

General hygienic precautions should be adopted. Clinically affected animals should be disposed of quickly and all introductions should be isolated and examined for signs of arthritis and endocarditis. All animals dying of the disease should be properly incinerated to avoid contamination of the environment.

Because of the difficulty of eradication biological prophylactic methods are in common use. Both hyperimmune serum and vaccines are used to control. The hyperimmune serum is given in repeated doses to suckling pigs in herd until they have attained 6 weeks. Repeated administration of the serum may cause anaphylaxis. Vaccines have proven successful for both swine and poultry. Two types of vaccines are available: a formalin killed culture with aluminium hydroxide gel adjuvant produced from strain of serotype 2. The strain is an efficient producer of the immunizing antigen (Wood 1992). Following a single vaccination at 6-10 weeks, significant protection upto market age is provided. However, a second booster at 2-4 weeks later is advisable.

Both inactivated and attenuated vaccines are available to prevent development of clinical signs of swine erysipelas. The ability of a live attenuated *E. rhusiopathiae* strain to become persistently established in pigs after intranasal exposure and its potential to cause clinical signs consistent with swine erysipelas after being administered directly into the nasopharynx of healthy pigs was evaluated (Newmann *et al.,* 2009). Five, *E. rhusiopathiae*-negative pigs were vaccinated by deep intranasal inoculation then followed for 14 days. Nasal swabs were collected daily for 5 days and clinical observations were made daily for 14 days post-vaccination. Nasal swabs were cultured for *E. rhusiopathiae* with the intent of back-passaging any recovered organisms into subsequent replicates. No organism was recovered from nasal swabs in the first vaccination replicate. A second replicate including 10 pigs was initiated and followed in an identical manner to that described above. Again, no *E. rhusiopathiae* was recovered from any pigs. No pigs in either replicate showed any signs of clinical swine erysipelas. The live attenuated *E. rhusiopathiae* strain evaluated in this study did not appear to become persistently established in pigs post-vaccination, did not cause any local or systemic signs consistent with swine erysipelas, and was therefore unlikely to revert to a virulent state when used in a field setting.

Recent studies have identified an antigen of approximately 65 kDa of *E.rhusiopathiae* as a protective antigen (Chin *et al.*, 1992; Kabayashi *et al.*, 1992) that elicit immunity against infection by a wide range of serotypes. Immunity is short lived and is protective against acute form of disease only (Wood 1992). Nazierbieke *et al* (2010) evaluated effects of a novel surface protective antigen A (SpaA) and its N protective domain against *E.rhusiopathiae* infection and reported that recombinant SpaA-N is a protective antigen of *E.rhusiopathiae* type 2 strain and might be a useful vaccine candidate. The use of live culture vaccines is prohibited in many countries due to the risk of variation in virulence of strain and the possibility of spreading the infection. None of the vaccine gives a life long protection from a single vaccination and the actual duration of immunity achieved following vaccination varies considerably. The use of a culture filtrate from the broth culture of an attenuated strain has been used. This vaccine reduces the cases of polyarthritis due to erysipelas but not arthritis, hence could not be popularized.

There are many reports on the characterization of protective antigens of *E. rhusiopathiae*. A mouse protective antigen was identified in culture supernatant and in 10 mM NaOH extracts of bacterial cells. Neuraminidase was also considered a protective antigen, because mice were protected by passive immunization with rabbit antiserum against *E. rhusiopathiae* neuraminidase. In 1 mM EDTA extract of T28 (serotype 2), one major polysaccharide capsular antigen of 14.4 to 22 kDa and two main protein antigens of 64 and 48 kDa were revealed by immunoblotting with rabbit antiserum. However, the protective activity of these antigens was not examined in the work reported. Groschup *et al.* (7) showed that protective antisera from pigs recognized prominent bands of 64 to 66 and 39 to 40 kDa in 1 mM EDTA and 10 mM NaOH extracts of T28. Both antigens were trypsin sensitive and contained no detectable polysaccharide. Mice immunized with preparations of the 64- to 66-kDa band were protected against challenge with Frankfurt XI (serotype N). They also described the enhanced production of these protective antigens in serum-free modified Feist broth. However, some questions remain as to whether the band of 64 to 66 kDa is the only protective antigen of the bacteria, this band contains only one kind of protective antigen, and this antigen can elicit protection in swine.

Galan and Timoney (1990) first identified a mouse protective antigen gene in a 5.4-kb *Eco*RI fragment of chromosomal DNA of virulent strain E1-6P (serotype 1a)). Guinea pig antiserum against the recombinant clone of this gene reacted with *E. rhusiopathiae* protein antigens of 66, 64, and 43 kDa. These proteins are of the same size as the protective proteins mentioned above. However, the DNA sequences of the gene were not described, and it is also not known whether the clone contained only one gene. Recently, a novel surface protective antigen (SpaA) of *E. rhusiopathiae* was identified from serotype 2 in a mouse model using a monoclonal antibody recognizing 64-kDa proteins of most serotypes of *E. rhusiopathiae*. Mice immunized with live recombinant *Escherichia coli* intraperitoneally survived after challenge with the same strain of *E. rhusiopathiae*. In this study, the presence of 20-amino-acids repeat units at the C terminus was shown to be essential for protection.

In contrast to protein antigens, 14.4- to 22-kDa capsular antigen appears to be not necessary for protection. A live acapsular mutant created by insertion and excision of Tn*916*, which is avirulent in mice, could confer complete protective immunity to mice.

The existence of a common protective antigen among serotypes of *E. rhusiopathiae* was identified experimentally and practically. Although killed vaccines are prepared from serotype 1a and live vaccines are from serotype 2, both vaccines can cross-protect pigs against challenge with strains of serotypes 1 and 2.

Little is known about the genetic properties of its protective antigens. Recently, a surface protective antigen (SpaA) gene was identified from serotype 2 in a mouse model. Imada *et al.*(1999) cloned spaA from virulent strain Fujisawa (serotype 1a) and determined that the N-terminal 342 amino acids without C-terminal repeats of 20 amino acids have the ability to elicit protection in mice. Fusions of 342 amino acids of Fujisawa SpaA and histidine hexamer (HisSpa1.0) protected pigs against challenge with both serotype 1 and serotype 2, the most important serotypes in the swine industry. Pigs immunized with HisSpa1.0 reacted well with both HisSpa1.0 and intact SpaA by enzyme-linked immunosorbent assay and immunoblotting. Serum collected at the time of challenge from a pig immunized with HisSpa1. 0 markedly enhanced the in vitro phagocytic and killing activity of pig neutrophils against the bacteria. DNA sequences of protective regions of spaA genes from five strains of serotypes 1 and 2 were almost identical. The full DNA sequences also seemed to be conserved among strains of all 12 serotype reference strains harboring the spaA gene by restriction fragment length polymorphism analysis of PCR products. These results indicates that SpaA is a common protective antigen of serotypes 1 and 2 of *E. rhusiopathiae* in swine and will be a useful tool for development of new types of vaccines and diagnostic tools for effective control of the disease.

The gene encoding a protective protein antigen of the gram-positive bacterium *Erysipelothrix* rhusiopathiae, an important veterinary pathogen responsible for erysipelas in swine and a variety of diseases in animals, was cloned and sequenced (Shimoji *et al.*, 1999). The gene encodes a polypeptide of 597 amino acids plus a putative signal sequence of 29 amino acids, resulting in a mature protein with a molecular mass of 69,017 Da. Sequence analysis of the gene product revealed a C-terminal region composed of nine tandem repeats of 20 amino acids and a total sequence that is nearly identical to that of the 64-kDa cell surface protein (SpaA) of the bacterium. Because of this similarity, the protein was designated SpaA.1. In this study, we examined whether the SpaA.1 protein could induce protective antibodies and whether we could identify the region involved in protective immunity. Both the mature SpaA.1 protein and its C-terminal repeat region, but not the N-terminal segment, were expressed in *Escherichia coli* and purified as a histidine-tagged fusion recombinant protein. Rabbit antiserum raised against the mature SpaA.1 protein passively protected mice from lethal challenge with a virulent homologous strain, Fujisawa-SmR, suggesting that protection is mediated by humoral antibodies. To determine which domain of the SpaA.1 protein is responsible for the observed protection, mice were actively immunized with either the mature SpaA. 1 protein or the C-terminal repeat region and then challenged with Fujisawa-SmR. The result showed that mice immunized with the mature SpaA.1 protein, but not the C-terminal repeat region, were protected, suggesting that the protection-eliciting epitope(s) is located within the N-terminal two-thirds of the SpaA.1 molecule. This was confirmed by passive immunization experiments in which the protective activity of rabbit antiserum, raised against mature SpaA. 1 protein, was not abolished by absorption with the purified recombinant C-terminal repeat region. In addition, antibodies specific for the C-terminal repeat region were unable to protect mice from lethal challenge. These results show that the N-terminal two-thirds of the SpaA.1 molecule may constitute a good vaccine candidate against erysipelas.

In one study, the authors cloned and sequenced spa genes from all E. rhusiopathiae serovar reference strains as well as from a serovar 18 strain which was not classified as any species in the genus Erysipelothrix (To and Nagai 2007). Sequence analysis revealed that the Spa proteins could be classified into three molecular species, including SpaA, which was previously found in serovars 1a and 2, and the newly designated SpaB and SpaC proteins.

The SpaA protein is produced by *E. rhusiopathiae* serovars 1a, 1b, 2, 5, 8, 9, 12, 15, 16, 17, and N, the SpaB protein is produced by *E. rhusiopathiae* serovars 4, 6, 11, 19, and 21, and the SpaC protein is produced only by serovar 18. The amino acid sequence similarity was high among members of each Spa type (96 to 99%) but low between different Spa types (approximately 60%). The greatest diversity in Spa proteins was found in the N-terminal half of the molecule (50 to 57% similarity), which was shown to be involved in immunoprotection. Coinciding with this, immunoblot analysis revealed that rabbit antisera specific to each Spa reacted strongly with the homologous Spa protein but weakly with heterologous Spa proteins. A mouse cross-protection study showed that the three recombinant Spa (rSpa) proteins elicited complete protection against challenge with homologous strains but that the level of protection against challenge with heterologous strains varied depending on the rSpa protein used for immunization. Our study is the first to demonstrate sequence and antigenic diversity in Spa proteins and to indicate that rSpaC may be the most promising antigen for use as a vaccine component because of its broad cross-protectiveness.

Although live-attenuated or bacterin vaccines are effective in protecting against erysipelas, the genetic construction of their active antigen has not been identified. To clarify the surface antigen(s) involved in protective and arthritic response, using monoclonal antibody I2A against the surface proteins of E. rhusiopathiae, Makino *et al.* (1998) identified a protective antigen, which consists of 606 amino acids. Analysis of deletion derivatives of the gene, spaA(surface protective antigen), showed that the SpaA protein binds tightly to the bacterial cell surface via eight repeat units with a GW-module consisting of 20 amino acids at the C-terminus. Although DeltaSpaA lacking their repeat units lost its ability to induce protection against E. rhusiopathiae infection, intact SpaA protein showed the protection. We conclude that the presence of repeat units is essential both for the binding of SpaA to the bacterial cell surface and for protection. It is believed that the repeat region at the C-terminus should be a candidate for a subunit vaccine against erysipelas.

In herds where sows are regularly vaccinated prior to farrowing, a persisting maternal passive immunity may require that piglet vaccination be delayed until 10-12 weeks of age for an effective active immunity.

References

Bender, J.S., Chen, H.G., Irwin, C.K., Schwarz, K.J. and Opriessnig, T. 2010. Characterization of erysipelothrix species isolated from clinically affected pigs, environmental samples and vaccine strains from six recent swine erysipelas outbreaks in the United State. Clin. Vaccine Immunol. **17:** 1605-1611.

Bender J.S., Irwin C.K., Shen H.G., Schwartz K.J., Opriessnig T.2011. *Erysipelothrix* spp. genotypes, serotypes, and surface protective antigen types associated with abattoir condemnations. J. Vet. Diagn. Invest. **23:** 139-142.

Bender, J.S., Kinyon, J.M., Kariyawasam, S., halbur, P.G. and Opriessnig, T. 2009. Comparison of conventional direct and enrichment culture methods for *Erysipelothrix* spp. from experimentally and naturally infected swine. J. Vet. Diagn. Invest. **21:** 863-868.

Chin, J.C., Twiner, B. and Eamens, G.J. 1992. Serological assay for swine erysipelas using nitrocellulose particles impregnated with an immunodominant 65 kDa antigen from *Erysipelothrix rhusiopathiae* Vet-Microbiol. **31:** 169-180.

Chuma, T., Kawamoto, T., Shahada, F., Fujimoto, H. and Okamoto, K. 2010. Antimicrobial susceptibility of *Erysipelothrix rhusiopathiae* isolated from pigs in Southern Japan with a modified agar dilution method. J. Vet. Med. Sci. **72:** 643-645.

Coutinho T.A. Imada Y. de Barcellos D.E., de Oliveira S.J. and Moreno A.M.2011.Genoyping of Brazilian *Erysipelothrix* spp. strains by amplified fragment length polymorphism. J..Microbiol. Methods. **84:** 27-32. Epub 2010 Oct 14.

Devi A.S., Ogawa Y., Shimoji Y. and Ponnuraj K.2010.Cloning, expression, purification, crystallization and preliminary X-ray diffraction analysis of the collagen-binding region of RspB from *Erysipelothrix rhusiopathiae*. Acta. Crystallogr. Sect F Struct. Biol. Cryst. Commun. **66:** 156-159. Epub 2010 Jan 27.

Eriksson H., Brännström S., Skarin H. and Chirico J.2010.Characterization of Erysipelothrix rhusiopathiae isolates from laying hens and poultry red mites (Dermanyssus gallinae) from an outbreak of erysipelas. Avian Pathol. **39:** 505-509.

Galan J E and Timoney J F.1990. Cloning and expression in *Escherichia coli* of a protective antigen of *Erysipelothrix rhusiopathiae*. Infect. Immun. **58:** 3116–3121.

Gyles, C.L. 1993. *Erysipelothrix rhusiopathiae*. In pathogenesis of bacterial diseases in animals. Ed. G.L. Gyles and C.O. Thoen. pp. 80-85. Ames: Iowa State University Press, U.S.A.

Imada Y., Goji N., Ishikawa H., Kishima M. and Sekizaki T.1999.Truncated surface protective antigen (SpaA) of *Erysipelothrix rhusiopathiae* serotype 1a elicits protection against challenge with serotypes 1a and 2b in pigs. Infect. Immun. **67:** 4376-4382.

Kabayashi, S., Sato, H., Hirose, K. and Saito, H. 1992. Immunological characterization of protective antigens prepared by alkaline treatments of whole cells and from the culture filtrate of *Erysipelothrix rhusiopathiae*. Vet. Microbiol. **30:** 75-85.

Lee J.J., Kim D.H., Lim J.J., Kim D.G., Chang H.H., Lee H.J., Kim S.H., Rhee M.H., Endale M., Imada Y., Kim O.J. and Kim S.2011.Characterization and identification of *Erysipelothrix rhusiopathiae* isolated from an unnatural host, a cat, with a clinical manifestation of depression. J. Vet. Med. Sci. **73:** 149-54. Epub 2010 Sep 8.

Makino S., Yamamoto K., Murakami S., Shirahata T., Uemura K., Sawada T., Wakamoto H., and Morita H.1998.Properties of repeat domain found in a novel protective antigen, SpaA, of *Erysipelothrix rhusiopathiae*. Microb. Pathog. **25:** 101-109.

Makino S.I., Yamamoto K., Asakura H.and Shirahata T.2000.Surface antigen, SpaA, of *Erysipelothrix rhusiopathiae* binds to Gram-positive bacterial cell surfaces. FEMS Microbiol. Lett. **186:** 313-317.

Muller, H.E. 1980. Neuraminidase and other enzymes of *Erysipelothrix rhusiopathiae* as possible pathogenic factors. In Arthritis: Models and Mechanisms. Ed. H. Deicher and L.C. Shulz. pp 58-67, New York: Springer-verlag, U.S.A.

Nazierbeke, W., Zhang, L., He, C., peng, Q. and Borrathybay, E. 2010. [Immunity of native Spa A and recombinant spa- N against *Erysipelothrix rhusiopathiae* infection in mice]. WeiShang Wu Xue Bao **4:** 367-372.

Neumann E,J., Grinberg A,, Bonistalli K,N,, Mack H,J, Lehrbach P,R, and Gibson N.2009.Safety of a live attenuated *Erysipelothrix rhusiopathiae* vaccine for swine. Vet, Microbiol. **135:** 297-303. Epub 2008 Sep 21.

Ogawa Y., Ooka T., Shi F., Ogura Y., Nakayama K., Hayashi T. and Shimoji Y.2011.The Genome of *Erysipelothrix rhusiopathiae*, the Causative Agent of Swine Erysipelas, Reveals New Insights into the Evolution of Firmicutes and the Organism's Intracellular Adaptations. J. Bacteriol. **193:** 2959-71. Epub 2011 Apr 8.

Opriessnig T., Bender J.S., and Halbur P.G.2010.Development and validation of an immunohistochemical method for rapid diagnosis of swine erysipelas in formalin-fixed, paraffin-embedded tissue samples. J .Vet. Diagn. Invest. **22:** 86-90.

Schulz, L.C., Ehard, H., Hermanns, W., Messow, C., Drommer, W., Langer, I. and Trantwein, G. 1980. The different phases of *Erysipelothrix rhusiopathiae* erysipelothrix polyarthritis: comparison with other microbial models. In Arthritis: Models and Mechanisms. Ed. H. Deischer and L.C. Shulz. pp. 12-23, New York; Spingerverlag, U.S.A.

Shen H.G., Bender J.S., and Opriessnig T.. 2010.Identification of surface protective antigen (spa) types in *Erysipelothrix* reference strains and diagnostic samples by spa multiplex real-time and conventional PCR assays. J. Appl. Microbiol. **109:** 1227-33. doi: 10.1111/j.1365-2672.2010.04746.x. Epub 2010 Aug 19.

Shimoji Y., Asato H., Sekizaki T., Mori Y. and Yokomizo Y.2002.Hyaluronidase is not essential for the lethality of *Erysipelothrix rhusiopathiae* infection in mice. J. Vet. Med. Sci. **64:** 173-176.

Shimoji Y., Ogawa Y., Osaki M., Kabeya H., Maruyama S., Mikami T. and Sekizaki T.2003.Adhesive surface proteins of *Erysipelothrix rhusiopathiae* bind to polystyrene, fibronectin, and type I and IV collagens. J. Bacteriol. **185:** 2739-2748.

Shimoji Y., Mori Y. and Fischetti V.A.1999.Immunological characterization of a protective antigen of *Erysipelothrix rhusiopathiae*: identification of the region responsible for protective immunity. Infect. Immun. **67:** 1646-1651.

Shimoji Y., Yokomizo Y., Sekizaki T., Mori Y. and Kubo M. 1994.Presence of a capsule in *Erysipelothrix rhusiopathiae* and its relationship to virulence for mice. Infect. Immun. **62:** 2806-2810.

Takahashi, T., Hirayama, N., Sawada, T., Tamura, Y. and Muramatsu, M. 1978a. Correlation between adherence of *Erysipelathrix rhusiopathiae* strains of serovar Ia to tissue culture cells originated from porcine kidney and their pathogenicity in mice and swine. Vet. Microbiol. **13:** 57-64.

Takahashi, T., Sawada, T., Muramatsu, M., Tamura, Y., Fujisawa, T., Benno, Y. and Mitsuoka, T. 1987b. Serotype, antimicrobial susceptibility and pathogenicity of *Erysipelothrix rhusiopathiae* isolates from tonsils of apparently healthy slaughter pigs. J.Clin. Microbiol. **25:** 536-539.

To H., and Nagai S.2007.Genetic and antigenic diversity of the surface protective antigen proteins of *Erysipelothrix rhusiopathiae*. Clin. Vaccine Immunol. **14:** 813-820. Epub 2007 May 2.

To H., Koyama T., Nagai S., . and Nunoya T.2009.Development of quantitative real-time polymerase chain reaction for detection of and discrimination between Erysipelothrix rhusiopathiae and other Erysipelothrix species. J. Vet. Diagn. Invest. **21:** 701-706.

Wang, Q., Chang, B.J. and Riley, T.V. 2009. *Erysipelothrix rhusiopathiae*. Vet. Microbiol. **140:** 405-417.

Wood, R.L. 1984. Swine erysipelas. A review of prevalence and research. J. Am. Vet. Med. Assoc. **184:** 944-949.

Wood, R.L. 1992. Erysipelas. In Disease of swine 7th Ed. Ed. A.D. Lama, B.E. Straw, W.L., Mengeling, S.D. 'Allaire and D.J. Taylor. pp 475-86. Ames: Iowa State University Press, U.S.A.

Yamazaki Y.2006.A multiplex polymerase chain reaction for discriminating *Erysipelothrix rhusiopathiae* from *Erysipelothrix* tonsillarum. J.Vet. Diagn. Invest. **18:** 384-387.

□□□

Chapter 17

Bordetella Infection

Dr. S.K. SRIVASTAVA
Former, Division of Bacteriology & Mycology
Indian Veterinary Research Institute, Izatnagar-243122
Bareilly (U.P.)

Bordetella Infection

The genus *Bordetella* contains several species, some of which are important pathogens of human and some of animals. The organisms are small, gram-negative rods and coccobacilli. The organisms are aerobic and non-spore forming. These are catalase and oxidase positive and do not ferment carbohydrates. There are both motile and non-motile species.

Important species of *Bordetella* are listed below;

- *Bordetella bronchiseptica* – Natural hosts are animals, causes respiratory disease including atrophic rhinitis of pigs.
- *Bordetella avium* – causes turkey coryza or avian bordetellosis.
- *Bordetella pertussis* – causes whooping cough in humans.
- *Bordetella parapertussis* – causes a mild form of whooping cough in humans.

Some less important species are *Bordetella hinzii, Bordetella holmesii, Bordetella petrii* and *Bordetella trematum* recovered from various animal species and birds causing various disease symptoms.

Bordetella *bronchiseptica*

B.bronchiseptica has been implicated in porcine atrophic rhinitis, kennel cough and bronchopneumonia in many species of animals. *B.bronchiseptica* has a capsule like envelope and pili and are motile by a peritichous flagella. It does not require blood agar to grow and growth is satisfactory in peptone water alone. They grow very well on MacConkey agar and cetrimide agar. None of the *Bordetella* spp. survives in environment outside host's body for a long time. The natural habitat of *Bordetella* is the respiratory tract of susceptible animals because of their preference of amino acids proline and glutamic acid which is present in respiratory secretions. Although the organism has simple growth requirement, they are readily killed by decreased oxidation / reduction (Eh) potential, UV irradiation, pH and temperature changes and many germicidals.

B.bronchiseptica gram stained

Bordetella spp. causes highly contagious respiratory disease of animals and is prevalent worldwide. Young animals are most commonly affected. The entire respiratory system may be affected with the pathogen resulting in acute exudative inflammation. The animal exhibits oculonasal discharge, coughing, sneezing, dyspnea, decreased weight gain and tracheal collapse. Most infections are probably asymptomatic or mildly symptomatic. In swine it is the causative agent of atrophic rhinitis. Toxigenic *Pasteurella multocida* may be involved in the disease condition resulting in progressive atrophic rhinitis Atrophic rhinitis is common in swine worldwide. *B. bronchiseptica* also causes infections in cats characterized by respiratory signs, fever, ocular discharge and lymphadenopathy (Egberiuk *et al.,* 2009).

The organism spread through direct contact to the susceptible host from the reservoir of infection. The most severe lesions occur in non-immune animals infected during the first week of life. Animals infected at 4 weeks develop less severe lesions while those infected at 10 weeks do not develop significant lesions. Accordingly, the clinical findings depend on the age as well as stage of the disease. In acute cases in piglets 3-9 weeks of age irritation of nasal mucosa causes sneezing, coughing and small amount of mucopurulent nasal discharge accompanied by watery ocular discharge. In severe cases dyspnea and cyanosis occur. The bleeding may also occur. In more chronic cases inspissated material may be expelled during paroxysms of sneezing. Often there is deformity of face. The nasal bones and premaxillae turn upwards and interfere with approximation of the invisor and to a less extent the molar teeth. Prehension and mastication become difficult. The condition may be unilateral or bilateral, developing most commonly in pigs of 8-10 weeks of age. There is high morbidity and low mortality in affected animals. Stress related occurrence is not uncommon under field situations.

Cell surface lipopolysaccharide-endotoxin of *B. broncisepticais* a potent virulence factor. In order to better characterize the endotoxin structure to virulence relationships, Basheer *et al.* (2011) studied the lipid A structures of B. bronchiseptica isolates from human and rabbit origins as a function of their virulence phases. Matrix-assisted laser desorption/ionization time-of-flight mass spectrometry (MALDI-TOF-MS) has been widely used for the structural characterization of bacterial endotoxins and their lipid A moieties. This method combined with chemical analytical methods proved to be essential for the characterization of small samples and discrete but essential structural modifications. The occurrence of palmitate (C(16)) in the *B. bronchiseptica* lipid A structures is shown for the first time at two sites. Their presence was also demonstrated for the first time in correlation with the virulence phase of *B. bronchiseptica* clinical isolates.

Besides swine, other animals infected with *Bordetta bronchiseptica* are dogs, cats, rabbits, horses and guinea pigs. In dogs it is the causative agent of a disease manifestation characterized by tracheobronchitis commonly known as kennel cough. Atypical *B.bronchiseptica* infections is causative agent of wound infections, abortion, bacteremia peritonitis etc. in immunocompromised human beings and domestic animals. *B.avium* infection is normally observed in turkey. The disease is called turkey coryza.

"Kennel cough" in dogs in animal shelters is readily transmissible, reduces adoption rates, and commonly leads to the euthanasia of affected dogs. In cats, tracheobronchitis, conjunctivitis, and pneumonia have been associated with *Bordetella bronchiseptica* infection-but most cases of upper-respiratory infection (URI) probably are caused by herpesvirus and calicivirus, and many *B. bronchiseptica* culture-positive cats are clinically normal (Foley *et al.*, 2002). The prospective observational study was undertaken to document the contribution of B. bronchiseptica to disease in cats and dogs from two animal shelters undergoing outbreaks of canine kennel cough, to evaluate whether cross-species transmission might have occurred, and to determine if the presence of infected cats represented a risk to dogs. Clinically defined cases of kennel cough in dogs and URI in cats were investigated in two shelters by calculating clinical-disease incidence, alveolar-lavage cytological examination, bacterial and viral cultures, antibiotic-susceptibility testing, and molecular fingerprinting by pulsed-field gel electrophoresis. In a 40-cat and 40-dog "no-kill" shelter, the prevalences of culture positivity were 47% for *B. bronchiseptica* and 36% for calicivirus at the same time as two resident dogs demonstrated clinical cough. When no dogs had kennel cough 3 months later, 10% of cats were *B. bronchiseptica*-culture-positive and 63% calicivirus positive. In a large traditional shelter, the incidence of kennel cough in dogs increased over 12 weeks to a maximum of 19 cases/week/120 dogs, during which time the culture prevalence was 23% for *B. bronchiseptica* in dogs and 47% in cats. Three to 6 months before the kennel-cough epidemic, no dogs or cats were *B. bronchiseptica* positive. Very little genetic variability was detected in isolates from these shelters; all isolates except one corresponded to a single strain type which was identical to the pattern in a vaccine used in these shelters. Isolates from other cats, a horse, a llama, and a sea otter were genetically distinct from the shelter isolates. There was widespread resistance to cephalosporins and ampicillin, but low or no resistance to amoxicillin/clavulanate, trimethoprim-sulfamethoxazole, tetracycline, and enrofloxacin. Greater percent resistance was observed in the traditional shelter than in the no-kill shelter and feline isolates were more likely to be resistant than canine isolates.

Colonization of hosts by *B. bronchiseptica* can lead to a range of diseases, from lethal pneumonia to asymptomatic infection, which is thought to be caused by differences in host immune status, polymicrobial infection, and/or bacterial strain variation. However, in inbred and specific-pathogen-free mice, the 50% lethal dose (LD_{50}) can still differ by up to 100,000-fold between bacterial strains, suggesting that substantial differences in virulence may be due to strain variation alone.

Pathogenesis

B.bronchiseptica has the tendency to bind the ciliated epithelium of the respiratory tract. This binding is preventable by neuraminidase treatment of host cells. It is followed by cilial paralysis and inflammation. The binding is mediated by an extracellular protein of 150 kDa in size. *B.avium* does not produce this protein designated as filamentous haemagglutinin (FHA). The FHA is secreted from cells but remains attached to the cells. In *B.pertussis,* there are 3 domains which are involved in adherence to eukaryotic cells: the arg-gly-asp (RGD) sequence, a carbohydrate - binding site and a heparin binding site (Relman *et al.,* 1989; Manozz *et al.,* 1991). The extracellular matrix proteins fibronectin, laminin and collagen remains attached to the RGD sequence and is recognized by integrin receptors. In FHA the RGD sequence is known to bind to 11 integrin CR3 on macrophages and promote phagocytosis (Relman *et al.,* 1990). FHA of *B.bronchiseptica* has the ability to bind bovine red blood cells and this property correlates with virulence of the organisms for pigs.

Similarly agglutination of guinea pigs erythrocytes correlates with pathogenecity of *B.avium* for turkeys. FHA is highly immunogenic and presence of antibodies against FHA is protective against respiratory challenge in mouse models. It has been postulaled that *B.bronchiseptica* and *B.avium* attach to sialoganglioside receptors in the respiratory tract whereas *B.pertussis* attaches to asialoglyco sphingolipids and sulfatides (Ishikawa and Isayama 1987; Brennan *et al.,* 1991).

Besides FHA another entity responsible for attachment is a 68-70 kDa outer membrane protein. It is encoded by a single gene and native protein is 93 kDa which is later modified to the mature form. It's RGD sequence located in the outer of passenger domain is chiefly responsible for *Bordetella pertussis* cells to bind to host cells (Leininger *et al.,* 1991) pertactin has been shown to be a protective antigen that can induce immunity to atrophic rhinitis in pigs and mice (Bemis and Burns, 1993).Pertactin is an auto-transporter protein produced by all members of *Bbronchiseptica* cluster. Two regions of the protein that contain sequence repeat (region ICRI and R2) show polymorphism. Pertactin plays a critical role in allowing bacteria to resist neutrophil mediated clearance (Inatsuka *et al.,* 2010). Both FHA and pertactin are necessary for optimal colonization of the swine respiratory tract (Nicholson *et al.,* 2009). Adherence is also mediated by the presence of fimbriae on cell surface. Fimbriae enhance the colonization of the bacteria to tracheal surface and for persistence of the bacteria on the surface on the surface (Mattoo *et al.,* 2000). Al least 2 fimbrial types exist in *B.bronchiseptica* and *B.avium* (Mooi *et al,* 1987). In *B.bronchiseptica,* the fimbriae is consisting of 3 proteins of molecular weights 21.5, 22 and 24 kDa whereas in *B.avium* 3 proteins 14.4, 17 and 24 kDa are present as fimbrial subunits (Bemis and Burns 1993). In *Bordetella pertussis* 4 genes, fim2, fim3 and fim X and fim A have been identified as single copy genes unlinked with chromosome. One of these fim2 is present in *B.brnchiseptica* but not *B.avium.* Genes coding accessory proteins involved in regulation and transport of fimbriae have also been identified as fim B, C and D (Willemms *et al,* 1992). Genetic makeup of *B.bronchiseptica* and *B.avium* need to be further characterized.

Bordetella species possess several other virulence factors besides the one described for the attachment. An 216 kDa adenylate cyclase toxin, also called cyclolysin, has been identified possessing both adenyl cyclase and hemolysin activity. This toxin contains 15 repeats of a 13 amino acid sequence and 5 repeats of a 9 amino acid sequence with C-terminal hemolysin portion of the molecule (Glaser *et al.,* 1988). The action of this toxin is to evade host immune system defences by thwarting phagocytosis. The toxin acts by building cAMP inside affected macrophages and prevent phagocytic activity of neutrophils by avoiding formation of phagolysosomes. It also has the property to escape into an endocytic compartment that does not lead to fusion with lysosome. Adenyl cyclase plays an important role during colonization of *B.bronchiseptica* to swine nasal cavity (Hibrand-Saint Oyant *et al.,* 2005). Adenylate cyclase in

B.pertussis is released from cells and enters the host cell helped by the hemolysin portion, through binding to glycolipid moeties on the cell surface which help in formation of pores (Gordon *et al.*, 1988). Soon after, it begins to catalyze the production of cAMP, probably by the action of calmodulin. The bacteria thus survive intracellularly because there is no respiratory burst of macrophages and neutrohils.

Bordetella produce an intracellular dermonectrotic toxin, ranging between 155 to 190 kDa. The toxin is an essential virulence factor of *B.bronchiseptica* responsible for causing atrophic rhinitis (Brockmeier *et al.*, 2002). The toxin is heat labile and is inactivated by heating at 56^{0}C. It is lethal for mice and known to inhibit the sodium potassium ATPase and cause contraction of smooth muscles surrounding peripheral blood vessels (Endoh *et al.*, 1990). It is a single chain peptide inactivated by trypsin, formalin and glutaraldehyde. It is lethal for mice. The toxin does not effect ciliary activity but damage the cultured swine nasal tissue. The degree of turbinate atrophy induced by *B.bronchiseptica* in pigs correlates with the level of dermonecrotic toxin produced. This necrotoxin impairs osteogenesis (Horiguchi *et al.*, 1991). Cultured osteoprogenitor cells exposed to the purified toxin show altered morphology and reduction in growth. The turbinate atrophy caused by *Bordetella* is due to the inhibition of osteogenesis (Bemis and Burns 1993).

To efficiently colonize and persist in the lower respiratory tract, bacteria must survive multiple host immune mechanisms. *Bordetella bronchiseptica* is a gram-negative respiratory pathogen that naturally infects mice and persists in the lower respiratory tract for up to 49 days postinoculation. Pilione *et al.* (2004) examined the effect of mutation of the *pagP* gene on the persistence of *B. bronchiseptica* in the lower respiratory tract of mice. The *pagP* gene encodes a palmitoyl transferase that is responsible for the addition of a palmitoyl group to the lipid A region of *B. bronchiseptica* lipopolysaccharide. Data presented here confirm that a *B. bronchiseptica* delta *pagP* mutant demonstrates defective persistence in the lower respiratory tract of wild-type mice. We hypothesized that the defective persistence of the B. bronchiseptica deltapagP mutant was due to an increased susceptibility of this mutant to a host immune response. *In vivo* data indicate that both B cells and the complement component C3 are required for the reduced bacterial numbers of the deltapagP mutant on day 14 postinoculation. In addition, an *in vitro* complement killing assay demonstrated that *B. bronchiseptica* exhibits pagP-dependent resistance to antibody-mediated complement killing at low concentrations of immune serum. Taken together, these results suggest that *pagP* is required for *B. bronchiseptica* to resist antibody-mediated complement lysis during respiratory infection.

The regulation of *Bordetella* virulence factors is primarily under the control of the BvgAS two-component regulatory system. In the Bvg⁺ phase, which is necessary and sufficient for respiratory tract infection, virulence factors such as adenylate cyclase toxin, filamentous hemagglutinin, pertactin, fimbriae, and a type III secretion system are expressed, while in the Bvg⁻ phase, believed to be involved in environmental survival, these genes are suppressed and other genes, such as those for flagellin, are expressed.

In addition to the known virulence factors already mentioned, the *wbm* and *pagP* genes, whose expression results in LPS modifications, are also regulated by BvgAS, suggesting they may be involved in the infectious process. The *pagP* gene encodes a palmitoyl transferase that is responsible for transferring a palmitate group to the lipid A region of LPS. Mutation of *pagP* homologues in *Salmonella enterica* serovar Typhimurium and *Legionella pneumophila* is associated with increased sensitivity to killing by cationic antimicrobial peptides. This suggests that the lipid A acylation state may influence outer membrane permeability. In addition, changes in lipid A acylation have been shown to affect complement activation and opsonization, as well as TLR-4 recognition *in vitro*. Despite these compelling data, the influence of lipid A acylation on *in vivo* host-pathogen interactions is not well understood.

The LPS structure of the wild-type RB50 strain of *B. bronchiseptica* is primarily hexa-acylated in the Bvg⁺ phase, while LPS from the Ä*pagP* mutant of this strain is penta-acylated in the Bvg⁺ phase due to the lack of a sixth palmitoyl group in the lipid A region. Mutation of the *pagP* gene results in a defect in the ability of *B. bronchiseptica* to persist in the lungs of wild-type mice. It is hypotesized that a functional *pagP* gene protects *B. bronchiseptica* against host immune responses that are responsible for the early clearance of the Ä*pagP* mutant.

The membrane-distal repeated carbohydrate structure of LPS, the O-antigen, can prevent antibody functions and may vary as a mechanism of immune evasion. Genes of the wbm locus are required for the assembly of O-antigen on the animal pathogen Bordetella bronchiseptica and the human pathogen *B. parapertussis*. However, the important human pathogen B. pertussis lacks these genes and a number of in vitro and in vivo characteristics associated with O-antigen in other organisms. To determine the specific functions of O-antigen in these closely related *Bordetella* subspecies, we compared wbm deletion (Deltawbm) mutants of *B. bronchiseptica* and B. parapertussis in a variety of assays relevant to natural respiratory tract infection. Complement was not activated or depleted by wild-type bordetellae expressing O-antigen, but both Deltawbm mutants activated complement and were highly sensitive to complement-mediated killing *in vitro*. Although the O-antigen structures appear to be substantially similar, the two mutants differed strikingly in their defects within the respiratory tract. The B. *parapertussis* Deltawbm mutant was severely defective in colonization of the tracheas and lungs of mice, while the *B. bronchiseptica* Deltawbm mutant showed almost no defect. While in vitro characteristics such as serum resistance may be attributable to O-antigen directly, the role of O-antigen during infection appears to be more complex, possibly involving factors differing among the closely related bordetellae or different interactions between each one and its host (Burns *et al.*, 2003).

Interestingly, differences between their abilities to infect, persist in, and cause disease in different hosts correlates with differences in their lipopolysaccharide (LPS) structures. Furthermore, It has been previously shown that mutants of these three bordetellae expressing truncated LPS have very different defects during in vivo infection, suggesting that their LPS structures play roles in infection that are specific to each organism. *B. pertussis* LPS comprises a lipid A domain and a branched-chain core oligosaccharide that together form the structure called band B. This may be further modified by the addition of a complex trisaccharide (band B plus trisaccharide) and called band A. *B. bronchiseptica* expresses band B and band A LPS but also expresses an O-antigen that is a homopolymer of 2,3-dideoxoy-2,3-di-*N*-acetylgalactosaminuronic acid and is attached somewhere in the core-trisaccharide region. While *B. parapertussis* expresses the same O antigen as *B. bronchiseptica*, it expresses a band B LPS that is electrophoretically distinguishable from that of *B. pertussis* and *B. bronchiseptica*, indicating that the *B. parapertussis* core is smaller than that of the other two species. *B. parapertussis* also does not express band A LPS, possibly because of a mutation in the *wlbH* gene involved in band A trisaccharide biosynthesis.

A *B. pertussis* strain with a deletion in the *wlb* locus (Ä*wlb*) expresses only band B LPS, indicating that these genes are required for the addition of the trisaccharide of band A. In *B. bronchiseptica*, this mutation results in the loss of both the band A trisaccharide and O antigen (presumably because of loss of the core acceptor site), leaving a lipid A-inner core molecule that was electrophoretically indistinguishable from that of the *B. pertussis* Ä*wlb* mutant.*B. parapertussis* Ä*wlb* mutants express an LPS molecule that lacks both band A trisaccharide and O antigen but is more electrophoretically mobile than that of the Ä*wlb* mutants of the other two subspecies because of the apparently smaller lipid A-inner core structures. Although the LPS structures of Ä*wlb* mutants of *B. pertussis* and *B. bronchiseptica* were similar and the LPS structures of both *B. parapertussis* and *B. bronchiseptica* Ä*wlb* mutants lack expression of the band A trisaccharide and O-antigen, there were substantial differences among the phenotypes of the three mutants in a mouse infection model. While the *B. pertussis* Ä*wlb* mutant was severely defective in colonization of the nasal cavities of BALB/c mice, neither of the other mutants showed any defect in the colonization of or persistence at this site. The *B. parapertussis* Ä*wlb* mutant was severely defective in colonizing the lungs, being recovered in numbers 1/10,000 of those of the wild-type strain by day 3 postinoculation. However, the *B. bronchiseptica* mutant was recovered from the lungs in numbers similar to those of the wild-type strain until day 7 postinoculation. The variety of defects of these three mutants was interpreted to reflect the diversity of functions of LPS in infection. It is interesting that resistance to serum complement, which has been attributed to O-antigen expression in other bacteria, was observed with wild-type *B. bronchiseptica* and *B. parapertussis*, which express O-antigen, but not with wild-type *B. pertussis* or the *wlb* mutants, which do not.

Adjacent to the *wlb* locus in both *B. bronchiseptica* and *B. parapertussis* is the *wbm* locus, which is responsible for the expression of the 2,3-dideoxy-2,3-di-*N*-acetylgalactosaminuronic acid homopolymeric O antigen. Deletion of *wbmB* through the N-terminal portion of *wbmE* (Ä*wbm*) in *B. bronchiseptica* and *B. parapertussis* leads to loss of O-antigen expression in these bacteria. Since *B. pertussis* naturally lacks O-antigen, it is worth noting that deletion of the *wbm* locus removes the major structural difference between the LPSs of *B. bronchiseptica* and *B. parapertussis* and that of *B. pertussis*.

Despite the fact that closely related bacteria can cause different levels of disease, the genetic changes that cause some isolates to be more pathogenic than others are generally not well understood. Buboltz *et al.* (2009) used a combination of approaches to determine which factors contribute to the increased virulence of a *Bordetella bronchiseptica* lineage. A strain isolated from a host with B. bronchiseptica-induced disease, strain 1289, was 60-fold more virulent in mice than one isolated from an asymptomatically infected host, strain RB50. Transcriptome analysis and quantitative reverse transcription-PCR showed that the type III secretion system (TTSS) genes were more highly expressed by strain 1289 than strain RB50. Compared to strain RB50, strain 1289 exhibited greater TTSS-mediated cytotoxicity of a mammalian cell line. Additionally, we show that the increase in virulence of strain 1289 compared to that of RB50 was partially attributable to the TTSS. Using multilocus sequence typing, we identified another strain from the same lineage as strain 1289. Similar to strain 1289, we implicate the TTSS in the increased virulence of this strain. Together, these data suggest that the TTSS is involved in the increased virulence of a *B. bronchiseptica* lineage which appears to be disproportionately associated with disease. These data are consistent with the view that *B. bronchiseptica* lineages can have different levels of virulence, which may contribute to this species' ability to cause different severities of respiratory disease.

Beta-defensins are cationic peptides which form part of the innate immune response of the respiratory epithelium (Erles and Brownlie 2010). Due to their antimicrobial properties and immunostimulatory activity, beta-defensins are potential tools for the treatment and prevention of respiratory disease. In dogs, infectious respiratory disease is a common problem, particularly in housed animals. This study aimed to assess the presence of four beta-defensins in the canine respiratory tract and to use quantitative real-time PCR to determine mRNA levels following microbial challenge. Three beta-defensins, CBD1, CBD103 and CBD108, were detected in respiratory cells. All three defensins were also readily expressed in skin samples, while their expression in lymphoid tissues and the kidney was low and inconsistent. Treatment of primary tracheal epithelial cells with lipopolysaccharide (LPS) or infection with canine respiratory coronavirus led to decreased expression of CBD103 and CBD108, while cells infected with canine parainfluenza virus had lower levels of CBD1 and CBD108. Furthermore CBD103 was demonstrated to have antimicrobial activity against the respiratory pathogen Bordetella bronchiseptica.

Components in cellular matrix regulate activities of various growth factors by binding and liberating them in response to alteration in the extracellular environment. The fibroneclin based extra-cellular matrix may function as a temporary storage system for the toxin enabling small amount of toxin to act (Fukui *et al.,* 2010). In atrophic rhinitis there is resorption and replacement fibrosis of the osseous core. Experimental infection with *B.broncheseptica* alone does not result in severe turbinate atrophy or twisting or shortening of the snout. The severe turbinate atrophy is caused by mixed infection with *B.bronchiseptica* and toxigenic *Pasteurella multocida.*

Besides the above toxin, a 921D tracheal cytotoxin (a muramyl peptide toxic to ciliated epithelium) has been identified in *Bordetella* spp. It causes destruction of ciliated cells and swelling of mitochondria. This loss of cilia causes mucous, bacteria and foreign particles to accumulate leading to coughing. The toxin also causes inhibition of DNA synthesis in epithelial cells. The binding site and mechanism of action for this toxin has not been described. Expression of nearly all these virulence factors is positively regulated by bVgAS locus. Bvg A and BvbS comprise a 2 component signal transduction system that mediate transition between at least 3 identifiable phases, avirulent (Bvg+) phase, an avirulent (Bvg-) phase and an intermediate phase (Mattoo *et al.,* 2001).

Other factors responsible for the damage to host by *Bordetella* are lipopolysaccharide, possessing lethality for galactosomine- sensitized mice. It is pyrogenic and mitogenic as well, activates macrophages and induction of tumor necrosis factor (Amano *et al.*, 1991). It is also a major chemotactic factor during infection. *Bordetella* also produces several outer membrane proteins that is important in virulence. One of these is a 40 kDa porin protein, similar to the GroEL proteins found in other species (Burns *et al.*, 1991).

Bordetella also produces iron binding siderophores, bordetellin, which may have role in virulence, even though it produces a receptor for iron-transferrin complexes. *Bordetella* are rarely detected in the blood stream or deep body tissues.

B.avium produces a histamine sensitizing factor resembling *B.pertussis* toxin, a cytotoxin, adhesion and a dermonecrotic toxin.

Bacterial virulence is influenced by the activity of two-component regulator systems (TCSs), which consist of membrane-bound sensor kinases that allow bacteria to sense the external environment and cytoplasmic, DNA-binding response regulator proteins that control appropriate gene expression. Respiratory pathogens of the Bordetella genus require the well-studied TCS BvgAS to control the expression of many genes required for colonization of the mammalian respiratory tract. Kaut *et al.*(2011) describe the identification of a novel gene in Bordetella bronchiseptica, plrS, the product of which shares sequence homology to several NtrY-family sensor kinases and is required for B. bronchiseptica to colonize and persist in the lower, but not upper, respiratory tract in rats and mice. The plrS gene is located immediately 5' to and presumably cotranscribed with a gene encoding a putative response regulator, supporting the idea that PlrS and the product of the downstream gene may compose a TCS. Consistent with this hypothesis, the PlrS-dependent colonization phenotype requires a conserved histidine that serves as the site of autophosphorylation in other sensor kinases, and in strains lacking plrS, the production and/or cellular localization of several immune-recognized proteins is altered in comparison to that in the wild-type strain. Because plrS is required for colonization and persistence only in the lower respiratory tract, a site where innate and adaptive immune mechanisms actively target infectious agents, the authors hypothesize that its role may be to allow Bordetella to resist the host immune response.

Diagnosis

Samples of choice are nasal swabs, sediment of transtracheal washes and tracheal swabs (Coryza of turkeys). The samples are cultured on blood and MacConkey agar and incubated aerobically. Small, circular, dewdrop colonies appear in 48 hours. On further incubation the colonies enlarge, becoming flat and glistening. Stained smears reveal small gram-negative rods or coccobacilli.

Bordetella bronchiseptica are motile and indole negative and does not produce H_2S. Urease is produced and tests for oxidase and catalase are positive. Carbohydrates are not fermented.

In Dutch laboratories molecular detection of B. pertussis and B. parapertussis is commonly based on insertion sequences IS481 and IS1001, respectively. Both IS elements are more widely spread among *Bordetella* species. Both *Bordetella holmesii,* and *B. bronchiseptica* can harbour IS481. Also, IS1001 is found among B. bronchiseptica. IS481, and IS1001 based PCR thus lacks specificity when used for detection of specific *Bordetella* spp.Roorda *et al.* (2011) designed a PCR based on IS1002, another IS element that is present among Bordetella species, and exploited it as a template in combination with PCR for IS481, and IS1001. In combining the PCRs for IS481, IS1001, and IS1002, and including an inhibition control, the workers were able to detect and discriminate all clinically relevant *Bordetella* species.The report indicates that an improved PCR method for specific detection of *B. pertussis, B. parapertussis, B. holmesii,* and *B. bronchiseptica* was developed.

Menard *et al.* (2007) describes a real-time PCR assay for the detection and identification of *Bordetella* pertussis and *Bordetella parapertussis.* The assay is based on amplification of a fragment from the repeat sequence regions IS481 and IS1001 found in *B. pertussis* and *B. parapertussis,* respectively, with subsequent species identification by melting curve analysis using SYBR Green chemistry. Discrimination between the two species was straightforward, as the corresponding melting points showed a significant difference of 7 degrees C. The assay was evaluated first with reference strains and retrospective human clinical samples, and then prospectively with 132 human clinical specimens received between March 2003 and December 2005. The assay allowed the rapid detection of 22 positive clinical samples, of which 15, including one fatal case, were not identified by standard culture techniques. The new assay was sensitive and specific, and can be implemented easily using any real-time PCR apparatus.

Treatment and Control

The atrophic rhinitis is not treatable. Preventive measures include maintenance of an aged sow herd with a low carrier rate; thorough disinfection and clean up of farrowing houses and nurseries after each use. Prophylactic use of sulfonamides in feed and water is useful. Continuous nasal swabbing is done to identify and eliminate carrier sows. If therapy is induced tylosin, oxytetracycline, ceftiofur given parenterally is useful. Repeated administration of the drug is required. Alternatively trimethoprin sulfonamide in the drinking water for 3 weeks may be administered. For treating kennel cough tetracycline and chloramphenicol are administered. Kanamycin is administered by aerosole to unresponsive dogs. Penicillin is not effective.

MICs for 349 *Bordetella bronchiseptica* isolates from respiratory tract infections of swine were determined by broth microdilution (Kadlec *et al.*2004). The lowest MIC at which 90% of isolates tested are inhibited (MIC90) was that of tetracycline and enrofloxacin (0.5 microg/ml), whereas the highest MIC90s were those of tilmicosin and cephalothin (32 microg/ml) as well as streptomycin (256 microg/ml). One hundred and 63 Bordetella bronchiseptica isolates from pigs, consisting of 65 isolated in 2003 and 98 isolated in 2007, were tested for antimicrobial susceptibility to 17 antimicrobial agents by the disk diffusion method. All 163 *B. bronchiseptica* isolates were sensitive to polymyxin B and cefoperazone/sulbactam; the majority of the strains were sensitive to amikacin (149/163; 91.4%), gentamicin (132/163; 81.0%), ampicillin/sulbactam (127/163; 77.9%) and ciprofloxacin (115/163; 70.6%). A high level of resistance was found for furazolidone (100%), ampicillin (90.2%), cefazolin (89.0%), streptomycin (87.7%), amoxicillin/clavulanic acid (74.2%) and tetracycline (64.4%). Comparison of the data revealed that isolates with multiresistance to at least six or eight of the 17 antimicrobials used became more frequent, with the proportions increasing from 32.3% or 16.9% in 2003 to 90.8% or 41.8% in 2007 (Zhao *et al.*, 2011).

Twenty florfenicol- and/or chloramphenicol-resistant *Bordetella bronchiseptica* isolates of porcine and feline origin were investigated for the presence of floR and cml genes and their location on plasmids (Kadlec *et al.*, 2007). The *B. bronchiseptica* isolates were investigated for their susceptibility to antimicrobial agents by broth micro- or macrodilution and for their plasmid content. Hybridization experiments and PCR assays were conducted to identify resistance genes. Transformation and conjugation studies were performed to show their transferability. Representatives of both types of genes including their flanking regions were sequenced. Moreover, inhibitor studies with the efflux pump inhibitor Phe-Arg-beta-naphthylamide (PAbetaN) were performed.The gene floR was found in the chromosomal DNA of 9 of the 18 florfenicol/chloramphenicol-resistant isolates. Sequence analysis revealed that the deduced FloR protein sequence differed by a single amino acid exchange from FloR of Vibrio cholerae. A chloramphenicol-resistant, but florfenicol-susceptible isolate carried a novel plasmid-borne cml gene, designated cmlB1. The CmlB1 protein revealed only 73.8-76.5% identity to known CmlA proteins. The gene cmlB1 was not part of a gene cassette. The results of inhibitor studies with PAbetaN suggested that a so-far unidentified efflux system might play a role in phenicol resistance of the remaining florfenicol- and/or chloramphenicol-resistant isolates.The identification of the first member of a new subclass of cml genes, cmlB1 from *B. bronchiseptica,* extends our knowledge on specific chloramphenicol exporters.

Control measures should aim at eliminating *B.bronchiseptica* and *P.multocida*. These control measures should include eradication, mass medication and vaccination. Adoption of hygienic measures also reduces the incidence of atrophic rhinitis. Bacterin toxoid preparations are given to sow before farrowing so that the colostrums contribute to protection against atrophic rhinitis. Piglets up to 4 weeks of age may also be vaccinated. Modified live intranasal vaccines prepared from the bacterial cells are administered to young pigs. For dogs bacterins and intranasal vaccines are used for controlling Kennel cough. Ellis *et al.* (2001) reported that a *B.bronchiseptica* vaccine given parenterally and intranasally was effective in puppies against *B.bronchiseptica* infection. A bivalent modified live vaccine against canine tracheobronchitis was given by intranasal route along with injectable trivalent vaccine against canine parvovirus, canine distemper virus and canine adenovirus. The vaccine performed well as far as production of antibodies in animals was concerned (Jacobs *et al.*, 2007).

Bordetella bronchiseptica is a Gram-negative bacterium that colonises the respiratory tract of mammals and is considered to be a primary pathogen of domestic cats. It is sensible to consider *B. bronchiseptica* as a rare cause of zoonotic infections. The bacterium is susceptible to common disinfectants. The bacterium is shed in oral and nasal secretions of infected cats. Dogs with respiratory disease are an infection risk for cats. The microorganism colonises the ciliated epithelium of the respiratory tract of the host, establishing chronic infections. A wide range of respiratory signs has been associated with B bronchiseptica infection, from a mild illness with fever, coughing, sneezing, ocular discharge and lymphadenopathy to severe pneumonia with dyspnoea, cyanosis and death. Bacterial culture and PCR lack sensitivity. Samples for isolation can be obtained from the oropharynx (swabs) or via transtracheal wash/ bronchoalveolar lavage. Antibacterial therapy is indicated, even if the signs are mild. Where sensitivity data are unavailable, tetracyclines are recommended. Doxycycline is the antimicrobial of choice. Cats with severe B bronchiseptica infection require supportive therapy and intensive nursing care. In some European countries an intranasal modified-live virus vaccine is available. The modified-live product is licensed for use as a single vaccination with annual boosters. Cats should not be routinely vaccinated against B bronchiseptica (non-core), since the infection generally causes only a mild disease.

To determine comparative efficacy of vaccines administered IM and intranasally, used alone or sequentially, to protect puppies from infection with *Bordetella bronchiseptica* and determine whether systemic or mucosal antibody response correlated with protection a study was undertaken by Ellis *et al.* (2001).A randomized controlled trial w2as designed. In 2 replicates of 25 dogs each, 14-week-old puppies that were vaccinated against canine distemper virus and parvovirus were vaccinated against *B. bronchiseptica* via intranasal, IM, intranasal-IM, or IM-intranasal administration or were unvaccinated controls. Puppies were challenge exposed via aerosol administration of *B. bronchiseptica* 2 weeks after final vaccination. Clinical variables and systemic and mucosal antibody responses were monitored for 10 days after challenge exposure. Puppies in replicate 1 were necropsied for histologic and immunohistochemical studies.Control puppies that were seronegative before challenge exposure developed paroxysmal coughing, signs of depression, anorexia, and fever. Vaccinated puppies (either vaccine) that were seronegative before challenge exposure had fewer clinical signs. Puppies that received both vaccines had the least severe clinical signs and fewest lesions in the respiratory tract. Vaccinated dogs had significantly higher concentrations of *B. bronchiseptica*-reactive antibodies in serum saliva before and after challenge. Antibody concentrations were negatively correlated with bacterial growth in nasal cavity and pharyngeal samples after challenge exposure. Parenterally and intranasally administered vaccines containing *B. bronchiseptica* may provide substantial protection from clinical signs of respiratory tract disease associated with infection by this bacterium. Administration of both types of vaccines in sequence afforded the greatest degree of protection against disease.

Healthy dogs with low antibody titer to *Bordetella bronchiseptica* were vaccinated intranasally with an avirulent live vaccine, subcutaneously with an antigen extract vaccine, or subcutaneously and intranasally with a placebo(Davis *et al.*, 2007). Intranasally vaccinated dogs developed *B. bronchiseptica*-specific IgA titers in nasal secretions that remained at high levels until the end of the study; dogs vaccinated subcutaneously with the antigen extract or placebo did not develop measurable antigen-specific IgA titers in nasal secretions. Dogs were challenged with virulent live *B. bronchiseptica* 63 days after vaccination. Intranasally vaccinated dogs had significantly lower cough scores (P < or =.0058) and shed significantly fewer challenge organisms (P <.0001) than dogs in either of the other groups. Cough scores of subcutaneously vaccinated dogs were not significantly different from placebo-vaccinated dogs.

Zhao *et al.* (2010) showed the immunogenicity and protective efficacy of five pertactin recombinants against *Bordetella bronchiseptica* (Bb) challenge. The complete coding sequence (2040 bp) of the prn gene (PRN) and its fragments,5'-terminal 1173 bp fragment (PN),3'-terminal 867 bp fragment (PC), two copies of region I (654 bp; PR I) in PN, and 2 copies of region II (678 bp; PR II) in PC, were separately cloned into the prokaryotic expression vector pGEX-KG, and expressed in the *Eschierichia coli* BL21 (DE3) using induction by isopropyl-beta-D-thiogalactopyranoside. The recombinant proteins were named GST-PRN, GST-PN, GST-PC, GST-2PR I and GST-2PR II. All five recombinant proteins showed immunological reactivity in the Western-blot analysis. Mice, immunized subcutaneously with two doses of the purified proteins mixed with an equal volume of Freund's adjuvant,produced robust PRN-specific IgG antibody levels. When challenged, 6 of 9 mice in GST-2PR I group and all 9 mice in the other groups survived intranasal challenge with three times the 50% lethal dose (LD50) of virulent Bb HH0809. After challenge with 10 LD50 7/9,3/9,6/9,1/10 and 6/10 of the mice survived. Furthermore, complete protection against intraperitoneal (i.p.) challenge with 10 LD50 of HH0809 was observed in mice that were injected i.p. with 0.5 ml rabbit anti-GST-PRN, GST-PN,GST-PC or GST-2PR II serum. Only 1 of 10 mice survived in the group of mice that received anti-GST-2PR I, and no survivors were noted in the group of mice that received PRN-absorbed rabbit antiserum (0/5). The authors concluded that all of five pertactin recombinants had differential immunogenicity and protective efficacy against Bb challenge. Mice immunized with GST-PC had better survival against fatal Bb challenge than did those immunized with GST-PN. In addition, GST-2PR II and GST-2PR I provided the similar results These data may have implications for the development of safe and efficacious subunit vaccines for the prevention of bordetellosis on the basis of these five pertactin recombinants.

References

Amano, K., Watanabe, M., Takimoto, H. and Kumazawa, Y. 1991. Structural and biological comparison of lipopolysaccharide (LPS) from *Bordetella* species. Dev. Biol. Stand. **73:** 193-199.

Bemis, D.A. and Burns, E.H. 1993. *Bordetella*: in pathogenesis of bacterial infections in animals. Pp. 201-215. Ed. C.L. Gyles and C.O. Thoen. IOWA State Univ. Press. Ames.

Basheer S.M, Guiso N., Tirsoaga A., Caroff M. and Novikov A..2011. Structural modifications occurring in lipid A of *Bordetella bronchiseptica* clinical isolates as demonstrated by matrix-assisted laser desorption/ionization time-of-flight mass spectrometry. Rapid Commun Mass Spectrom. **25:** 1075-1081. doi: 10.1002/rcm.4960. Epub 2011 Mar 29.

Brennan, M.J., Hannah, J.H. and Leininger, E. 1991. Adhesion of *Bordetella pertussis* to sulfatides and to the Gal-NAC-beta 4-Gal sequence found in glycosphingolipids. J. Biol. Chem. **266:** 18827-18831.

Brockmeier, S.L., Register, K.B., Magyar, T., LaxA. J., Pullinger, G.D. and Kunkle, R.A. 2002. Role of dermonecrotic toxin of *Bordetella bronchiseptica* in the pathogenesis of respiratory diseases in swine. Infect. Immun. **70:** 481-490.

Buboltz A.M., Nicholson T.L., Weyrich L.S. and Harvill E.T.2009.Role of the type III secretion system in a hypervirulent lineage of *Bordetella bronchiseptica*. Infect. Immun. **77:** 3969-3977. Epub 2009 Jul 13.

Burns, D., Gould-Kostka, J., Kessel, M. and Achiniega, J. 1991. Purification and immunological characterization of a GroEL like protein from *Bordetella pertussis*. Infect. Immun. **59:** 1417-1422.

Burns V.C., Pishko E.J., Preston A., Maskell D.J. and Harvill E.T.2003.Role of *Bordetella* O-antigen in respiratory tract infection. Infect Immun. **71:** 86-94.

Davis R., Jayappa H., Abdelmagid O.Y., Armstrong R., Sweeney D. and Lehr C.2007.Comparison of the mucosal immune response in dogs vaccinated with either an intranasal avirulent live culture or a subcutaneous antigen extract vaccine of *Bordetella bronchiseptica*. Vet. Ther. **8:** 32-40.

Egberink, H., Addie, D., Belak, S., Boucrant-Baralon, C., Frymus, T., Gruffydd-Jones, T. *et al.*, 2009. *Bordetella bronchiseptica* infection in cats. A B C D guidelines on prevention and management. J. Feline. Med. Surg. **11:** 610-614.

Ellis, J.A., Haines, D.M., West, K.H., Burr, J.H., Dayton, A., Townsend, H.G., Kanara, E.W., Konoby, C., Crichlow, A., Martin, K. and Headrick, G. 2001. Effect of vaccination on experimental infection with *Bordetella bronchiseptica* in dogs. J. Am. Vet. Med. Assoc. **218:** 367-375.

Endoh, M., Nagai, M., Burns, D.L., Nakase, Y. and Mandark, C.R. 1990. Effect of exogenous agents on the action of *Bordetella* heat-labile toxin. Proc. 5th Int. Symp. Pertussis. Pp. 30-36, Bethesda.

Erles K., Brownlic J.2010.Expression of beta-defensins in the canine respiratory tract and antimicrobial activity against *Bordetella bronchiseptica*. Vet. Immunol. Immunopathol. **135:** 12-19. Epub 2009 Oct 29.

Foley J.E., Rand C., Bannasch M.J., Norris C.R and Milan J.2002.Molecular epidemiology of feline *Bordetellosis* in two animal shelters in California, USA. Prev. Vet. Med. **54:** 141-156.

Fukui, M.A., Kumitani, S., Miyake, M. and Horiguchi, Y. 2010. Association of *Bordetella bronchiseptica* toxin with the extracellular matrix. BMC Microbiol. **10:** 247-249.

Glaser, P., Dandim, A., Lardant, D., Barzu, O. and Ullman, A. 1988. *Bordetella pertussis* adenylate cyclase: The gene and the protein. Tokai J. Exp. Clin. Med. 13 (Suppl.) 239-252.

Gordon, V., Leppla, S. and Hewlett, E. 1988. Inhibitor of receptor mediated endocytosis block to entry of *Bacillus anthracis* adenylate cyclase toxin but not that of *Bordetella pertussis* adenylate cycle toxin. Infect. Immun. **56:** 1066-1069.

Hibrand-Saint Oyant, L., Bourges, D., Chivaleyre, C., Raze, D., Locht, C. and Salmon, H. 2005. Role of *Bordetella bronchiseptica* adenylate cyclase in nasal colonization and in development of local and systemic immune responses in piglets. Vet. Res. **36:** 63-77.

Horiguchi, Y., Nakai, T. and Kume, K. 1991. Effects of *Brodetella bronchiseptica* dermonecrotizing toxin on the structure and function of osteoblastic clone MC373-E1 cells. Infect. Immun. **59:** 1112-1116.

Inatsuka, C.S., XuQ., Vujkovic-Cvijin, I., Wong, S., Stibitz, S., Miller, J.F. and Cotter, P.A. 2010. Pertactin is required for *Bordetella* species to resist neutrophil- mediated clearance. Infect. Immun. **78:** 2901-2909.

Ishikawa, H. and Isayama, Y. 1987. Evidence for Sialyl conjugates as receptors for *Brodetella bronchiseptica* on swine nasal mucosa. Infect. Immun. **55:** 1607-1609.

Jacobs, A.A., Bergman, J.G., Theelen, R.P., Jasper, R., Helps, J.M., Horspool, L.J. and Paul, G. 2007. Compatibility of a bivalent modified live vaccine against *Bordetella bronchiseptica* and CPiV and a trivalent modified live vaccine against CPV, CDV and CAV-2. Vet. Rec. **160:** 41-45.

Kadlec K., Kehrenberg C. and Schwarz S.2007.Efflux-mediated resistance to florfenicol and/or chloramphenicol in *Bordetella bronchiseptica*: identification of a novel chloramphenicol exporter. J. Antimicrob. Chemother. **59:** 191-196. Epub 2007 Jan 15.

Kadlec K., Kehrenberg C., Wallmann J. and Schwarz S.2004.Antimicrobial susceptibility of *Bordetella bronchiseptica* isolates from porcine respiratory tract infections. Antimicrob Agents Chemother. **48:** 4903-4906.

Kaut C.S., Duncan M.D., Kim J.Y., Maclaren J.J., Cochran K.T. and Julio S.M. 2011.A Novel Sensor Kinase Is Required for *Bordetella bronchiseptica* To Colonize the Lower Respiratory Tract. Infect. Immun. **79:** 3216-3228. Epub 2011 May 23.

Leininger, E., Roberts, M., Kenimer, J., Charles, I., Fairweather, N. Novotny, P. and Brennan, M. 1991. Pertactin, an arg-gly-asp containing *Bordetalla pertussis* surface protein that promotes adherence of mammalian cells. Proc. Nat. Acad. Sci. USA, **88:** 345-349.

Mattoo, S., foreman - Wykert, A.K., Cotter, P.A. and Miller, J.F. 2001. Mechanisms of *Bordetella* pathogenesis. Front Biosci. **6:** 168-186.

Mattoo, S., Miller, J.F. and Cotter, P.A. 2000. Role of *Bordetella bronchiseptica* fimbriae in tracheal colonization and development of humoral immune response. Infect. Immun. **68:** 2024-2033.

Menozzi, F.D., Gangiez, C. and Locht, C. 1991. Interactions of the *Bordetella pertussis* filamentous haemagglutinin with heparin. Fed. Eur. Microbial. Soc. Microbiol. Lett. **62:** 59-64.

Ménard A., Lehours P., Sarlangue J., Bébéar C., Mégraud F., and de Barbeyrac B. 2007.Development of a real-time PCR for the identification of *Bordetella pertussis* and *Bordetella parapertussis*. Clin. Microbiol. Infect. **13:** 419-423.

Mooi, F., Vander, Heide, H., terA vest, A., Welinder, K., Livey, I., Vander Zeist, B. and Gaastra, W. 1987. Characterization of fimbrial subunits from *Bordetella* species. Microb. Pathog. **2:** 473-484.

Nicholson, T.L., Brockmeier, S.L. and Loving, C.L. 2009. Contribution of *Bordetella bronchiseptica* filamentous hemagglutinin and pertactin to respiratory disease in swine. Infect. Immun. **77:** 2136-2146.

Pilione M.R., Pishko E.J., Preston A., Maskell D.J. and Harvill E.T.2004.pagP is required for resistance to antibody-mediated complement lysis during *Bordetella bronchiseptica* respiratory infection. Infect. Immun. **72:** 2837-2842.

Roorda L., Buitenwerf J., Ossewaarde J.M., and van der Zee A.2011.A real-time PCR assay with improved specificity for detection and discrimination of all clinically relevant *Bordetella* species by the presence and distribution of three Insertion Sequence elements. BMC Res Notes. **4:** 11.

Zhao Z., Wang C., Xue Y., Ding K., Zhang C., Cheng X., Li Y., Liu Y. and Wu T.2010. Immunogenicity and protective efficacy of pertactin recombinants against *Bordetella bronchiseptica* challenge]. Wei. Sheng. Wu Xue. Bao. **50:** 1239-45. [Article in Chinese]

Zhao Z., Xue Y., Wang C., Ding K., Wu B., He Q., Cheng X. and Chen H.2011.Antimicrobial susceptibility of *Bordetella bronchiseptica* isolates from pigs with respiratory diseases on farms in China. J. Vet. Med. Sci. **73:** 103-106. Epub 2010 Aug 20.

□□□

Chapter 18

Moraxella Infection

Dr. S.K. SRIVASTAVA
Former, Division of Bacteriology & Mycology
Indian Veterinary Research Institute, Izatnagar-243122
Bareilly (U.P.)

Moraxella Infection

Moraxella are small, gram negative, aerobic, non motile rods or coccobacilli comprising of at least 10 species but only *Moraxella bovis* is responsible for a significant disease in animals, namely, infectious bovine keratoconjunctivitis (IBK), also known as Pink eye (Chandler *et al.*, 1979). A coccoid Moraxella, *Moraxella boviculi* has been isolated from eyes of calves affected with 1BK (Angelos *et al.*, 2007b). Nine lactating dairy cows were evaluated because of eye lesions (Galvao and Angelos 2010). Examination revealed mild to severe ulceration of the lower and/or upper eyelids, mild to severe swelling surrounding affected eyes, and profuse lacrimation. Lesions typically affected 1 eye, and involved the eyelid skin and conjunctiva. *Moraxella bovoculi* was isolated from affected cases. Oxytetracycline treatment led to cure within 2 wk.Moraxella are catalase and oxidase positive, do not use carbohydrates and do not require X or V factors. Typically, freshly isolated colonies are haemolytic on blood agar, flat and friable and produce a pitting of the agar. Capsule may be present in fresh isolates.

Some species and the animals from which they are recovered are as follows:

M.bovis	:	Cattle and horses
M.canis	:	Dogs and cats, human bite wounds
M.boviculi	:	1BK- like disease in cattle

M.caprae	:	Goats
M.cuniculi	:	Rabbits
M.ovis	:	Sheep and goats
M.boevrei	:	Goats
M.lacunata	:	Many animal species and humans, equine abortions, septicaemia in goats
M.phenolpyruvica	:	Cattle, sheep, swine, goats
M.caviae	:	Guinea pigs

With the exception of *M.bovis* and *M.lacunata,* none other is pathogenic, however, they are encountered in clinical specimens. All the species, including *M.bovis,* occurs commensal frequently on the skin and mucous membrane of upper respiratory tract.

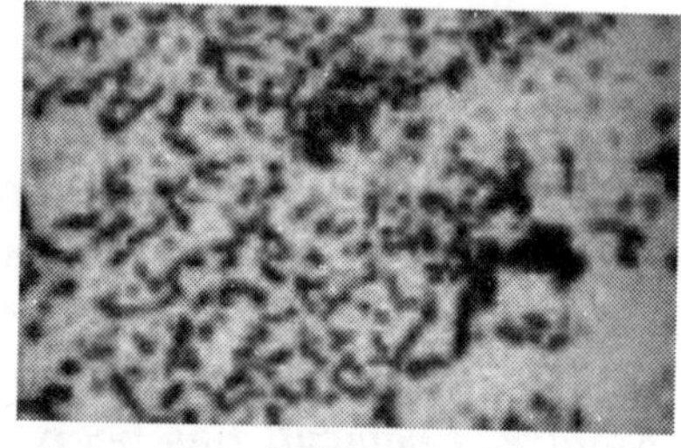

M.bovis

1BK is economically a very important disease throughout the world and spreads very rapidly among the herd. Cattle can carry *M.bovis* in eye, nasal cavity or vagina. Source of infection are usually the carrier animals. The disease is characterized by keratitis and conjunctivitis with purulent discharge. Photophobia, blepharospasm and profuse lacrimation are also seen. In several cases the cornea may perforate and become opaque followed by blindness. In some animals there is early regression of lesions. Complication characterized by corneal ulcer and meningitis is common. One or both the eyes are affected. Weight loss and declined milk yield are frequently noticed. *M.bovis* spread most commonly by flies but it can also spread by direct contact. It is most prevalent during summer and autumn in European countries and Americas and both young and adult cattle are susceptible. The prevalence with in the herd varies from year to year. The dry dusty environment and grazing in tall grass predisposes the animals to the infection. Other predisposing factors include prolonged exposure to sunlight, breed susceptibility vitamin A deficiency and concurrent viral infection, particularly the bovine rhinotracheitis virus. The disease is more severe when the calves are concurrently given a modified live infectious bovine rhinotracheitis virus vaccine. Mycoplasma and Ureaplasmal infection also predisposes the animal to the disease. Increased colonization of *M.bovis* in Mycoplasma boviculi infection has been observed.

M.bovis, stained smear

Following the infection, animals develop pilus specific antibodies that neutralize the haemolytic activity. These antibodies also inhibit the pilus mediated adherence of the cells. (Moore and Rutter 1989). Both systemic and local immune response develop. However, local cell mediated immunity is believed to provide protection against the disease.

Pathogenesis

Most of the virulent *M.bovis* strains posses the ability to produce an RTXlike haemolysin and polar pili (Pederson *et al.*, 1972; Punch and Slatter 1984). Virulent strains exhibit different plasmid profile than non-virulent strains (Brown *et al.*, 1998). The RTX operon is absent in non-haemolytic strains (Angelos *et al.*, 2003). Haemolysin is a heat labile, calcium dependent protein responsible for production of transmembrane pores in red blood cells (Clinkenbeard and Thiessen 1991). Haemolysin probably acts similar to siderophore, trapping the iron from lyzed red blood cells and supplying to the organism. Therefore the haemolysin contributes in the establishment of infection. Haemolysin also damages bovine neutrophil membrane but not human neutrophils (Hoien-Dalen *et al.*, 1990; Kagonyera *et al.*, 1989) the hemolysin also cause direct damage through the release of neutrophil granules into the tissues resulting in corneal damage through the action of collagenases and other proteolytic enzymes. Leukotoxicity for macrophages by haemolytic strains has been described. *M.bovis* cells and culture supernatant both are capable of killing bovine corneal epithelial cells *in vitro*.

In the eye, the haemolysin (Cytolysin) may be responsible for most of the pathological changes. A cytolysin-enriched vaccine has been reported to confer some protection in cattle against IBK (George *et al.*, 2005). This vaccine contained 4 protein ranging from 65 to 91 Kd and contaminated with endotoxin. Recent studies have shown that *M.bovis* may utilize host iron sources via iron-repressible outer membrane proteins and siderophores for growth.

Pili produced by *M.bovis* are classified as type 4 pili. The pili are thin with N-methylphenylalanine as the first amino acid and having a highly homologous hydrophobic N-terminal. The pilin protein possessed by different *M.bovis* are of different molecular weight and more than one type of pilin may be present on one strain. Pili on several isolates has been placed in 7 serogroups (A to G) (Moore and Lepper 1991). Piliated to non-piliated phase variation occurs due to inversion of the pilin encoding gene. It is the principal virulence factor of *M.bovis*. The loss of piliation renders the strain non virulent. Phenotypic characteristic associated with the piliated strains are autoagglutination, haemagglutination and formation of pellicle in broth cultures. Presence of pili is associated with the virulence of bacteria as non-piliated strains are of reduced virulence. Pili formation is soon lost after sub-culturing of the strain. Pili are responsible for the adherence of bacteria to bovine corneal and conjunctival epithelium followed by colonization of cells and production of disease. Pili also stimulate type specific protective immunity. Emergence of new *M.bovis* strains having serologically different pili often leads to the outbreak of disease.

Previous infection appears to confer a significant immunity which lasts through to the next season when further reinfection usually with minimal clinical disease, confers further immunity. Lacrimal secretions have high concentration IgA antibodies than IgG or IgM.

M.bovis organisms have a capsular polysaccharide characterized as unmodified chondroitin disaccharide repeat unit (Wilson *et al.*, 2005). It's contribution in pathogenicity of the organisms has not been worked out, however, it appears to confer resistance against phagocytosis as with other capsular bacteria.

The cell wall fractions of *M.bovis* possess a dermonecrotic activity, besides an exotoxin reported to be present in cell sap preparations (Pugh *et al.*, 1973). Lipopolysacharide may also contribute towards the pathogenicity. Hyaluronidase and collegenase produced by the organisms may also play a role in disease. Proteins that bind lactoferrin and transferring have been found and are probably involved with iron acquisition.

Several factors that contribute to development and spread of disease are animal breed due to degree of pigmentation of the eye of the breeds and the presence of number of flies. High number of flies, especially the face flies (Musca autumnalis) increases the chances of spread of the disease.

The disease begins with invasion of conjunctiva and cornea resulting in oedema and predominantly neutrophilic inflammation. Microscopic corneal erosions are present with in 12 hours of infection before the inflammatory response is visible suggesting that some exotoxin is responsible for this condition. Corneal opacity and vascularization may result followed by ulceration and rupture leading to uveal prolapse and panopthalmitis. The disease is self limiting but may take weeks to months to cure. The animal may loose weight as it is unable to forage due to blindness.

Laboratory Diagnosis

Luxurient growth appears on the blood or serum upon inoculation of eye discharges or swab. The organisms grow aerobically. The colonies are round, translucent and grayish white with size varying from 1 to 2 mm in diameter. A narrow zone of haemolysis is evident around the colonies.

Stained smears reveal gram-negative or gram-varriable coccobacilli usually occurring in pairs. Chain formation is rare. *M.bovis* is non-mobile, non-spore forming and encapsulated. Specific fluorescent antibody conjugates can be applied directly to suspect colonies on plates for identification.

Precise identification of the strains requires biochemical characterization. The organism does not ferment carbohydrates. Litmus milk becomes alkaline, nitrates are not reduced and indole is not formed. Proteolytic activity is demonstrated by gelatin liquefaction test.

A fluorescent antibody test is also used for rapid identification of the organisms in the tears and ocular discharges and from cultures.

Treatment and Control

Early acute cases respond well to treatment with ophthalmic solutions containing antibiotics such as furazolidone, oxytetracycline, ampicillin, gentamicin, kanamycin. Antibiotic can be injected sub conjunctivally. The aim of the systemic treatment is to achieve an effective concentration of antibiotics in tears. *M.bovis* is also susceptible to sulfonamides, erythromycin, Ceftiofur, tilmicosin and tylosin. Repeated treatment is required. Severe cases should be placed in a dark shelter out of direct sunlight. When corneal vascularization is extensive, the injection of a mixture of corticosteroid and antibiotic under the bulbar conjunctivae is recommended to promote healing. Recovery may require 3-4 weeks.

In a herd of 70 bull calves (4-5 months of age) kept on pasture, 56 (80%) animals showed, after natural infection with *Moraxella bovis* (*M. bovis*), typical clinical signs of infectious bovine keratoconjunctivitis (IBK)(Starke *et al.*, 2007). Eyes with epiphora, photophobia, blepharospasm and/or a corneal ulcer with a diameter of less than 5 mm were considered as moderately affected. Those with a corneal ulcer > 5 mm diameter and/or even more profound findings were considered as severely affected. The objective was to study in IBK affected calves in a prospective randomized case control study the therapeutic efficacy of intrapalpebral (i.p.) injections of oxytetracycline (OTC) (200 mg OTC-hydrochloride 10% in the upper eyelid of moderately affected and in both eyelids of severely affected eyes) and intramuscular (i.m.) treatment (long-acting OTC-dihydrate; 20 mg/kg body weight for both moderately and severely affected patients). 29 animals (20 moderately affected, 9 severely affected) were treated i.p. and 27 animals (19 moderately, 8 severely affected) were treated i.m.. For fly control, deltamethrin was applied to all bulls at d 0. The OTC-treatment was repeated at intervals of 3-8 d until recovery. All animals recovered within 42 days. The mean number of treatments per animal and the interval between diagnosis and assessment of healing were not affected by the method of OTC administration; the latter averaged out at about 10 d for moderately affected and 17 d for severely affected eyes. Significantly less medication was required per animal for i.p. than for i.m. treatments (moderately affected: 281 vs. 2033 mg; severely affected: 1156 vs. 3982 mg). In conclusion, both methods of OTC administration were found to be similarly effective for the treatment of IBK in calves.

Lane *et al.* (2006) evaluated the clinical efficacy of a single injection of tulathromycin, compared with saline (0.9% NaCl) solution-treated control calves, for treatment of induced infectious bovine keratoconjunctivitis in calves.30 Holstein bull calves ranging from 5 to 6 months old and 75 to 200 kg (165 to 440 lb) with no history of Moraxella bovis infections, no history of *M. bovis* vaccination, and negative results for *M. bovis* on 3 consecutive ocular bacterial cultures. Both eyes of each calf were infected with 1 X 10(10) colony-forming units of piliated *M. bovis* for 3 consecutive days prior to the trial. On day 0, ocular lesion scores were determined for each calf and the calves were weighed and assigned to a treatment (2.5 mg/kg [1.14 mg/lb] of body weight, SC) or control group according to a stratified random allocation based on weight and lesion score. Eyes were stained with fluorescein and photographed daily to record healing. Eyes were evaluated bacteriologically for *M. bovis* on days 0 to 6 and at 3-day intervals thereafter.Median time to ulcer resolution in calves treated with tulathromycin was 9.1 days. More than 50% of control calves still had ulcers at the end of the trial (21 days). *Moraxella* sp was isolated less often from the eyes of treated calves than from the control calves. By day 10, the treated calves had lower ocular lesion scores than control calves. In conclusion a single dose of tulathromycin (SC) was an effective treatment of calves with experimentally induced infectious bovine keratoconjunctivitis. The long serum half-life of tulathromycin, along with the results of this trial, suggests that tulathromycin may be a rational choice as a single-injection treatment for infectious bovine keratoconjunctivitis.

Eastman *et al.* (1998) determined whether combined parenteral and oral administration of oxytetracycline would ameliorate a herd outbreak of infectious bovine keratoconjunctivitis (IBK) and to compare efficacy of this regimen with that of subconjunctival administration of procaine penicillin G.Randomized field trial was designed. Using 119 Hereford calves in a herd undergoing a naturally occurring outbreak of IBK. Calves were randomly assigned to 1 of the following 3 groups: oxytetracycline treatment, procaine penicillin G treatment, and control. After initial treatment, calves were examined 3 times/wk for 7 weeks. The surface area of all corneal ulcers was measured during each examination. Ocular secretions were collected from all calves at least weekly and were tested for *Moraxella bovis*. Calves treated with oxytetracycline had a lower prevalence of IBK than did calves treated with procaine penicillin G or control calves and required fewer additional treatments than did calves treated with procaine penicillin G. Mean time for healing of corneal ulcers was significantly less for calves that received oxytetracycline or procaine penicillin G than for control calves. Calves treated with oxytetracycline developed fewer corneal ulcers and fewer recurrent ulcers than did calves in the other groups. *Moraxella bovis* was isolated less often from ocular secretions collected from calves in the oxytetracycline group than from calves in the other groups.Combined parenteral and oral administration of oxytetracycline appears to be an effective method of reducing severity of a herd outbreak of IBK and may be superior to treatment of affected animals with procaine penicillin G.

IBK is difficult to prevent considering its mode of spread. As soon as an animal is detected to be suffering with pink eye, it should be separated and treated with adequate antibiotics. Measures to reduce face flies and other insects should be adopted. This includes use of insecticides ear tags. Housing of animals in the shady areas is helpful in reducing the cases. Reducing other predisposing factor alongwith a close surveillance of animals is of considerable advantage. Carrier animals must be identified and removed from the herd (Brown *et al.,* 1998).

Immunoprophylaxis against 1BK involve use of a commercial bacterin comprising of killed whole cells of *M.bovis*. Repeated vaccinations are required for achieving satisfactory immunity. The immunity is not augmented by the addition of adjuvant in the vaccine. Ribosome vaccine and disrupted cells have failed to stimulate protective immunity. Live vaccine has induced some protection against challenge with the homologous strains but the immunity against heterologous strains has been weak.

Although it has been reported that the low efficacy of whole cell vaccines against IBK is mainly due to the difficulties in keeping the cellular piliation level of *M. bovis* during the growth of bacteria in stirred bioreactors, the problem has not yet been overcome because the mechanisms involved in the loss of piliation are still not fully clarified. In this work Prieto *et al*(2008) found that during the culture of *M. bovis* in liquid media, around 15% of the cells changed from piliated to non-piliated phenotypes at the end of the growth. Nevertheless, it was demonstrated that the main cause of cellular piliation loss in *M. bovis* growing in stirred and/or sparged bioreactors is due to shear forces, which are a function of the volumetric gassed power drawn [P(g)V(-1)]. Therefore, the authors tested here the use of bubble column bioreactors to protect *M. bovis* cell-bound pili from mechanical agitation damage effects.

These bioreactors operated at a superficial air velocity of 0.0065 m s(-1) yielded a cellular piliation level of 25%, in contrast to 1% obtained for stirred bioreactors. The addition of carboxymethylcellulose (CMC) at 0.10% [w v(-1)] to culture medium proved to be suitable to improve the final piliation level (65%). It was demonstrated by FT-IR spectroscopy and ELISA technique, that this chemical additive has a pili protective role interacting with the cells but without affecting pili antigenic properties.

Vaccines containing pilus antigens with or without corneal degrading enzymes antigen have shown the ability to protect against challenge with homologous strains of *M.bovis.* Administration of pilus vaccine into the sub-conjunctiva results in enhanced protection as compared with the systemic administration in calves (Pugh *et al.,* 1985). Antibodies that neutralize the pilus mediated adherence are pilus S-type specific (Lepper 1988). Following vaccination of animals with the pilus vaccine, the anti-pilus antibodies are detected in colostrum which provide passive immunity to new born calves. Pilus vaccines appears to be the most effective vaccine against pink eye in cattle, eliciting a high level of IgA secretary antibodies in the lacrimal fluid. Pili (fimbriae) were prepared from *Moraxella bovis* strain Dalton 2d (Dal2d) and from a derivative of *Pseudomonas aeruginosa* K/2PfS that contained a plasmid-borne Dal2d pilin gene and produced pili having serogroup-specific identity to Dal2d (Lepper *et al.,* 1993). Nine calves were vaccinated with two doses each of 30 micrograms authentic M. bovis Dal2d pili in oil adjuvant and 10 calves were vaccinated with a similar dose of P. aeruginosa-derived Dal2d pili in the same formulation. All 19 calves and 10 non-vaccinated controls were challenged by instillation of 1 x 10(9) virulent M. bovis Dal2d cells into both conjunctival sacs 19 days after the second vaccine dose. The serological response to vaccination and the degree of protection against experimentally induced infectious bovine keratoconjunctivitis (IBK) were assessed. None of the nine calves vaccinated with authentic M. bovis Dal2d pili developed IBK while two of those vaccinated with *P. aeruginosa*-derived Dal2d pili developed lesions which accounted for a mean group lesion score of 0.3. In contrast, 9 of the 10 non-vaccinated calves developed IBK lesions, the majority of which were progressive, required early treatment and accounted for a mean group lesion score of 1.5. These results demonstrate the potential of a relatively low dose of pili produced by recombinant DNA technology for development of an effective vaccine against IBK. Calves were vaccinated with cloned *Moraxella bovis* pili of serogroup C (experiment 1) or B (experiment 2) either as a monovalent formulation or as part of a multivalent preparation with pili of six other serogroups (Lepper *et al.,* 1995). Within 4 weeks of the second vaccine dose vaccinated calves and non-vaccinated controls were challenged via the ocular route with either virulent *M. bovis* strain Dal2d (serogroup C) or M. bovis strain 3WO7 (serogroup B) in experiments 1 and 2, respectively. Calves vaccinated with multivalent vaccines had significantly lower antibody titres than those vaccinated with monovalent preparations. Nevertheless, the levels of protection against infectious bovine keratoconjunctivitis (IBK) achieved with multivalent vaccines were 72% and 83% for the groups challenged with *M. bovis* strains of serogroups B and C, respectively. The serogroup C monovalent vaccine gave 100% protection against experimentally induced IBK and *M. bovis* isolates cultured from the eyes 6 days post-challenge were identified as belonging solely to serogroup C. Unexpectedly, only 25% protection was achieved against homologous strain challenge of calves that received the monovalent serogroup B vaccine. Furthermore, the majority of *M. bovis* isolates recovered from calves in this group belonged to serogroup C, as did half of those isolates cultured from the multivalent vaccinates. The remaining bacterial isolates from the latter group, together with all isolates from the non-vaccinated controls, belonged to serogroup B. Results are consistent with the hypothesis that derivatives of the serogroup B challenge inoculum had expressed serogroup C pilus antigen within 6 days of the challenge, possibly as a result of pilus gene inversion occurring in response to the presence of specific antibody in eye tissues and tears.

A successful vaccine containing all 7 antigenic types will prove most effective in preventing the disease. In order to further improve quality of vaccine, a recombinant pilin or pilin-*M.bovis* cytotoxin subunit vaccine has been developed and used as a ISCOM matrix adjuvant vaccine (Lepper *et al.*, *1993;* Angelos *et al.*, 2007a). Vaccinated animals exhibit high level of antibodies to pilin and cytotoxin. The use of pilin-cytotoxin proved superior to cytotoxin vaccine alone. Vaccine containing pilin alone was also effective . Although surface pili or cytolysins have been used for the development of vaccine, however, other virulence determinants that include protease fibrinolysin and phospholipases may be used. A phospholipase B from *M.bovis* was characterized by Farn *et al.* (2001) as a vaccine candidate. The gene for this protein encodes a protein of 616 amino acids with a MW of 65.8 kDa. The analysis of FT-IR spectra of piliated, nonpiliated and sheared Moraxella bovis cells, together with purified pili suspensions spectra, allowed the identification of 3 IR regions associated to spectroscopic markers of Type-IV pili: 1750-1600, 1450-1350 and 1280-950 cm(-1)(Bosch *et al.*, 2010). Such IR-specific markers were found for piliated cells grown in different culture systems (liquid or solid media), independently of the strain or pili serotype. They were also sensitive to pili expression levels. Therefore, on the basis of these specific spectral features, an FT-IR ANN-based model was developed to classify piliation levels in 5 distinct groups. An overall classification rate of almost

90% demonstrates the strong potential of the ANN system developed to monitor *M. bovis* cultures in vaccine production.

George *et al.* (2005) determined the immunogenicity of a *Moraxella bovis* cytolysin-enriched vaccine for prevention of infectious bovine keratoconjunctivitis (IBK).104 mixed-breed beef calves ranging between 4 and 8 months of age were usedVaccines were prepared by the diafiltration of broth culture supernatant from hemolytic *M. bovis* or sterile media. The diafiltered retentate was combined with Quil A adjuvant. Calves were randomly assigned to receive either the cytolysin vaccine (n = 35) or, as controls, adjuvant (35) or saline (0.9% NaCl) solution (34). Eyes of all calves were examined weekly for signs of IBK for 15 weeks. Calves that developed severe IBK were treated SC with florfenicol. Cytolysin vaccine contained 4 proteins with molecular masses ranging between 65 and 90 kd. Cytolysin-vaccinated calves had fewer instances of IBK than control calves. The time of onset of corneal lesions in cytolysin-vaccinated calves that developed IBK was delayed, compared with that of calves in either control group. The cytolysin-Quil A vaccine contained endotoxin, but calves did not have clinical signs of illness after vaccination. In conclusion calves that were vaccinated with a cytolysin-enriched vaccine had some resistance to IBK. Vaccines containing concentrated diafiltered *M. bovis* cytolysin could protect beef calves against IBK.

Other cell surface components such as outer membrane proteins should be studied as possible vaccine candidates (Mc Connel and House 2005). Kukuda *et al.* (2003) had earlier reported that a 79 kDa iron-repressible outer membrane protein of *M.bovis* as a possible vaccine candidate.

Parenterally administered immunogens used to prevent the disease do not offer complete protection possibly because they stimulate a poor ocular mucosal secretory response, in which locally secreted immunoglobulin-A (sIgA) is one of the main components. The principal aim of one study was to evaluate by an indirect enzyme linked immunosorbent assay (ELISA), the local ocular mucosal sIgA response against Mb purified pili, produced after intranasal inoculation of experimental vaccines (Zbrun *et al.*2011). Pili were adjuvanted by several different adjuvants (QuilA, Marcol Arlacel, Marcol Span, microencapsulated pili with PLGA polymers). Results were compared to sIgA response produced by adjuvant placebo inoculations and by IBK natural infection. Significantly higher anti-pili IgA response ($p<0.05$) was detected in calves vaccinated intranasally with pili QuilA and pili Marcol Span compared to control calves, although this specific immune response did not seem to be related to protection against Mb infection or typical IBK lesion development.

The efficacy of a recombinant Moraxella bovis cytotoxin subunit vaccine to prevent naturally occurring infectious bovine keratoconjunctivitis (IBK) was evaluated in a randomized, blinded, controlled field trial (Angelos *et al.*, 2004). Ninety-three cross bred beef calves were vaccinated with either saline, ISCOM matrix (adjuvant control), or a recombinant *M. bovis* cytotoxin carboxy terminus peptide plus ISCOM matrix and boostered 21 days later. Ocular examinations were performed once weekly for 20 weeks. At week 12, the cumulative proportion of calves with ulcerated eyes in the recombinant vaccine group was significantly lower than in the saline control group. Throughout the 20 week trial, the cumulative proportion of ulcerated calves remained lowest in the recombinant vaccine group. By week 7, nonulcerated calves in the recombinant vaccine group had significantly higher changes in serum neutralizing titers and cytotoxin specific to total IgG ratios in serum and tears as compared to calves in the control groups. The trend for a reduced cumulative proportion of IBK in the vaccinated calves over the 20 week trial suggests that a recombinant *M. bovis* cytotoxin vaccine may be beneficial in helping to prevent naturally occurring IBK.

To evaluate the efficacy of a recombinant Moraxella bovis pilin-M. bovis cytotoxin subunit vaccine to prevent naturally occurring infectious bovine keratoconjunctivitis (IBK; pinkeye), a randomized, blinded, controlled field trial was conducted in a herd of beef cattle (Angelos *et al.*, 2007). One hundred and one steers were vaccinated with ISCOM matrix (adjuvant control), recombinant M. bovis cytotoxin carboxy terminus+ISCOM matrix (MbxA), or recombinant *M. bovis* pilin-cytotoxin carboxy terminus+ISCOM matrix (pilin-MbxA); calves received secondary vaccinations 21 days later. Calves were examined once weekly for 18 weeks for the development of corneal ulcers associated with IBK. Overall, the pilin-MbxA vaccinated group had the lowest overall cumulative proportion of ulcerated calves. Calves that received MbxA, whether alone or with pilin had significantly higher M. bovis cytotoxin serum neutralizing titers as compared to control calves. Results of ocular cultures suggested that vaccination with an M. bovis antigen affected organism type isolated from an ulcer: *M. bovis* was cultured more often from the eyes of control calves than from the eyes of calves vaccinated with MbxA and pilin-MbxA. In addition, vaccination of calves with MbxA and pilin-MbxA resulted in a higher prevalence of *Moraxella bovoculi* sp. nov. in ocular cultures. While no significant difference was observed between a cytotoxin versus pilin+cytotoxin vaccine against IBK, the reduced cumulative proportion of IBK in the pilin-cytotoxin vaccinated calves suggests it may provide an advantage over a cytotoxin vaccine alone. Efficacy of an *M. bovis* vaccine may be reduced in herds where IBK is associated with *M. bovoculi* sp. nov.

References

Angelos, J.A., Bonifacio, R.G., Ball, L.M. and Hess, J.F. 2007a. Prevention of naturally occurring infectious bovine keratoconjunctivitis with a recombinant *Moraxella bovis* pilin-*Moraxella bovine* cytotoxin-ISCOM matrix adjuvanted vaccine. Vet. Microbiol. **125:** 274-283.

Angelos, J.A., Hess, J.F. and George, L.W. 2003. An RTX operon in hemolytic *Moraxella bovis* is absent from non-haemolytic strains. Vet. Microbiol. **92:** 363-377.

Angelos J.A., Hess J.F. and George L.W.2004.revention of naturally occurring infectious bovine keratoconjunctivitis with a recombinant *Moraxella bovis* cytotoxin-ISCOM matrix adjuvanted vaccine. Vaccine. **23:** 537-545.

Angelo, J.A., Spinks, P.Q., Ball, L.M. and George, L.W. 2007b. *Moraxella boviculi* sp. nov. isolated from calves with infectious bovine keratoconjunctivitis. Int. J. Syst. Evol. Microbiol. **57:** 789-795.

Bosch A., Prieto C., Serra D.O., Martina P., Stämmbler M., Naumann D., Schmitt J. and Yantorno O.2010.Type-IV pili spectroscopic markers: applications in the quantification of piliation levels in *Moraxella bovis* cells by a FT-IR ANN-based model. J Biophotonics. **3:** 522-533.

Brown, M.H., Brightman, A.H., Fenwich, B.W. and Rider, M.A. 1998. Infectious bovine keratoconjunctivitis: a review. J. Vet. Intern. Med. **12:** 259-266.

Chandler, R.L., Baptists, P.J.H.P. and Turfrey, B. 1979. Studies on the pathogenicity of *Moraxella bovis* in relation to infectious bovine kerato conjunctivitis. J. Comp. pathol. **89:** 441-448.

Clinkenbeard, K.D. and Thiessen, A.E. 1991. Mechanism of action of *Moraxella bovis* haemolysin. Infect Immun. **59:** 1148-1152.

Eastman T.G., George L.W., Hird D.W. and Thurmond M.C.1998.Combined parenteral and oral administration of oxytetracycline for control of infectious bovine keratoconjunctivitis. J. Am. Vet. Med. Assoc. **212:** 560-563.

Farn, J.L., Strugnell, R.A., Hoyne, P.A., Michalski, W.P. and Tennent, J.M. 2001. Molecular characterization of a secreted enzyme with phospholipase B activity from *Moraxella bovis*. J. Bacteriol. **183:** 6717-6720.

Galvão K.N. and Angelos J.A.2010.Ulcerative blepharitis and conjunctivitis in adult dairy cows and association with *Moraxella bovoculi*. Can. Vet. J. **51:** 400-402.

George, L.W., Borrowman, A.J. and Angelos, J.A. 2005. Effectiveness of a cytolysin-enriched vaccine for protection of cattle against infectious bovine keratoconjunctivitis. Am. J. Vet. Res. **66:** 136-142.

Hoien-Dalen, P.S., Rosenbusch, R.F. and Roth, J.A. 1990. Comparative characterization of the leukocidic and haemolytic activity of *Moraxella bovis*. Am. J. Vet. Res. **51:** 191-196.

Kagonyera, G.M., George, L. and Miller, M. 1989. Effects of *Moraxella bovis* and culture filtrates on ^{51}Cr-labeled bovine neutropils. Am. J. Vet. Res. **50:** 18-21.

Lane V.M., George L.W. and Cleaver D.M.2006.Efficacy of tulathromycin for treatment of cattle with acute ocular *Moraxella bovis* infections. J. Am. Vet. Med. Assoc. **229:** 557-561.

Kakuda, T., Oishi, D., Tsubaki, S. and Takai, S. 2003. Molecular cloning and characterization of a 79-kDa iron-repressible outer membrane protein of *Moraxella bovis* FEMS microbiol. Lett. **225:** 279-284.

Lepper, A.W. 1988. Vaccination against bovine keratoconjunctivitis: Protective efficacy and antibody response induced by pili of homologous and heterologous strains of *Moraxella bovis*. Aust. Vet. J. **65:** 310-316.

Lepper A.W., Atwell J.L., Lehrbach P.R., Schwartzkoff C.L., Egerton J.R. and Tennent J.M.1995.The protective efficacy of cloned *Moraxella bovis* pili in monovalent and multivalent vaccine formulations against experimentally induced infectious bovine keratoconjunctivitis (IBK). Vet. Microbiol. **45:** 129-138.

Lepper, A.W., Elleman, T.C., Hoyne, P.C., Lehrbach, P.R., Atwell, J.L., Schwartz koff, C.L., Egerton, J.R. and Tennent, J.M. 1993. A *Moraxella bovis* pili vaccine produced by recombinant DNA technology for the prevention of infectious bovine keratoconjunctivitis. Vet. Microbiol. **36:** 175-183.

McConnel, C.S. and House, J.K. 2005. Infectious bovine keratoconjunctivitis vaccine development. Aust. Vet. J. **83:** 506-510.

Moore, L.J. and Lepper, A.W.D. 1991. A unified serotyping scheme for *Moraxella bovis*. Vet. Microbiol. **29:** 75-83.

Moore, L.J. and Rutter, J.M. 1989. Attachment of *Moraxella bovis* to calf corneal cells and inhibition by antiserum. Aust. Vet. J. **66:** 39-42.

Pedersen, K.B., Froholm, L.O. and Bovre, K. 1972. Fimbriation and colony type of *Moraxella bovis* in relation to conjunctivae colonization and development of keratoconjunctivitis in cattle. Acta. Pathol. Microbiol. Scand (B). **80:** 911-918.

Prieto C.I., Bosch A., Zielinski G., Cúneo J. and Yantorno O.M.2008.Vaccine against infectious bovine keratoconjunctivitis: a new approach to optimize the production of highly piliated *Moraxella bovis* cells. Vaccine. **26:** 6542-6549.

Pugh, G.W., Hughes, D.E. and Schulz, V.D. 1973. The pathophysiological effect of *Moraxella bovis* toxins on cattle, mice and guinea pigs. Can. J. Comp. Med. **37:** 70-78.

Pugh, G.W., Kopecky, K.E. and McDonald, T.J. 1985. Infectious bovine kerato conjunctivitis: Sub conjunctival administration of a *Moraxella bovis* pilus preparation enhances immunogenicity. Am. J. Vet. Res. **46:** 811-815.

Punch, P.I. and Slatter D.H. 1984. Review of infectious bovine keratoconjunctivitis. Vet. Bull **54:** 193-207.

Starke A., Eule C., Meyer H., Im Winkel C., Verspohl J. and Rehage J.2007.Efficacy of intrapalpebral and intramuscular application of oxytetracycline in a natural outbreak of infectious bovine kertoconjunctivitis (IBK) in calves. Dtsch .Tierarztl. Wochenschr. **114:** 219-224.

Wilson, J.C., Hitchen, P.G., Frank, M., Peak, I.R., Collins, P.M., Morris, H.R., Dell, A. and Grice, I.D. 2005. Identification of a capsular polysaccharide from *Moraxella bovis*. Carbohydra. Res. **340:** 765-769.

Zbrun MV, Zielinski GC, Piscitelli HC, Descarga C, Urbani LA, Defain Tesoriero MV, Hermida L2011Evaluation of anti-*Moraxella bovis* pili immunoglobulin-A in tears following intranasal vaccination of cattle. Res Vet Sci. 2011 Jun 9. [http://www.ncbi.nlm.nih.gov/pubmed/21664636].

□□□

Chapter 19

Haemophilus

Dr. S.K. SRIVASTAVA
Former, Division of Bacteriology & Mycology
Indian Veterinary Research Institute, Izatnagar-243122
Bareilly (U.P.)

Haemophilus

Species of genus Haemophilus are small, pleomorphic, gram-negative rods. They are oxidase positive, non-motile and facultatively anaerobic bacteria. They require either X factor (hemin) or V factor (Nicotinamine adenine dinucleotide). The organisms are present as commensels on mucous membrane of genital, upper digestive and respiratory tract. The important species of Haemophilus from Veterinary disease point of are:

1. *Haemophilus parasuis* – Glasser's disease in swine; requires V factor.
2. *Haemophilus paragallinarum* – Infectious coryza in chicken; requires V factor but not X factor for growth.
3. *Haemophilus somnus* – Various infections in cattle and sheep; does not require X or V factor.
4. *Haemophilus haemoglobinophilus* – Cystitis and genital infections in dogs; requires X factor but not V factor for growth.

Other *Haemophilus* spp. of lower importance are as listed below :

1. *Haemophilus felis* – It is commensal of the nasopharynx of apparently normal cats. It requires CO_2 and V factor for growth.
2. *Haemophilus influenzae murium* – Causes cystitis and respiratory infections in mice. It requires X factor.

3. *Haemophilus paracuniculus* – Isolated from intestine of rabbits. It requires V factor.

Haemophilus spp. are readily killed by heat and die rapidly in culture and storage until freeze dried or stored at -70⁰C. Serotypes may differ in pathogenicity and geographical prevalence. There are variability in serotypes; 3 of *H.paragallinauim* and at least 15 of *H. parasuis*. In addition several non-virulent strains also occur which interfere in laboratory diagnosis of the disease.

Haemophilus parasuis

It is the causative agent of Glasser's disease (porcine polyserositis) in pigs. The organism has also been isolated from wild boars (Aragon *et al.*, 2010). The disease has world wide occurrence. Reports mainly have originated from Europe and America. Nasal swabs are examined to ascertain the status of the *Haemophilus* infection in pigs (Turni and Blackall 2010). The disease was first described by Glasser in 1910. Post mortem lesions seen in Glasser's disease may range from no gross observable lesions to large depositions of fibrin in joints and on any or all of the serosal surfaces of the body (Macinnes and Smart, 1993). The disease occurs as sporadic outbreaks usually in weanlings to 4 months old pigs exposed to various stresses. The onset is rapid and occurs within 2-7 days of the initiating stress. The case fatality rate is high if the cases are left untreated. A respiratory carrier state is believed to occur and stress leads to the occurrence of the disease. Piglets are most susceptible to the infection but are protected due to the presence of maternal antibodies.

Haemophilus parasuis is a common upper respiratory tract commensal that can be isolated from conventionally raised pigs of all ages. In these animals, it causes a sporadic stress-associated disease. In high health status herds, *H. parasuis* can also be associated with high morbidity and mortality rates in pigs of all ages. To date, 15 serovars have been described , but, depending on the geographic region and the typing method used, up to 25% of isolates may be nontypable.

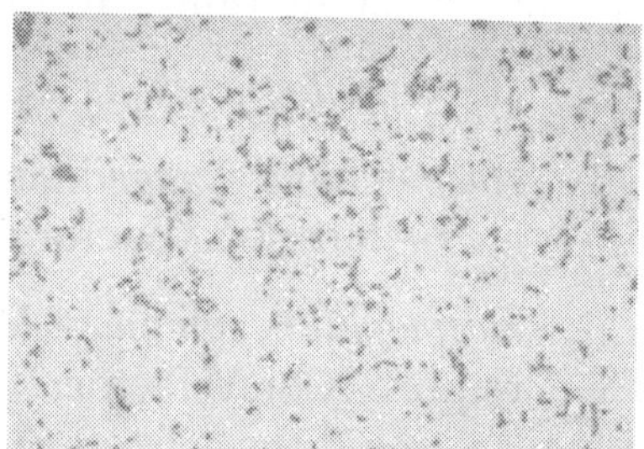

H.parasuis gram stained

From a limited number of challenge studies in pigs and guinea pigs, serovars 1, 5, 10, and 12 to 14 appear to be associated with a high virulence potential and serovars 2, 4, and 15 with intermediate virulence; serovars 3, 6 to 9, and 11 are reported to be avirulent. Consistent with these findings, Oliveira *et al* reported that serovars 1, 2, 5, 12 to 14, and nontypable isolates are the most frequently recovered from systemic sites, whereas serovar 3 and nontypable strains are present in the upper respiratory tract of healthy swine in the United States. Serovars 2, 4, 5, 12, 14, and nontypable *H. parasuis* disease isolates have also been reported in Australia, China, Japan, Germany, and Spain. That said, no clear correlation between virulence and serovar has been demonstrated, and by a variety of methods considerable genetic heterogeneity can be detected, not only between but also within serovars.

It is suggested that causative organism is common in most herds and the disease occurs only when pigs from an uninfected herd are introduced to a contaminated environment especially if exposed to a stress.

The disease is characterized by a sudden onset with a moderate to high fever, anorexia, dyspnoea meningitis and coughing. The joints are swollen and fluid swelling of the tendon sheathes may be clinically evident. Death occurs with in 2-5 days after the onset of the illness. Animals which have survived may develop chronic arthritis, pleuritis and obstruction due to peritoneal adhesion. The disease is most common in SPF pigs.

Since the variability in virulence is supported by serotyping and genotyping (particularly, multilocus sequence typing [MLST]), Aragon *et al* (2010) examined the relationship between the classification of 8 field strains by these methods and their capacity to cause disease in snatch-farrowed, colostrum-deprived piglets. The severity of clinical signs and lesions produced by the different strains correlated with the quantity of H. parasuis recovered from the lesions. However, the virulence of the strains in the animal model did not show a total correlation with their serovar or their classification by MLST. More studies are needed to identify a virulence marker that could substitute animal experimentation in H. parasuis. In addition, the authors reproduced disease in domestic pigs with a strain isolated from the nasal cavity of wild boars. This result indicates the existence of virulent strains of H. parasuis in wild suids, which could produce disease under appropriate circumstances, and suggests a possible source of infection for domestic pigs.

Pathogenesis

The virulence mechanism is largely unknown. To date, numerous attempts have been made to identify virulence factors or even virulence markers for virulent strains. Several putative virulence factors have been suggested, including fimbriae, neuraminidase, and transferrin-binding proteins, but, in the absence of genetic tools, their precise roles have yet to be confirmed. Furthermore, neuraminidase and likely fimbriae and the transferrinbinding proteins appear to be present in strains of all serovars of *H. parasuis*. Polyacrylamide gel electrophoresis profiles, particularly proteins of 36 to 38 kDa, have been suggested to be a marker for virulent strains, but, again, their role in virulence, if any, is unknown . The identification of genes that can be used to differentiate between harmless commensal *H. parasuis* strains and those with higher virulence potential is crucial for the effective management of Glasser's disease.

The bacteria probably adhere to the upper respiratory tract most probably through pili, the expression of which depends on the growth conditions. The spread is haematogenous although the invasive mechanism is not known. A total of 15 serovars were described by kielstein and Rapp-Gabrielson (1992), however, 26% of the 243 isolates studied were non-typable. There are evidence that serovars differ in their pathogenicity and accordingly pathogenesis also varies. However, there are conflicting reports on this hypothesis. Virulence factors include encapsulation, outer membrane protein profile and whole cell protein profile. Endotoxin, outer membrane lipopolysaccharide may be one of the virulence factor. Upon binding of LPS to protein in the host, release of some proinflammatory cytokines (IL-1 and TNF) is evident. Pigs dying of acute Glasser's disease show septicaemia, cyanosis and renal glomerular necrosis with microthrombi in other tissues (Peet *et al.*, 1983). The superoxide dismutase produced by *H.parasuis* might help from killing cells. Besides, the capsule is antiphagocytic. Virulent strains isolated from systemic diseases are more antiphagocytic than from healthy animals (Olvera *et al.*, 2009). Sack and Baltes (2009) identified a putative hemolysin operon in virulent strains but not in non-virulent strains of *H.parasuis* suggesting a role of haemolysin in virulence.

Haemophilus (H.) parasuis is best known as the cause of Glässer's disease, a potentially fatal polyserositis in pigs. The mechanisms underlying virulence differences on the molecular level are largely unknown to date. Sacks and Baltes (2009) have compared the serotype 5 (causes polyserositis) and 11 (described as avirulent) reference strains by modified representational difference analysis, and identified five potentially virulence associated factors present in the invasive serotype 5 strain, but not in the avirulent serotype 11 strain. Among these, a putative hemolysin operon, hhdBA, was identified, which is also present in half of the serotype reference strains described as virulent, but not in those reference strains that were reported to cause no disease in animal infection experiments. The presence of all identified genes was investigated in serotype reference strains as well as in 26 field isolates from clinically ill pigs.

Although *Haemophilus parasuis* is an important bacterial pathogen of swine, little is known about its pathogenesis or why some strains seem to be more virulent than others. Therefore, Hill *et al.* (2003) used differential display reverse transcription-polymerase chain reaction (DDRT-PCR) to search for virulence-associated genes in a pathogenic serotype 5 strain, *H. parasuis* 1185. Gene expression was evaluated following growth in conditions chosen to begin to approximate those found in the upper respiratory tract and those encountered by the organism during acute infection. Seven different differentially expressed gene fragments were identified in cells grown at 40 degrees C in both the presence and absence of swine serum. Based on the deduced amino acid sequences, the most strongly up-regulated genes were homologs of fadD (a fatty acyl-CoA synthetase), apaH (diadenosine tetraphosphatase), pstI (enzyme I of the phosphoenolpyruvate-protein phosphotransferase system), and cysK (cysteine synthetase). Homologs of Std (Na(+)- and Cl(-)-dependent ion transporter), HSPG (a mammalian basement membrane-specific heparin sulphate core protein precursor) and PntB (pyridine nucleotide transhydrogenase) were also up-regulated, but to a much lower extent. Sequences homologous to all of the differentially expressed genes were detected in the reference strains of all 15 *H. parasuis* serotypes.

Using differential-display reverse-transcriptase-mediated polymerase chain reaction, Metcalf and MacInnes (2007) found that homologues of genes encoding fructose bisphosphate aldolase (fba), adenylosuccinate synthetase (purA), 2',3'-cyclic nucleotide phosphodiesterase (cpdB), lipoprotein signal peptidase (lspA), pyrophosphate reductase (lytB), superoxide dismutase (sodC), tyrosyl t-RNA synthetase (tyrS), cysteine synthetase (cysK), an unknown protein, and a homologue of a hydrolase of the haloacid dehydrogenase superfamily were upregulated in response to iron restriction. In addition, the purA, cpdB, lspA, lytB, and sodC homologues, cDNAs homologous with a Na+/alanine symporter, fatty acid ligase (fadD), diadenosine tetraphosphatase (apaH), and an unknown protein were upregulated in response to CSF. In screening for the presence of these differentially expressed genes to assess their usefulness as diagnostic markers of high virulence potential, the authors detected homologues of all of these genes in all of the reference strains of the 15 established serovars. The hydrolase homologue, however, was expressed only in representative *H. parasuis* strains associated with a high virulence potential, suggesting that this enzyme may play a role in pathogenesis.

Haemophilus parasuis is a commensal bacterium in the swine upper respiratory tract, but virulent strains can invade host and cause Glässer's disease under certain conditions. In order to explore the virulence difference in *H. parasuis* strains, a virulent isolate, SH0165 (serotype 5), and an avirulent isolate, 7140 (serotype 4), were selected to investigate genetic differences by genomic subtraction. A total of 560 clones were screened by dot-blot and PCR, and 33 fragments present in SH0165 but absent from 7140 were identified. They encode eight gene categories, the sclB family, restriction modification system, phage products, transport system, outer membrane proteins, metabolism, and DNA synthesis and insertion sequences. We investigated the distribution of 21 fragments in 15 reference strains. Six fragments were more prevalent in virulent strains than avirulent strains based on statistical analysis; three fragments were SH0165-specific, and the remaining 12 were diversely distributed. Having analyzed these significantly differential fragments, including the sclB family, ABC-type transporter, fhuA and nhaC, it is presumed that these genes are associated with virulence in H. parasuis (Wang *et al.*2011).

As virulence factors are known to be regulated during disease, the objective of one study was to identify genes of a virulent serovar 5 strain with altered expression after iron restriction or in the presence of porcine cerebrospinal fluid (CSF), conditions that reflect *in-vivo* growth conditions. Using differential-display reverse-transcriptase-mediated polymerase chain reaction, we found that homologues of genes encoding fructose bisphosphate aldolase (fba), adenylosuccinate synthetase (purA), 2',3'-cyclic nucleotide phosphodiesterase (cpdB), lipoprotein signal peptidase (lspA), pyrophosphate reductase (lytB), superoxide dismutase (sodC), tyrosyl t-RNA synthetase (tyrS), cysteine synthetase (cysK), an unknown protein, and a homologue of a hydrolase of the haloacid dehydrogenase superfamily were upregulated in response to iron restriction. In addition, the purA, cpdB, lspA, lytB, and sodC homologues, cDNAs homologous with a Na+/alanine symporter, fatty acid ligase (fadD), diadenosine tetraphosphatase (apaH), and an unknown protein were upregulated in response to CSF. In screening for the presence of these differentially expressed genes to assess their usefulness as diagnostic markers of high virulence potential, we detected homologues of all of these genes in all of the reference strains of the 15 established serovars. The hydrolase homologue, however, was expressed only in representative *H. parasuis* strains associated with a high virulence potential, suggesting that this enzyme may play a role in pathogenesis.

Diagnosis

A total of 15 serovars of *H. parasuis* have been defined, and some strains are cannot be typed by serotyping. This serovar diversity and lack of extensive cross-reaction between serovars makes it difficult to diagnose and control *H. parasuis* infections. Several molecular methods, including PCR, in-situ hybridization, improved species specific PCR [1] and real-time PCR, have been developed for rapid detection of *H. parasuis*. In addition, some serological methods have also been developed for antibody detection after *H. parasuis* infection, including the indirect hemagglutination test (IHA), enzyme-linked immunoassay and the complement fixation test. However, a universal serological method for detecting this pathogen has not been developed to date. Despite the lack of extensive cross-reaction between serovars, weak cross-reactions were still observed between some strains with different serovars.

Clinical specimens are collected and streaked on blood agar with a staphylococcus streak for providing the V factor. Blood agar supplies hemin, if *Haemophilus* is X dependent. Chocolate agar provides X and V factors. Small dew drop colonies develop alongwith staphylococcal streak after 24-48 hours. Identification is based on morphological, biochemical and colonial characteristics and V factor requirement. Recently, genotyping methods have been developed with the goal of correlating genotype with the degree of virulence of *H.parasuis* strains (Olvera *et al.,* 2007).

Direct examination of the clinical specimen for gram-negative rods prior to the cultural examination may suggest *Haemophilus* infections. It is difficult to develop a universal serological method for detection of this pathogen. Guo *et al.*(2010) reported a universal plate-agglutination test for detecting H. parasuis. Diagnostic antisera were prepared by mixing antisera of serovars 4, 5, 12, 13 and 14 in the optimized ratio. The results of the plate-agglutination test showed that the diagnostic antisera could agglutinate with all 15 reference strains of *H. parasuis* and 74/75 clinical isolates. Further, the specificity of the method was validated with 22 bacterial strains from 12 related species.

Various forms of polymerase chain reactions have been standardized including RT-PCR for diagnosis of *H.parasuis* in pigs (Turni *et al.,* 2010). A PCR test for identification of *Haemophilus parasuis* was optimized using the 16S rDNA sequences of the 15 serotype reference strains of *H. parasuis* (Angen *et al.,* 2007). The test was evaluated on a collection of 218 Danish field isolates as well as on 81 representatives of 27 other species, including genetically affiliated species within Pasteurellaceae. In addition, DNA preparations from 56 H. parasuis isolates from North America were included. To obtain a test that was specific for *H. parasuis,* a multiplex PCR using 3 different primers was developed. The PCR test produced an amplicon of approximately 1090 bp only with representatives of *H. parasuis.* The test was further evaluated on 55 clinical samples from 16 Danish pigs suspected for being infected with *H. parasuis,* showing polyserositis or septicemia at autopsy as well as on 492 nasal swabs. The test was compared with the performance of a PCR test earlier published by Oliveira *et al.* [Oliveira, S., Galina, L., Pijoan, C., 2001. Development of a PCR test to diagnose Haemophilus parasuis infections. J. Vet. Diagn. Invest. 13, 495-501]. The sensitivity of the present PCR test was found to be slightly lower when applied on clinical samples from diseased pigs and 10-fold lower when tested on pure cultures of H. parasuis (5CFU and 0.5CFU/PCR reaction, respectively). Addition of 1.4 x 10(5) Escherichia coli to each PCR tube did not alter the sensitivity of the tests. No difference in sensitivity of the tests was observed when tested on purified DNA. On the other hand, the present PCR test was found to be 100% species specific for *H. parasuis,* in contrast to the PCR test of Oliveira *et al.,* which also tested positive for strains belonging to *A. indolicus, A. porcinus,* and *A. minor,* species commonly occurring in the upper respiratory tract. However, when the PCR test of Oliveira *et al.* is used on samples from systemic locations the chances for false positive results are apparently low. The present PCR test represents a rapid and reliable method for genetically based identification of *H. parasuis.* The high species specificity of the test makes it suitable for detection of *H. parasuis* in clinical samples, regardless of the presence of affiliated species and contaminating flora. As the two PCR tests differ in sensitivity and specificity, the use of both PCR tests for different purposes is a possibility.

Treatment and Control

Treatment with penicillin, trimethoprim-sulfadoxine ceftiofur, enrofloxacin or oxytetracycline is effective in the early stages of the disease. If possible, susceptibility testing should be carried out as many strains are resistant to several antibiotics. Avoidance of stress is important. *H. parasuis* isolates (n=112) from pigs were tested for antimicrobial susceptibility against 23 antimicrobial agents by the disk diffusion method(Xu *et al.*2011). All isolates were sensitive to Florfenico and most strains were sensitive to Cefotaxime (103/112; 92%), Ceftazidime (99/112; 88.4%), Chloramphenicol (90/112; 80.4%) and Gentamicin (85/112; 75.9%). High resistance levels to Nalidixic acid (84.8%), TMP (67.9%) and Trimethoprim+Sulfamethoxazole (58%) were observed. Genomic DNA extracted from 52 isolates resistant to at least seven antimicrobial agents was analyzed by PFGE and 46 distinct PFGE patterns identified. Diverse variation was observed between the drug-resistant H. parasuis isolates examined, suggesting that resistance traits were acquired independently by the respective isolates.

For control purpose prophylactic dosing at the time of shipping and medication of feed on drinking water on animal with a suitable drug may be of value. A formalin killed bacterin administered before weaning has proven highly effective. Several commercial bacterins contain more than one strain because of cross protection between selected strains of *H.parasuis.* Immunity is chiefly humoral.

The influence of age and maternal antibodies on the development and duration of postvaccinal antibody response against Glässer's disease were investigated 9 Pomorska *et al.,* 2011). Pigs born to immune (MDA-positive) and non-immune (MDA-negative) sows were vaccinated with inactivated vaccine. Vaccination was done according to three different protocols: at 1 and 4, at 2 and 5 or at 4 and 7 weeks of age. There were also two control groups for MDA-negative and MDA-positive pigs. The level of *Haemophilus parasuis* (Hps) specific antibodies were determined using commercial ELISA test. No serological responses were seen in any of the groups after the first vaccination. Maternally derived antibodies (MDA) against Hps were above the positive level until approximately 3 weeks of life in MDA-positive pigs. In those pigs the strongest postvaccinal humoral response was observed in piglets vaccinated at 4 and 7 weeks of age. In the remaining MDA-positive piglets only slight seroconversion was noted but levels of antibodies never exceeded values considered as positive. All MDA-negative pigs produced Hps-specific antibodies after the second vaccination. The results of the present study indicated that MDA may alter the development and duration of active postvaccinal antibody response. Age of pigs at the moment of vaccination was not associated with the significant differences in the magnitude of antibody response, however influenced the kinetics of decline of Hps-specific antibodies.

The outer membrane protein of *H.parasuis* serovar 5 has been demonstrated to be consisting of 15 proteins (Zhou *et al.*, 2009). The native transferring binding outer membrane protein of *H.parasuis* serovar 5 strain was used experimentally to assess its role in protecting pigs against the infection. Ability to protect strongly against challenge infection was demonstrated (Frandoloso *et al.*, 2010). In contrast the recombinant protein vaccine against death did not protect due to the challenge infection.

The recently completed genome sequence of *Haemophilus parasuis* strain SH0165 allowed the workers to screen putative OMPs for the development of recombinant vaccines. The objective of this study was to evaluate the immunogenicity and protective efficacy of three OMPs of *H. parasuis*. Three putative OMPs (SmpA, YgiW and FOG) were cloned, expressed and purified by Ni affinity chromatography using nitriloacetic acid resin. Mice were immunized either individually (individual protein, IP) or synergistically (synergistic protein, SP) with the recombinant proteins. A significant increase in IgG titer was detected in all protein-immunized mice. Isotyping studies revealed that the antibodies produced were predominantly IgG2a-type, indicating a predominant Th1 response. A significant increase was observed in IL-2, IL-4 and IFN-γ levels in the culture supernatants of splenocytes isolated from immunized mice. Furthermore, mice were challenged intraperitoneally with 6×10(9)CFU (5×LD(50)) of highly virulent homologous serovar 5 strain (SH0165) or 7.0×10(9)CFU (5×LD(50)) of the heterologous serovar 4 strain (MD0322) at fourteen days after the last immunization. All of the recombinant proteins enhanced survival and reduced histopathological lesions(Yuan *et al.*, 2011).

The lack of a vaccine against a broad spectrum of strains has limited the control of the disease. Recently, virulence associated trimeric autotransporters (VtaA) were described as antigenic proteins of *H. parasuis* (Olvera *et al.*, 2011). In this study 6 VtaA were produced as recombinant proteins and used to immunize snatch-farrowed, colostrum-deprived piglets. Immunized animals developed specific systemic and mucosal antibodies. The protective capacity of the anti-VtaA antibodies was evaluated by the inoculation of 3 × 10(8) or 6 × 10(6) colony forming units (CFU) of the highly virulent strain Nagasaki. Vaccinated animals had a delayed course of disease and 33 or 57%, respectively, of the animals survived the lethal challenge. The partial protection achieved with the recombinant VtaA supports their potential as candidates to be included in future vaccine formulations against *H. parasuis.*

Haemophilus (Avibacterium) paragallinarum

H.paragallinarum is the causative agent of infectious coryza. It is an acute, contagious upper respiratory tract infection and affects chicken of practically all ages. The sign include nasal discharge, swelling of sinuses, facial oedema and conjunctivitis. Air sac and lung involvement is also observed. Loss of productivity may cause considerable economic losses particularly at multi age farms. The disease appears in both acute and chronic form. The morbidity rate is high and the mortality rate low. It typically varies from 20% to 50% and 5-20%, respectively. Recovered chicken may shed the organisms for a long time. Apparently healthy carrier state also occurs. The bacterium is host specific and its survival in the environment is for a short duration only. The disease is world wide in occurrence. In India, the disease has been reported during 35 outbreaks which occurred in poultry in North India (Jaswinder Kaur *et al.*, 2004). Page (1962) described that 3 serogroups (I, II & III) are responsible for outbreaks in birds. Subsequently, Blackall *et al.* (1990) designated these serogroups as serogroups A, C, B, respectively and included 4 serovars to each of A and C. The serovars differs in their virulence for chickens (Soriano *et al.*, 2004). New variants of these serovars also occur (Blackall 1999). The bacterins should preferably contain the serovars likely to be encounterd.

The enterobacterial repetitive intergenic consensus polymerase chain reaction (ERIC-PCR) technique was used for fingerprinting of reference strains and Mexican isolates of *Haemophilus paragallinarum.* A total of nine ERIC patterns were given by the nine serovar reference strains of this bacteria. Two Modesto (C-2) reference strains from different sources showed the same ERIC pattern. Seventeen ERIC patterns were obtained among 29 Mexican isolates included in the study, belonging to serovars prevalent in Mexico (A-1, A-2, B-1, and C-2). Obtained results indicate that the ERIC-PCR technique could be used as a molecular laboratory tool for subtyping of *H. paragallinarum* (Soriano *et al.,* 2004).

Pathogenesis

Several virulence factors have been described. These include haemagglutinating antigen present on outer membrane protein required for colonization of the bacteria in the host. It is suggested that there occurs at least 3 haemagglutinins for adhesion during infection. Haemagglutinins are heat sensitive, trypsin sensitive and serovar specific. Barnard *et al.* (2008) demonstrated that this protein show similarities with other types of adhesions found in gram-negative bacterins. Transferrin binding protein production, as a result of growth of the organism in the iron deficient conditions, has been described (Ogunnariwo and Schryvers 1992), and has a role in virulence of the organisms.

The organisms also possess an antiphagocytic hyaluronic acid capsule. The endotoxin (LPS) is toxic and responsible for hydropericardium in chickens. Rivero-Garcia *et al.* (2005) reported that *H.paragallinarum* strains secrete a 100 kDa metallo protease into culture media lacking serum. The activity was inhibited by EDTA and inactivated by calcium. The secreted protein partially degrade chicken immunoglobulins G. It is postulated that this protein could play a role in the disease process in chickens.

It is suggested that *Haemophilus paragallinarum* requires at least three haemagglutinins for adhesion during infection. Barnard *et al.* (2008) reports the partial purification and characterization of the HA-L haemagglutinin from *H. paragallinarum* strain 46-C3, a heat sensitive, trypsin sensitive haemagglutinin that has been shown to be the serovar specific haemagglutinin in this organism. Using the pl and molecular mass obtained, it was shown that this protein shares similarities with other types of adhesins found in Gram-negative bacteria. The haemagglutination assay conditions were optimized at pH 7.5 at 37 degrees C. It was also shown that activity is enhanced by the addition of Ca2+ and Mn2+ ions.

The gene encoding a haemagglutinin of H. paragallinarum, hagA, has been identified and the full-length nucleotide sequence determined. An approximately 39 kDa protein, recognized by an anti-haemagglutinin monoclonal antibody, mAb4D, was purified from H. paragallinarum strain 0083 and the N-terminal sequence obtained(Hobb *et al.*2002). The full-length nucleotide sequence was obtained by inverse PCR and the deduced amino acid sequence of the protein encoded was shown to be similar to other outer-membrane proteins of closely related organisms in the HAP group (Haemophilus, Actinobacillus, Pasteurella), especially the P5 protein of

Haemophilus influenzae. The hagA gene was cloned into a His-tag expression vector and overexpressed in *Escherichia coli* strain M15(pREP4). The identity of the purified recombinant protein as a *H. paragallinarum* haemagglutinin was confirmed by haemagglutination of chicken red blood cells and reactivity, in a Western blot, with the monoclonal antibody specific for the serovar A haemagglutinin.

When *Avibacterium paragallinarum* reference strain 0083 (serovar A) was grown in an iron-restricted culture medium, the expression of the 60, 68 and 93 kDa outer membrane proteins increased as compared with normal media. Sera of chickens experimentally infected with *Av. paragallinarum* recognized these iron-restriction induced proteins, suggesting their expression in vivo. The three outer membrane proteins were identified as transferrin receptor and iron transport proteins by mass spectroscopy and a search in sequence databases. As these proteins have been reported to be regulated by the Fur protein in many bacteria, Abascal *et al.* (2009) investigated, through molecular methods, the presence of the fur gene in *Av. paragallinarum*. A candidate fur gene of *Av. paragallinarum* was amplified by polymerase chain reaction using complementary primers to conserved regions of fur gene sequences from members of the Pasteurellaceae family. The nucleotide sequence of the cloned gene, from ATG to TAA stop codon, was 453 base pairs in length and the deduced amino acid sequence showed 94% identity with Fur sequences of Actinobacillus pleuropneumoniae and Haemophilus ducreyi. The Av. paragallinarum deduced Fur protein (17.8 kDa) amino acid sequence contains the N-terminal helix-turn-helix DNA-binding domain and the two iron-binding sites in the C-terminal end, typical of other described Fur proteins. The study of iron-restriction-induced proteins and the mechanism regulating their expression could lead to an understanding of the responses of *Av. paragallinarum* to survive in an iron-restricted environment on host mucosal surfaces. *Haemophilus paragallinarum* secretes metalloproteases into different culture media lacking serum. Secreted proteins, concentrated by precipitation with 70% ammonium sulphate ((NH(4))(2)SO(4)) or methanol, displayed proteolytic activity at >100 kDa molecular mass in 10% polyacrylamide gels co-polymerized with porcine gelatin (0.1%). They were active in a broad pH range (4-9); pH 7.5 being the optimum. Protease activity was inhibited by 20 mmol EDTA/L and reactivated by calcium. The proteolytic activity was heat-stable at 40, 50, and 60 degrees C, but its activity diminished at 70 degrees C or higher. Secreted proteins partially degraded chicken immunoglobulin G (IgG) and cross-reacted with a polyclonal serum against a high molecular mass protease secreted by Actinobacillus pleuropneumoniae. Extracellular proteases could play a role in infectious coryza caused by *H. paragallinarum* (Rivero-Garcia *et al.,* 2005).

Diagnosis is based on bacteriological isolation of the organism as described for other *Haemophilus*. The organism is extremely fastidious requiring specific growth conditions for isolation. Serologically, agglutination, agar gel diffusion and haemagglutination inhibition tests are used for diagnosis. A PCR has been described for identifying DNA for diagnosing the disease (Blackall, 1999, Jaswinder Kaur 2004).

The application of a recently described PCR test for the detection of *Haemophilus paragallinarum* in China is described. The test was used to examine a total of 127 chickens sourced from a challenge trial (38 chickens), a respiratory disease-free experimental chicken farm (50 chickens) and eight farms with suspect infectious coryza (IC) outbreaks (39 chickens). The PCR results were compared with traditional culture (Chen *et al.*, 1998). The PCR detected 14/14 infected birds in the challenge trial as compared with 13/14 for culture. The 50 chickens from the disease-free experimental farm were all negative by both PCR and culture. PCR yielded 15/39 birds and 6/8 commercial farms positive as compared with 8/39 birds and 4/8 farms positive by culture. All farms positive by PCR had chickens showing the typical clinical signs of IC, indicating that culture failed to confirm coryza on two farms that had the typical clinical signs of the disease. Although chickens on two commercial farms were thought initially to be suffering from coryza, detailed clinical examination yielded no birds with typical clinical signs. The 12 chickens examined from these two farms were negative by both PCR and culture. The results suggest that the PCR test for *H. paragallinarum* is a suitable alternative to culture even under the typical field and laboratory conditions

The ability of blocking ELISAs and haemagglutination-inhibition (HI) tests to detect antibodies in sera from chickens challenged with either Avibacterium (*Haemophilus*) *paragallinarum* isolate Hp8 (serovar A) or H668 (serovar C) was compared. Serum samples were examined weekly over the 9 weeks following infection. The results showed that the positive rate of serovar A specific antibody in the B-ELISA remained at 100% from the second week to the ninth week. In chickens given the serovar C challenge, the highest positive rate of serovar C specific antibody in the B-ELISA appeared at the seventh week (60% positive) and was then followed by a rapid decrease. The B-ELISA gave significantly more positives at weeks 2, 3, 7, 8 and 9 post-infection for serovar A and at week 7 post-infection for serovar C. In qualitative terms, for both serovar A and serovar C infections, the HI tests gave a lower percentage of positive sera at all time points except at 9 weeks post-infection with serovar C. The highest positive rate for serovar A HI antibodies was 70% of sera at the fourth and fifth weeks post-infection. The highest rate of serovar C HI antibodies was 20% at the fifth and sixth weeks post-infection. The results have provided further evidence of the suitability of the serovar A and C B-ELISAs for the diagnosis of infectious coryza (Sun *et al.*, 2007).

Treatment and Control

The organism is susceptible to various antibiotics and can be used for treatment of affected cases. In one study, 18 *Avibacterium paragallinarum* isolates collected in Taiwan from 1990 to 2003 were serotyped and tested for resistance to antimicrobial agents (Hsu *et al.*2007). Serotyping revealed that 13 isolates were Page serovar A and 5 isolates were Page serovar C. More than 75% of the isolates were resistant to neomycin, streptomycin and erythromycin. The most common resistance pattern (15 isolates, 83.3%) was neomycin-streptomycin. Furthermore, 88.9% of the isolates were resistant to two or more antibiotics. About 72% of isolates contained plasmids (pYMH5 and/or pA14). Plasmid pYMH5 encoded functional streptomycin, sulfonamide, kanamycin and neomycin resistance genes and revealed significant homology to a broad host-range plasmid, pLS88. Plasmid pA14 encoded a putative MglA protein and RNase II, both of which might be associated with virulence. Furthermore, seven isolates showed haemocin activity. Plasmid pYMH5 is the first multidrug-resistance plasmid reported in *A. paragallinarum* and it may facilitate the spread of antibiotic-resistance genes between bacteria. The putative virulence plasmid pA14 and haemocin-like activity in *A. paragallinarum* indicate two possible mechanisms which might be responsible for the pathogenesis.

Bacterins are available for control of the disease. Bivalent and trivalent infectious coryza vaccines have proven to be useful in controlling the disease (Fernandez *et al.*, 2005).

Soriano *et al.* (2004) carried out cross protection studies in chicken vaccinated with one of the nine currently recognized Kume haemagglutinis serovars. The results confirmed that serogroups A, B and C represent 3 district immunovars. Within Kume serogroup A there was generally good cross protection among all 4 serovars, but with serogroup C there was a reduced level of cross-protection between some of the four serovars. Results suggested that the vaccine failures in some instances may be due to lack of cross protection between the vaccine strains and the field strains.

A study was carried out to test whether a commercially available coryza vaccine (Nobilis Coryza, Intervet International BV) could protect chickens against challenge with recent NAD-independent isolates. SPF chickens were vaccinated twice at 3 and 7 weeks of age and were challenged at 9 weeks of age with 5 different NAD-independent isolates of serotype A or C-3. The results after challenge show that the coryza vaccine induces good protection against challenge with the different South African NAD-independent isolates of *H. paragallinarum,* including serotype C-3(Jacobs and Van der Werf 2000). The protection and level of hemagglutination-inhibition (HI) antibodies conferred in infectious coryza bivalent- and trivalent-immunized chickens against *Avibacterium paragallinarum* field isolates of the prevalent serovars in Mexico (A-1, A-2, B-1, and C-2) were investigated. The bivalent bacterin (A-1 and C-1) conferred significant protection and increased HI antibodies against isolates of serovars A-1, A-2, and C-2, but not against a serovar B-1 isolate. The trivalent bacterin (A-1, B-1, and C-2) conferred protection and increased HI antibodies against all four of the isolates. The results confirmed that in poultry areas where serovar B-1 is prevalent, the inclusion of this serovar in bacterins is needed to confer protection against infectious coryza caused by *A. paragallinarum* isolates of serovar B-1 (Fernandez *et al.,* 2005).

A study was designed to assess and compare three different formulations of the new Onderstepoort infectious coryza (IC) quadrivalent vaccine, which contain an NAD-independent strain of Avibacterium paragallinarum (previously known as *Haemophilus paragallinarum*)(Dungu *et al.,* 2009), and a commercial IC vaccine, not containing an NAD-independent strain, for their safety and ability to protect chickens of varying ages against virulent challenges with four different serovars of *A. paragallinarum,* including the NAD-independent strain of the C-3 serovar. Four groups of 140 chickens each were vaccinated at the age of 17 weeks and revaccinated at the age of 19 weeks with each of the four vaccine formulations. A similar sized group of non-vaccinated chickens was used as control. Two rounds of challenge were conducted: a group of chicken in each vaccination group was challenged between 31 and 35 weeks of age, while another group was challenged between 51 and 55 weeks of age. The "in-contact" challenge model was used in this experiment. For each vaccination group, the four challenge strains representing four local serovars were used in each challenge round. The efficacy of the vaccines was compared based on overall protection levels obtained and the duration of protection. The safety of the different vaccines was determined by the severity of post-vaccination reactions. The need for the incorporation of the NAD-independent strain in the vaccine was evidenced by the low protection level against NAD-independent challenge recorded in the group of birds vaccinated with the commercial vaccine. The results obtained confirmed not only the variation in virulence of different South African serovars, with serovar C-3 being the most virulent and serovar B having almost no virulence but also the age related increase in susceptibility.

Inactivated vaccines of Avibacterium paragallinarum provide protection and reduce the economic losses caused by infectious coryza. However, inactivated bacterins provide protection only against the Page serovars included in the vaccine. Hsu *et al.* (2007) investigated the immunological properties of a functional recombinant haemagglutinin protein (rHagA) derived from a Taiwan isolate strain A9 as the immunogen for vaccination. The rHagA subunit vaccine protected 71% of immunized chickens against 10(10) colony-forming units (CFU) of viable A9. Vaccinated chickens which showed no clinical signs of coryza developed haemagglutination inhibition (HI) titers of 1:10 or greater. Haemagglutination (HA) of serovars A and C was not affected by the presence of rHagA specific antiserum. The HA of rHagA could only be induced against formaldehyde-fixed chicken red blood cells (FA-RBCs). These results suggested that HagA is a moderate immunogen and might not be a major haemagglutinin *in-vivo*. However, HagA might be involved in haemagglutination when treated serovar C aggregates fixed RBCs in vitro.

In one study, the disease profiles caused by the NAD-dependent isolates of H. paragallinarum in vaccinated chickens were studied (Bragg *et al*., 2005). It was shown that the clinical signs induced in the vaccinated chickens were substantially less severe than were those in unvaccinated chickens, as was expected. However, due to the high virulence of the serovar C-3 isolates, clinical signs in the vaccinated chickens challenged with this isolate were still detected. These were as severe as those occurring in unvaccinated chickens challenged with serovar B-1 isolates. Although the clinical signs induced in unvaccinated birds challenged with serovar A-1 were more severe than those occurring when vaccinated birds were challenged with serovar C-3, the overall disease profiles were similar. Substantial clinical signs were recorded in vaccinated birds challenged with serovar C-3. This could be interpreted as vaccination failure if the disease profile obtained in unvaccinated birds is not considered. It was found that a high level of protection was provided by this vaccine against challenge by serovar C-3. The high virulence of this serovar resulted in the development of clinical signs in vaccinated birds. These findings could possibly explain the large number of so-called vaccination failures that are reported in South Africa and elsewhere.

Haemophilus somnus (Histophilus somni)

H.somnus in cattle causes a variety of disease symptoms. The four principal syndromes that characterize the *H.somnus* disease complex are:

1. Respiratory involvement, characterized by fibrinopurulent broncho-pneumonia and septicaemia. Tracheitis may also be seen.
2. Thromboembolic meningoencephalitis resulting from vasculitis of meningeal vessels, death of the animal.
3. Fimbrinous pleuritis and arthritis.
4. Endometritis, Vulvovaginitis and cervicitis.

One or more syndrome may be seen in the same animal. Besides several other syndromes such as mastitis and abortions, conjunctivitis otitis, and myocardial and muscular necrosis may be observed. The organism has been isolated from udder secretions of cattle with naturally occurring mastitis. The disease usually occurs in feed lot cattle hence it is not of much importance to India. Young and unexposed animals are most susceptible to the infection. The morbidity of the nervous form of disease in a susceptible group of calves is low and average about 2% but may be up to 10% in some outbreaks. The mortality is high. The nervous form of disease occurs most commonly in feed lot cattle from 6 to 12 months of age. A septicaemia leading to thrombolic meningo encepthalitis and infarts in brain and cerebellum is very characteristic. The prencephalitic stage is marked by high fever. The disease complex most commonly encountered is characterized by pleuritis, pneumonia and myocardial infarction including myocarditis.

The neural and septicaemic form is usually fatal. *Haemophilus somnus* is also considered to be a cause of various forms of reproductive failures causing significant losses to the farmer. The organism has been isolated from semen of bulls used for artificial insemination resulting in disease in inseminated cows (Atyabi *et al.,* 2005). The organism can be isolated from the respiratory and reproductive tract of normal animals. Usually in association with other organisms such as *Pasteurella* spp. in bulls, the organism has been isolated from semen and preputial orifice, preputial cavity, urinary bladder, accessory sex glands and the preputial washings of steers. Consequently the organisms are present is urine. Most bulls harbour the infection in the prepuce. The organism has also been isolated from vagina, cervix, uterus and bladder of cows and may be the cause of vaginitis and cervicitis. The calves following respiratory infection become nasal carrier of the organisms. The method of transmission is presumed to be by contact with infective respiratory and reproductive secretions or by aerosol transmission.

H.somnus is an intracellular pathogen and posses several virulence factors. Howard *et al.* (2004) postulated that *H.somnus* significantly reduces the superoxide anion. (O_2^-) by bovine alveolar macrophages and PMN cells and this may be an important virulence factor. These virulence mechanisms have been characterized as adherence to the host epithelial cells and serum resistance. A heparin binding protein on the bacterial cells could serve as initial adhesin to sulfate proteoglycans on the endothelial cell surface (Behling-Kelly *et al.,* 2006). The organism posses an antiphagocytic exopolysaccharide (slime layer) and lepooligosaccharide (LOS) released in membrane fibrils and blebs which has been observed to trigger capsule activation and stimulate opoptosis in bovine endothelial cells. This effect is associated with the production of reactive oxygen and nitrogen intermediates and is amplified by platelets. Colonization of mucous membrane is the first step in development of the disease. Subsequently the organisms involve the circulatory system and cause septicaemia with localization in many tissues and organs. Marked leucopenia & neutropemia is also seen. This causes vasculitis, most probably due to the formation of immune complexes suggesting type III hyersensitivity. The common site of localization is the brain causing a thrombomeningoenphalitis. It is possible that previous exposure to *H.somnus* infection is necessary for typical brain lesions to develop. Several areas of necrosis marked with haemorrhages may occur. Localization in synoviae results in polysynovitis. Disseminated intravascular coagulation may be the feature as a result of immunopathological lesion caused due to the endotoxin. Animals dying of nervous symptoms usually do not show pneumonia without fibrin deposition. If pneumonia occurs as a result of entry of organisms through the upper respiratory tract it is characteristically sub acute or chronic in nature. The lesion in lung with pneumonia comprise of suppurative to necrotizing bronchiolitis. Laryngitis and polypoid tracheitis has also been seen in *H.somnus* infection. The LOS undergoes a phenomenon known as antigenic phase variation which is thought to aid in the ability of the bacterium to evade the host immune response. It is composed of 3 main components, endotoxin lipid A, an inner core and an outer core. The outer core is species specific. LOS is similar to LPS except that it does not contain component O antigen. LOS is less hydrophilic making it suitable for mucosal environment (Howard 1998). *H.somnus* produces an antibody binding protein which has a preference for binding IgG2 isotype in cattle. *H.somnus* also exherts toxicity for several bovine cells. Attachment or adherence of cells is prerequisite to colonization which in carrier animals does not produce any symptoms. The adherence of cells to vascular endothelial cells may lead to vasculitis and thromsosis. The lipopolysaccharide present on the outer surface may be the precipitating factor in this phenomenon.

H.somnus cells posses F c receptom on their surface and mediate binding to bovine cells through this structure. Four immunoglobulin binding proteins have been observed in *H.somnus*. Three of these are 350,270 and 120 kDa and strongly bind to bovine immunoglobulin G, IgA and IgM. A 41 kDa receptor bind these immunoglobulins. All 4 receptors are antigenic related and the 41 kDa receptor seem to be a subunit of the 350, 270 and 120kDa proteins. *H.somnus* also contains 2 bacterial transferring receptors (105 & 73 kDa in size) which contributes to its virulence by binding to bovine transferrin. Transferrin binding proteins are present on the surface of outer membrane protein (OMP) (Ogunnariwo *et al.*, 1990). Outer membrane protein genes and subsequent factors are also responsible for survival of the organism in the serum and the virulence of the cells (Cole *et al.*, 1992). The organisms also possess plasmid but their role in virulence is not known. Drug resistance plasmids have been demonstrated in *Haemophilus somnus*. One of the OMP considered to be important from pathogenicity point of view is a protective 40 kDa OMP (Corbeil *et al.*, 1991).

Diagnosis

Specimen are collected from various lesions and subjected to bacteriological isolation. Organisms can be recovered from semen samples and preputial washing of healthy bulls. For isolation, blood and yeast agar is used and the plates are incubated at 37ºC and 10% CO_2. It does not require X or V factor. Various biochemical tests are performed to identify the organism.

Treatment and Control

Antimicrobials such as oxytetracycline is usually effective. Other drugs of choice are penicillin G, ampicillin, colistin and novobiocin. In case of outbreaks mass medication of feed and water supplies may be indicated.

A killed bacterin containing whole bacteria in an aluminum hydroxide adjuvant is practiced in several countries. The vaccine is well immunogenic and protective. Serum antibody titers appear unrelated to the occurrence of infection.

The bacterin may also be used in face of an outbreak. New cases may be treated with suitable antibiotics. Vaccination failures may occur due to the infection if a serotype is not present in the vaccine. Circulating antibodies are protective. Role of cell mediated immunity is unknown.

References

Abascal E.N., Guerra A.C., Vázquez A.S., Tenorio V.R., Cruz C.V., Zenteno E., Contreras G.P., and Pacheco S.V.2009.Identification of iron-acquisition proteins of *Avibacterium paragallinarum*. Avian Pathol. **38:** 209-213.

Angen O., Oliveira S., Ahrens P., Svensmark B. and Leser T.D.2007.Development of an improved species specific PCR test for detection of *Haemophilus parasuis*. Vet. Microbiol. **119:** 266-276. Epub 2006 Nov 20.

Aragon, V., Cerdacuellar, M., Fraile, L., Mombarg, M., Nofrasias, M., Olvers, A., Sibila, M., Solanes, D. and Segales, J. 2010. Correlation between clino-pathological outcome and typing of *Haemophilus parasuis* field strains. Vet. Microbiol. **142:** 387-393.

Atyabi, N., Havarashti, P., Vojgani, M., Tajeek, P. and Vandyosefi, J. 2005. Antificial insemination encountered with *Haemophilus somnus* infection in cattle. Iranian J. Vet. Res. **6:** 62-65.

Barnard T.G., Van Heerden E., Bragg R.R. and Albertyn J.2008. *Haemophilus paragallinarum* haemagglutinin: role in adhesion, serotyping and pathogenicity. Onderstepoort J. Vet. Res. **75:** 11-16.

Behling-Kelly, E., Volnderheid, H., Kim, K.S., Corbeil, L.B. and Czupriynski, C.J. 2006. Roles of cellular activation and sulfated glycans in *Haemophilus somnus* adherence to bovine brain microvascular endothelial cells. Infect. Immun. **74:** 5311-5318.

Blackall, P.J. 1999. Infectious coryza: Overview of the disease and new diagnostic options. Clin. Microbiol. Rev. **12:** 627-632.

Blackall, P.J., Christensen, H., Beckenham, T., Blackall, L.L. and Bisgaard, M. 2005. Reclassification of *Pasteurella gallinarum*, *(Haemophilus) paragallinarum*, *Pasteurella avium* and *Pasteurella volantium* as *Avibacterium gallinarum* gen. nov., comb. Nov., *Avibacterium paragallinarum* comb. Nov., *Avibacterium avium*. Comb. Nov. and *Avibacterium volantium* comb. nov. Int. J. Syst. Evol. Microbiol. **55:** 353-362.

Bragg R.R.2005.Effects of differences in virulence of different serovars of *Haemophilus paragallinarum* on perceived vaccine efficacy. Onderstepoort J. Vet. Res. **72:** 1-6.

Chen X., Chen Q., Zhang P., Feng W. and Blackall P.J.1998.Evaluation of a PCR test for the detection of *Haemophilus paragallinarum* in China. Avian Pathol. **27:** 296-300.

Cole, S.P., Guiney, D.G. and Corbeil, L.B. 1992. Two linked genes for outer membrane protein are absent in four non-disease strains of *H.somnus*. Mol. Microbiol. **6:** 1895-1902.

Corbeil, L.B., Kania, S.A. and Gogolewski, R.P. 1991. Characterization of immuno dominant surface antigens of *Haemophilus somnus*. Infect. Immun. **59:** 4295-4301.

Czuprynski, C.J., Leite, F., Sylte, M., Kuckleburg, C., Schultz, R., Inzana, T., Behling-Kelly, E. and Corbeil, L. 2004. Complexities of the pathogenesis of *Mannheimia haemolytica* and *Haemophilus somnus* infections: challenges and potential opportunities for prevention. In proceedings of the 3rd Int. Vet. Vaccines and Diag. Conf., Univ. of Guelph, Canada 13-18 July, 2003.

Dungu B., Brett B., MacDonald R., Deville S., Dupuis L., Theron J. and Bragg R.R.2009.Study on the efficacy and safety of different antigens and oil formulations of infectious coryza vaccines containing an NAD-independent strain of *Avibacterium paragallinarum*. Onderstepoort J. Vet. Res. **76:** 299-309.

Fernendez, R.P., Collindress, H.L., Velasquez, Q.E., Soriano, V.E. and Blackall, P.J. 2005. Protection conferred by bivalent and trivalent infectious coryza bacterins against prevalent serovars of *Avibacterium (Haemophilus) paragallinarum* in Mexico. Avian Dis. **49:** 585-587.

Frandolvso, R., Martinez, S., Rodrignez-Ferri, E.F., Garcia-Iglesias, M.J., Perez-Martinez, C., Martinez Fernandez, B. and Gutierrez-Martin, C.B. 2010. Development and characterization of protective *Haemophilus parasuis* subunit vaccines, based on native proteins with affinity to porcine transferrin and their comparison with other subunit and commercial vaccines. Clin. Vaccine Immunol. [http://www.ncbi.nlm.nih.gov/pubmet/2026701].

Guo D., Tang C., Hai Q., Shao G. and Yue H.2010.Development of a universal plate-agglutination test for detecting *Haemophilus parasuis*. J. Vet. Sci. **11:** 355-357.

Hill C.E., Metcalf D.S. and MacInnes J.I.2003.A search for virulence genes of *Haemophilus parasuis* using differential display RT-PCR. Vet. Microbiol. **96:** 189-202.

Hsu Y.M., Shieh H.K., Chen W.H., Shiang J.H. and Chang P.C.2007.Immunogenicity and haemagglutination of recombinant *Avibacterium paragallinarum* HagA. Vet. Microbiol. **122:** 280-289. Epub 2007 Jan 23.

Hsu Y.M., Shieh H.K., Chen W.H., Sun T.Y. and Shiang J.H.2007.Antimicrobial susceptibility, plasmid profiles and haemocin activities of *Avibacterium paragallinarum* strains. Vet. Microbiol. **124:** 209-218.

Hobb R.I., Tseng H.J., Downes J.E., Terry T.D., Blackall P.J., Takagi M. and Jennings M.P.2002.Molecular analysis of a haemagglutinin of *Haemophilus paragallinarum*. Microbiology. **148:** 2171-2179.

Howard, M.D., Boone, J.H., Buechner-Maxwell, V., Schurig, G.G. and Inzana, T.J. 2004. Inhibition of bovine macrophages and poly-morphonuclear leukocytes superoxide anion production by *Haemophilus somnus*. Microbial. Pathogene. **37:** 263-271.

Howard, Michael, D. 1998. Antigenic characterization of *Haemophilus somnus* lipooligosaccharide. [http://scholar.lib.vt.edu/thesis/available/etc. 101398081516/unrestricted/etd.paf].

Jacobs A.A. and van der Werf J.2000.Efficacy of a commercially available coryza vaccine against challenge with recent South African NAD-independent isolates of *Haemophilus paragallinarum* in chickens. J. S. Afr. Vet. Assoc. **71:** 109-110.

Kaur, Jaswinder, Sharma, N.S., Gupta, Kuldip and Singh, A. 2004. Indian J. Anim. Sci. **74:** 462-465.

Kielstein, P. and Rapp-Gabrielsen, V.J. 1992. Designation of 15 serovars of *Haemophilus parasuis* on the basis of immunodiffusion using heat-stable antigen extracts. J. Clin. Microbiol. **30:** 315-320.

MacInnes, J.I. and Smart, N.L. 1993. *Actinobacillus* and *Haemophilus*: In pathogenesis of bacterial infections in animals. Ed. C.L. Gyles and C.O. Thoen pp. 188-200. Ames. IOWA State University Press, USA.

Metcalf D.S. and MacInnes J.I..2007.Differential expression of *Haemophilus parasuis* genes in response to iron restriction and cerebrospinal fluid. Can. J. Vet. Res. **71:** 181-188.

Ogunnariwo, J.A. and Schryvers, A.B. 1992. Correlation between the ability of *Haemophilus paragallinarum* to acquire ovo transferring bound iron and the expression of Ovo-transferrin-specific receptors. Avian Dis. **36:** 655-663.

Ogunnariwo, J.A., Cheng, C., Ford, J. and Schryner, A.B. 1990. Response of *Haemophilus somnus* to iron limitation: Expression and identification of bovine specific transferring receptor. Microb. Pathog. **9:** 397-406.

Olvera, A., Ballester, M., Nofrarias, M., Sibila, M. and Aragon, V. 2009. Differences in phagocytosis susceptibility in *Haemophilus parasuis* strains. Vet. Res. **40:** 24-28.

Olvera A., Pina S., Pérez-Simó M., Aragón V., Segalés J. and Bensaid A. 2011.Immunogenicity and protection against *Haemophilus parasuis* infection after vaccination with recombinant virulence associated trimeric autotransporters (VtaA). Vaccine. **29:** 2797-2802. Epub 2011 Feb 12.

Olvera, A., Segales, J. and Aragon, V. 2007. Update on the diagnosis of *Haemophis parasuis* infection in pigs and novel genotyping methods. Vet. J. **174:** 522-529.

Page, L.A. 1962. *Haemophilus* infections in chickens. Characteristics of 12 *Haemophilus* isolates recovered from diseased chickens. Am. J. Vet. Res. **23:** 85-95.

Peet, R.L., Fry, J., Lloyd, J., Henderson, J., Curran, J. and Moir, D. 1983. *Haemophilus parasuis* septicaemia in pigs. Aust. Vet. J. **60:** 187.

Pomorska-Mól M., Markowska-Daniel I., Rachubik J. and Pejsak Z.2011.Effect of maternal antibodies and pig age on the antibody response after vaccination against Glässers disease. Vet .Res. Commun. **35:** 337-343. Epub 2011 May 17.

Rivero-Garcia, P.C. Cruz, C.V., Alonso, P.S., Vaca, S. and Negrete-Abascal, E. 2005. *Haemophilus paragallinarum* secretes metalloproteases. Can. J. Microbiol. **51:** 893-896.

Sack, M. and Baltes, N. 2009. Identification of novel potential virulence associated factors in *Haemophilus parasuis*. Vet. Microbiol. **136:** 382-386.

Soriano, E.V., Longinos, G.M., Tellez, G., Fernendes, R.P., Suarez-Guemes, F. and Blackall, P.J. 2004. Cross protection study of the serovars of *Haemophilus paragallinarum* in the kume haemagglutinin scheme. Avian Pathol. **33:** 506-551.

Soriono, V.E., Langinos, G.M., Fernandez, R.P., Velasquez, Q.E., Ciprian, C.A., Salazar-Garcia, F. and Blackall, P.J. 2004. Virulence of the nine serovar reference strains of *Haemophilus paragallinarum*. Avian Dis. **48:** 886-889.

Sun H., Miao D., Zhang P., Gong Y., Blackall P.J.2007.A comparison of a blocking ELISA and a haemagglutination inhibition assay for the detection of antibodies to Avibacterium (*Haemophilus*) *paragallinarum* in sera from artificially infected chickens. Biologicals. **35:** 317-320. Epub 2007 Jul 26.

Turni, C. and Blackall, P.J. 2010. Serovar profiling of *Haemophilus parasuis* on Australian farms by sampling line pigs. Aust. Vet. J. **88:** 255-259.

Turni, C., Pyke, M. and Blackall, P.J. 2010. Validation of a real time PCR for *Haemophilus parasuis*. J. App. Microbiol. **108:** 1323-1331.

Wang X., Xu X., Zhang S., Guo F., Cai X. and Chen H.2011.Identification and analysis of potential virulence-associated genes in *Haemophilus parasuis* based on genomic subtraction. Microb. Pathog. **51:** 291-296.

Xu C., Zhang J., Zhao Z., Guo L., Zhang B., Feng S., Zhang L. and Liao M. 2011. Antimicrobial Susceptibility and PFGE Genotyping of *Haemophilus parasuis* Isolates from Pigs in South China (2008-2010). J. Vet. Med. Sci. 2011 Apr 4.[http://www.ncbi.nlm.nih.gov/pubmed/21467759].

Yuan F., Fu S., Hu J., Li J., Chang H., Hu L., Chen H., Tian Y. and Bei W.2011.Evaluation of recombinant proteins of *Haemophilus parasuis* strain SH0165 as vaccine candidates in a mouse model. Res. Vet .Sci. May 17[http://www.ncbi.nlm.nih.gov/pubmed/21596404].

Zhou, M., Guo, Y., Zhao, J., HuQ, Hu Y., Zhang, A., Chen, H. and Jin, M. 2009. Identification and characterization of novel immunogenic outer membrane proteins of *Haemophilus parasuis* serovar 5. Vaccine **27:** 5271-5277.

□□□

Chapter 20

Fusobacterium necrophorum

Dr. S.K. SRIVASTAVA
Former, Division of Bacteriology & Mycology
Indian Veterinary Research Institute, Izatnagar-243122
Bareilly (U.P.)

Fusobacterium necrophorum

F.necrophorum is an anaerobic, gram-negative bacillus with filamentous forms occurring occasionally. The species occurs world wide. The organisms usually reside as commensal in the alimentary tract and on mucous membranes. The organism has been divided into 4 biovars based on the haemagglutinating activity. The biovars are designated as A, B, AB and C. Biotypes A and B have been isolated from abscesses involving bovine liver and a variety of other infections. Biotype A is more virulent than biotype B. Biotype AB is rarely isolated from animals. Biotype C has been named as Fusobacterium pseudonecrophorum which has been recently changed to F.varium. Several bio variation from sheep have been described (Zhou *et al.,* 2010). The etiological agent is associated with a variety of necrotic purulent infections in animals and humans. Included are diseases of cattle such as liver abscesses and foot rot, which have economically important consequences for the cattle industry.

Based on several characteristic and DNA analysis biotype A and B are designated as subspecies necrophorum and funduliforme, respectively, of F.necrophorum (Shinjo *et al.,* 1991). These differ morphologically, biochemically and biologically. Subsp. necrophorum is more virulent than subsp. funduliforme, which is present in the alimentary tract as a part of commensal flora. Subspecies funduliforme is present in ruminal lesions. Subsp. necrophorum is usually found in pure cultures in the liver abscesses whereas funduliforme is present in mixed cultures.

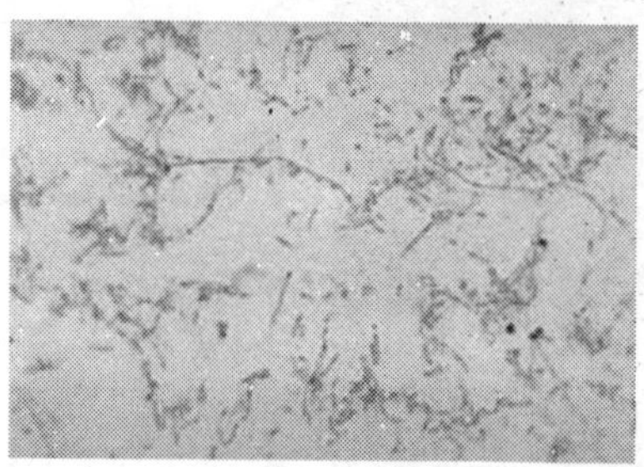

F.necrophorum gram stained

In cattle, *F.necrophorum* is associated with nitritis, cellulites, mastitis and calf diphtheria and is found in necrotic foci in necrotic larynsitis and foot rot. In calves it is also associated with stomatitis, enteritis and granulocytopenia *F.necrophorum* is also associated with papillomatous digital dermatitis in dairy cattle. *F. necrophorum* is the causal agent of hepatic abscesses, foot rot, necrotic laryngitis (calf diphtheria), and other necrotic lesions in cattle. Liver abscesses in feedlot cattle and foot rot in beef and dairy cattle are of significant economic importance to the cattle industry. Historically, *F. necrophorum* has been classified into four biotypes or biovars: A, B, AB, and C. Biotype C, now called *Fusobacterium pseudonecrophorum*, and biotype AB are rarely encountered in liver abscesses. Biotypes A and B, the most frequent types encountered in hepatic abscesses, have been assigned subspecies status: *F. necrophorum* subsp. necrophorum and *F. necrophorum* subsp. funduliforme, respectively. *F. necrophorum* subsp. necrophorum is more virulent, produces more leukotoxin and hemagglutinin, and is isolated more frequently from hepatic abscesses in cattle than *F. necrophorum* subsp. funduliforme. In a study, it was found that animals suffering with PDD had the presence of IgG antibodies in the serum against the organism suggesting that the antibody detection could be of diagnostic value (Moe *et al.*, 2010). It is the primary cause of liver abscess (necrobaccillosis) and foot rot. The disease is of greater importance in feeder cattle where it occurs secondarily to rumenitis. In these animals there is considerable financial loss due to condemnation of livers. In lambs, navel infection may occur at birth or through ruminal ulcers. Some of the common conditions in which Fusobacterium spp. are found as secondary invadors are navel ill and hepatic necrobacillosis in sheep and cattle and in pneumonia of calves. In necrobacillosis there is usually no lesions unless the abscesses are very large and result in acute or chronic illness. In acute cases there is fever, anorexia, depression, fall in milk production and weakness. The affected animals show arching of the back and reluctance to move or lie down. In chronic cases there are no localizing signs but anorexia, emaciation and intermittent diarrhea and constipation occur. A high leukocytosis with a marked neutrophils may be present with a large or multiple liver abscess. During the development of the abscesses blood level of sialic acid is elevated. Death is uncommon but may result if an abscess erodes through a portal vein and sudden shedding of the organisms in the body.

Liver abscesses in slaughtered beef cattle result from aggressive grain-feeding programs. The incidence, averaging from 12 to 32% in most feedlots, is influenced by a number of dietary and management factors. Liver abscesses represent a major economic liability to producers, packers, and ultimately consumers. Besides liver condemnation, economic impacts include reduced feed intake, reduced weight gain, decreased feed efficiency, and decreased carcass yield. *Fusobacterium necrophorum*, a member of the ruminal anaerobic bacterial flora, is the primary etiologic agent. Actinomyces pyogenes is the second most frequently isolated pathogen. Ruminal lesions resulting from acidosis generally are accepted as the predisposing factors for liver abscesses.

In cattle, infection is often associated with Arcanobacterium pyogenes and other anaerobes. It is of central importance in foot rot in cattle, sheep, goats and deer in which it causes disease in association with Dichelobacter nodosus. It is a normal inhabitant of rumen of cattle which adhere to ruminal wall and causes ruminitis.

Pathogenesis

F. necrophorum is a normal inhabitant of the gastrointestinal tracts of animals and humans. Virulence factors and pathogenic mechanisms that contribute to the transition of this otherwise commensal organism to a pathogen are poorly understood. A leukotoxin, endotoxin, hemolysin, hemagglutinin, and several enzymes such as DNase and proteases have been suggested as possible virulence factors. However, several studies implicate leukotoxin, a protein cytotoxic to ruminant polymorphonuclear cells, as the major virulence factor. The importance of leukotoxin as a virulence factor in F. necrophorum infections is indicated by a correlation between toxin production and ability to induce abscesses in laboratory animals (5), an inability of non-leukotoxin-producing strains to induce foot abscesses in cattle following intradermal inoculation , and a relationship between antileukotoxin antibody titers and protection against infection in experimental challenge studies.

Bacterial leukotoxins and cytotoxins generally have molecular masses of less than 200 kDa. This includes characterized leukotoxins of Mannheimia (Pasteurella) haemolytica (104,000 Da) , Staphylococcus aureus (38,000 and 32,000 Da), and Actinobacillus actinomycetemcomitans (114,000 Da) and other pore-forming toxins of gram-negative bacteria (103,000 to 198,000 Da). However, leukotoxin secreted by F. necrophorum was shown to be approximately 300 kDa in size based on Sephadex column purification and sodium dodecyl sulfate-polyacrylamide gel electrophoresis (SDS-PAGE) analyses.

The organism is in ruminal contents and adherent to the ruminal wall. Its role in ruminal fermentation is to metabolize lactic acid and degrade feed and epithelial proteins. The ruminal concentration is higher in grain-fed than forage-fed cattle. From the rumen, the organism gains entry into the portal circulation and is trapped in the liver to cause abscesses. The organism is an opportunistic pathogen and a primary causative agent of liver abscesses, an economically important disease of grain-fed cattle. Liver abscesses are often secondary to ruminal acidosis and rumenitis in grain-fed cattle. Two subspecies of *F. necrophorum*, subsp. necrophorum (biotype A) and subsp. funduliforme (biotype B), are recognized that can be differentiated based on morphological, biochemical, biological and molecular characteristics. The subsp. necrophorum is more virulent and is isolated more frequently from infections than the subsp. funduliforme. Several toxins or secreted products have been implicated as virulence factors. The major factors contributing to ruminal colonization and invasion into the liver are hemagglutinin, endotoxin and leukotoxin, of which leukotoxin is the protective antigen. In some conditions, the organism synergistically interacts with Arcanobacterium pyogenes, a facultative anaerobic organism and a secondary etiologic agent, to cause liver abscesses.Vascular damage from the primary or other lesions leads to localization of organisms in the liver and development of the lesions. The organisms invades and multiplies in the anaerobic environment provided by damaged tissues. It is frequently a secondary invader which grows at low Eh. Neutrophils are the predominant phagocytes in the lesions later on macrophages predominate. A 103 kDa dimeric protein leukotoxin (leukocidin) is responsible for ability of the microbes to resist the phagocytic activity of the neutrophils (Emery *et al.*, 1986) and is a major virulence factor. The leucocidin may be identical to haemolysin and posses phospholipase A activity. DNA sequencing and sequence assembly analysis has led to a 7.45 Kb sequence which include the putative hly gene of haemolysin (Miao *et al.*, 2010). The lukotoxin operon of *F.necrophorum* consists of 3 genes. The promoter regions of 2 subspecies of *F.necrophorum* differ in sequence, in length of the sequence between the upstream determinant and the first gene of the leukotoxin operon and in *E.coli* host cells (Zhang *et al.*, 2006). Okamoto *et al.* (2007) reported a collagenolytic cell wall components (CCWC) of *F.necrophorum* subsp. necrophorum damage the cell surface, forming tiny holes on the cell membranes deformation of hepatocellular vimetin. CCWC could be an important pathogenic factor in the development of hepatic. The bacteria·LPS is responsible for the endotoxic shock syndrome, although, in some instances the lesions are too small to produce clinical signs. *F.necrophorum* produces a variety of expacellular products eg. haemagglutinin, adhesins, PAF, Protease and DNAse. Their significance in disease process is not known. Haematogenous spread from hepatic lesions may result in multiple lesions in many organs and rapidly fetal termination. (Radostitis *et al.*, 1994) LPS is non-protective. Other surface characteristics of the organism (fimbriae, capsule) have been described in detail although the organism posses a pili.

Capsular strains of *F.necrophorum* are more virulent for mice than non-capsulated strains. Capsules induces abscess formation. Role of peptidoglycans is not known clearly.

The cell wall antigens of *F.necrophorum* possess some common antigens and circulating antibodies have no effect in immunity. Synergy occurs between facultative aerobic and anaerobic microorganisms. The facultative aerobic bacteria induces capsule formation, scavenges oxygen, curtail phagocytosis of the anaerobic bacteria. They also produce beta-lactamases which protect a penicillin sensitive obligate anaerobic partner.

The major virulence factor of this bacterium is leukotoxin, a secreted protein of high molecular weight active against leukocytes from ruminants. The screening of a genomic DNA library with polyclonal antisera raised against native affinity-purified leukotoxin and further extension of the sequence using inverse PCR led to the cloning of the entire leukotoxin gene. The leukotoxin gene open reading frame (ORF; lktA) consists of 9,726 bp and encodes a protein of 3,241 amino acids with an overall molecular weight of 335,956. The leukotoxin does not have sequence similarity with any other bacterial leukotoxin. Five truncated overlapping polypeptides covering the whole lktA ORF were used to immunize rabbits. In Western blot assays, polyclonal antisera raised against all five truncated polypeptides recognized affinity-purified leukotoxin from *F. necrophorum* culture supernatant in a Western blot assay. Antisera directed against two of the five polypeptides had neutralizing activity against the toxin. The entire leukotoxin ORF was expressed in Escherichia coli. Flow-cytometric analysis showed that the recombinant leukotoxin was active against bovine polymorphonuclear leukocytes and was inhibited with antiserum raised against the *F. necrophorum* leukotoxin. Southern blot hybridization analysis revealed different patterns of lktA hybridizing bands between isolates of the two subspecies of *F. necrophorum*. The gene encoding the leukotoxin (lktA) in *F. necrophorum* has been cloned, sequenced and expressed in *Escherichia coli*. Because of low expression levels, problems associated with purifying full-length recombinant protein, and of the physical instability of the protein, five overlapping leukotoxin gene truncations were constructed (Narayanan *et al.*2001). The recombinant polypeptides (BSBSE, SX, GAS, SH, and FINAL) were expressed in *E. coli* and purified by nickel-affinity chromatography. The objectives were to investigate the effectiveness of the purified truncated polypeptides to induce protective immunity in mice challenged with *F. necrophorum*. The polypeptides, individually or in combination, and inactivated native leukotoxin or culture supernatant of F. necrophorum were homogenized with an adjuvant and injected into mice on days 0 and 21. Blood samples were collected to measure serum anti-leukotoxin antibody titers on days 0, 21 and 42 and on day 42, mice were experimentally challenged with F. necrophorum. All polypeptides were immunogenic, with GAS polypeptide eliciting the least antibody response. Two polypeptides (BSBSE and SH) induced significant protection in mice against *F. necrophorum* infection. Protection was better than the full-length native leukotoxin or inactivated supernatant.The study demonstrated that the leukotoxin of *F. necrophorum* carries epitopes that induce protective immunity against experimental fusobacterial infection, thus providing further evidence to the importance of leukotoxin as a major virulence factor (Narayanan *et al.*2003).

Diagnosis

The organism is a strict anaerobe and grows best on enrichment medium. Thioglycolate broth is used for culturing pus. Various primary media are used; one with hemin and menodione, blood agar and selective media to suppress facultative anaerobes. Two to four days of incubation is required. Many strains produce L-form of initial isolation making it difficult to maintain colonies which are small, smooth, convex and whitish yellow in colour with a narrow zone of alpha or beta haemolysis. Pleomorphic rods are visible. The specimen include the lesions from liver and other organs and the organism can be recovered almost in pure form from the pus from bovine liver abscesses.

The clinical material may have a very pungent odour if anaerobes are present. Besides culturing a direct gram staining is attempted to demonstrate the organisms involved.

Colony morphology, pigmentation, fluorescence and antimicrobial susceptibility may indicate the genus involved. Biochemical test, gas liquid chromatography and DNA probes are used for identification. An ELISA has been described for diagnosis of cattle foot rot using leukotoxin protein as the antigen (Guo *et al.*, 2010). In this report serodiagnostic ELISA (rL-ELISA) using recombinant truncated leukotoxin protein PL2 (aa 311-644) of *Fusobacterium necrophorum* as antigen was developed for detection of antibodies against *F. necrophorum* from cattle footrot. In rL-ELISA, the recombinant diagnostic antigen showed no cross-reaction with antisera against bovine foot and mouth disease virus, bovine rhinotracheitis virus, bovine viral diarrhea virus, bovine rotavirus type A, bovine *Escherichia coli*, and bovine Salmonella. The rL-ELISA could confirm the existence of antibodies against *F. necrophorum* at day 7 after infection. Detection of the field samples indicated relative sensitivity of rL-ELISA to nL-ELISA using the purified native leukotoxin A as antigen was 96.43%, and relative specificity of rL-ELISA to nL-ELISA was 94.26%. These data demonstrated the rL-ELISA would have a potential use for early diagnosis of cattle footrot caused by *F. necrophorum.*

An enzyme-linked-immunosorbent assay (ELISA) with HCl heat-extracted antigen of *Fusobacterium necrophorum* was conducted to detect specific immunoglobulins G and M in infected cattle. The ELISA revealed an increase (> 0.40) in specific IgG in most of the animals with hepatic abscesses but not that in specific IgM. All the lesions were positive for *F. necrophorum*. These findings indicated that the ELISA for immunoglobulin G detection may prove to be a useful tool for predictive serodiagnosis of F. necrophorum infection in cattle (Kanoe *et al.*, 1996).

Differences in biological activities (hemagglutination, hemolytic, leukotoxic, and virulence) and ribotypes between the two subspecies of Fusobacterium necrophorum of bovine ruminal and liver abscess origins were investigated (Okwumabua *et al.*1996). Hemagglutination activity was present in all hepatic, but only some ruminal, strains of Fusobacterium necrophorum subsp. necrophorum. Ruminal *F. necrophorum* subsp. necrophorum had low leukotoxin titers yet was virulent in mice. *Fusobacterium necrophorum* subsp. funduliforme of hepatic or ruminal origin had no hemagglutination activity, had low hemolytic and leukotoxic activities, and was less virulent to mice. For ribotyping, chromosomal DNAs of 10 *F. necrophorum* subsp. necrophorum and 11 F. necrophorum subsp. funduliforme isolates were digested with restriction endonucleases (EcoRI, EcoRV, SalI, PstI, and HaeIII) and examined by restriction fragment length polymorphisms after hybridizing with a digoxigenin-labeled cDNA probe transcribed from a mixture of 16 and 23S rRNAs from *Escherichia coli*. The most discriminating restriction endonuclease enzyme for ribotyping was EcoRI. The presence or absence of two distinct bands of 2.6 and 4.3 kb differentiated the two subspecies. Regardless of the origin, only *F. necrophorum* subsp. necrophorum, a virulent subspecies, had a ca. 2.6-kb band, whereas *F. necrophorum* subsp. funduliforme, a less virulent subspecies, had a ca. 4.3-kb band. Ribotyping appears to be a useful technique to genetically differentiate the two subspecies of F. necrophorum.

Treatment and Control

Common antibiotics used are penicillin, chloramphenicol, tetracycline, metronidazole and clindamycin. Trimethoprim-sulfonamides are of unpredicable utility due to the presence of thymidine in necrotic materials. The obligate anaerobes are resistant to all the aminoglycosides.

Hepatic abscesses in feedlot cattle can be reduced by the feeding of a low proportion of grain in the ration. Feeding chlortetracycline throughout the fattening period may reduce the number of hepatic abscesses. Feeding tylosin daily to young cattle can also reduce the occurrence of liver abscesses and improve weight gain and feed conversion. In sheep the disease can be controlled by navel disinfection and proper hygiene.

A toxoid provide a satisfactory immunity among young cattle. The serum antileukotoxin antibody response and protection against subsequent experimental challenge with *Fusobacterium necrophorum* were investigated in 30 steers vaccinated with crude *F. necrophorum* leukotoxoid (Saginala *et al.* 1996). Culture supernatant of *F. necrophorum*, strain 25, containing leukotoxoid was concentrated. The steers were assigned randomly to six groups (n = 5): PBS control with Stimulon adjuvant; vaccinated with concentrated supernatant diluted to provide 2.5, 5.0, 10.0, or 20.0 ml with the water-soluble Stimulon adjuvant; and 5.0 ml with the Ribi oil-emulsion adjuvant. The steers were injected subcutaneously on days 0 and 21. Blood samples were collected at weekly intervals to monitor serum antileukotoxin antibody titres. On day 42, all the steers were challenged intraportally with *F. necrophorum* culture. Three weeks later (day 63), the steers were killed and necropsied for examination of their livers and assessment of protection. Steers vaccinated with crude leukotoxoid tended to have higher antileukotoxin titres than the controls, but the difference was not significant. Also, the antibody titre did not appear to be dose-dependent. In the control group, 3 out of 5 steers developed liver abscesses. The incidence of liver abscesses in steers vaccinated with Stimulon adjuvant was not dose related; however, only 8 of the 25 vaccinated steers developed abscesses. None of the steers vaccinated with the 5.0 ml dose with Ribi had any abscesses. Evidence for a relationship between antileukotoxin antibody and protection was shown by the lower titre in those steers that developed abscesses compared to those that did not. It was concluded that antileukotoxin antibody titres probably provided some degree of protection against experimentally induced liver abscesses, but further dose-titration studies using Ribi or possibly another more effective adjuvant will be needed to confirm this.

The efficacy and the optimum dose of *Fusobacterium necrophorum* crude leukotoxoid vaccine required to immunize and protect steers against experimentally induced liver abscesses were evaluated(Saginala *et al.*1997). The vaccine consisted of cell-free culture supernatant of a high leukotoxin-producing strain of *F. necrophorum*, inactivated with formalin and homogenized with an adjuvant. Twenty-five steers were assigned randomly to the following five treatment groups: control; three doses (1.0, 2.0, and 5.0 mL) of the culture supernatant; and 2.25 mL of the concentrated supernatant (equivalent to 5 mL of the original supernatant). Vaccine was injected subcutaneously on d 0 and 21. Blood samples were collected weekly to monitor antileukotoxin antibody titers. Three weeks after the second vaccination (d 42), all steers were injected intraportally with *F. necrophorum* culture to induce liver abscesses. Three weeks later (d 63), steers were euthanatized and necropsied; livers were examined and protection assessed. Antileukotoxin antibody titers in the control steers generally did not differ from the baseline (wk 0) titers. The titers in the vaccinated groups increased, more so after the second injection, and the increase was generally dose-dependent. Necropsy examination revealed that all steers in the control group had abscesses in the liver. In the vaccinated groups, two of five steers in the 1.0-mL group and one each in the 2.0-, 5.0-, and 2.25-mL (concentrated) groups had liver abscesses. Antileukotoxin antibody titers were higher ($P < .05$) in steers that did not develop abscesses than in steers that developed abscesses. The difference suggested a protective effect of antileukotoxin antibodies against experimentally induced liver abscesses.Recombinant leukotoxin when injected in mice have proven to provide immunity against challenge infection (Narayanan *et al.*, 2003). Bacterins and other cytoplasmic components are immunogens but none have provided protective immunity (Tan *et al.*, 1996).

References

Emery, D.L., Edwards, R.D. and Rathel, J.S. 1986. Studies on the purification of leucocidin of *Fusobacterium necrophorum* and its neutralization by specific antisera. Vet. Microbiol. **11:** 357-372.

Guo, D.H., Sun, D.B., Wu, R., Yang, H.M., Zhang, J.S., Fan, C.L., Sun, B. and Wang, J.F. 2010. An indirect ELISA for serodiagnosis of cattle foot rot caused by *Fusobacterium necrophorum*. Anaerobe. **16:** 317-320.

Kanoe M., Hirabayashi T., Matsuoka Y., Inoue M., Uraoka Y., Taguchi S. and Motoyoshi S.1996.Use of enzyme-linked-immunosorbent assay for detection of IgG and IgM antibodies to *Fusobacterium necrophorum* in cattle. Microbios. **87:** 257-262.

Miao, L., Liu, Y. Li, Q., Wang, Z., Li, H. and Zheng, G. 2010. Screening and sequence analysis of hemolysin gene of *Fusobacterium necrophorum*. Anaerobe. **16:** 402-404.

Moe, K.K., Yan, T., Misumi, K., Kubota, C., Nibe, K., Yamazaki, W., Muruguma, M. and Misawa, N. 2010. Detection of antibodies against *Fusobacterium necrophorum* and Porphyromonas levii- like species in dairy cattle with papillomatous digital dermatitis. Microbiol. Immunol. **54:** 338-346.

Narayanan, S.K., Chengappa, M.M., Stewart, G.C. and Nagaraja, T.G. 2003. Immunogenicity and protective effects of truncated recombinant leukotoxin proteins of *Fusobacterium necrophorum* in mice. Vet. Microbiol. **93:** 335-347.

Narayanan S.K., Nagaraja T.G., Chengappa M.M. and Stewart G.C.2001.Cloning, sequencing, and expression of the leukotoxin gene from *Fusobacterium necrophorum*. Infect. Immun. **69:** 5447-5455.

Okamoto, K., Kanoe, M., Yaguchi, Y., Watanabe, T. and Inoue, T. 2007. Effects of the colleagenotytic cell wall components of *Fusobacterium necrophorum* subsp. necrophorum on bovine hepatocytes. Res. Vet. Sci. **82:** 166-168.

Okwumabua O., Tan Z., Staats J., Oberst R.D., Chengappa M.M. and Nagaraja T.G.1996Ribotyping to differentiate *Fusobacterium necrophorum* subsp. *necrophorum* and *F. necrophorum* subsp. funduliforme isolated from bovine ruminal contents and liver abscesses. Appl. Environ. Microbiol. **62:** 469-472.

Radostitis, O.M., Blood, D.C. and Gay, C.C. 1994. Veterinary Medicine. A text book of the disease of cattle, sheep, pigs, goats and horses. Bailliere Tindall; The bath Press, Avon, Great Britain.

Saginala S., Nagaraja T.G., Lechtenberg K.F., Chengappa M.M., Kemp K.E. and Hine P.M.1997.Effect of *Fusobacterium necrophorum* leukotoxoid vaccine on susceptibility to experimentally induced liver abscesses in cattle. J. Anim. Sci. **75:** 1160-1166.

Saginala S., Nagaraja T.G., Tan Z.L., Lechtenberg K.F., Chengappa M.M. and Hine P.M..1996.The serum neutralizing antibody response in cattle to *Fusobacterium necrophorum* leukotoxoid and possible protection against experimentally induced hepatic abscesses. Vet. Res. Commun. **20:** 493-504.

Shinjo, T., Fujisawa, T. and Mitsuoka, T. 1991. Proposal of two subspecies of Fusobacterium necrophorum (Flugge) Moore and Hobleman: *Fusobacterium necrophorum* subsp. *necrophorum* subsp. nov. nom. Rev. (ex Flugge 1886) and Fusobacterium necrophorum subsp. funduliforme subsp. nov., nom. Rev (ex Halle 1898). Int. J. Syst. Bacteriol. **41:** 395-397.

Tan, Z.L., Nagaraja, T.G. and Chengappa, M.M. 1996. Fusobacterium necrophorum infections: virulence factors, pathogenic mechanisms and control measures. Vet. Res. Commun. **20:** 173-140.

Zhang, F., Nagaraja, T.G., George, D. and Stewart, G.C. 2006. The two major subspecies of *Fusobacterium necrophorum* have distinct leukotoxin operon promoter regions. Vet. Microbiol. **112:** 73-78.

Zhou, H., Bennett, G., Buller, N. and Hickford, J.G. 2010. Isolation of two novel *Fusobacterium necrophorum* variants from sheep in Australia. Vet. Microbiol. [http://www.ncbi.nlm.nih.gov/pubmed/20869818].

□□□

Chapter 21

Pathogenic Actinomycetes (Nacardia and Actinomyces)

Dr. S.K. SRIVASTAVA
Former, Division of Bacteriology & Mycology
Indian Veterinary Research Institute, Izatnagar-243122
Bareilly (U.P.)

Pathogenic Actinomycetes (Nocardia and Actinomyces)

Actinomycetes are gram positive bacteria showing branching filaments when grown *in vitro*. Both the genera resemble in their pathogenicity pattern. However, there are some differential characteristics as shown in the table below:

Characteristics	**Actinomyces**	**Nocardia**
Source	Endogenous	Exogenous
Gaseous requirement	Anaerobic/micoraero philic	Aerobic
Catalase	- or +	+
Acid fastness	-	+
Penicillin	Susceptible	Resistant except *N.nova*
Lymphnode involvement	Rare	Common
Sulfur granules	Common	Rare
Growth on sabouraud's Agar	-	+
Mycolic acid* in cell wall	-	+

* Nocardiomycolic Acid

Nocardia is present in most of the environmental conditions. It has 3 main species.

N. asteroids	-	Infects domestic animals and human
N. brasiliensis	-	Infect humans
N. otididiscaviarum	-	Infects the guinea pigs and human and causes bovine mastitis

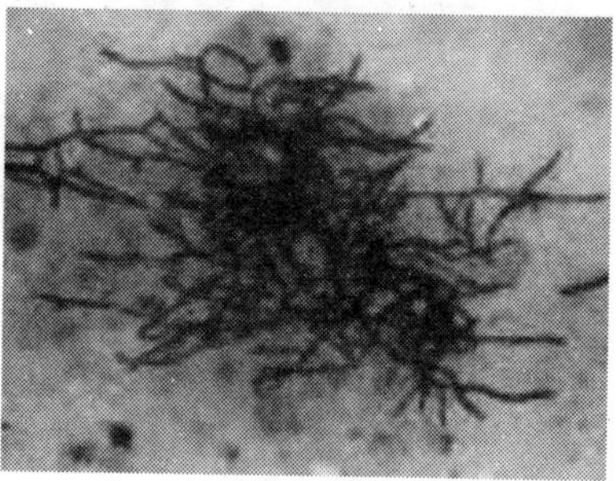
N. asteroid gram stained

Although some, controversy exists concerning the specific number of valid species of *Nocardia*, the genus *Nocardia* currently contains more than 50 species that have been characterized by phenotypic and molecular methods. However, not all of these species have been subjected to the same level of analysis. Further work may reveal that a few of these species are not indeed "valid." Among the currently accepted species, approximately half are recognized human and/or animal pathogens. Manifestations of disease range from cutaneous infection caused by traumatic inoculation of the organism in a normal host to severe pulmonary or central nervous system (CNS) disease in an immunocompromised host.

The species of the genus *Nocardia* in the family *Nocardiaceae* form a homogenous cluster among the *Corynebacteriaceae*, a suborder of the order *Actinomycetales*. The present and generally accepted definition of *Nocardia* is based mainly on molecular phylogenetic information, notably that from 16S rRNA gene sequences (180). Like members of the genus *Mycobacterium*, the nocardiae contain tuberculostearic acids, but in contrast to mycobacteria, they also possess short-chain (40- to 60-carbon) mycolic acids and usually exhibit characteristic branching on Gram staining. The nocardiae also have a peptidoglycan cell wall composed of *meso*-diaminopimelic acid, arabinose, and galactose. Nocardiae are ubiquitous in the environment and can be found worldwide as saprophytic components in fresh- and saltwater, soil, dust, decaying vegetation, and decaying fecal deposits from animals. Some species are more prevalent in geographical locations with a specific climate. For example, *Nocardia brasiliensis*, usually associated with cutaneous infection and mycetoma, is more commonly isolated in areas with tropical or subtropical climates and is often encountered in the southwestern or southeastern United States.

Health care-associated transmission or acquisition of the nocardiae has been documented but is relatively rare. However, nocardial infections are not considered to be communicable from person to person, although this may relate to the relative infrequency of close association of high-risk patients

Of these *N.asteroides* accounts for the most of the cases and has been recovered from lesion in humans, dog, cats, cattle, goat, horses & pigs (Walton and Libke, 1974; Orchard 1979). It is a heterogenous collection of nocardiae. It is now called as complex *N.nova* is a part of this collection and most frequently isolated from affected cats and dogs. All animals are susceptible to the infection. The cell wall architecture and constituents are typical of the coryneform group. The organisms occur worldwide as saprophytes in soil and water and the infection is picked up from these sources. What has been referred to as *N.asteroides* is now considered a complex made up of *N.asteroides, N.farcinica* and *Nocardia nova.* Of these, *N.asteroides* is the principal pathogen. Nocardiosis is usually a chronic progressive disease characterized by suppurating, granulomatous lesions. Sporadic infection occurs in many animals species. In cattle, it causes an acute or chronic mastitis with granulomatous lesions and draining fistulous tracts. Mastitis occurs in the form of large outbreaks. Sporadically abortions also occur. The tropical disease bovine farcy was initially attributed to *N.farcinica* but its precise role is unknown. It is probably *N.asteroides* (Minniken *et al.*, 1977). The disease is characterized by suppurative lesions mainly involving neck and limbs. It begins in the skin and may involve the superficial lymph vessels and nodes. Bovine farcy is also called as mycotic lymphangitis and bovine nocardiosis. Subsequent studies on bovine farcy have incriminated *Mycobacterium farcinogenes* and *Mycobacterium senegalese* with the disease.

In most of the cases the infection originates from organisms aspirated into the respiratory tract or introduced into skin wounds, leading to the development of necrotizing pneumonia or superficial skin lesions. The organisms may also be ingested with the dissemination hematogenously. Subsequently osteomyelitis and widespread abscess formation may occur. Central nervous system involvement is rare in animals Macneill *et al.* (2010) for the first time reported Nocardia infection in disseminated form in a dog showing fever, anorexia and multiple subcutaneous masses. The characteristic Nocardia lesion is an abscess or cluster of abscesses localized by minimal amount of fibrous tissues. Thus the spread of infection to adjacent tissues is possible through haematogenous route. *N.asteroides* does not produce granuloma. In case of infection with *N.brasilensis* and *N.caviae,* granules are produced in tissues.

Pathogenesis

The virulence factors of *Nocardia* have been poorly understood, however, the amount of peptidoglycan in the cell wall has been proposed to be related to virulence (Beadles *et al.,* 1980). Strain to strain variation in the thickness of peptidoglycan has been incriminated with the virulence of Nocardia. It is suggested that increased amount of peptidoglycan could cause resistance to degradation by phagosomal hydrolytic enzymes especially the lysozyme. Beadles *et al.* (1980) postulated that a longer lag phase *in vitro* could be incriminated with greater susceptibility of some strains to normal host defense mechanisms. This is further augmented by the fact that *N.asteroides* cells at stationary phase are less virulent than log phase cells. Cells of *N.brasillensis* do not show this difference (Conde *et al.,* 1982).

Both peptidoglycan and mycolic acid of *N.asteroides* may be responsible for this effect. These structures are possibly also necessary for inhibiting the phagosome - lysosome fusion and resist the microbicidal effect of polymorphonuclear leukocytes (PMNS). No toxin has been found to be produced but some enzymes of *N.asteroides* such as catalase and superoxide dismutase plays a role in virulence. The nordiae contain the toxic and immunostimulating glycolipid trehalose dimycolate (cord factor) in their cell walls, which has been found to play a major role in macrophage activation (Silva and Faccioli 1992). It influences the release of tumor necrosis factor which is important in host resistance to infection. *Nocardia* infection can be regional or disseminated depending on various host and pathogen related factors. It may extend to regional lymph nodes or spread by contiguousness. Dissemination occurs to liver, kidneys, bows, joints and rarely the central nervous system.

The nocardial mastitis rarely occurs in cattle. It occurs as a acute or subacute disease and is accompanied by lesions characterized by extensive granuloma. The organisms invade the mammary gland through the teat canal and fever and anorexia develop and later stage is characterized by circumscribed abscess and fibrosis. The spread is from lobule to lobule until all the lobules are infected. The organisms are visible on cultures of milk. Small specks are visible in the milk due to the formation of mycelia. Grossly diffuse fibrosis and granulomatous lesions containing pus are present in mammary tissues. Only a few sporadic cases have been reported in horses, pigs, and cattle. In all previous reports, of nocardial abortion, the causative agent was identified as *Nocardia asteroides.* The current report describes an aborted bovine fetus that was infected with *Nocardia farcinica.* Placenta, abomasal fluid, lung, liver, and kidney specimens from a late-term bovine abortion were submitted to the clinical laboratory. The gross findings included purulent exudate in the placenta and numerous abscesses in lung (Bawa *et al.,* 2010). Histologically, there was necrotizing and suppurative placentitis, pyogranulomatous pneumonia, and nephritis with numerous intralesional branching and filamentous, Gram-positive bacteria. Nocardia farcinica was isolated by bacteriology, and the bacteriology result was confirmed by 2 established polymerase chain reaction protocols and by DNA sequencing.

Nineteen putative *Nocardia farcinica* isolates epidemiologically associated with intramammary products containing neomycin were obtained from clinical cases in a Canada-wide mastitis epizootic (Brown *et al.*2007). Epidemiologic investigations were unable to identify the mechanism for transmission. To evaluate the hypotheses generated (intrinsic versus extrinsic contamination) and to confirm the identity of *N. farcinica,* the authors compared these isolates phenotypically (biochemicals and antimicrobial susceptibility studies) and genotypically (16S rRNA gene sequencing analysis, chromosomal DNA and ribotyping profiles) with the type and reference strains of *N. farcinica.* Results of biochemical studies and 16S rRNA gene sequencing identified the isolates as *N. farcinica.* Results of chromosomal DNA and ribotyping profiles and antimicrobial resistance to amikacin indicated all were a unique clone of *N. farcinica* that differed from the control isolates. The study suggests the epizootic was caused by transmission of a unique clone of *N. farcinica* through intrinsically contaminated dry cow intramammary products rather than an extrinsic source.

A stillborn calf at 259 days of gestation was examined. The dam showed no clinical signs of disease, and the stillbirth was occurred sporadically and were characterized by focal necrosis surrounded by infiltration of the cells such as macrophages and multinucleated giant cells. The lesions were observed systemically. The hyphae were visible by Grocott's stain and they were positive by immunohistochemical stain using serum of a rabbit immunized with the isolated organism (Saito *et al.*2009). The isolated bacteria were determined to be *Nocardia farcinica* by bacteriological and molecular analysis and was confirmed that the stillbirth was caused by infection with and proliferation of *Nocardia farcinica.* This is the first report of a bovine stillbirth caused by this organism.

Diagnosis

Gram positive, acid fast with beaded filaments along with shorter coccobacillary forms are visible in smears prepared from the Nocardia infected samples. Granules occur in *N.brasiliensis* and *N.otitidiscaviarum* but rarely in *N.asteroides.* The acid fast staining show some retention of carbol fuchsin stain indicating partial acid fastness. Some strains are not acid fast at all.

The organisms grow on an enrichment medium. On blood agar and sabouraud's agar at 25^{0}C or 37^{0}C. Folded, raised or smooth or granular colonies are visible in 4 or 5 days. The yellow pigmented or white colonies are visible. The mycelia are readily visible in slide cultures on sabourand agar.

A presumptive diagnosis is based on the demonstration of typical organisms in clinical material and on colonial, cultural, morphologic and staining characteristics. *Nocardiae* reduces nitrate and are catalase positive.

The recent explosion of newly described species of *Nocardia* results from the impact in the last decade of newer molecular technology, including PCR restriction enzyme analysis and 16S rRNA sequencing. These molecular techniques have revolutionized the identification of the *nocardiae* by providing rapid and accurate identification of recognized *nocardiae* and, at the same time, revealing new species and a number of yet-to-be-described species. There are currently more than 30 species of nocardiae of human and veterinary clinical significance, with the majority of isolates being N. nova complex, *N. abscessus, N. transvalensis* complex, *N. farcinica, N. asteroides* type VI (*N. cyriacigeorgica*), and *N. brasiliensis*. These species cause a wide variety of diseases and have variable drug susceptibilities. Accurate identification often requires referral to a reference laboratory with molecular capabilities, as many newer species are genetically distinct from established species yet have few or no distinguishing phenotypic characteristics. Correct identification is important in deciding the clinical relevance of a species and in the clinical management and treatment of patients with nocardial disease.

Treatment and Control

Surgical removal and drainage of the lesions are attempted. Trimethoprim - sulfonamides are effective. Antimicrobial treatment has to be continued for at least 12 weeks. Alternative drugs include aminocycline and doxycycline. Nocardiae are resistant to fluoroquinolones. *Nocardia nova* responds to the penicillins and macrolides and tetracyclines. Veterinary isolates of *Nocardia nova* (n=18), *Nocardia farcinica* (n=3) and *Nocardia cyriacigeorgica* (n=1) underwent microbroth dilution testing to ciprofloxacin, enrofloxacin and pradofloxacin (Gvendir *et al.*2011). The MIC(50) and MIC(90) of pradofloxacin, ciprofloxacin and enrofloxacin that inhibited growth of *Nocardia nova* isolates were 2 (4), 8 (16), 16 (32) ìg/mL, respectively. The tentative ECOFF values for pradofloxacin and ciprofloxacin were 32ìg/mL and for enrofloxacin 64ìg/mL. The MIC or MIC range for the three *N. farcinica* isolates of pradofloxacin, ciprofloxacin and enrofloxacin were 0.25-0.5, 2 and 2ìg/mL and for the single N. cyriacigeorgica isolate were 1, 4 and 4ìg/mL, respectively. On the basis on these results, fluoroquinolones appear to have limited therapeutic potential for most Nocardia infections.

Fluoroquinolones have several properties that make them potentially attractive candidates for the treatment of *Nocardia* infections, but information regarding their in vitro activity is limited. Minimum inhibitory concentrations (MIC) of five fluoroquinolones and other antimicrobials were determined by the reference broth dilution and E-test methods for 33 consecutive clinical isolates of Nocardia speciated by 16S rRNA gene sequences(Hansen *et al.* 2011). The isolates included: *Nocardia cyriacigeorgica* (n = 6), *N. nova* (n = 8), *N. farcinica* (n = 8), *N. brasiliensis* (n = 3), *N. asteroides* (n = 4), and *N. veterana* (n = 4). MIC50/MIC90 results for ciprofloxacin, gatifloxacin, gemifloxacin, levofloxacin, and moxifloxacin by broth dilution were 32/32, 2/4, 1/4, 32/32, and 2/2 microg/ml, respectively. The MICs by broth dilution and E-test were within a two-fold doubling dilution for 94%, 97%, 97%, 100%, and 100% of isolates for ciprofloxacin, gatifloxacin, gemifloxacin, levofloxacin, and moxifloxacin, respectively. For ciprofloxacin, the E-test results showed either complete categorical agreement or minor error compared to the reference broth dilution method for 97% (32/33) of the isolates. For other fluoroquinolones, using Streptococcus pneumoniae breakpoints, 94% (124/132) of MIC results by E-test showed either complete agreement or minor error compared to the reference broth dilution method. Fluoroquinolones show variable in vitro activity against clinical isolates of *Nocardia* spp., and MICs determined by the E-test show reasonable agreement with those determined by the reference broth dilution method.

Phenotypic characteristics, antimicrobial susceptibility profile, and clinical-epidemiological features of 28 Nocardia strains isolated from 19 cases of bovine mastitis, eight cutaneous-subcutaneous lesions and one case of pneumonia in dogs were evaluated. Microbiological, biochemical, cytological and scanning electron microscopy methods were used in diagnosis. Nocardia asteroides type IV, *Nocardia otitidiscaviarum,Nocardia nova* (type III) and *Nocardia farcinica* (type V) were isolated from bovine milk, bronchial lavage and/or cutaneous-subcutaneous abscesses in dogs. Nocardial bovine mastitis was diagnosed predominantly in clinical cases, in dairy herds with poor environmental hygienic conditions between milking and inappropriate intramammary therapy. Canine nocardiosis was observed commonly in animals co-infected with distemper virus. Sulphamethoxazole-trimethoprim (92.8%), amikacin (92.8%) and ceftiofur (92.8%) were the most effective drugs in 28 isolates. Multiple drug resistance to three or more and five or more antimicrobials was observed in ten (35.7%) and three (10.7%) strains, respectively, predominantly with use of cloxaxillin, cefoperazone and ampicillin (Ribeiro *et al.*, 2008).

Antimicrobial therapy of nocardiae mastitis may produce temporary clinical relief and cessation of shedding. Control requires removal of infected animals from rest of the animals and general hygienic measures should be adopted. Thorough disinfection of premises and equipments is required.

Actinomyces

Organisms belonging to the genus Actinomyces are gram-positive diphtheroid or filamentous rods. Branching filaments are visible in pathologic specimen whereas in culture diphtheroid form predominates. Actinomyces have distinct cell wall constituents as given in the table. The organism are non-motile & non-spore forming; microaeerophilic or anaerobic except for *Actinomyces viscosus* and *Actinomyces naislundii* which are facultatively anaerobic. The organisms are catalase negative (except *A. viscosus*) and fermentative.

Important species of Actinomyces are given below:-

1. *Actinomyces bovis* - Actinomycosis, Lumpy Jaw in cattle
2. *A.viscosus* - Pneumonia, pyothorax and subcutaneous infection in dogs.
3. *A. naeslundii* - Infrequent infection in animals.
4. *Actinomyces suis* - Pyrogranulomatous mastitis in sows. Also recovered from purulent vaginal discharges in sows.
5. *Actinomyces israelii* - Actinomycosis in human; lesions may involve jaw, thorax or abdomen.

Members of Actinomyces require enriched medium for growth and Co_2 further stimulates the growth. These are oral commensals that only occasionally invade damaged tissues. Secondarily they are present in gastro intestinal tract. Most actinomycotic infections are endogenous. Bites are another means of transmission but it is rarely caused.

The disease causes development of granuloma characterized by the presence of "sulphur granules". Upon crushing of the granules, gram positive branching filaments, short rods and cocci are visible. The sulphur granules are composed of bacterial filaments and mineralized calcium phosphate. A calcium phosphate protein complex encapsulates the organisms as a result of phosphatase activity in response to inflammation (Gyles 1993). The development of antibodies form a complex with actinomyces antigen which are deposited in tissues in the form of clubs, most commonly formed with infection with *A.bovis.*

"Lumpy Jaw" is the disease caused by *A.bovis* in cattle. The organisms invade the tissues as a result of trauma and produce localized lesions in bones. This causes interference in prehension and mastication leading to emaciation. When the alimentary tract is involved there is physical interference with rumination and ruminal movement and digestion resulting in partial starvation. Rarely localization occurs in other organs caused by hematogenous spread from the primary lesions.

A.bovis is a common inhabitant of the bovine mouth and infection is presumed to occur through wounds to the buccal mucosa caused by sharp pieces of feed or foreign material. Infection may also occur through dental alveoli. Infection of the alimentary tract wall is probably related to laceration by sharp foreign bodies.

Lumpy Jaw occurs only sporadically in affected herds, it is of importance because of treatment. It has been recorded from most part of the world.

In the Lumpy Jaw, the Jaw bones develop osteomyelitis. Lesions are granulomatous in nature.

Actinomycosis of Jaw commences as a painless bony swelling which appear on mandible or maxilla usually at the level of the central molar tooth. The enlargement may be diffuse or discrete. Some lesions enlarge rapidly with in a few week whereas others slowly over a period of months. The swelling are hard and painful to touch. They usually break through the skin and discharge through one or more openings, the sinuses often heal and new open. In severe cases spread to contiguous soft tissues may be extensive and involve the muscle and facia of the throat. Excessive swelling of maxilla may cause dyspnea.

The soft tissue involved in the disease is the esophageal groove region which spread to the lower esophagus and the anterior wall of reticulum leading to impaired digestion characterized by diarrhoea. Less common lesions of soft tissues include orchitis in bulls, the trachea causing partial obstruction and abscess in the brain. Actinomyces is also incriminated with otitis externa in cattle (Duarte & Hamden 2004).

A goat with neurologic signs had multifocal abscesses containing sulfur granules in the right brain and temporal bone(Hirai *et al.*2007). Histologically, the lesions consisted of pyogranulomas with several radiating bacterial colonies of various sizes. A tangled mass of filamentous and gram-positive bacteria was recognized in the central part of the colony. Actinomyces naeslundii antigen was detected in the colonies of bacteria in the brain and neighboring bone tissue by immunohistochemistry. Actinomycosis involving the central nervous system (CNS) and temporal bone is rare in animals. Cerebral infection with *A. naeslundii* may have resulted from direct extension from cervicofacial regions because the CNS lesions were distributed asymmetrically and were continuous with the right temporal bone.

A.viscosus is mostly associated with infection is dogs (Davenport *et al.*, 1975; Ehler 1977). The disease may be in the form of abscesses at various organs but thorasic infections are most common. The lesions are similar to that produced by *Nocardia* species and lack the presence of sulphur granules (Pine and Oherman 1966).

Actinomyces pyogenes is the second most frequently encountered pathogen, next only to *Fusobacterium necrophorum*, in liver abscesses of feedlot cattle. Ninety-one isolates, presumptively identified as *A. pyogenes*, isolated from liver abscesses of cattle were studied(Narayanan *et al.*, 1998) characteristics by the API 20 Strep kit were similar to those reported previously for *A. pyogenes* isolated from other infections, except that 18% of isolates hydrolyzed esculin. Nine isolates that resembled *A. pyogenes* in morphology and in certain biochemical characteristics, but fermented mannitol and/or raffinose, were called *A. pyogenes*-like (APL) organisms. The five antimicrobial agents, bacitracin, chlortetracycline, oxytetracycline, tylosin, and virginiamycin were inhibitory to all strains of *A. pyogenes* and APLs. Generally, APL organisms had higher mean hemolytic and leukotoxic activities than *A. pyogenes*. All isolates of *A. pyogenes* and APLs produced proteases and neuraminidases. Ribotyping with endonucleases, including BstEII, ClaI, EcoRI, EcoRV, HaeIII, MboI, PvuII, SalI, and SmaI alone or in combinations, showed considerable genetic heterogeneity in both *A. pyogenes* and APLs. No specific ribopattern characteristic of each group was observed with any of the endonuclease used. The origin of *A. pyogenes* and APLs and the relative importance of APLs in causing liver abscesses in feedlot cattle are not known.

In a four-year-old male cat, a subcutaneous phyma about 3.5 cm in diameter was surgically removed from the left inframandibular region. Histopathologically, the phyma was found to be the swollen medial retropharyngeal lymph node containing an actinomycotic abscess. The filamentous organisms in the abscess stained positively by the Gram's, Grocott's and periodic acid-Schiff methods, and were negative by the Ziehl-Neelsen method. By the immunoperoxidase method, the organisms were specifically identified as *Actinomyces viscosus* serotype 2 by its antiserum absorbed with *A. viscosus* serotype 1 antigen(Murakami *et al.*1997).

The characteristics, history, clinical signs, treatment and outcome of nine horses with abscesses caused by *Actinomyces* species were reviewed. DNA sequencing was used to determine the species of one of the isolates (Fielding *et al.*, 2008). The horses were one to 11 years of age, and the abscesses were most commonly located in the submandibular and retropharyngeal regions. The bacterium was usually cultured as the sole isolate and the horses were most often affected in the autumn. Most of the abscesses were treated with antimicrobials and drainage, but some of them recurred. The horses with submandibular abscesses had residual scar tissue that in some cases did not resolve.

The tonsils of eleven pigs and the mammary glands of a sow were used to investigate actinomycotic lesions due to *Actinomyces* sp. Infection (Murakami *et al.*1998). At necropsy, there was no abnormality on these tonsils, on the other hand, numerous abscesses containing sulfur granules were found in the mammary. Histopathologically, the *Actinomyces* sp. lesions were noted as crypt abscesses in the tonsils and as pus-forming granulomas in the mammary glands. The microorganisms in both lesions were composed of bead-like cocci, bacillary cells and short, branching filaments, those cells being positive by the Gram's and Grocott's methods. Clubs were formed around the microbial clumps in these lesions. Immunohistochemically, there were cross-reactions between antibodies of *Actinomyces* sp. Chiba 101 (101) and swine actinomycetes of 7 species: *A. bovis, A. hyovaginalis, A. israeli, A. naeslundii, A. pyogenes, A. suis* (formerly Eubacterium suits) and *A. viscosus.* However it was possible to differentiate *Actinomyces* sp. 101 from them by absorption and dilution of the antiserum, then the microorganisms in the tonsillar crypt abscesses and the granulomatous mastitis were labelled with an immunoperoxidase technique using the absorbed *Actinomyces* sp. 101 antiserum. Thus, these immunolabelling properties are suggestive of the presence of *'A. suis'* (Grässer) Franke 1973. An unusual Actinomyces-like bacterium originating from a pig with mastitis was subjected to a polyphasic taxonomic investigation(Hoyles *et al.*2001). The morphological and biochemical characteristics of the organism were consistent with its preliminary assignment to the genus Actinomyces but it did not appear to correspond to any recognized species. PAGE analysis of whole-cell proteins confirmed the phenotypic distinctiveness of the bacterium and 16S rRNA gene sequence analysis demonstrated that it represents a hitherto unknown sub-line amongst a cluster of *Actinomyces* species which embraces *Actinomyces canis, Actinomyces georgiae, Actinomyces hyovaginalis, Actinomyces meyeri,* Actinomyces odontolyticus, Actinomyces radingae and Actinomyces turicensis. Based on phylogenetic and phenotypic evidence, it is proposed that the unknown bacterium isolated from pig mastitis be classified as *Actinomyces suimastitidis* sp. nov. The type strain of *Actinomyces suimastitidis* is CCUG 39279T (= CIP 106779T).

Actinomyces produces toxin or enzyme that could be incriminated as virulence factor. *Actinomyces pyogenes,* an important pathogen of the bovine udder, was mainly characterized by production of the enzymes protease and neuraminidase. Both enzymes could be isolated and further analyzed. In addition *A. pyogenes* demonstrated lectin-like surface structures which caused hemagglutination reactions of neuraminidase treated erythrocytes. Further surface antigens of *A. pyogenes* which characteristically cross reacted with antisera against group polysaccharide antigens of streptococci of serological group G allowed an additional serological identification of this species(Lammler 1990). A. pyogenes further demonstrated binding properties for the plasma proteins alpha 2-macroglobulin, haptoglobin and fibrinogen and bacteriocin-like activities which caused growth inhibition of micrococci and staphylococci.

Twenty-two *Actinomyces pyogenes* isolates were recovered from hepatic abscesses in cattle and evaluated for hemolysin production (Funk *et al.*, 1996). Hemolysin was collected from supernatant of cultures grown in 6% CO_2 in brain heart infusion (BHI) broth. The effect of oxidizing and reducing agents, enzymes, temperatures and pH on hemolytic activity were studied using sheep erythrocytes as the target cells. This study showed that A. pyogenes hemolysin is oxygen stable; sensitive to treatment by protease, trypsin, and amylase; and destroyed by treatment at extreme temperatures (56 and 100 degrees C) and pH (pH 3 and 11). Production of hemolysin was studied in BHI, RPMI-1640, and a defined serum-free *A. pyogenes* medium under aerobic and anaerobic conditions. Maximum hemolysin was produced in BHI incubated aerobically in 6% CO_2 and to a lesser degree anaerobically in RPMI-1640. No hemolysin was produced in the defined *A. pyogenes* medium. Differential filtration, isoelectric focusing and sodium dodecyl sulfate polyacrylamide gel electrophoresis identified two hemolysin proteins with pI values of 3.40 and 9.45 and estimated molecular masses of 62 and 58 kDa, respectively. Cell-free supernatant samples positive for hemolysin activity also were screened for leukotoxin activity. Significant levels of leukotoxin were detected in all samples screened. Rabbit antisera raised against somatic antigens from two strains of *Actinomyces pyogenes* reacted specifically in a peroxidase anti-peroxidase technique which was developed for the location of the bacteria in formalin-fixed tissues(Leifsson *et al.*1995). The technique was applied on experimental murine and spontaneous bovine lesions caused by *A. pyogenes*. By electron microscopy and immunohistochemistry it was demonstrated that pulmonary intravascular macrophages play a role in the uptake of *A. pyogenes* from the blood, and in the production of pyaemic pulmonary lesions.

Trauma and possibly some other disruption in the tissues or immune response are required to initiate disease by the endogenous bacteria. Anaerobic conditions prevailing in the wounds support the growth of bacteria. Some unknown cellular factors of *A.viscosus* are responsible for chemotactic behaviour towards human polymorphonuclear cells and stimulate host immune cells to produce mediators of inflammation (Engel *et al.*, 1976, 1977).

A.viscosus produces slime that is helpful in the adherence on tooth surfaces subsequently leading to the formation of dental plaque. Additionally 2 distinct types of fimbrae are present on surface, type 1 adheres to salivary rich protein on tooth surfaces whereas type 2 is responsible for binding to lactose-sensitive moiety present on certain streptococci and to buccal epithelial cells (Cisar *et al.*, 1979). The role, if any, of these fimbrae in disease process in animals is not known. Interbacterial interactions between oral streptococci and actinomyces and their adherence to tooth surface and the associated host cells are key early events that promote development of the complex oral biofilm referred to as dental plaque. In *Actinomyces oris* these interactions depends on lactin like activity or type Z fimbriae, the shaft and tip fimbrillins, Fim A and fim B, respectively. The lectin like activity resides only in shaft fim A and not fim B (Mishra *et al.,* 2010). Yeung (1992) demonstated the existence and expression by divergent Actinomyces groups of genomic sequence that are closely related to the type I fimbrae of *A.viscosus* strain T14V.

In mice, *A.naeslundii* produces more severe acute form of disease than *A.israelii* or *A.viscosus* (Behbehani and Jordan 1982). During the chronic stage, *A.israelii* persisted and produced severe disease whereas the other 2 species were eliminated. During the early stage of infection the Actinomyces exherts a chemotastic effect on polymorphonuclear cells but these cells were unable to penetrate the central granules in the *A.israelii* lesions probably due to the very dense nature of the lesions (Behbehani *et al.,* 1983). Besides, the surface capsule produced by *A.israelii* may be the factor. It was noted by Behbehani *et al.*(1983) that eoginophilic rim at the edge of the *A.israelii* lesions may be due to arginine-rich proteins and the release of lysosomal enzymes. In contrast *A.viscosus* and *A.naeslundii* in the core of lesions are destroyed due to complement activation.

Diagnosis

Organisms are demonstrated in lesions. Suspected exudates are examined for "sulfur granules", which appear as yellowish particles varying in firmness, upto several millimeters in diameter. Granules are washed in saline and placed under a coverslip and gently pressed. The rosettes formation, with filaments extended into clubbed frings are suggestive of actinomyces.

Crushed granules, exudates or tissue impressions are stained with gram and acid-fast stain. Branching, gram-positive, beaded, non-acid fast filaments suggest *Actinomyces* spp.

Crushed granules or exudates are inoculated on enrichment medium and incubated at 37^{0}C under 10% CO_2 tension. Colonies develop in 48 hrs. or more. *Actinomycs bovis* forms granular to smooth microcolonies with in 24 hrs. *Actinomyces viscosus* produces smooth to granular colonies up to 2mm in diameter. Some unclassified animals derived Actinomyces show pattern of the type species *A.israelii* of humans. Haemolysis is rare.

Treatment and Control

The effective treatment of actinomycosis has been recorded as administering isoniazid orally for a month or treatment must be interrupted when signs of toxicity appears such as hypersalivation, anorexia, vomiting and development of dandruff. The treatment can be restarted when the symptoms have subsided. Long term penicillin derivate therapy is required in dogs and cats. Aminoglycosides and fluoroquinolones are ineffective. Other broad spectrum antibiotics can also be tested. The treatment will not cure the bone structure. Soft tissue lesions can be drained off. Lavage of lesions with iodine is effective both in cattle and dogs. Oral or intraveneous dosing of iodide may be given. Abortion may occur in cattle following the treatment. Occasionally animal shows distress, restlessness, dyspnea, tachycardia and staggering. Roentgenological tests have been used extensively but are of doubtful permanent value.

A 12-year-old Arabian stallion was evaluated for a refractory skin problem of 2 years' duration. Skin nodules and pustules, which would rupture, had developed over the right lumbar muscles. Anaerobic culturing from the pustules yielded *Actinomyces viscosus*, and histologic examination of biopsy specimens revealed globular eosinophilic structures. Concomitant treatment with isoniazid (8 mg/kg of body weight, q 24 h for 8 weeks), trimethoprim-sulfadiazine (30 mg/kg, q 24 h for 8 weeks), and sodium iodide solution (66 mg/kg, every 1, 2, or 4 weeks, for 32 weeks) resolved the condition. (Specht *et al.*, 1991).

Control of the spread of the disease is effective through the prevention of contamination of pasture and feed utensil and segregation of affected animals is useful in containing the further spread of the disease. Hygienic measures adopted on routine basis are effective in controlling the disease.

References

Bawa B., Bai J., Whitehair M., Purvis T. and Debey B.M.2010.Bovine abortion associated with *Nocardia farcinica*. J. Vet. Diagn. Invest. **22:** 108-111.

Beadles, T.A., Land, G.A. and Knezek, D.J. 1980. An ultrastructural comparison of cell envelopes of *Nocardia arteroides* and *Nocardia brasiliensis*. Mycopathologia **70:**25-32.

Behbehan, M.J. and Jordan, H.V. 1982. Comparative pathogenicity of *Actinomyces* species in mice. J. Med. Microbiol. **15:** 465-473.

Behbehan, M.J., Heeley, J.D. and Jordan, H.V. 1983. Comparative histopathology of lesions produced by *Actinomyces israelii, Actinomyces naeslundii* and *Actinomyces viscosus* in mice. Am. J. Pathol. **110:** 267-274.

Brown J.M., Cowley K.D., Manninen K.I. and McNeil M.M.2007.Phenotypic and molecular epidemiologic evaluation of a *Nocardia farcinica* mastitis epizootic. Vet. Microbiol. **125:** 66-72. Epub 2007 May 6.

Cisar, J.O., Kolenbrander, P.E. and McIntire, F.C. 1979. Secificity of coaggregation reactions between human oral streptococci and strains of *Actinomyces viscosus* or *Actinomyces naeslundii*. Infect. Immun. **24:** 742-752.

Conde, C., Melendro, E.I., Fresan, M. and Ortiz-Ortiz, L. 1982. *Nocardia brasiliensis*: Mycetoma induction and growth cycle. Infect. Immun. **38:** 1291-1295.

Davenport, A.A., Carter, G.R. and Benekey, E. 1975. *Actinomyces viscosus* in relation to other Actinomyces and actinomycosis. Vet. Bull. **45:** 313-316.

Duarte, E.R. and Hamdem, J.S. 2004. Otitis in cattle, an aetiological review. J. Vet. Med. B Infect. Dis. Vet. Public Health. **51:** 1-7.

Ehler, W.J. 1977. Actinomycosis in dog. Canine Pract. **4:** 15-17.

Engel, D.G., Clagett, J., Page, R. and Williams, B. 1977. Mitogenic activity of *Actinomyces viscosus*. I. Effect on murine B and T lymphocytes and partial characterization. J. Immunol. **118:** 1466-1471.

Engle, D.G., Epps, E. and Clagget, J. 1976. *In vivo* and *in vitro* studies on possible pathogenic mechanisms of *Actinomyces viscosus*. Infect. Immun. **14:** 548-554.

Fielding C.L., Magdesian K.G., Morgan R.A., Ruby R.E. and Sprayberry K.A. 2008. *Actinomyces species* as a cause of abscesses in nine horses. Vet. Rec. **162:** 18-20.

Funk P.G., Staats J.J., Howe M., Nagaraja T.G. and Chengappa M.M.1996.Identification and partial characterization of an *Actinomyces pyogenes* hemolysin. Vet. Microbiol. **50:** 129-142.

Govendir M., Norris J.M., Hansen T., Wigney D.I., Muscatello G., Trott D.J. and Malik R.2011.Susceptibility of rapidly growing mycobacteria and Nocardia isolates from cats and dogs to pradofloxacin. Vet. Microbiol. 15.[http://www.ncbi.nlm.nih.gov/pubmed/21726965]

Gyles, C.L. 1993. *Nocardia: Actinomyces*: dermatophilus. In pathogenesis of bacterial infections in animals. Pp.124-132. Ed. C.L. Gyles and C.O. Thoen, Ames: IOWA State University Press, USA.

Hansen G., Swanzy S., Gupta R., Cookson B. aznd Limaye A.P.2008.In vitro activity of fluoroquinolones against clinical isolates of *Nocardia* identified by partial 16S rRNA sequencing. Eur. J. Clin. Microbiol. Infect. Dis. **27**(2): 115-20. Epub 2007 Nov 9.

Hirai T., Nunoya T. and Azuma R.2007.*Actinomycosis* of the brain and temporal bone in a goat. J. Vet. Med. Sci. **69:** 641-643.

Hoyles L., Falsen E., Holmström G., Persson A., Sjödén B. and Collins M.D.2001. *Actinomyces suimastitidis* sp. nov., isolated from pig mastitis. Int. J. Syst. Evol. Microbiol. **51**(Pt 4): 1323-1326.

Lämmler C. 1990. [The possible pathogenic factors of *Actinomyces pyogenes*. A review]. Berl. Munch. Tierarztl. Wochenschr. **103:** 121-125.

Leifsson PS. Basse A. Jensen HE. Bloch B. Aalbaek B.1995.Pulmonary intravascular macrophages in the pathogenesis of bovine pulmonary lesions caused by *Actinomyces pyogenes*. J.Comp.Pathol. **112:** 197-206.

Macneill, A.L., Steeil, J.C., Dossin, O., Hoien-Dalen, P.S. and Maddox, C.W. 2010. Disseminated nocardiosis caused by *Nocardia abscesses* in a dog. Vet. Clin. Pathol. [http://www.ncbi.nlm.nih.gov/pubmed/20698939].

Minnikem, D.E., Patel, P.V., Alshamaony, L. and Goodfellow, M. 1977. Polar lipid composition in the classification of *Nocardia* and related species. Int. J. Syst. Bacteriol. **27:** 104-117.

Mishra, A., WuC, YangJ., Cisar, J.O., Das, A. and Tom-That, H. 2010. The *Actinomyces ovis* type 2 fimbrial shaft fim A mediates coaggregation with oral streptococii, adherence to red blood cells and biofilm development. Mol. Microbiol. [http://www.ncbi.nlm.nih.gov/pubmed/20545853].

MurakamiS., Yamanishi M.W. and Azuma R. 1997.Lymph node abscess due to *Actinomyces viscosus* in a cat. J. Vet. Med. Sci. **59:** 1079-1080.

Murakami S., Azuma R., Koeda T., Oomi H., Watanabe T. and Fujiwara H. 1998. Immunohistochemical detection for *Actinomyces* sp. in swine tonsillar abscess and granulomatous mastitis. Mycopathologia. **141:** 15-19.

Narayanan S. Nagaraja TG.,Staats J.,Chengappa MMaOberst RD.1998.Biochemical and biological characterizations and ribotyping of *Actinomyces pyogenes* and *Actinomyces pyogenes*-like organisms from liver abscesses in cattle. Vet Microbiol. 1998 Apr 15; **61**(4): 289-303.

Orchard, V.A. 1979. Nocardial infections of animals in New Zealand. 1976-78. N.Z. Vet. J. **27:** 159-165.

Pine, L. and Overman, J.R. 1966. Differentiation of capsule and hyphae clubs of bovine sulphur granules. Sabouraudia. **5:** 141-143.

Ribeiro M.G., Salerno T., Mattos-Guaraldi A.L., Camello T.C., Langoni H., Siqueira A.K., Paes A.C., Fernandes M.C. AND Lara G.H.2008.*Nocardiosis*: an overview and additional report of 28 cases in cattle and dogs. Rev. Inst. Med. Trop. Sao. Paulo **50:** 177-185. Epub 2008 May 14.

Saito S., Nishimura T., Kamata H., Takamatsu D. and Sato M.2009.Bovine stillbirth due to *Nocardia farcinica*. J. Vet. Med. Sci. **71:** 1665-1668.

Silva, C.L. and Faccioli, L.H. 1992. Tumor necrosis factor and macrophage activation are important in clearance of *Nocardia brasilinsis* from livers and spleens of mice. Infect. Immun. **60:** 3566-3570.

Specht T.E., Breuhaus B.A., Manning T.O., Miller R.T. and Cochrane R.B.1991.Skin pustules and nodules caused by *Actinomyces viscosus* in a horse. J. Am. Vet. Med. Assoc. **198:** 457-459.

Walton, A.M. and Libke, K.G. 1974. *Nocardiosis* in animals. Vet. Med. Small Anim. Clin. **69:** 1105-1107.

Yeung, M.K. 1992. Conservation of an *Actinomyces viscosus* T14V type 1 fimbrial subunit homolog among divergent groups of *Actinomyces* spp. Infect. Immun. **60:** 1047-1054.

□□□

Chapter 22

Chlamydia

Dr. S.K. SRIVASTAVA
Former, Division of Bacteriology & Mycology
Indian Veterinary Research Institute, Izatnagar-243122
Bareilly (U.P.)

Chlamydia

Chlamydiae are gram negative pleomorphic, obligate intracellular bacteria placed in genera *Chlamydia* and *Chlamydophila* based upon 16S and 23S rRNA ribotyping. The organism lack peptidoglycan. A trilaminar outer membrane consists of protein and genus specific lipopolysaccharide. Proteins confer species and type-specificity and may act as adhesins. These are unable to synthesize energy source (ATP). Therefore, for energy they have to depend on host's metabolic pathways in order to reproduce. Their life cycle alternates between non-infectious proliferative stages and infectious non-proliferative stages. The infectious stage consists of condensed elementary bodies (EB), 200-400 nm in size. These are capable of entering host epithelium mucosa or phagocytic cells via phagocytosis/endocytosis. The elementary bodies are metabolically very sluggish. These elementary bodies change into non-infectious, metabolically active, reticulate bodies (RB) measuring 600 to 15 nm, that generate by binary fission, a new crop of elementary bodies that are released upon cell lysis. In the host they form intracytoplasmic membrane limited inclusions with in the phagocytic vacuoles. Besides intermediate forms are often seen and vary from 300-500 nm. These are often called dispersing forms or condensing forms depending on whether they are EB or RB or vice versa. Elementary bodies appear red by macchiavello's stain and reddish purple by Giemsa stain while reticulate bodies stain blue, green, reddish and blue, respectively. Chlamydiae do not grown on cell-free media. They require living cells such as Yolksac and tissue culture. The following species have been recognized.

- *Chlamydophila psittaci* : Heterogenous; causes avian chlamydiosis and bovine abortion.
- *Chlamydophila pecorum* : It has been recovered from cattle and sheep with conditions, namely sporadic bovine encephalitis, encephalitis, infectious poly-arthritis, pneumonia and diarrhea.
- *Chlamydophila suis* : Intestinal infections in pigs.
- *Chlamydophila caviae* : Inclusion conjunctivitis in guinea pigs.
- *Chlamydophila pneumonia* : One serovar; causes variety of respiratory infections in humans and possibly in horses; subclinical disease in sheep, goat and cattle.
- *Chlamydophila abortus* : Enzootic abortion of sheep and goats; abortion in cattle, pigs and goats; bovine mastitis.
- *Chlamydia felis* : Conjunctivitis in cats.
- *Chlamydia trachomatis* : Many serovars; causes trachoma, conjunctivitis in infants, lymphogranuloma venereum; organisms similar to this isolated from swine.
- *Chlamydia muridarum* : Respiratory infection in mice.

Because of diversity of results obtained by DNA probes and restriction endonuclease analysis of Chlamydiae isolates it seems probable that there are a large number of subgroups of *Chlamydia psittaci*. Though various genetically diverse Chlamydiae may cause avian chlamydiosis only a few *C.psittaci* strains are highly prevalent and frequently associated with clinical infections (Chahota *et al.*, 2006).

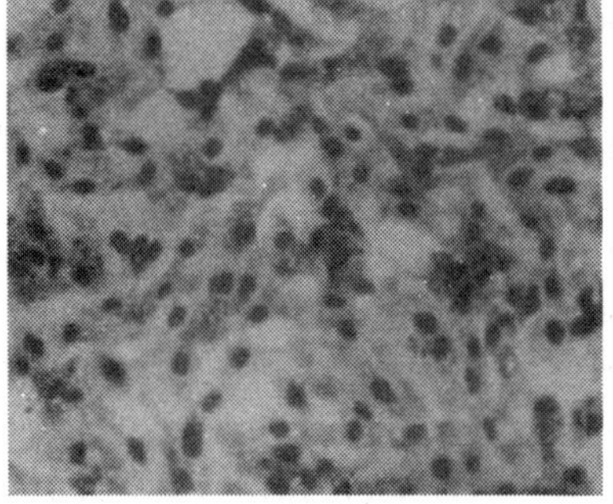

C.psittaci gram stained

The genome size, $6.6X10^8$ Da is among the smallest in prokaryotes. The genome sequence of *Chlamydophila abortus* shows a high level of conservation in both sequence and overall gene content in comparison to other *Chlamydiaceae*. The 1,144,377 bp genome contains 961 predicted coding sequences, 842 of which are conserved with those of *Chlamydophila caviae* and *C.pneumoniae*. In *C.abortus* several regions of variation have been identified which in code highly variable protein families responsible for tissue tropism (Thomson *et al.*, 2005). There is much RNA in the reticulate but little in elementary bodies. In the reticulate body, electron dense material is fairly uniformly dispersed throughout the cell interior whereas in the elementary body it is like a compact nucleoid. Reticulate bodies transport adenosine triphosphate (ATP) into cells and adenosine diphosphate (ADP) out of cells. In the presence of ATP, peptides are synthesized.

Chlamydiae is recognized world wide including some parts of India such as H.P. Mostly *C.psittaci* has been reported, however, it may have been *C.pecorum*. Host species predilection is related to immunotypes and DNA endonuclease digestion pattern. *Chlamydiae* infect the mucous membrane of the respiratory and gastrointestinal tracts of many normal animals including avian species. The organisms (elementary bodies) are shed in secretions and feces in small numbers from asymptomatic animals, which constitute significant reservoirs of infection. *Chlamydiae* can survive for long periods in soil and feces.

Pastures and the environment are generally contaminated by vaginal discharges, placenta and aborted fetuses. Inhalation and ingestion of the infective bodies are the common route of acquiring the infection. There are evidences that arthropod borne infections may take place. Avian Chlamydiosis (Psittacosis) is manifested in a latent, sub acute or chromic form. The respiratory and digestive tracts are affected and the infections become systemic. Signs of avian disease include ocular and nasal discharges, conjunctivitis, weakness and nasal discharge, sinusitis, conjunctivitis, weakness and loss of condition. At necropsy there may be serofibrinous polyserositis, enlargement of spleen and liver and characteristic multifocal necrosis of the spleen and liver. Large intracytoplasmic basophilic inclusions may be seen in infected tissue.

In both animals and birds, the severity of the disease may vary from clinically in apparent infection to serve systemic infections. An asymptomatic carrier state is now thought to be a common sequel, if infection is not properly treated. The organisms are transmitted from animals to birds and vice-versa. Transmission from animals to wild life also occurs in some cases (Lemus *et al.*, 2010).

Enzootic abortion of ewes has been recognized for a century but the causal agent was not identified as *Chlamydiae* until 1950 (Stamp *et al.*, 1950). Abortion occurs sporadically in cattle and rarely in other species. The ovine abortion strain (Immunotype I) of *C.psittaci* produces abortion or weak young in sheep, goats and cattle and a few cases of abortion in human beings. Ewes abort typically late in pregnancy without premonitory signs or after effects except for a vulvar discharge and occasionally retained placenta. Bovine abortion follow similar pattern. Most of intestinal isolates from sheep and goats are Immuno-type 2 (poly arthritis- conjunctivitis).

Sporadic bovine encephalomyelitis (SBE) is a febrile disease predominantly of young cattle producing locomotor, postural and behavioral disturbances. There may be mild cough, nasal discharge and diarrhea.

Clinical intestinal infections are seen in young calves and may be phases of systemic Chlamydiosis (SBE, polyarthritis).

Chlamydial polyarthritis involves synovial tissues of most joints of the lambs. Affected lambs exhibit various clinical signs characterized by stiffness, lameness and anorexia. Polyarthritis is caused by immunotype 2 of *C.pecorum*. Morbidity may go upto 80% but the mortality rate is less than 1%.

Highly virulent strains can cause death in turkeys (Grimes and Wyrick 1991). These Chlamydiae strains occasionally cause disease in chickens, pigeons or sparrow. Human infections have been observed. Chlamydiosis is a common, chronic infection of psittacine birds and pigeons characterized by enteritis, airsacculitis, pneumonitis and hepatosplenomegaly. Clinical signs include conjunctivitis, blepharitis and rhinitis. Onset of the disease is insidious and may occur weeks after exposure. Egg production is dropped. Severity varies with strain virulence. Morbidity may range from 5% to 80% whereas mortality may vary from 1% to 30%.

Pathogenesis

The virulence factors of the Chlamydiae comprise of Lipopolysaccharide (LPS) that stimulates inflammatory responses by the host that can lead to endotoxic shock in animals and man. Lipid A of LPS possess endotoxic properties.

Another virulence attribute of the Chlamydiae is the production of CPAF (Chlamydiae protease- or proteasome – like activity factor). This factor enables the bacteria to escape T cell recognition thus permits the bacteria to complete its life cycle repeatedly within the host. CPAF degrades the host transcription factor associated with the production of major histocompatability complex molecules.

Chlamydiae also possess type III secretion apparatus which provides a "pore" in the vacuole membrane and allows the transport of products into the cytosol of host cells. Toxins have not been demonstrated.

The *Chlamydiae* have a predilection for epithelial cells. The EB attach to and are endocytosed by epithelial cells, where they multiply due to somewhat altered phagolysosomal fusion by trafficking to endosomes that do not readily fuse to lysosomes. Most probably the prevention of acidification of endosomes has this effect. Researches have shown that live *Chlamydia* prevents acidification (Andersen 1993). Synthesis of host DNA, RNA and protein ceases and cells eventually disintegrate through host enzyme action. Microbial toxicity and tissue damage elicit inflammatory response.

The placental and fetal infections in ruminants in characterized by abortion during the last week of gestation. Animals acquire the infection through ingestion or inhalation of the causative organism, including sheep showing placental infections. It has been suggested that the infection is first established in tonsils of sheep. (Jones and Andersen, 1988) from where it is disseminated hematogenously to various organs. Then a low grade of infection is caused due to persistent *Chlamydiae* in a latent form. In *C.abortus* infection placenta is involved resulting in tissue damage & inflammation. Placental infection usually becomes established between 60 to 90 days of infection. The cells then migrate to from the placenta to fetus resulting in abortion. *Chlamydiae* in the material circulation have a direct content with the chorionic epithelium resulting in information of hematomas.

Some unexplained endocrinological or related immune relate changes may play a significant role in the formation of hematomas (Buxton *et al.*, 1990). The initial lesions in the placenta involve the limbus of the placentomas in the hilar region, where chlamydiae inclusions are seen in the trophoblast (Buxton *et al.*, 1990). With the progression of the infection involving loss of the cotyledonary and intercotyledonary placental epithelial cells, a mixed cell inflammatory reaction develops. This is followed by the development of purulent arteritis in the thickened placental mesenchyme underlying the lesions. During the later stage severe necrosis and sloughing of the endometrial epithelium occur. Secondary infection involves infection of the fetus, in which necrotic foci are present in most fetal organs and tissues. Characteristic lesions are multifocal cotyledonary necrosis and red brown intercotyledonary exudates. The popliteal and mesenteric lymph nodes are enlarged. In enzootic abortion of sheep caused by *Chlamydophila abortus*, the organism replicates in trophoblast cells leading to their destruction and dissemination of the organisms to the fetal organs. The amniotic and allantoic fluid of affected ewes contains immunoglobulins (IgG) directed against outer membrane protein and macrophage infectivity potentiator protein (Marques *et al.*, 2010). Intracellular *Chlamydial* infections are controlled by TC (H) 1- type CD4 (+ve) T cells in bovine. Indoleamine 2, 3-dioxygenase is expressed in the placenta to prevent immunological rejection of semiallogeneic fetus (Entrican *et al.*, 2010).

The polyarthritis – polyserositis in ruminants is acquired through ingestion or parenterally. The subsequent multiplication results in diarrhea and Chlamydemia. The organisms are subsequently distributed throughout the body including joints. There is joint enlargement with accumulation of synovial fluid. In severe cases, tendon sheaths may contain excessive fluids (Andersen 1993).

During the Chlamydial infection the immune response develop resulting in high level of antibodies directed against lipopolysaccharide and other antigens. The protective antibodies are thought to be directed against the major serovar specific outer membrane protein. Many such proteins are of high molecular weight (Cavenini *et al.*, 1991).

Laboratory Diagnosis

For diagnosis of enzootic abortion of sheep and goats, examination of placenta and fetus (es) is carried out by fluorescent antibody staining. Modified Ziehl Neelsen, Giemsa or Gimenez staining is also carried out. Isolation of Chlamydia is attempted using chicken eggs or cell cultures (L-cells). Characteristic large intra-cytoplasmic inclusions are seen in cell culture. Decontamination of suspected feces, placentas, urine, semen and conjunctival fluid can be accomplished by treatment with combination of gentamicin (50mg/ml), vancomycin (75 mg/ml) and nystatin (500 units/ml). With tissue cultures, centrifugation of the inoculum onto the monolayer is beneficial. Eggs are inoculated into the yolk sac and candled daily thereafter. Yolk sac of embryos dying 3 or more days after inoculation are examined for Chlamydial inclusion. Serological diagnosis can be carried out by complement fixation test (CFT) or ELISA. A four fold rise in antibody types between paired serum samples is indicative of the ongoing infection.

Chlamydophila abortus infection can be diagnosed using an outer membrane antigen based ELISA. The CFT lacks sensitivity and specificity because of cross reactivity with many gram-negative bacteria (Longbottom *et al.*, 2002).

An ELISA to differentiate between *C.abortus* and *C.pecorum* in ewes has been described (Longbottom *et al.*, 2002). The impression smears of stained tissues stained by Giemsa and Gimenez procedure is effective for diagnosis of *C.psittaci* infection. ELISA based kits are available for antigen detection in feces. They are sensitive and specific but false positives are encountered. Paired serum samples from *C.psittaci* affected birds may be subjected to complement fixation, latex agglutination and ELISA procedure for detecting rise in antibody titres.

For disease involving brain (sporadic bovine encephalomyelitis) of cattle, smears, culture and histo-pathological examination of brain samples from affected and non affected cattle from same herd is used. The finding of Chlamydia from characteristic lesions is highly presumptive. The characteristic histopathological changes which include a purulent inflammation of the meninges and parenchyma of the brain, is also indicative.

A four fold increase in titer of paired serum samples in the complement fixation test is highly suggestive of the occurrence of the disease. A moderate to high titer in a sick or recovered animal with low or negative titers in an affected titres supports a diagnosis of the sporadic bovine encephamyelitis. A definitive diagnosis depends on the isolation and identification of the causative organism (*Chlamydophila pecorum*).

Infections caused by members of the Chlamydiaceae family have long been underestimated due to the requirement of special laboratory facilities for the detection of this group of intracellular pathogens. Furthermore, new studies of this group of intracellular pathogens have revealed that host specificity of different species is not as clear as recently believed. As most members of the genus Chlamydophila have shown to be transmissible from animals to humans, sensitive and fast detection methods are required. In this study, SYBR green-based real-time assays were developed that detect all members of Chlamydiaceae and differentiate the most prevalent veterinary Chlamydophila species: *Cp. psittaci, Cp. abortus, Cp. felis,* and *Cp. caviae*. By adding bovine serum albumin to the master mixes, target DNA could be detected directly in crude lysates of enzymatically digested conjunctival or pharyngeal swabs or tissue specimens from heart, liver, and spleen without further purification. The assays were evaluated on veterinary specimens where all samples were screened using a family-specific PCR, and positive samples were further tested using species-specific PCRs. *Cp. psittaci* was detected in 47 birds, *Cp. felis* was found in 10 cats, *Cp. caviae* was found in one guinea pig, and Cp. abortus was detected in one sheep. The screening assay appeared more sensitive than traditional microscopical examination of stained tissue smears. By combining a fast, robust, and cost-effective method for sample preparation with a highly sensitive family-specific PCR, the authors were able to screen for *Chlamydiaceae* in veterinary specimens and confirm the species in positive samples with additional PCR assays (Nordentoft *et al.*, 2011)

Using a species specific real time PCR all *Chlamydophila* and *Chlamydia* spp. could be identified in animals (Pantchev *et al.*, 2010). *Chlamydophila psittaci* species specific and genus-specific PCRs targeting the rDNA ribosomal spacer and OMP gene have been described (Geens *et al.*, 2005). The PCR have been reported to be useful in detection of pathogens in turkeys.

Treatment and Control

Tetracycline has been the drug of choice in the treatment of Chlamydial infection. Tylosin at high dose level is effective if administered early in the disease. Administration in carried out for 2-3 weeks. Sulfonamides are also effective for *Chlamydia trachomatis* as these organisms synthesize their own folic acid from the host cells. In contrast *Chlamydophila psittaci* required preformed folic acid and thus is not inhibited by sulfonamides.

Penicillin treatment may give rise to the development of intracellular spheroblasts and therefore not recommended for the treatment. In birds, flock treatment involves incorporating the drug in feed. Moderate doses (200g/ ton) are adequate for disease control in turkey. To limit outbreaks of the disease in ewes, intramuscular inoculations (20mg/kg) of long acting antibiotics are given at 2 week intervals. Tetracycline is given orally to lambs (150 to 200 mg/kg) to prevent arthritis. For pet birds, tetracycline - containing millet (0.5mg/kg) is available in some countries.

Vaccines composed of killed organisms (formalin treated) have been available for some years to prevent abortions in ewes and goats. The addition of adjuvants in the vaccine improves the efficacy of the vaccine. A subcellular vaccine (major outer membrane protein) for ovine abortion has provided good protection (Tan *et al.*, 1990). This vaccine reduces immune response to LPS which is not related to the protection. A live attenuated vaccine for feline pneumonitis in cats is available. The vaccine reduces or eliminates clinical signs but do not prevent infection. Therapeutic vaccinatio against *C.abortus* and *C.pecorum* induced mastitis in cattle has been tested and found to hold potential for temporary improvement of Chlamydial disease (BiesenKamp *et al.*, 2007). Vaccination against *C.psittaci* infections provides variable results. Vaccine for avian Chlamydiosis is not available.

Vaccination is the best approach for controlling the spread of chlamydial infections, in animal and human populations. The ultimate goal of vaccine research is to develop efficacious vaccines that induce sterile, long-lasting, heterotypic protective immune responses. To date, the greatest success has been in developing whole organism based killed or live attenuated vaccines against the animal pathogens Chlamydophila abortus and Chlamydophila felis. However, similar approaches have proved unsuccessful in combating human chlamydial infections. More recently, emphasis has been placed on the development of subunit or multicomponent vaccines, as cheaper, safer and more stable alternatives. Central to this is a need to identify candidate vaccine antigens, which is being aided by the sequencing of representative genomes of all of the chlamydial species. In addition, it is necessary to identify suitable adjuvants and develop methods for antigen delivery that are capable of eliciting mucosal and systemic cellular and humoral immune responses. DNA vaccination in particular holds much promise, particularly in terms of safety and stability, although it has so far been less effective in humans and large animals than in mice. Thus, much research still needs to be done to improve the delivery of plasmid DNA, as well as the expression and presentation of antigens to ensure that effective immune responses are induced.

The protective effect of DNA vaccination with the gene encoding the major outer-membrane protein (MOMP) of *Chlamydophila abortus* has been studied in non-pregnant and pregnant mouse models after chlamydial challenge (Hechard *et al.*, 2003). OF1 outbred mice were vaccinated intramuscularly three times every 3 weeks, mated and challenged with C. abortus 2 weeks after the last injection of DNA. In non-pregnant mice, the MOMP DNA vaccine elicited a specific humoral response with predominantly IgG2a antibodies, suggesting a Th1-type immune response. The induced antibodies showed no in vitro neutralizing effect on *C. abortus* infectivity. Moreover, immunization with the momp gene showed no reduction in the mean splenic bacterial counts of non-pregnant or pregnant mice or in the mean placental bacterial counts of pregnant mice after the *C. abortus* challenge. Nevertheless, the MOMP DNA immunization induced a non-specific and partial protection in fetuses against challenge. The immunogenicity and protective effect of a DNA vaccine encoding the heat-shock protein (Hsp) GroEL of *Chlamydophila abortus* AB7, an obligate intracellular bacterium that causes abortion in sheep, was evaluated in pregnant and non-pregnant mouse models. The C. abortus groEL gene was cloned by screening a genomic library constructed in lambdaFIX II arms with a nucleic acid probe corresponding to the central portion of the groEL gene from C. *abortus*. Sequence analysis of a positive clone revealed an open reading frame of 1632 bp encoding a 544 amino acid polypeptide with a predicted molecular mass of 58 256 Da and highly similar to GroEL of *Chlamydia trachomatis* (93%) and *Chlamydophila pneumoniae* (94%). As observed in other sequenced chlamydial genomes, the groEL gene belongs to an operon comprising another gene encoding the Hsp GroES. OF1 outbred mice were immunized intramuscularly with plasmid DNA carrying the groEL gene three times at 3 week intervals and challenged 2 weeks after the last DNA injection. In pregnant mice, no reduction in abortion was observed and the DNA vaccination failed to reduce the bacterial infection in the placenta and spleen of mice. Nevertheless, partial protection of fetuses was obtained. Immunization of non-pregnant mice with the groEL gene resulted in a specific humoral response with the predominant IgG2a isotype, suggesting a Th1-type immune response. The anti-GroEL antibodies showed no neutralizing effect *in vitro* on C. abortus infectivity. Although the DNA vaccine induced a delayed-type hypersensitivity response, it failed to elicit an efficient cellular immune response since the mice were not protected against bacterial challenge (Hechard *et al.*, 2004).

Chlamydophila abortus is the causative agent of abortion in pigs and pregnant women. Seroconversion rates were arranged from 11% to 80% in piglets and sows in China. These very high rates illustrate the scale of the problem in China and highlight the urgent need for the development of a C. abortus vaccine. An efficacious anti-chlamydial vaccine should induce not only strong mucosal and systemic T-helper type 1 (Th1) immune response but also give a humoral response that enhances Th1 activation following infection. In order to evaluate an active immune response of a combination of the major outer membrane protein (MOMP) DNA- and protein-based vaccines, 54 BALB/c mice were randomly assigned to six groups and inoculated intramuscularly with: (i) 100 microg pcDNA::MOMP, (ii) 10 microg r-MOMP, (iii) primed with 100 microg pcDNA::MOMP and boosted with 10 microg r-MOMP, (iv) primed-boosted with a combination of pcDNA::MOMP and r-MOMP simultaneously, (v) live-attenuated 1B vaccine, (vi) 100 microg pcDNA3.1 vector. All animals were vaccinated two times at 14 days intervals. Results showed that mice given DNA and r-MOMP induced higher antibody levels, higher T cells proliferation and an elevated level of chlamydial clearance in spleen, which was equivalent to the clearance of 1B vaccine. Mice administrated the DNA-primed/MOMP-boosted approach elicited moderate antibody levels, less T-lymphocyte proliferation and lower chlamydial clearance as compared with 1B vaccine. Co-immunization with DNA- and r-MOMP vaccine may provide novel ways for active immunization strategy against swine *C. abortus* (Zhang *et al.*, 2009).

A bacteriophage-delivered DNA vaccine against *Chlamydophila abortus* was constructed by cloning a eukaryotic cassette containing the ompA gene (which expresses the Major Outer Membrane Protein) into a bacteriophage lambda vector Ling *et al.*, 2011). Four groups, each of 20 BALB/c mice were inoculated separately with the phage vaccine, a conventional DNA vaccine based on the same ompA expression cassette, a live attenuated vaccine (strain 1B) or the empty phage vector. The phage and DNA vaccines and empty phage vector were administered intramuscularly on days 0, 14 and 28; the attenuated vaccine was given once on day 0. Half the animals in each group were challenged on day 42 by intraperitoneal injection of live C. abortus and sacrificed on day 49. Phage-vaccinated mice developed moderate antibody levels against *C. abortus* and yielded higher levels of IFN-γ and IL-2 compared with the attenuated live vaccine group. Clearance of chlamydiae from spleens was significantly better in the attenuated vaccine group compared with the phage vaccine group, while both groups were significantly superior to the DNA vaccine and control groups ($p<0.01$). Although levels of protection in the mouse model were lower in phage-vaccinated animals, than in 1B vaccinated animals, phage vaccines offer several other advantages, such as easier handling and safety, potentially cheaper production and no chance of reversion to virulence. Although these are preliminary results in a model system, it is possible that with further optimisation immunization with phage vaccines may provide a novel way to improve protection against *C. abortus* infection and trials in large animals are currently being initiated.

Prompt disposal of infected material and segregation of affected animals is helpful in control of ovine abortion. Young turkey poults should be placed in clean quarters, with no access to infected droppings and unexposed to potentially contaminated air currents.

References

Andersen, A.A. 1993. *Chlamydia*. In pathogenesis of Bacterial Infections in Animals. Pp. 312-320. Ed. C.A. Gyles and C.O. Thoen. Ames: IOWA State University Press, USA.

Biesenkemp - Uhe, C., Li Y; Hehnen, H.R., Sachse, K. and Kaltenboeck, B. 2007. Therapeutic *Chlamydophila abortus* and *C.pecorum* vaccination transiently reduces bovine mastitis associated with *Chlamydophila* infection. Infect. Immun. **75:** 870-877.

Buxton, D., Barlow, R.M., Finlayson, J., Anderson, I.E. and MacKellar, A. 1990. Observations on the pathogenesis of *Chlamydia psittaci* infection of pregnant sheep. J. Comp. Pathol. **102:** 221-237.

Canenini, R., Donati, M., Brocchi, E., Desimone, F. and LaPlaca, M. 1991. Partial characterization of an 89 kDa highly immunoreactive protein from *Chlamydia psittaci* Ap-2 causing ovine abortion. Fed. Eur. Microbiol. Soc. **81:** 111-116.

Chahota, R., Ogawa, H., Mitsuhashi, Y., Ohyak, Yamaguchi, T., Fukushi, H. 2006. Genetic diversity and epizootiology ot *Chlamydophila psittacii* prevalent among the captive and feral avian species based on VD 2 region of ompA gene. Microbiol. Immunol. **50:** 663-678.

Entrican, G., Wattegedera, S., Wheelhouse, N., Allan, A. and Rocchi, M. 2010. Immunological paradigm and the pathogenesis of ovine *Chlamydial abortion*. Am. J. Reprod. Immunol. **64:** 287-294.

Geens, T., Dewitte, A., Boon, N. and Vanrompay, D. 2005. Development of *Chlamydophila psittaci* species-specific and genotype specific real time PCR. Vet. Res. **36:** 787-797.

Grimes, J.D. and Wyrick, P.B. 1991. *Chlamydiosis* (ornithosis). In Diseases of poultry, 9th Ed. Ed. B.W. Calnek, H.J. Barves, C.W. Beard, W.M. Reid and H.W. Joder, Jr. Ames: IOWA State University Press, USA.

Héchard C., Grépinet O., Rodolakis A..2003.Evaluation of protection against *Chlamydophila abortus* challenge after DNA immunization with the major outer-membrane protein-encoding gene in pregnant and non-pregnant mice. J. Med. Microbiol. **52**(Pt 1): 35-40.

Héchard C., Grépinet O. and Rodolakis A.2004.Molecular cloning of the *Chlamydophila abortus* groEL gene and evaluation of its protective efficacy in a murine model by genetic vaccination.J. Med. Microbiol. **53**(Pt 9): 861-8.

Jones, G.E. and Anderson, I.E. 1988. *Chlamydia psittaci* : Is tonsillar tissue the portal of entry in ovine enzootic abortion? Res. Vet. Sci. **44:** 260-61.

Lemus, J.A., Fargallo, J.A., Vergara, P., Parejo, D., and Banda, E. 2010. Natural cross *Chlamydial* infection between livestock and free living bird species. PLOS one. 5:ref. 13512.

Ling Y., Liu W., Clark J.R., March J.B., Yang J. and He C.2011.Protection of mice against Chlamydophila abortus infection with a bacteriophage-mediated DNA vaccine expressing the major outer membrane protein. Vet. Immunol. Immunopathol. 2011 Aug 9.[http://www.ncbi.nlm.nih.gov/pubmed/21872342]

Longbottom, D., Fairley, S., Champan, S., Psarrou, E., Vreton, E. and Livingstone, M. 2002. Serological diagnosis of ovine enzootic abortion by enzyme linked immunosorbant assay with a recombinant protein fragment of the polymorphic outer membrane protein POMP90 of *Chlamydophila abortus*. J. Clin. Microbiol. **40:** 4235-4243.

Marques, P.X., O'Donovan, J., Souda, P., Gutierrez, J., Williams, E.J., Worrall, S., McElroy, M., Proctor, A., Brady, C., Sammin, D., Basset, H., White legge, J.P., Markey, B.K. and Nally, J.E. 2010. Amniotic and allantoic fluid from experimentally infected sheep contain immunoglobulin specific for *Chlamydophila abortus*. Vet. Immunol. Immunopathol, 13 (http://www.ncbi.nlm.nih.gov/pubmed/ 21126774).

Nordentoft S., Kabell S. and Pedersen K. 2011.Real-Time Detection and Identification of *Chlamydophila* Species in Veterinary Specimens by Using SYBR Green-Based PCR Assays. Appl. Environ. Microbiol. **77:** 6323-6330. Epub 2011 Jul 15.

Pantchev, A., Sting, R., Bauerfeind, R., Tyczka, J. and Sachse, K. 2010. Detection of all *Chlamydophila* and *Chlamydia* spp. of veterinary interest using species- specific real-time PCR assay. Comp. Immunol. Microbiol. Infect. Dis. **33:** 473-484.

Stamp, J.T., McEwen, A.D., Watt, J.A.A. and Nisbet, D.J. 1950. Enzootic abortion in ewes I. Transmission of the disease. Vet. Rec. **62:** 251-254.

Tan, T.W., Herring, A.J., Anderson, I.E. and Jone, G.E. 1990. Protection of sheep against *Chlamydia psittaci* infection with a subcellular vaccine containing the major outer membrane protein. Infect. Immun. **58:** 3101-3108.

Thomson, N.R., Yeats, C., Bellk, Holdn, M.T., Bently, S.D., Livingstone, M. and Cerdeno-Tarraga, A.M. 2005. The *Chlamydophila abortus* gene sequence reveal an array of variable proteins that contribute to interspecies variation. Genome Res. **15:** 629-640.

Zhang F., Li S., Yang J., Yang L. and He C. 2009.Induction of a protective immune response against swine *Chlamydophila abortus* infection in mice following co-vaccination of omp-1 DNA with recombinant MOMP. Zoonoses Public Health. **56:** 71-76. Epub 2008 Aug 20.

□□□

Chapter 23

Q Fever

Dr. S.K. SRIVASTAVA
Former, Division of Bacteriology & Mycology
Indian Veterinary Research Institute, Izatnagar-243122
Bareilly (U.P.)

Q fever, an important global occupational zoonotic problem has a worldwide distribution with notable exception of New Zealand (Hilbink *et al.,* 1993 and Norlander, 2000). The disease is also known as query fever, abattoir fever, Nine-mile fever, coxiellosis and Burnet's rickettsiosis. 'Q fever' or 'query fever' was first recognized as a new clinical entity as a result of study of an outbreak of febrile disease among abattoir workers in Brisbane, Australia in 1935. The organism was later isolated from Derrick's patients by Burnet and Freeman. In 1938, these organisms were named as *Coxiella burnetii.* Presently, the infection is endemic in many areas and its prevalence has been confirmed in at least 51 countries including India. The available reports indicate wide prevalence of Q fever infection among man and animals in India (Malik and Yadav, 2002).

Global scenario

Occurrence in man: Human coxiellosis appears in the form of sporadic cases or outbreaks. The human infection is often asymptomatic, and its mild form can be mistaken for other febrile diseases. Q. fever is usually benign, but mortality occurs in 1 to 11% of patients with chronic Q. fever (Raoult, 1990). It has been estimated that the patients persistently infected with *C.burnetii* will develop chronic Q fever in 1-16% of reported patients worldwide (Siegman-Igra *et al.,* 1997), which is most commonly endocarditis, but can also manifest as an infection of vascular grafts or aneurysms, osteomyelitis, or hepatitis. In southern France, 5 to 8% of cases of endocarditis are due to *Coxiella burnetii* (Tissot-Dupont *et al.*, 1994).

Occurrence in animals: Infection in domestic animals is usually chronic, dormant but it may cause abortions in sheep and goats (Lang, 1990), and in cattle usually along with infertility and other reproductive problems (To *et al.*, 1998). The infection has been found in almost all species of domestic animals and many wild animals, including birds. Serological surveys conducted in endemic areas have revealed a sizable proportion of reactors in the bovine, ovine and a caprine population.

Indian scenario

Pasricha was the first to suspect the occurrence of Q fever in India (Kumar *et al.*, 1981). Extensive serosurveys and isolation studies conducted in the past, mostly in the animals clearly indicated that high prevalence of this infection in human and animal populations in different states, with notable high prevalence in Punjab, Haryana, Rajasthan, UP, M.P. and Karnataka (Malik and Yadav, 2002). The seroprevalence studies conducted in the country have shown the disease to be widely prevalent among human beings (2.7-26%) and domestic animals namely sheep (6.2-14.41%), goats (14.26-17.5%), cattle (14-98%), buffalo (14.5-15.22%), equines (20.1%), swine (14.67%), dog (16%) and poultry (11.87%). Moreover, the antibodies against the agent has also been detected in the milk of humans (3.09% &, 14.37%) and animals cow (8.54%), buffalo (5.68%) and goat (10.16%) (Malik *et al.*, 2000).

Occurrence in Man: In India, the first confirmed human case has been reported way back in 1954 (Anderson and Kalra, 1954, Acha *et al.*, 2003). The first outbreak of Q fever in India was recorded among Gurkhas stationed at Dehradun. A possibility of human milk as a source of Q fever infection in breastfed Indian babies became evident when 5 out of 97 (5.2%) samples of human milk were found to be positive either for *C.burnetii* and/or its antibody by capillary agglutination test (CAT) (Kumar *et al.*, 1981). The isolation of *C.burnetii* from aborted human placenta by specific seroconversion in guinea pigs was first reported in India by Prasad *et al.*, (1986), who also detected antibodies against the agent in 14.37% of 153 human milk samples by CAT.

Occurrence in Animals: Among the animals, cattle, sheep, goats and equines seem to serve as major reservoir of the infection. The excretion of *C.burnetii* in the milk of domestic animals has also been recorded in India (Sethi *et al.*, 1978). Serological investigations have indicated that *C.burnetii* infection is endemic among domestic animals in India (Malik and Yadav, 2002). The sero-reactors to *Coxiella burnetii* were noticed to be highest (17.51%) in goats followed by buffaloes (14.54), sheep (6.25%) and none in case of dogs in Bareilly

(UP) and Delhi region (Kumar *et al.*, 1999). In India, 1.2% of 342 birds and 14.3% of 91 wild land animals tested were positive for *C. burnetii* (Yadav and Sethi, 1980). In view of the detection of antibodies against *C.burnetii* in several species of birds (Rarotra *et al.*, 1978), the free living birds could play some role in the epidemiology of Q fever as they frequently visit human as well as animal habitats. With the isolation of pathogen from rodents, insectivores, poikilotherms and a python, the involvement of these species as reservoirs of *C.burnetii* has been reported in India (Yadav and Sethi, 1980).

Etiology

Coxiella burnetii is a gram-negative obligate intracellular bacterium, highly pleomorphic coccobacillus (0.2 to 0.4 μm wide, 0.4 to 1.0 μm long). The casual agent is widely found in nature and responsible for infection in humans, domestic and wild animals, pets, birds, poikilotherms and arthropods. The economic losses due to *C.burnetii* infection in farm animals may be associated with abortions and the birth of dead or weak offspring.

C.burnetii, like *Chlamydia,* has a complex life cycle with at least two forms; a metabolically active large cell variant (LCV) comparable to the *Chlamydia* sp. Reticulate body and a spore-like small cell variant (SCV) comparable to the *Chlamydia* sp. elementary body. Unlike *Chlamydia,* both cell forms are infectious. Further, the SCV (or another resilient form) can survive in the environment outside a host for years while remaining infectious, and is small enough to be carried and dispersed for miles by wind. The disease is manly transmitted through infectious aerosols and it has been estimated that even a single organism can cause the disease.

Source of Infection and Mode of Transmission:

In **human infections**, the most commonly identified sources are farm animals, especially cattle, goats and sheep (Lang, 1990; Raoult and Marrie, 1995; Maurin and Raoult, 1999) shedding large quantities of infectious agent into the environment during on abortion or normal delivery, not only in the birth fluids, placenta and fetal membranes but also in the urine and faeces (McQuiston and Childs, 2002). Therefore, in man, the most important route of infection is thought to be through the inhalation of aerosols that have been contaminated with the products of parturition of infected animals (Tissot-Dupont and Raoult, 1993). In abattoir, aerosols are generated by the handling fetuses, placentas, uteruses, hide and wool. It has been estimated that 1 gram of infected placental tissue can contain as many as one billion organisms (Welsh *et al.*, 1985). According to a recent report, the sexual transmission of Q. fever occurred in a man with occupationally acquired Q fever to his wife (Millazzo *et al.*, 2001). Although *C.burnetii* was originally isolated from ticks and has been identified in at least 40 species of ticks (Lee *et al.*, 2004; Maurin and Raoult, 1999), the role ticks play in transmission of the agent to animals is not completely defined and tick transmission to humans is rare. Humans have also been infected by eating contaminated milk products (Fishbein and Raoult, 1992).

In animals, two cycles of infection are distinguished in nature; one in domestic animals (mainly cattle, sheep and goat) and the other in natural foci, where the agents circulates between wild animals and their ectoparasites, especially ticks. The domestic animals are the main reservoirs responsible for transmission of the agent to human (Nolander, 2000). The most common mode by which the infection is transmitted between domestic animals is through the inhalation of aerosols from contaminated placental material, amniotic fluid and excreta. The placenta of the infected animals can contain as much as 10^9g of the causative agent, which can be transported long distances via inert material. Because of the strong resistance, the agent can be isolated from soil as log as six months after infected animals have left the area. New foci of infection are created when an infected animals joins a disease-free herd. *C. burnetii* was found in 57 bulls semen used for A.I. (Kruszewska and Tylewska-Wierzbanowska, 1997).

Infection caused by *C.burnetii* in animals is usually asymptomatic. Clinical signs of acute infection, including fever, loss of appetite, mild cough, rhinitis and rapid respiration rate, have been reported in sheep experimentally inoculated with *C.burnetii*, but these signs are non-specific, and they have not been described in natural infections (Belchev and Pavlov, 1997 and Martinov *et al.*, 1989). The symptoms are visible at birth of full-term dead or weak, lower weight offspring (Berri *et al.*, 2000, Ho *et al.*, 1995, Martinov *et al.*, 1989, Moeller, 2001, Palmer *et al.*, 1983; To *et al.*, 1998). Abortions typically occur over a 2 to 4 week period and may affect 5 to 50% of the flock. In a study Q fever was reported to cause in 9 percent (19 cases) of the abortions (Moeller, 2001). Most of the abortions occurred in the last trimester of pregnancy or near term. Goats naturally infected with *C.burnetii* may abort without apparent clinical signs, but anorexia and depression for 1 to 2 days before abortions have been observed. In some affected does there is placental retention for 2 to 5 days, and agalactia may occur within 1 week of abortion (Waldham *et al.*, 1978). In cattle, *C.burnetii* has been implicated as the cause of fertility problems, including abortions and increased frequency of return to service (Sting *et al.*, 2000; To *et al.*, 1998). Both dogs and cats may have weak or stillborn offspring as a result of *C.burnetii* infection (Buhariwala *et al.*, 1996; Marrie *et al.*, 1988a).

Pathogenesis

Cows, goats and sheep are generally infected with *C.burnetii*. *C. burnetii* infected animals usually do not experience symptomatic infection. The organisms enter the blood in the acute phase and subsequently the organisms can be demonstrated in blood, lungs, spleen and liver. Fever may or may not develop *C.burnetii* infection often becomes chronic with persistent shedding of *C.burnetii* in feces and urine. In such chronic infections, uterus and mammary glands are primary sites of infection (Babudieri 1959). Organisms are also shed in the milk of cows, sheep and goats, cows remain asymptomatic however, in goats abortions may be evident. The shedding of *C.burnetii* into the environment occurs mainly during parturition. Placenta is heavily contaminated. Abortions are common in cattle, sheep and goats (Waldham *et al.*, 1978; Palmer *et al.*, 1983). The route of infection, the inoculating dose, the bacterial strain and several host factors may determine the pathogenesis. In animals, cardiac valve defect, immuno-suppression or pregnancy may encourage the development of infection.

C.burnetii infection may be induced in a number of laboratory animals, including mice, rats, rabbits, guinea pigs and monkeys. The infection in laboratory animals may be totally asymptomatic, induce fever and granuloma formation or be fatal especially when heavy *C.burnetii* inocula are used.

T. cell immunity is effective in containing the infection but not completely, thus many animals develop chronic infection. The intracellular survival of *C.burnetii* and establishment of persistent infection probably correspond to subversion of microbicidal functions of macrophages as well as impairment of T-cell immune response (Mege *et al.*, 1997). During natural infection *C.burnetii* resists the killing action of monocytes-macrophages by producing superoxide dismutase and catalase. Surprisingly, virulent phase 1 *C.burnetii* strongly stimulates the synthesis of tumor necrosis factor (TNF) by human monocytes (Capo *et al.*, 1996), thereby enhancing the microbicidal activity of infected monocytes. TNF-α may also enhance ingestion of the poorly internalized phase I *C.burnetii* by monocytes-macrophages by upregulating adhesion receptors on these cells.

Immunocompetent patients with acute Q fever develop a transient bacteremia with *C.burnetii* found inside the circulating monocytes. Such infected monocytes in blood may attach to the damaged endothelial surfaces of valvular tissues leading to colonization of cardiac valves and endocarditis (Mege *et al.*, 1997).

Since few circulating *C.burnetii* infected monocytes are detected during Q fever endocarditis, additional factors are likely to be involved in the pathogenesis of Q fever, including immune complexes which are constant during chronic Q fever.

The *C.burnetii* lipopolysaccharide may contribute to the infection leading to disseminated intravascular coagulation in affected individuals (Athanassopoulou *et al.*, 2011). *C.burnetii* also contains an outer membrane proteins and certain proteins of this OMP might play a role in virulence of the organism. *C.burnetii* exhibit a biphasic development cycle whereby highly resistant small cell variant are generated from large cell variant is considered fundamental to the virulence of *C.burnetii*. Various antigens have been identified in these 2 types of cells which may be important in the pathogenesis and induction of protective immunity in hosts (Coleman *et al.*, 2007).

Diagnosis

Diagnosis of Q fever is complicated by the fact that many acute infections of Q fever are either asymptomatic, mild, or resemble influenza symptoms (Maurin and Raoult, 1999). *C.burnetii* is a biohazard level III zoonotic agent and should be handled very carefully in the laboratory as well as when collecting samples from infected animals.

(a) *Isolation*: The isolation of *C.burnetii* from acute blood or placental tissue requires the inoculation of samples into 6-7 day old embryonated chicken eggs through yolk sac, guinea pigs or mice (Schopf *et al.*, 1991; Spyridaki *et al.*, 1998; To *et al.*, 1998). A number of cells lines can be used for invitro cultures. Animal inoculation is hazardous because animals shed *C.burnetii* in the feces and urine (Raoult, 1990), therefore, extreme care should be taken while handling the infected laboratory animals. The pathogen is best visualized in impression smears of infected yolk sac/ guinea pig spleen stained with Gimenez's stain. If at all required, clinical samples are injected intraperitoneally into guinea pigs which become febrile and are sacrificed 5 to 8 days later. Spleen extracts from infected animals are used for isolation of *C.burnetii*..

(b) *Serological diagnosis*: Serological methods are simple and safe, with most commonly employed methods being capillary agglutination test (CAT), complement fixation test (CFT), fluorescent antibody technique (FAT) and enzyme immunoassay (EIA). Of these, the CAT and CFT show considerable cross reactivity. Antibodies are mostly detected only after 2 to 3 weeks from the onset of the disease. Q fever patients" sera have been reported to show considerable cross-reactivity against *Bartonella hanselae* in more than 50% cases (Scola and Raoult, 1996), *Legionella micdadei* in 34.5% cases (Musso and Raoult, 1997), Chlamydiae (Schopf *et al.*, 1991) and human immunodeficiency virus (Calle *et al.*, 1998). The serological methods are used commonly but lack of standardization, particularly the ELISA may give confounding results. ELISA and micro immunofluorescence test give similar results with cow sera. ELISA is less sensitive in animal than man. Furthermore, *C.burnetii* and *Chlamydia psittaci* mixed infections have been shown to occur in cases of abortion in goats (Schof *et al.*, 1991). Therefore, identification of *C.burnetii* infected animals may require the use of additional confirmatory tests like polymerase chain reaction (PCR). The CFT tests still the OIE reference test inspite of its weaknesses such as weak sensitivity. Moreover, CFT fail to detect recent Q fever infection.

(c) *Detection by PCR*: Of late, PCR has become a useful tool for the detection of *C.burnetii* in biological samples (Yuasa *et al.*, 1996; Lorenz *et al.*, 1998). Specific fragments of *C.burnetii* DNA can be amplified from fresh or frozen samples, including serum, buffy coats, milk, cerebral spinal fluid, bone marrow, placenta, liver, cardiac valve, fetal tissue, vaginal swabs, feces, and other biological specimens. Primers derived from htpAB associated sequence have been employed in a PCR assay for detection of *C.burnetii* in cow's milk (Willems *et al.*, 1994). Further, primers based on a repetitive transposon like element (trans-PCR) proved highly specific and sensitive (Willems *et al.*, 1994). PCR is most useful for detection of shedders. Only PCR allows detection of metritis in ewes (Berri *et al.*, 2000). Vaidya *et al.*, (2000) carried out PCR targeting 1S1111, the repetitive transposon like region of *C.burnetii* and a real time PR for detection of *C.burnetii* in samples collected from women. Both PCR were sensitive than pathogen isolation. The PCR were also specific. A real time PCR has been reported to detect *C.burnetii* in ruminant placenta and aborted fetuses targeting insertion sequence IS IIII gene (Jones *et al.*, 2010).

Treatment & Control

Antibacterial agents such as oxytetracycline, and aureomycin are most effective. Doxycycline remains the preferred antibiotic in the treatment of acute Q fever (Kovacova & Kazar 2002). Erythromycin has been used successfully to treat pneumonia in man, however, reports contrary to this are available in the literature. Penicillin has no inhibitory effect so is the case with chloramphenicol and erythromycin. Rifampicin and ofloxacin are also preferred in certain instances such as acute infections. Recently clarithromycin has been shown to be the most effective macrolide compound against *C.burnetii* strains. For carrying out the antibiotic susceptibility several animal models and cell culture models are used since *C.burnetii* do not grow in artificial media. To test the efficacy of the antibiotic against chronic infections, cell culture models chronically infected with *C.burnetii* are employed. Using this model, antibiotics such as difloxacin, ciprofloxacin, oxolinic acid and rifampin have been found effective. These data do not corroborate with clinical findings. However, clinically, administration of two injection of oxytetracycline (20 mg per kg body weight) during the last month of gestation in ruminants is effective in treating the abortions. In known infected herds administration of tetracycline (8 mg/kg day) prophylactically in the water supply prior to parturition may reduce spread of the organisms.

For control of the disease specific caution must be taken when introducing a new animal into a Q.fever free flock. A serological investigation should be performed in the animals before mixing with the Q.fever free animal. Since parturition is critical for the transmission of the disease, in the infected flocks, birth must take place in a specific location away from the animal housing and the place should be disinfected alongwith the utensils and equipments used. Placentas and fetuses must be picked up and destroyed as soon as possible in order to prevent ingestion by domestic or carnivores. Gloves, boots, masks etc. should be used by the workers.

Pasteurization at 72^{0}C for 15 seconds or sterilization of milk from injected flock is regularly recommended even if the oral route is not the main one. Awareness among the veterinarians, laboratory workers and attendants about the symptoms of the disease is essential. Vaccination of uninfected flocks with an efficient vaccine is useful in controlling the disease (Kovacova and Kazar 2002; Serbezov *et al.,* 1999).

Current vaccines used in humans and animals include formalin- killed whole cell vaccine preparations and chloroform methanol extracted bacterial residue. For preparation of whole cell vaccine bacteria in phase I are used. Adverse reactions with formalin killed vaccine have been observed. This vaccine is also used for vaccinating human beings. In Russia, a live attenuated human vaccine is produced with the attenuated M-44 strain of *C.burnetii* (Freylikhman *et al.,* 2003). The use of vaccine in human is still debated.

In animals formalin killed whole cell phase 1 bacterin has been found to reduce shedding of bacteria in placentas and milk in vaccinated goats ewes and cows following natural infection. However, contradictions are available suggesting that the vaccine can protect only the uninfected animals but is not able to treat infected animals. Goats vaccinated with inactivated vaccine have been found to shed vaccine strain of *C.burnetii* in milk (Hermans *et al.,* 2011). This may jeopardise the control programme based on the detection of the organisms in the milk of vaccinated animals. In contrast the phase II vaccine is not effective in protecting livestock against *C.burnetii* infection (Durand *et al.,* 1993; Arrican *et al.,* 2005). This phase II vaccine fails to prevent human, animal and environmental contaminations. Vaccines can prevent abortion in animals and phase I vaccine must be used to control the disease.

There is no test that allows distinguishing vaccinated animals from animals infected with *C.burnetii.*

Several proteins and lipopolysaccharide have been tested to serve as vaccines against Q.fever. Recombinant fusion proteins have been used but these have not induced significant protection although purified natural proteins may induce full protection in both guinea pigs and mice (Williams *et al.,* 1981; Zhang and Samuel, 2003). New immunodominant antigens have been cloned for development of novel diagnostic assays and subunit vaccines against Q fever (Zhang *et al.,* 2004). These studies, mostly conducted in laboratory animals, have shown that the vaccines allow strong reduction of the shedding of *C.burnetii.*

References

Acha, P.N. and Szytres, B. 2003. Chlamydiosis, Rickettsiosis and Vibriosis. In: Zoonoses and Communicable diseases common to man. 3rd edn. Pan American Health Organization, pp. 16-27.

Anderson, R.K. and Kalra, S.L. 1954. Q. fever studies in India: A case of Q.fever. Indian J. Med. Res., **42:** 307-311.

Arrican- Bouvery, N., Sourian, A., Bodier, C., Dufour, P., Rousset, E. and Rodolakis, S. 2005. Effect of vaccination with phase I and phase II coxiella burnetii vaccines in pregnant goats. Vaccine. **23:** 4392-4402.

Athanassopoulou, P., Liatsos, G., Pirounaki, M., Skounakis, M. and Moulakakis, A. 2011. Disseminated intravascular coagulation as the laboratory hallmark of acute Q. fever. Diagn. Microbiol. Infect. Dis. **69:** 210-212.

Ayres, J.G.; Flint, N., Smith, E.G., Tunnicliffe, W.S., Fletcher, T.J., Hammond, K., Ward, D. and Marmion, B.P. 1998. Post-infection fatigue syndrome following Q.fever. Qjm., **91:** 105-123.

Babudieri, B. 1959. Q.fever: A zoonoses. Adv. Vet. Sci., **5:** 81-182.

Belchev, L. and N. Pavlov. 1997. Histopathology of *Q rickettsiosis* in sheep. Vet. Med. Nauki, **14:** 43-49.

Berri, M., Laroncau, K. and Rodolakis, A. 2000. The detection of *Coxiella burnetii* from ovine genital swabs, milk and fecal samples by the use of a single touch down polymerase chain reaction. Vet. Microbiol. **72:** 285-293.

Berri, M., Laroucau, K. and Rodolakis, A. 2000. The detection of *Coxiella burnetii* from ovine genital swabs, milk and fecal samples by the use of a single touchdown polymerase chain reaction. Vet. Microbiol., **72:** 285-293.

Buhariwalla, F., Cann, B. and Marrie, T.J. 1996. A dog related outbreak of Q.fever. Clin. Infect. Dis., **23:** 753-755.

Calle, De la N., Yebra, M., Portero, F. and Lopez, E. 1998. False positivity of antibodies against immunodeficiency virus in a case of Q. fever. Rev. Clin. Esp. **198:** 401-404.

Capo, C., Zugun, F., Stein, A., Tardei, G., Lepidi, D., Raoult, D. and Mege, J.F. 1996. Upregulation of tumor necrosis factor and interleukin- 1â IN Q. fever endocarditis. Infect. Immun. **64:** 1638-1642.

Coleman, S.A., Fischer, E.R., Cockrell, D.C., Voth, D.E., Howe, D., Mead, D.J., Samuel, J.E. and Heinzen, R.A. 2007. Proteome and antigen profiling of *C.burnetii* developmental forms. Infect. Immun. **75:** 290-298.

Durand, M.P. 1993 [L'excretion lacteeet placentaire de *Coxiella burnetii* agent de la fievre Q, Chez, la vache. Importance et prevention] Bull. Acad. Natl. Med. **177:** 935-945.

Fishbein, D.B. and Raoult, D. 1992. A cluster of *Coxiella burnetii* infection associated with exposure to vaccinated goats and unpasteurized dairy products. Am. J. Troph. Med. Hyg. **47:** 35-40.

Fournier, P. and Raoult, D. 1998. Diagnosis of Q. fever. J. Clin. Microbiol., **36:** 1823-1834.

Freylikhman, O., Tokarevick, N., Suvorov, A., Vorobiova, E. and Totolian, A. 2003. *Coxiella burnetii* persistence in three generations of mice after application of live attenuated human M-44 vaccine against Q. fever. Ann. NY Acad. Sci. **990:** 496-499.

Harris, R.J., Storm, P.A., Lloyd, A., Arens, M. and Marmion, B.P. 2000. Long-term persistence of *Coxiella burnetii* in the host after primary Q.fever. Epid. Infect. **124:** 543-549.

Hermans, M.H., Huijsmans, C.R., Schellekens, J.J., Savelkoul, P.H. and Wever, P.C. 2011. *Coxiella burnetii* DNA in goat milk after vaccination with coxevac Vaccine. Feb. 12 [http://www.ncbi.nlm.nih.gov/pubmed/21320538]

Hilbink, F., Penrose, M., Kovacova, E. and Kazar, J. 1993. A fever is absent from New Zealand. Int. J. Epidemiol. **22:** 945-949.

Ho, T., Htwe, K.K., Yamasaki, N., Zhang, G.Q., Ogawa, M., Yamaguchi, T., Fukushi, H. and Hirai, K. 1995. Isolation of *Coxiella burnetii* from dairy cattle and ticks and some characteristics of the isolates in Japan. Microbiol. Immunol. **39:** 663-671.

Jones, R.M.Twomey, D.F., Hannon, S., Errington, J., Bitchart, G.C. and Sawyer, S. 2010. Detection of *Coxiella burnetii* in placenta and abortion samples from British ruminants using real time PCR. Vet. Rec. **167:** 965-967.

Kovacova, E. and Kazar, J. 2002. Q. fever- still a query and undestimated infectious disease. Acta Virol. **46:** 193-210.

Kruszewska, D. and S. Tylewskawierzbanowska. 1997. Isolation of *Coxiella burnetii* from bull semen. Res. Vet. Sci. **62:** 299-300.

Kumar, A. Yadav, M.P. and Kakkar, S. 1981. Human milk as a source of Q. fever infection in breast-fed babies. Indian J. Med. Res. **73:** 510-512.

Kumar, A., Malik, S.V.S. and Bachhil, V.N. 1999. Seroprevalence of coxeillosis in domestic animals in Bareilly (U.P.) and Delhi. Indian J. Comp. Microbiol. Immunol. Infect. Dis. **20:** 132-133.

Lang, G.H. 1990. Coxiellosis in animals. In: Q.fever- the disease, (ed. T.J. Marrie), pp. 23-48. CRC Press, Boca Raton, FLA.

Langley, J.M., Marrie, T.J., Leblanc, J.C., Almudevar, A., Resch, L. and Raoult, D. 2003. *Coxiella burnetii* seropositivity in parturient women is associated with adverse pregnancy outcomes. Am. J. Obstet. Gynecol. **189:** 228-232.

Lee, J.H., Park, H.S., Jang, W.J. *et al.* 2004. Identification of the *Coxiella* Sp. detected from Haemaphysalis longicornis Ticks in Korea. Microbiol. Immunol. **48:** 125-130.

Lorenz, H., Jager, C., Willems, H. and Balger, G. 1998. PCR detection of *Coxiella burnetii* from different clinical specimens, especially bovine milk on the basis of DNA preparation with silica matrix. Appl. and Environ. Microbiol. **64:** 4234-4237.

Malik, S.V.S. and Yadav, M.P. 2002. Status of Q.fever in India. In: Meeting of the Task Force on Rickettsioses, April 12, ICMR Headquarters Office, New Delhi, LCD projections (28 slides).

Marrie, T.J., Buron, J.V., Fraser, J., Eileen, V. Haldan, M.B. and Faulkner, R.S. 1985. Seroepidemiology of Q. fever among domestic animals in Nova Scotia. A.J. P.H. **75**(7): 763-766.

Marrie, T.J., Durant, H., Williams, J.C., Mintz, E. and Waag, D.M. 1988. Exposure to parturient cats is a risk factor for acquisition of Q. fever in Maritime Canada. J. Infect. Dis. **158:** 101-108.

Marrie, T.J., MacDonald, A., Durant, H., Yates, L. and McCormick, L. 1988b. An outbreak of Q.fever probably due to contact with a parturient cat. Chest. **93:** 98-103.

Martinov, S.P., Neikov, P. and Popov, G.V. 1989. Experimental Q. fever in sheep. Europ. J. Epidemiol. **5:** 431-434.

Maurin, M. and Raoult, D. 1999. Q. fever. Clin. Microbiol. Rev. **12:** 518-553.

McQuiston, J.H. and Childs, J.E. 2002. Q. fever in humans and animals in the United States. Vector borne and zoonotic diseases **2**(3): 179-91.

Mege, J.L., Maurin, M., Capo, C. and Raoult, D. 1997. *Coxiella burnetii*: the 'query' fever bacterium. A model of immune subversion by a strictly intracellular microorganism. FEMS Microbiol. Rev. **19:** 209-217.

Millazzo, A., Hall, R., Storm, P.A., Harris, R.J., Winslow, W. and Marmion, B.P. 2001. Sexually transmitted Q. fever. Clin. Infect. Dis. **33**(3): 399-402.

Moeller, R.B. 2001. Causes of caprine abortion: diagnostic assessment of 211 cases (1991-1998). J. Vet. Diagnost. Invest. **13:** 265-270.

Musso and Raoult, D. 1997. Serological cross-reactions between *Coxiella burnetii* and *Legionella micdadei*. Clin. Diagn. Lab. Immunol. **4:** 208-212.

Norlander, L. 2000. Q. fever epidemiology and pathogenesis. Microbes and Infection, **2:** 17-424.

Palmer, N.C., Kierstead, M., Key, D.W., Williams, J.C., Peacock, M.G. and Vellend, H. 1983. Placentitis and abortion in goats and sheep in Ontario caused by *Coxiella burnetii*. Can. Vet. J. **24:** 60-61.

Prasad, B., Chandiramani, N. and Wagle, A. 1986. Isolation of *Coxiella burnetii* from human sources. Int. J. Zoonoses. **13:** 112-117.

Raoult, D. 1990. Host factor in the severity of Q. fever. Ann. N.Y. Acad. Sci. **590:** 33-38.

Raoult, D. and Marrie, T. 1995. Q. fever. Clin. Infect. Dis. **20:** 489-496.

Raoult, D., Tissot-Dupont, H., Foucault, C., Gouvernet, J., Fournier, P.E., Bernit, E., Stein, A., Nesri, M., Harle, J.R. and Weiller, P.J. 2000. Q. fever 1985-1998-Clinical and epidemiologic features of 1,383 infections. Medicine. **79:** 109-123.

Rarotra, J.R., Yadav, M.P. and Sethi, M.S. 1978. Seroepidemiology of Q. fever in poultry. Avian Dis. **1:** 167-169.

Ruppanner, R., Brooks, D., Franti C.E., Behmen, D.E., Morrish, D. and Spineli, J. 1982. Q. fever hazards from sheep and goats used in research. Arch. Environ. Health. **37:** 103-110.

Schopf, K., Khaschabi and Dackau. 1991. Enzootic abortion in a goat herd caused by mixed infection with *Coxiella burnetii* and Chlamydia psittasi. Case report. Tierarz. Prax. **19:** 630-634.

Scola, B.L. and Raoult, D. 1996. Serological cross-reaction between *Bortonella Quintana, Bartonella henselae* and *Coxiella burnetii*. J. Clin. Microbiol. **34**(9): 2270-2274.

Serbezov, V.S., Kazar, J., Novkirishki, V., Gatcheva, N., Kovacova, E. and Voynova, V. 1999. Q. fever in Bulgaria and Slovakia. Emerg. Infect. Dis. **5:** 388-394.

Sethi, M.S., Bhupender-Singh, Yadav, M.P. 1978. Experimental infection of *Coxiella burnetii* in chicken. Clinical symptoms, serologic response and transmission through egg. Avian Diseases, **22**(3): 391-395.

Siegman-Igra, Y., Kaufman, O, Keysary, A., Rzotkiewicz, and Shalit, I. 1997. Q. fever endocarditis in Israel and a worldwide review. Scand. J. Infect. Dis. **29:** 41-49.

Spyridaki, I., Gikas, A., Kofteridis, D., Psaroulaki, A. and Tselentis, Y. 1998. Q. fever in the Greek island of Crete: detection, isolation and molecular identification of eight strains of *Coxiella burnetii* from clinical samples. J. Clin. Microbiol. **36:** 2063-2067.

Stein, A. and Roult, D. 1998. Q. fever during pregnancy: a public health problem in southern France. Clin. Infect. Dis. **27:** 592-596.

Sting, R., Simmert, J., Mandl, J., Seemann, G., Bay, F., Muller, K.F., Schmitt, K. and Mentrup, T. 2000. *Coxiella burnetii* infections and infections with bacteria of the genus Chlamydia in dairy cattle. Berl. Munch. Tieratz. Wochens. **113:** 423-430.

Thapliyal, D.C. 1999. Q. fever In: Diseases of animals transmissible to man. 1st edition. Pp. 204-207. Eds. International Book Distributing Company.

Tigertt, W.D., Benenson, A.S. and Gochenour, W.S. 1961. Airborne Q. fever. Bacteriol. Rev. **25:** 285-293.

Tissot-Dupont, H. and Raoult, D. 1993. Epidemiologic de la fievre. Q Bull. Epidemiol. Hebd. **5:** 17-18.

Tissot-Dupont, H., Thirion, X. and Raoult, D. 1994. Q. fever serology: cutoff determination for microimmunofluorescence. Clin. Diagn. Lab. Immunol. **1:** 189-196.

To, H., Htwe, K., Kako, N., Kim, H., Yamaguchi, T., Fukushi, H. and Hirai, K. 1998. Prevalence of *Coxiella burnetii* infection in dairy cattle with reproductive disorders. J. Vet. Med. Sci. 60:859-861.

Vaidya, V.M., Malik, S.V.S., Kaur, S., Satish Kumar and Barbuddhe, S.B., 2008. Comparison of PCR, immunofluorescence assay and pathogen isolation for diagnosis of Q. fever in humans with spontaneous abortions Jr. Clin. Microbiol. 46:2038-44.

Waldhalm, D.G., Stoenner, H.G., Simmons, R.E. and Thomas, L.A. 1978. Abortion associated with *Coxiella burnetii* infection in dairy goats. J. Am. Vet. Med. Assoc. 173:1580-81.

Welsh, H.H., Lennette, Abhinanti, F.R. and Winn, J.F. 1985. Air-borne transmission of Q. fever: the role of parturition in the generation of infective aerosols. Ann. N.Y. Acad. Sci. 70:528-40.

Willems, H., Thiele, D., Frolech-Retter, R. and Krauss, H. 1994. Detection of *Coxiella burnetii* in cow's milk using the polymerase chain reaction. J. Vet. Med. B. 41:580-7.

Williams, J.C., Peacock, M.G. and McCaul, T.F. 1981. Immunological and biological characterization of *Coxiella burnetii* phases I and II separated from host components. Infect. Immun. 32:840-51.

Yadav, M.P. and Sethi, M.S. 1980. A study on the reservoir status of Q. fever in avi fauna, wild mammals and poilkilotherms in Uttar Pradesh (India). Int. J. Zoonoses, 7: 85-9.

Yuasa, Y., Yoshiie, K., Takasaki, T., Yushida, H. and Oda, H. 1996. Retrospective survey of chronic Q. fever in Japan by using PCR to detect *Coxiella burnetii* DNA in Paraffin embedded clinical samples. J. Clin. Microbiol. 34:824-7.

Zhang, C.Q. and Samuel, J.E. 2003. Identification and cloning potentially protective antigens of *Coxiella burnetii* using sera from mice experimentally infected with Nine Mile phase I. Ann. N.Y. Acad. Sci. 990:510-20.

Zhang, G., Kiss, K., Seshadri, R., Hendrix, L.R. and Samuel, J.E. 2004. Identification and cloning of immunodominant antigens of *Coxiella burnetii*. Infect. Immun. 72: 844-52.

□□□

Chapter 24

Glanders : A Fatal Zoonotic Diseases

S.K. KHURANA
National Research Centre on Equines, Hisar, Haryana

Glanders is a highly contagious disease primarily of equids particularly horses, donkeys and mules. It is a disease of high zoonotic importance and with significant human health risk. It is caused by the gram-negative bacillus *Burkholderia mallei* (the name changed from *Pseudomonas mallei* and was previously classified variously as *Pfeifferella, Loefflerella, Malleomyces or Actinobacillus*). The disease is notifiable in India. In humans, this usually results in fatal disease. Considering that the disease in India is restricted to certain pockets with sporadic cases, and thus if any case of glanders is diagnosed in the field on clinical symptoms, it needs a timely confirmation for applying early mitigation and control strategy. Wernery *et al.* (2011) confirmed a natural infection of dromedaries with glanders. Multilocus variable number tandem repeat analysis of a Burkholderia mallei strain isolated from a diseased dromedary in Bahrain revealed close genetic proximity to strain Dubai 7, which caused an outbreak of glanders in horses in the United Arab Emirates in 2004.

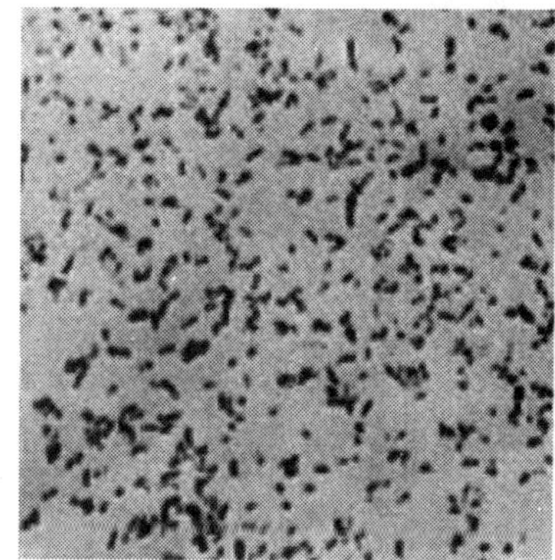

B.mallei gram stained

Burkholderia mallei is the primary bacteria that causes glanders in horses and other animals and occasionally, in humans. Glanders is difficult to diagnose and often fatal. The types of infection include localized, pus forming cutaneous infections, pulmonary infections, bloodstream infections and chronic supportive infections of the skin (CDC,2002). For localized infections, the ulceration will develop within 1 to 5 days at the site where the bacteria entered the body. Swollen lymph nodes may also appear. More mucus will be produced from the infected sites when bacteria enter into the eyes, nose or respiratory tract. Different infections may have different symptoms. In the case of a pulmonary infection, pneumonia, pulmonary abscess, and pleural effusion can occur. For bloodstream infections, it is fatal within 7 to 10 days. For chronic infections, multiple abscesses form within the muscles of the arms and legs, spleen, or live

Glanders organism has also been used in biological warfare. Glanders is believed to have been used during World War I to infect horses and mules that carried supplies and during World War II on horses and humans. Thus the organism has got a clear scope of bio-terrorism in the present day scenario. Hence we need to be prepared for its diagnosis with more sensitive, specific and less time consuming assay system.

Glanders is primarily a disease of equids particularly horses, donkeys and mules. Donkeys generally experience the acute form of disease and horses a more chronic form, while mules intermediate form in susceptibility. Carnivores are susceptible to disease if they consume glandered meat, felids appear to be more susceptible than canids. Outbreaks of glanders in captive wild felids have been reported. Several laboratory animals including hamsters and guinea pigs are susceptible. Humans are also susceptible to infection with glanders, which is important occupational disease of veterinarians, farriers, animal workers as well as laboratory workers. Swine and cattle are resistant to infection with *Burkholderia mallei,* but goats can be infected.

A collection of 147 isolates of Burkholderia pseudomallei, B. mallei, and B. thailandensis was characterized by multilocus sequence typing (MLST). The 128 isolates of B. pseudomallei, the causative agent of melioidosis, were obtained from diverse geographic locations, from humans and animals with disease, and from the environment and were resolved into 71 sequence types (Godoy *et al.*, 2003). The utility of the MLST scheme for epidemiological investigations was established by analyzing isolates from captive marine mammals and birds and from humans in Hong Kong with melioidosis. MLST gave a level of resolution similar to that given by pulsed-field gel electrophoresis and identified the same three clones causing disease in animals, each of which was also associated with disease in humans. The average divergence between the alleles of *B. thailandensis* and *B. pseudomallei* was 3.2%, and there was no sharing of alleles between these species. Trees constructed from differences in the allelic profiles of the isolates and from the concatenated sequences of the seven loci showed that the *B. pseudomallei* isolates formed a cluster of closely related lineages that were fully resolved from the cluster of B. thailandensis isolates, confirming their separate species status. However, isolates of *B. mallei*, the causative agent of glanders, recovered from three continents over a 30-year period had identical allelic profiles, and the *B. mallei* isolates clustered within the *B. pseudomallei* group of isolates. Alleles at six of the seven loci in *B. mallei* were also present within *B. pseudomallei* isolates, and B. mallei is a clone of *B. pseudomallei* that, on population genetics grounds, should not be given separate species status.

The genus *Burkholderia* was created by Yabuuchi et al. to accommodate the former rRNA group II *Pseudomonads*, excluding *Pseudomonas pickettii* and *Pseudomonas solanacearum*, which were transferred to the genus *Ralstonia.* Traditionally, the *Burkholderia* species are often known as plant pathogens and soil bacteria with two important exceptions, *B. mallei* and *B.* pseudomallei, *which can cause glander and melioidosis respectively in* humans and animals (Coenye and Vandamme, 2003). Once they enter the host, synthesis and release of certain toxin occur. Small amounts of toxin will not cause disease, but if a large quantity of the organism is incorporated, the amount of toxin is sufficient to cause specific symptoms (Thibault, 2004). *Burkholderia mallei* is a nonmotile, aerobic Gram-negative coccobacilus, which may or may not be oxidase positive or have growth potential on MacConkey agar. *Burkholderia pseudomallei,* on the other hand, is an oxidase positive, aerobic Gram-negative bacillus that is either straight or slightly curved (Newbauer, 2005).

Genome structure

'The genome of *B. mallei* consisits of two circular chromosomes. Chromosome 1 contains 3,510,148 bp, and chromosome 2 contains 2,325,379 bp. A total of 5,535 predicted protein-encoding ORFs are identified in the genome.' (Nierman *et al.*, 2004). The genome of this organism carries a large number of insertion sequences as compared to the related *Burkholderia pseudomallei*, with a large number of simple sequence repeats that may function in antigenic variation of cell surface proteins. (NCBI Genome Project).

Cell structure and metabolism

Burkholderia mallei is a genus of Gram-negative bacillus,width of the organism is 0.3 to 0.5 um and the length is 0.7 to 5.0 um, between rod and coccus shaped bacteria of the family *Pseudomonadaceae*, comprising animal and plant pathogens formerly classified in group II of the genus *Pseudomonas.* (Nierman, 2004).

The genome sequences of several strains of *B. mallei* and *B. pseudomallei* have revealed that *B. mallei* is a deletion clone of *B. pseudomallei* which lost >1,000 genes. Many of the gene deletions appear to have been caused by insertion sequence-mediated events and likely explain the many physiological differences that led to the classification of these two pathogens as separate species. Nearly all genes retained by *B. mallei* share ~99.5% DNA-DNA sequence identity with their *B. pseudomallei* homologs.

Geographic Distribution

Glanders is currently limited to parts of Asia and Africa, possibly the Balkan states, former Soviet republics, Mexico and South America. Asian countries affected are Turkey, Syria, Iraq, Iran, Pakistan, India, Burma, Indonesia, Philippines, China and Mangolia. Although glanders was once widespread throughout the world, it has been eradicated from many countries by diligent test and slaughter programs.

In India re-emergence of the disesease has been reported. NRCE had reported Re-emergence of Glanders in Maharashtra, Punjab, Uttarakhand and U.P. in 2006-07 after about a decade.During 2007-08 glanders was reported from Uttarakhand, A.P., H.P. and Haryana During 2009-10 glanders was reported from Chhattisgarh.During 2010-11 glanders was reported from Uttar Pradesh and Himachal Pradesh.

Transmission

The disease is introduced into horse populations by diseased or latently infected animals. Major route of infection in glanders is ingestion of pathogen present in secretions of infected animals. Inhalation of the organism is less likely to cause typical disease. Invasion by way of skin lesion is considered of minor importance in natural spread of disease. Close proximity alone may not usually be sufficient for transmission of glanders. Transmission is facilitated if the animals share feeding troughs and watering facilities.Artificial infection results in a fever 41 C in about 3 days and clinical signs within a week. In natural conditions manifestations of disease becoming apparent may take weeks or months. Such latent infections are a feature of epidemiology of glanders.

Pathogenesis

A well-studied aspect of pathogenesis by these closely-related bacteria is their ability to invade and multiply within eukaryotic cells. In contrast, the means by which *B. pseudomallei* and *B. mallei* adhere to cells are poorly defined. The purpose of the study of Balder *et al.* (2010) was to identify adherence factors expressed by these organisms. Comparative sequence analyses identified a gene product in the published genome of *B. mallei* strain ATCC23344 (locus # BMAA0649) that resembles the well-characterized Yersinia enterocolitica autotransporter adhesin YadA. The gene encoding this *B. mallei* protein, designated boaA, was expressed in *Escherichia coli* and shown to significantly increase adherence to human epithelial cell lines, specifically HEp2 (laryngeal cells) and A549 (type II pneumocytes), as well as to cultures of normal human bronchial epithelium (NHBE). Consistent with these findings, disruption of the boaA gene in B. mallei ATCC23344 reduced adherence to all three cell types by ~50%. The genomes of the *B. pseudomallei* strains K96243 and DD503 were also found to contain boaA and inactivation of the gene in DD503 considerably decreased binding to monolayers of HEp2 and A549 cells and to NHBE cultures.A second YadA-like gene product highly similar to BoaA (65% identity) was identified in the published genomic sequence of *B. pseudomallei* strain K96243 (locus # BPSL1705). The gene specifying this protein, termed boaB, appears to be *B. pseudomallei*-specific. Quantitative attachment assays demonstrated that recombinant *E. coli* expressing BoaB displayed greater binding to A549 pneumocytes, HEp2 cells and NHBE cultures. Moreover, a boaB mutant of *B. pseudomallei* DD503 showed decreased adherence to these respiratory cells. Additionally, a *B. pseudomallei* strain lacking expression of both boaA and boaB was impaired in its ability to thrive inside J774A.1 murine macrophages, suggesting a possible role for these proteins in survival within professional phagocytic cells.In conclusion the boaA and boaB genes specify adhesins that mediate adherence to epithelial cells of the human respiratory tract. The boaA gene product is shared by *B. pseudomallei* and *B. mallei* whereas BoaB appears to be a B. pseudomallei-specific adherence factor.

Using bacteriophage-mediated immunoscreening Tiyawisutsri *et al.* (2007) identified genes expressed in vivo during experimental equine glanders infection. A family of immunodominant antigens were identified that share protein domain architectures with hemagglutinins and invasins. These have been designated *Burkholderia* Hep_Hag autotransporter (BuHA) proteins. A total of 110/207 positive clones (53%) of a *B. mallei* expression library screened with sera from two infected horses belonged to this family. This contrasted with 6/189 positive clones (3%) of a *B. pseudomallei* expression library screened with serum from 21 patients with culture-proven melioidosis.In conclusion members of the BuHA proteins are found in other Gram-negative bacteria and have been shown to have important roles related to virulence. Compared with other bacterial species, the genomes of both *B. mallei* and *B. pseudomallei* contain a relative abundance of this family of proteins. The domain structures of these proteins suggest that they function as multimeric surface proteins that modulate interactions of the cell with the host and environment.

The antibiotic resistance profile and ability to infect via aerosol of these organisms and the absence of protective vaccines have led to their classification as major biothreats and select agents. Although documented infections by these bacteria date back over 100 years, relatively little is known about their virulence and pathogenicity mechanisms. Schell et al. (2008) used in silico genomic subtraction to generate their virulome, a set of 650 putative virulence-related genes shared by *B. pseudomallei* and *B. mallei* but not present in five closely related nonpathogenic *Burkholderia* species. Although most of these genes are clustered in putative operons, the number of targets for mutant construction and verification of reduced virulence in animal models is formidable. Therefore, *Galleria mellonella* (wax moth) larvae were evaluated as a surrogate host; we found that *B. pseudomallei* and *B. mallei*, but not other phylogenetically related bacteria, were highly pathogenic for this insect. More importantly, four previously characterized *B. mallei* mutants with reduced virulence in hamsters or mice had similarly reduced virulence in *G. mellonella* larvae. Site-specific inactivation of selected genes in the computationally derived virulome identified three new potential virulence genes, each of which was required for rapid and efficient killing of larvae. Thus, this approach may provide a means to quickly identify high-probability virulence genes in *B. pseudomallei*, *B. mallei*, and other pathogens.

The disease caused by *B. mallei*, glanders, is not well studied as there have been few well-documented cases since 1950. For both pathogens, infection usually occurs through wounds, aspiration, and possibly inhalation. Studies of intraperitoneally infected animals have shown that *B. pseudomallei* and *B. mallei* can rapidly migrate to the spleen and liver, where they multiply extensively within membrane-bound phagosomes and form abscesses. Untreated infections are often fatal.

Small-animal models are available for studying the pathogenesis of *B. pseudomallei* and *B. mallei*. These models include a sensitive (50% lethal dose, <10 cells) Syrian hamster model utilizing intraperitoneal injection and two mouse models utilizing C57BL/6 or BALB/c mice and aerosol, intranasal, or intraperitoneal infection. However, these models are expensive, cumbersome, and hazardous due to biosafety and biosecurity issues. A *Caenorhabditis elegans* nematode infection model for *B. pseudomallei* has been described, although it may have limited sensitivity due to the extremely high doses required for killing.

Compared to other bacterial pathogens, little is known about the virulence factors of *B. mallei* and *B. pseudomallei* or the molecular basis of the pathogenicity of these organisms. The only verified virulence factors for these pathogens are those that are well known and shared by most, if not all, animal and plant pathogens: exopolysaccharide capsule (CAP), type III secretion systems (T3SS), and lipopolysaccharide O antigen (LPS). Type II secretion, type IV pili, and flagella have been implicated in *B. pseudomallei* pathogenesis. Recently, a type VI secretion (T6S) gene cluster was shown to be required for the virulence of *B. mallei*. Several putative virulence factors, including two proteases, a hemolysin, a rhamnolipid, predicted transporter proteins, and three hypothetical proteins, have been identified using either nematode killing assays or biochemical analysis. However, these factors are yet to be verified by animal experiments. Recently, Tuanyok et al. identified a phospholipase C and a two-component regulator which are required for full virulence of *B. pseudomallei*.

The genome sequences of >25 *Burkholderiaceae* isolates representing >12 species and four genera are available (http://www.genomesonline.org/). These isolates occupy a wide diversity of ecological niches, yet they share a common core genome comprised of long syntenic regions containing >2,500 shared "housekeeping" genes whose products share >60% amino acid sequence identity. Of greater interest are the species- or isolate-specific genes, such as those found only in human-pathogenic *Burkholderia* spp. Therefore, we used in silico genomic subtraction to derive a set of 650 genes that are present in both *B. pseudomallei* and *B. mallei* but are not present in the sequenced nonpathogenic members of the *Burkholderiaceae*. This set is predicted to be highly enriched in novel virulence genes and has been designated the Bm-Bp virulome. Workers have investigated this virulome by selecting genes likely to encode novel virulence factors, inactivating them, and testing the corresponding mutants to determine whether they exhibited reduced virulence in wax moth larvae, a surrogate model that we adapted and verified as correlating with the hamster model commonly used to test *B. mallei* virulence.

The genus *Burkholderia* was created by Yabuuchi et al. to accommodate the former rRNA group II *Pseudomonads*, excluding *Pseudomonas pickettii* and *Pseudomonas solanacearum*, which were transferred to the genus *Ralstonia*. Traditionally, the *Burkholderia* species are often known as plant pathogens and soil bacteria with two important exceptions, *B. mallei* and *B.* pseudomallei, *which can cause glander and melioidosis respectively in* humans and animals (Coenye and Vandamme, 2003). Once they enter the host, synthesis and release of certain toxin occur. Small amounts of toxin will not cause disease, but if a large quantity of the organism is incorporated, the amount of toxin is sufficient to cause specific symptoms (Thibault, 2004). *Burkholderia mallei* is a nonmotile, aerobic Gram-negative coccobacilus, which may or may not be oxidase positive or have growth potential on MacConkey agar. *Burkholderia pseudomallei*, on the other hand, is an oxidase positive, aerobic Gram-negative bacillus that is either straight or slightly curved (Newbauer, 2005).

Ecology

Burkholderia mallei is not found in the United States and Western Europe due to a program of compulsory slaughter of infected horses or other animals. It is a highly adapted parasite of horses and cannot persist in nature outside of its host. However, it is still commonly seen among domestic animals in Africa, Asia, the Middle East, and Central and South America.(Godoy et al.,2003) *Burkholderia mallei* is quite sensitive to heat, UV light, desiccation and common disinfectants. In outbreaks, one must bury or burn all contaminated bedding and foodstuffs to prevent infection of accessible animals. Stalls and harness equipment should be thoroughly sterilized. Contact with infected animals, especially horses, should also be avoided. (Gilbert, 1992)

Pathology

Burkholderia mallei is the primary bacteria that causes glanders in horses and other animals and occasionally, in humans. Glanders is difficult to diagnose and often fatal. The types of infection include localized, pus forming cutaneous infections, pulmonary infections, bloodstream infections and chronic supportive infections of the skin. (CDC,2002) For localized infections, the ulceration will develop within 1 to 5 days at the site where the bacteria entered the body. Swollen lymph nodes may also appear. More mucus will be produced from the infected sites when bacteria enter into the eyes, nose or respiratory tract. Different infections may have different symptoms. In the case of a pulmonary infection, pneumonia, pulmonary abscess, and pleural effusion can occur. For bloodstream infections, it is fatal within 7 to 10 days. For chronic infections, multiple abscesses form within the muscles of the arms and legs, spleen, or liver.(Thibault et al 2004) There are no vaccines for glanders. However, the traditional veterinary treatment of streptomycin and sulfadiazine is somewhat effective.(Goody, 2003) *B. mallei* is less resistant to antibiotics comparing to many other *Pseudomonas* and it may be treated with sulfamethoxazole-trimethoprim, ceftazidime, and doxycycline.(CDC,2002)

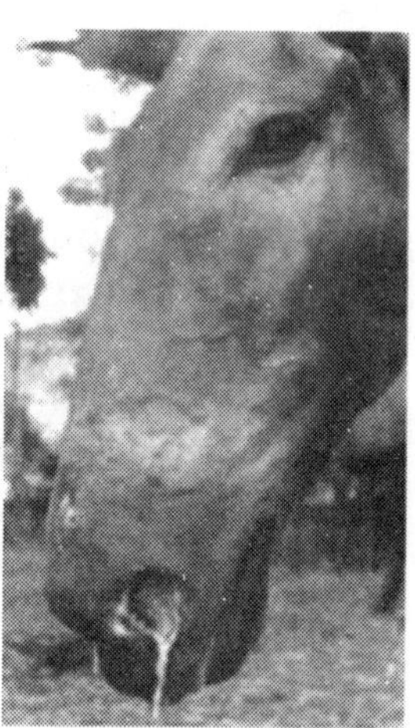

Horse infected by *B. mallei* (12)

Diagnosis

1. Clinical Signs and symptoms

Glanders is a contagious and fatal disease of horses, donkeys, and mules. The disease causes nodules and ulcerations in the upper respiratory tract and lungs. Typical nodules, ulcers, scars, and a debilitated condition can be sufficient to diagnose glanders. Unfortunately, many cases of glanders are latent and clinically inapparent. Therefore, systematic testing is essential to identify all infected animals in an outbreak. Glanders (from Middle English *glaundres* or Old French *glandres*, both meaning glands)[1] (Latin: *Malleus* German: *Rotz*) (also known as "Equinia," "Farcy," and "Malleus"[2]:282) is an infectious disease that occurs primarily in horses, mules, and donkeys. It can be contracted by other animals such as dogs, cats and goats. It is caused by infection with the bacterium *Burkholderia mallei*, usually by ingestion of contaminated food or water. Symptoms of glanders include the formation of nodular lesions in the lungs and ulceration of the mucous membranes in the upper respiratory tract. The acute form results in coughing, fever and the release of an infectious nasal discharge, followed by septicaemia and death within days. In the chronic form, nasal and subcutaneous nodules develop, eventually ulcerating. Death can occur within months, while survivors act as carriers.

Glanders is endemic in Africa, Asia, the Middle East, Central and South America. It has been eradicated from North America, Australia and most of Europe through surveillance and destruction of affected animals, and import restrictions.

The disease is commonly classified into three types:

1. *Pulmonary glanders*: This form is characterized by formation of round, grayish or white, firm, encapsulated nodules throughout the lung tissue. The nodules contain yellowish, cheesy pus.
2. *Nasal glanders*: There is typical formation of nodules in mucous membrane of nasal cavity, particularly of septum. Many of these nodules rupture and liberate mucopurulent exudates which become mixed with the serous or mucopurulent exudates already discharging from the nostrils. This yellowish green exudate is highly infectious. The ruptured nodules form ulcers with irregular, raised and hyperemic borders. The ulcers heal slowly to form a stellate scar. Both nodules and ulcers may be seen simultaneously. Regional lymph nodes are commonly swollen.
3. *Cutaneous glanders or Farcy*: Multiple glanders nodules form along the lymph vessels between affected lymph nodes. These nodules often rupture through skin to discharge yellowish exudate and form deep ulcers which heal slowly. Typical cutaneous lymphatic vessels may be referred to as Farcy pipes.

In most outbreaks, these forms may not be clearly distinct and may occur simultaneously in an animal. Chronic forms are more common though, the acute form typically progresses to death within about a week. The acute form is more common in donkeys and mules than in horses.

2. The mallein test (a prescribed test for international trade)

The mallein test has been the main test of field diagnosis. Mallein PPD is a lysate (solution of water-soluble protein fractions of heat-treated *B. mallei*) containing both endotoxins and exotoxins elaborated by the organism. Infected animals are allergic/ hypersensitive to mallein and exhibit local and systemic hypersensitivity after mallein inoculation similar to that exhibited in tuberculin testing. Inoculation with mallein may trigger a humoral serologic reaction to the complement fixation test. This seroconversion is thought to be transient but may be permanent if the animal undergoes repeated mallein testing. This is extremely important to consider if samples from the animals are destined for complement fixation test. Further, advanced clinical cases in horses and acute cases in donkeys and mules may give inconclusive results requiring additional methods of diagnosis to be employed.

The intradermo-palpebral test

This is the most sensitive, reliable and specific test. The preferred method of application of mallein is intradermo-palpebral. The concentrated mallein PPD (0.1 ml) is injected intradermally into the lower eyelid. The test is usually read at 24 and 48 hours after injection.

A positive reaction is visualized by marked oedematous swelling of the eyelid, and there may be a purulent discharge from the inner canthus or conjunctiva accompanied with photophobia, pain, and depression within 12 to 72 hours. There is usually a rise in temperature. In a negative response, there is usually no reaction or only a little swelling of the lower lid.

The ophthalmic test

This is less reliable than the intradermo-palpebral test. A few drops of mallein are instilled into the eye at the canthus. In an infected animal, the eyelids, and sometimes the side of the face, become swollen. Development of severe conjunctivitis within 6-12 hrs may also be evident. The reaction may also occur to a lesser extent in the opposite eye.

The subcutaneous test

This test interferes with subsequent serological diagnosis. The horse's temperature has to be under 102°F (38.8°C) on the day before the test, at the time of the injection, and at 9, 12 and 15 hours after the injection. A 10 cm square skin patch in the middle of the neck is clipped and disinfected; 2.5 ml of dilute mallein are injected subcutaneously into the centre of the patch. With a positive test, the horse develops a pyrexia of 104°F (40.0°C) or over during the first 15 hours, and a firm painful swelling with raised edges develops within 24 hours at the injection site. In nonglandered horses, there is no, or minimal, transient local swelling. Doubtful reactors may be retested after 14 days using a double dose of mallein.

A whole or section of a lesion, swabs of the exudates and a serum sample may be collected aseptically. The samples are required to be shipped to laboratory under refrigeration as soon as possible. Air-dried smears of exudate on glass slides may also be submitted for microscopic examination.

The causative organism may be cultured from samples from fresh lesions or lymph nodes. It may also be demonstrated microscopically in films made from this material.

The organisms are fairly numerous in smears from fresh lesions, but in older lesions they are scanty. The organisms are mainly extracellular, fairly straight Gram-negative rods with rounded ends, 2-5 µm long and 0.3-0.8 µm wide with granular inclusions of various size, often stain irregularly and do not have capsules or form spores. Unlike other organisms in the *Pseudomonas* group, *Burkholderia mallei* have no flagellae and are therefore non-motile. The organisms are difficult to demonstrate in tissue sections, where they may have a beaded appearance. In culture media, they vary in appearance depending on the age of the culture and type of medium. In older cultures, there is much pleomorphism. Branching filaments form on the surface of broth cultures.

Cultural characteristics

It is preferable to attempt isolation from unopened uncontaminated lesions. The organism is aerobic and facultatively anaerobic only in the presence of nitrate, growing optimally at 37°C. It grows well, but slowly, on ordinary culture media, 48-hour incubation of cultures is recommended; glycerol enrichment is particularly useful. After a few days on glycerol agar, there is a confluent, slightly cream-coloured growth that is smooth, moist, and viscid. With continued incubation, the growth thickens and becomes dark brown and tough. It also grows well on glycerol potato agar and in glycerol broth, on which a slimy pellicle forms. On plain nutrient agar, the growth is much less luxuriant, and growth is poor on gelatin. Glycerin-dextrose agar (GDA) containing 5% glycerin, 1% dextrose in nutrient agar is described as suitable for isolation by Verma (1989). In contaminated samples, supplementation of media with substances that inhibit the growth of Gram-positive organisms (e.g. crystal violet, proflavine) has proved useful, as has pretreatment with penicillin (1000 units/ml for 3 hours at 37°C).

Alterations to characteristics may occur *in vitro,* so fresh isolates should be used for identification reactions. The organism reduces nitrates. Although some workers have claimed that glucose is the only carbohydrate that is fermented (slowly and inconstantly), other workers have shown that if an appropriate medium and indicator are used, glucose and other carbohydrates, such as arabinose, fructose, galactose and mannose, are consistently fermented by *B. mallei.* Indole is not produced, horse blood is not haemolysed and no diffusible pigments are produced in cultures. Lack of motility is of special relevance.

Laboratory animal inoculation

Guinea-pigs, hamsters and cats have been used for diagnosis when necessary. The Strauss reaction is observed when infectious material from glanders patients is injected intraperitoneally into male guinea pigs. In positive cases, the guinea pig develops localized peritonitis involving the scrotal sac. Glanderous orchitis follows with painful enlargement of the testes. The testis becomes enlarged and painful and ultimately necrotic and is discharged through the scrotal skin. Individual resistance variations have been reported. The number of organisms and their virulence determines the severity of the lesions. The Strauss reaction is not specific for glanders, and other organisms can elicit it. Bacteriological examination of infected testes should confirm the specificity of the response obtained.

Serological Tests

A variety of serologic tests for glanders have been developed. They are superior to mallein testing in sensitivity and specificity.

Complement fixation test (a prescribed test for international trade)

The complement fixation test is widely used. Although not as sensitive as the mallein test, the CF test is an accurate serological test that has been used for glanders diagnosis for many years. It is reported to be about 95% accurate, serum being positive within 1 week of infection and remaining positive in the case of exacerbation of the chronic process.

Enzyme-linked immunosorbent assays

Recently a dot enzyme-linked immunosorbent assay has been developed and found to be superior to all previously described tests in its sensitivity. This test is inexpensive, rapid, and easy to perform and is not influenced by anticomplement activity. Both plate and membrane (blot) enzyme-linked immunosorbent assays (ELISAs) have been reported for the serodiagnosis of glanders, but none of these procedures has been shown to differentiate serologically between *B. mallei* and *B. pseudomallei*. Blotting approaches have involved both dipstick dot-blot and electrophoretically separated and transferred western blot methods. A competitive ELISA that uses an anti-lipopolysaccharide monoclonal antibody has also been developed and found to be similar to the CF test in performance. Continuing development of monoclonal antibody reagents specific for *B. mallei* antigenic components offers the potential for more specific ELISAs in the foreseeable future that will help resolve questionable test results of quarantined imported horses. At this time, none of these tests has been validated.

The avidin-biotin dot ELISA has been described, but has not yet been widely used or validated. The antigen is heat-inactivated bacterial culture that has been concentrated and purified. A dot of this antigen is placed on a nitrocellulose dipstick that is then used to test for antibody against *B. mallei* in equine serum. Using antigen-dotted, preblocked dipsticks, the test can be completed in approximately 1 hour. Serum or whole blood can be used for the test, and partial haemolysis does not impart any background colour to the antigen-coated area on the nitrocellulose.

Other methods

A counter-immunoelectrophoresis test has been described. The rose bengal plate agglutination test (RBT) has been described for the diagnosis of glanders in horses and other susceptible animals; the test has been validated in Russia only. The antigen is a heat-inactivated bacterial suspension coloured with rose bengal, which is used in a plate agglutination test.

The accuracy of other agglutination tests and precipitin is unsatisfactory for use in control programmes. Horses with chronic glanders and those in a debilitated condition give negative or inconclusive results. Cross-reactions with *B. pseudomallei,* the cause of melioidosis, are features of all of the serological tests for glanders. Therefore, these tests will result in false positive reactions in animals from areas where melioidosis is endemic.

A Western blot assay making use of a partly purified lipopolysaccaride (LPS) containing antigen of three Burkholderia mallei strains was developed (Elscnner et al.2011). The test was validated investigating a comprehensive set of positive and negative sera obtained from horses and mules from endemic and non endemic areas.The developed Western blot assay showed a markedly higher diagnostic specificity when compared to the prescribed CFT and therefore can be used as a confirmatory test. However, the CFT remains the test of choice for routine testing of glanders due to its high sensitivity, its feasibility using standard laboratory equipment and its worldwide distribution in diagnostic laboratories.The CFT should be amended by the newly validated

Western blot to increase the positive likelihood ratio of glanders serodiagnosis in non endemic areas or areas with low glanders prevalence. Its use for international trade of horses and mules should be implemented by the OIE. A polysaccharide microarray platform was prepared by immobilizing *Burkholderia pseudomallei* and Burkholderia mallei polysaccharides. This polysaccharide array was tested with success for detecting *B. pseudomallei* and B. mallei serum (human and animal) antibodies. The advantages of this microarray technology over the current serodiagnosis of the above bacterial tests is evident (Parathasarthy *et al.*, 2006).

PCR

There have been recent advances in the application of molecular biological techniques to the detection of glanders. A polymerase chain reaction (PCR) for the specific detection of *B. mallei* DNA has been developed that allows differentiation between *B. mallei* and *B. pseudomallei*. Most recently, two *B. mallei*-specific real-time PCR assays targeting the *B. mallei* $bimA_{ma}$ gene (*Burkholderia* intracellular motility A; BMAA0749), which encodes a protein involved in actin polymerization, were developed. The PCR primer and probe sets were tested for specificity against a collection of *B. mallei* and *B. pseudomallei* isolates obtained from numerous clinical and environmental (*B. pseudomallei* only) sources. The assays were also tested for cross-reactivity using template DNA from 14 closely related *Burkholderia* species. The relative limit of detection for the assays was found to be 1 pg or 424 genome equivalents. The authors also analyzed the applicability of assays to detect *B. mallei* within infected BALB/c mouse tissues. Beginning 1 h post aerosol exposure, *B. mallei* was successfully identified within the lungs, and starting at 24 h postexposure, in the spleen and liver. Surprisingly, *B. mallei* was not detected in the blood of acutely infected animals. This investigation provides two real-time PCR assays for the rapid and specific identification of *B. mallei.*

The technique has not yet been fully validated or gained wide acceptance. However, PCR has the potential to be a safe, fast method to confirm infection. Methods to differentiate between *B.mallei* and *B. pseudomallei* are important as this cannot be reliably accomplished by the current serological tests.

Burkholderia pseudomallei, may be differentiated from closely related species of Burkholderia mallei that causes glanders and non-pathogenic species of *Burkholderia thailandensis* by multiplex PCR (Lee *et al.*, 2005). The multiplex PCR consists of primers that flank a 10-bp repetitive element in *B. pseudomallei* and B. mallei amplifying PCR fragment of varying sizes between 400-700 bp, a unique sequence in *B. thailandensis* amplifying a PCR fragment of 308 bp and the metalloprotease gene amplifying a PCR fragment of 245 bp in *B. pseudomallei* and *B. thailandensis*. The multiplex PCR not only can differentiate the three *Burkholderia* species but can also be used for epidemiological typing of *B. pseudomallei* and *B. mallei* strains.

Kumar *et al.* (2011) expressed a novel recombinant *Burkholderia* intracellular motility A (rBimA) protein in E. coli for diagnosis of equine glanders. Purified rBimA was used in indirect ELISA format. All the 21 true positive sera samples used in the study tested positive whereas only 17 of the 1524 potentially negative sera tested positive by indirect ELISA, thus exhibiting 100% sensitivity and 98.88% specificity. Also, rBimA protein did not react with melioidosis patient and normal healthy human sera samples showing its high specificity. The developed assay can be used as a simple and rapid tool for diagnosis of glanders in equine sera samples.

Differential Diagnosis

Cases for specific glanders investigation should be differentiated on clinical grounds from other chronic infections of the nasal mucosae or sinuses, and from strangles (*Streptococcus equi* infection), ulcerative lymphangitis (*Corynebacterium pseudotuberculosis*), pseudotuberculosis (*Yersinia pseudotuberculosis*), sporotrichosis (*Sporotrichium* spp.) and other forms of pneumonia. Glanders should be excluded positively from suspected cases of epizootic lymphangitis (caused by *Histoplasma farciminosum*), with which it has many clinical similarities. In humans in particular, glanders should be distinguished from melioidosis (*B. pseudomallei* infection), which is caused by an organism with close similarities to *B. mallei.*

Purulent sinusitis, guttural pouch empyema, and other causes of nasal catarrh should also be considered. Skin lesions may be similar to those of dermatophilosis or dermatomycoses such as sporotrichosis. Knowledge of the progressive debilitating nature of glanders and application of serological or mallein tests will serve to distinguish glanders from other similar diseases.

Strangles is caused by *Streptococcus equi*. It is characterized by fever, anorexia, and depression with swollen submandibular lymph nodes and mucopurulent nasal discharge. The nasal discharge is usually bilateral, whereas it is most often unilateral in cases of glanders. Skin nodules and typical lung lesions are absent. Animals with strangles will not react to mallein testing or serological tests for glanders. *S. equi* is readily demonstrable. Strangles does not develop into a chronic, debilitating condition, and most infected horses recover within a few weeks.

Epizootic lymphangitis (caused by *Histoplasma farciminosum*) is characterized by cutaneous nodules originating from superficial lymph vessels. In epizootic lymphangitis, conjunctivitis is a common lesion. Demonstration of the infectious agent and application of the mallein test and serological testing will help distinguish between these diseases.

Ulcerative lymphangitis (caused by *Corynebacterium pseudotuberculosis*) is characterized by dermatitis and abscess formation predominantly in the pectoral and ventral abdominal regions. Standard diagnostic tests are again valuable in distinguishing this disease from glanders.

Melioidosis (caused by *B. pseudomallei*) is characterized by multiple abscesses in a variety of tissues and organs. Unlike glanders, it is not specifically a disease of equids and occurs most often in sheep, goats, and swine. It is characterized by dyspnea and lameness, but a wide array of clinical signs may be elicited. Diagnosis is confirmed by isolation of the causative organism. Serological cross-reactions occur with *B. mallei.*

Treatment and control

The scarcity of glanders in most countries in the world over the past 50–60 years means there is scant knowledge, with the exception of a few principally Russian sources, of the antimicrobial susceptibility of *B. mallei*, particularly to modern antimicrobials. Likewise, the *in vivo* efficacy of modern antimicrobials against *B. mallei* is not well known and few *in vitro* antibiotic susceptibility studies for *B. mallei* have been performed. The antibiotic susceptibility pattern of *B. mallei* is similar to that of *B. pseudomallei*, with *B. mallei* exhibiting resistance to a number of antibiotics. In some studies, doxycycline showed good *in vitro* activity against *B. mallei* . Both *B. mallei* and *B. pseudomallei* are sensitive to imipenem, and most strains are also susceptible to ceftazidime, ciprofloxacin and piperacillin. Furthermore, *B. mallei* is susceptible to aminoglycosides because it lacks the AmrAB–OprA efflux pump, which confers high-level aminoglycoside resistance to *B. pseudomallei* .

There are little data on the efficacy of antibiotics for the treatment of human glanders but current treatment options include a mixed antibiotic regimen that is often only partially effective, and assumes an early and accurate diagnosis. Single-drug antibiotic therapy is only partially effective and combinations of antibiotics must be used for extended periods. For example, a researcher who developed glanders following accidental laboratory exposure was treated with imipenem and doxycycline for 2 weeks, followed by treatment with azithromycin and doxycycline for an additional 6 months. An additional problem is that even more antibiotic-resistant variants of *B. mallei* have been reported and surgical drainage of abscesses may be required in some cases. Glanders prophylaxis has not yet been studied in detail, although approaches similar to those recommended below for melioidosis may be feasible. Moreover, there is no prophylactic or therapeutic vaccine for *B. mallei* infection available for humans or animals.

There is a need to develop an effective vaccine for individuals at risk of exposure from deliberate release, and understanding the immune response elicited during infection with *B. mallei* is central to this process. The relative importance of cellular versus humoral responses in the development of protective immunity against *B. mallei* is under investigation. Experimental evidence indicates that both play a role, but that stimulation of a Th1-like immune response may be important for protection. One study of murine monoclonal antibodies (mAbs) against *B. mallei* administered to mice prior to a lethal aerosol challenge reported non-sterilizing protection. Passive protection in the mouse model has also been described for the highly related *B. pseudomallei* using murine mAbs specific for *B. pseudomallei* polysaccharide. Humoral immune response profiling to infection is a logical approach to the evaluation of immunogenic antigens, and has the ability to define novel targets for both diagnostics and vaccines. Profiling using proteome microarrays has been described for a vaccinia virus proteome consisting of 185 individual viral proteins and used to determine Ab profiles in serum from vaccinia virus-immunized humans, primates, and mice. This technology has not been described in the literature to date for antibody profiling in response to infection with *B. mallei* or *B. pseudomallei*, although polysaccharide microarray technology has been described for the detection of *B. pseudomallei* and *B. mallei* antibodies to capsular antibodies. An alternative strategy for immunoscreening is the use of a bacteriophage expression library. This has recently been used to detect *in vivo* expressed antigens of *Staphylococcus aureus* and to utilize this information to develop a vaccine to protect against experimental nasal carriage. Although complex molecules such as LPS will not be represented, this technique offers an immediately available, rapid and simple means of identifying and testing putative candidate vaccines and targets for serological diagnostic tests.

There is currently no vaccine available for the prevention of disease. Sarkar-Tyson *et al.* (2009) report the protective efficacy of heat-inactivated *Burkholderia thailandensis, B. mallei* or *B. pseudomallei* cells as vaccines against murine melioidosis and glanders. Immunisation with heat-inactivated B. pseudomallei cells provided the highest levels of protection against either melioidosis or glanders. These studies indicate the longer term potential for heat-inactivated bacteria to be developed as vaccines against melioidosis and glanders.

Further Reading

Anonymous. 2006. Glanders *In*: Manual of Diagnostic Tests and Vaccines for Terrestrial Animals. http://www.oie.int/eng/normes/MMANUAL/A_00086.htm.

Jana, A.M., Gupta, A.K., Pandya, G., Verma, R.D., and Rao, K.M. 1982. Rapid diagnosis of glanders in equines by counter-immunoelectrophoresis. ***Indian Vet. J.*, 59:** 5-9.

Melanie P. Ulrich, David A. Norwood, Deanna R. Christensen and Ricky L. Ulrich. 2006. Using real-time PCR to specifically detect *Burkholderia mallei* . *J Med Microbiol.*, **55:** 551-559.

The USAHA gray book (Foreign Animal Diseases). 1998. http://www.vet.uga.edu/vpp/gray_book02/fad/gla.php (Sixth edition).

Verma, R.D. 1981. Glanders in India with special reference to incidence and epidemiology. ***Indian Vet. J.***, **58:** 177-183.

Verma, R.D., Sharma, J.K., Venkateswaran K.S., and Batra, H.V. 1990. Development of an avidin – biotin dot enzyme-linked immunosorbent assay and its comparison with other serological tests for diagnosis of glanders in equines. *Vet. Microbiol.*, **25:** 77-85.

Verma, R.D.1989. Research on epizootic, diagnosis and control of glanders with a view to eradicate the disease from India. Project Report, ICAR Research Scheme. 54 p.

References

Balder R., Lipski S., Lazarus J.J., Grose W., Wooten R.M., Hogan R.J., Woods D.E., and Lafontaine E.R.2010.Identification of *Burkholderia mallei* and *Burkholderia pseudomallei* adhesins for human respiratory epithelial cells. BMC Microbiol. **10:** 250.

Elschner M.C., Scholz H.C., Melzer F., Saqib M., Marten P., Rassbach A., Dietzsch M., Schmoock G., de Assis Santana V.L., de Souza M.M., Wernery R., Wernery U., and Neubauer H.2011.Use of a Western blot technique for the serodiagnosis of glanders. BMC Vet. Res. Jan 19; **7:** 4.

Godoy D., Randle G., Simpson A.J., Aanensen D.M., Pitt T.L., Kinoshita R. and Spratt B.G.2003.Multilocus sequence typing and evolutionary relationships among the causative agents of melioidosis and glanders, *Burkholderia pseudomallei* and Burkholderia mallei. J .Clin. Microbiol. **41:** 2068-2079.

Kumar S., Malik P., Verma S.K., Pal V., Gautam V., Mukhopadhyay C. and Rai G.P.2011.A recombinant *Burkholderia* intracellular motility A (BimA) protein for immunodiagnosis of glanders. Clin. Vaccine Immunol. 2011 Jul 13.[http://www.ncbi.nlm.nih.gov/pubmed/21752949].

Lee M.A., Wang D. and Yap E.H. 2005.Detection and differentiation of Burkholderia pseudomallei, *Burkholderia mallei* and *Burkholderia thailandensis* by multiplex PCR. FEMS Immunol. Med. Microbiol. **43:** 413-417.

Parthasarathy N., DeShazer D., England M. and Waag D.M.2006.Polysaccharide microarray technology for the detection of *Burkholderia pseudomallei* and *Burkholderia mallei* antibodies. Diagn. Microbiol. Infect. Dis. **56:** 329-332. Epub 2006 Jun 12.

Sarkar-Tyson M., Smither S.J., Harding S.V., Atkins T.P. and Titball R.W.2009.Protective efficacy of heat-inactivated *B. thailandensis, B. mallei* or *B. pseudomallei* against experimental melioidosis and glanders. Vaccine. **27:** 4447-4451. Epub 2009 May 31.

Schell M.A., Lipscomb L. and DeShazer D.2008.Comparative genomics and an insect model rapidly identify novel virulence genes of *Burkholderia mallei*. J. Bacteriol. **190:** 2306-2313. Epub 2008 Jan 25.

Tiyawisutsri R., Holden M.T., Tumapa S., Rengpipat S., Clarke S.R., Foster S.J. Nierman W.C, Day N.P and Peacock S.J.2007. *Burkholderia* Hep_Hag autotransporter (BuHA) proteins elicit a strong antibody response during experimental glanders but not human *melioidosis*. BMC Microbiol. 15; **7:** 19.

Wernery U., Wernery R., Joseph M., Al-Salloom F., Johnson B., Kinne J., Jose S., Jose S., Tappendorf B., Hornstra H. and Scholz H.C.2011.Natural *Burkholderia mallei* Infection in Dromedary, Bahrain. Emerg. Infect. Dis. **17:** 1277-1279.

□□□

Chapter 25

Campylobacter

R.S. RATHORE
IVRI, Izatnagar, Bareilly

Introduction

Bovine genital *Campylobacter*iosis is a venereally transmitted bacterial disease caused by *Campylobacter fetus* subsp *venerealis*. The disease is characterized by temporary infertility of female cattle as a result of a subacute diffuse mucopurulent cervicitis, endometritis, early embryonic death and salpingitis. Abortion occurs in a small percentage of infected cows, months after initial infection. Infected bulls show no clinical signs but many become carriers and subsequently infect females at service (Hum, 1994). All breeds of cattle are susceptible. The disease is often suspected in herds in which infertility or abortions occur. *Campylobacter fetus*, comprising two subspecies, *C. fetus* subsp. *fetus* and *C. fetus* subsp. *venerealis*, are important pathogens of humans and animals. It can be isolated from the genital tract of cattle (e.g. preputial smegma, vaginal mucus) or internal organs of aborted *fetus*es. Infections of veterinary importance are manifest as two distinct diseases of breeding: *C. fetus* subsp. *venerealis* causes enzootic infertility in cattle, while *C. fetus* subsp. *fetus* is associated with sporadic epizootic abortion in cattle and sheep (Garcia *et al.*, 1983; Skirrow, 1994). Ovine abortion is a worldwide problem, of particular importance in those countries where lamb is the predominant meat food source or is of economic significance (Aldomy, 1992; Orr, 1994). About 11% of ovine abortions diagnosed in Great Britain are *Campylobacter* related, mostly *C. fetus* associated. The natural route of transmission is considered to be fecal-oral, and asymptomatic intestinal carriage is believed to occur frequently (Smibert, 1965). In humans,

C. fetus subsp. *fetus* may cause an acute intestinal illness, or systemic disease, especially in immune-compromised hosts (Blaser, 1998). In developing countries like India, acute diarrhoeal diseases are major cause of childhood morbidity and mortality. *C. jejuni* has been established as an agent of bacterial enteritis in developed countries and is also reported from some developing countries like India. The organism is known to cause invasive type of bloody diarrhoea, watery diarrhoea or even a biphasic illness beginning with watery diarrhoea followed by bloody diarrhoea. Various species within the genus *Campylobacter* have emerged over the last three decades as important clinical pathogens of human and veterinary concern, where the majority of acute bacterial enteritis in human beings in the western countries is caused by these organisms, particularly due to thermo tolerant *Campylobacters* (Frost, 2001). The most frequently identified organism associated with diarrhoeal infections in humans is *Campylobacter jejuni*. According to the USDA –Economic Research Service, *C. jejuni* and *C. coli* cause approximately 1.3-1.75 million cases of food borne illness and 100-511 deaths annually in the USA (Allos, 1997; Buzby *et al.*, 1997). Apart from enteritis, zoonotic *Campylobacters* have been found to be associated with potentially life threatening complications like Guillain-Bare syndrome, reactive arthritis, abortion, hemolytic uraemic syndrome, meningitis etc. (Stern and Line, 2000; Stanfford and Tenkate, 2001). Other species of the genus such as *C. lari* and *C. fetus* appear to cause human disease less frequently than *C. jejuni*. But these figures underestimate the true incidence of *Campylobacter*iosis because most cases are relatively mild and are never seen in clinic or hospital settings, particularly in developing countries like India where no systematic studies have been done.

In the recent past, the number of human enteritis cases due to Campylobacters have been exceeded those of caused by *Salmonella* and *Shigella*, especially in developed world (WHO, 2002). Overall, the high incidence of clinical diseases associated with this organism, its low infective dose in humans and its potentially serious squeal, confirms its importance as a significant public health hazard worldwide (Tauxe, 2002).

Campylobacter spp. are found in the intestinal tract of many warm blooded mammals and birds. Many domestic and pet animals have been recognized as source of infection for human beings, like cattle, sheep, goat, pigs, dogs and poultry. Infection can also occur through consumption of contaminated drinking water, unpasteurized milk and raw or inadequately cooked meats such as beef, pork and mutton as well as seafood. Poultry has been documented as the main source of *C. jejuni* infection in human beings. *C. fetus* subsp. *fetus* was primarily regarded as an animal pathogen but it also has the potential to cause sporadic and epidemic food-borne disease.

Etiology

The family *Campylobacteriaceae* comprises genus *Campylobacter* and *Arcobacter*. *Campylobacter* genus comprises *of* small (0.2–0.9 ìm wide and 0.2–5.0 ìm long), spiral formed, Gram-negative bacteria with 18 species, six sub-species and two biovars. They are very different from other pathogens associated with food-borne disease in that they are essentially microaerophilic, growing best in an atmosphere containing approximately 10% CO_2 and approximately 5% O_2. The species pathogenic to man have a narrow temperature range for growth with a maximum of 42ºC and a minimum of 30ºC. These are classified as thermophilic *Campylobacters*. *Campylobacter* spp. are recognized as one of the most important cause of acute diarrhoeal disease in humans throughout the world. The three species most commonly involved in *Campylobacter* enteritis are *Campylobacter jejuni*, *Campylobacter coli* and *Campylobacter lari*. The thermotolerant *Campylobacter* spp. are closely related and hence differentiating *C. jejuni* and *C. coli* is difficult and solely based on the hippurate hydrolysis test. Table 1 shows the zoonotic members of the family *Campylobacteriaceae*. *Campylobacter* spp. are found in a wide range of sites in animals with some causing infections of the reproductive tract of certain domestic animals, which can lead to either abortion or infertility. Most infections are caused by *Campylobacter jejuni* and *C. coli*, although in the developing world *C. upsaliensis* is also important. *C. jejuni* and *C. coli* present an interesting dilemma. They can cause severe disease in infected people but are carried in the intestinal tracts of all types of domestic and many wild animals, almost always without any harmful effects. This carriage has major consequences for human health in terms of food-borne disease. The differences in pathogen behaviour in man and animals are not yet fully understood but are likely to be due to differential bacterial gene expression in different hosts. Bovine genital *Campylobacter*iosis (BGC, also known as bovine venereal *Campylobacter*iosis (BVC)) is a venereal disease characterised by infertility, early embryonic death, and abortion in cattle. The causal agent of this sexually transmissible disease is *Campylobacter fetus* subsp. *venerealis*. It can be isolated from the genital tract of cattle (e.g. preputial smegma, vaginal mucus) or internal organs of aborted *fetus*es (OIE, 2008).

Genus *Arcobacter*, is relatively new, proposed by Vandamme and De ley (1991), belonging to the family *Campylobacteraceae*, which encompasses a group of fastidious Gram-negative bacterium, spirally curved to 'S'-shaped rods, formerly known as 'aerotolerent *Campylobacters*'. Arcobacters can grow aerobically at lower temperatures, which is a distinctive feature that differentiates arcobacters from *Campylobacters*. To date, there are eleven recognized species, namely *Arcobacter butzleri*, *A. cryaerophilus*, *A. skirrowii*, *A. cibarius*, *A. nitrofigilis*, *A. halophilus*, *A. sulfidicus*, *A. mytili* sp. nov., *A.*

thereius sp. nov., *A. marinus* sp. nov. and *A. trophiarium* sp. nov. (Amare *et al.*, 2011). Amongst these *A. butzleri, A. cryaerophilus, A. skirrowii, and A. cibarus* are considered as emerging food-borne pathogens (Houf and Stephan, 2007). More predominantly, the species *viz., A. butzleri, A. cryaerophilus* and *A. skirrowii* have been found in farm animals and recognized as pathogenic for humans.

Table 1 : Zoonotic *Campylobacter* species

Family Member	Known source(s)	Disease associations Human	Veterinary
C. fetus subsp. *fetus*	Cattle, Sheep	Septicemia, Gastroenteritis Abortion, Meningitis	Bovine and ovine spontaneous abortion
C. fetus subsp. *venerealis*	Cattle	Septicemia	Bovine infectious infertility
C. jejuni	Poultry, Pig, Cattle, Sheep, Dogs, Cats, Water, Birds, Mink, Rabbit,	Gastroenteritis, septicemia, Abortion, Meningitis, Proctitis, Guillain-barre syndrome	Gastroenteritis, Avian hepatitis
C. coli	Pig, Poultry, Cattle, Sheep, Birds	Gastroenteritis, Septicemia	Gastroenteritis
C. lari	Birds, Water, Dogs, Monkey, Horses, Seal	Gastroenteritis, Septicemia	Avian gastroenteritis
C. upsaliensis	Dogs, Cats	Gastroenteritis, Septicemia, Abscesses.	Canine and feline gastroenteritis

History

Campylobacters were observed in stools of diarrhoeic infants in Germany as early as 1880, but first recognized identification of the organism was made in 1913 in association with abortion in sheep and confirmatory tests were carried out in 1918 when similar organisms were isolated from aborted bovine *fetus*es (McFadyean and Stockman, 1913; Smith, 1918). The organisms were originally assigned to the genus Vibrio, due to their spiral appearance and were named as *Vibrio fetus* (Smith and Taylor, 1919). However, it was not until 1947 that the human infection was first associated with the micro-aerophilic vibrios, which was associated with a pregnancy-related infection, where the *fetus* died (Moore *et al.*, 2005). Jones *et al.* (1931) named the bacterium causing enterocolitis in calves as *Vibrio jejuni*. Doyle in 1944 reported enterocolitis in Swine and named the organisms as *Vibrio coli*.

The genus *Campylobacter* was proposed in 1963, as it was realized that the organisms were not able to utilize sugars and had a different G+C content to that of Vibrio spp. (Sebald and Veron, 1963). *C. jejuni* and *C. coli* were named by Veron and Chatelian (1973) which cause enterocolitis. The genus *Campylobacter* is now classified under family *Campylobacteriaceae* (Vandamme and Delay, 1991).

Arcobacters were first described in the 1970s by Ellis and colleagues, who isolated them from aborted bovine fetal tissues and later porcine foetuses (Ellis *et al.*, 1977; 1978). *Arcobacters* were formerly referred as 'aerotolerant *Campylobacters*' due to their phenotypic and genotypic similarities to the genus *Campylobacter*. The genus *Arcobacter* was proposed to encompass these 'aerotolerant *Campylobacters*' by Vandamme *et al.* (1991).

Virulence factors and Pathogenesis

Campylobacter fetus subspecies *venerealis* and *C. fetus* subspecies *fetus* are structurally unusual in that they possess a microcapsule or S layer, which consists of high molecular weight proteins arranged in a lattice formation. This S layer confers resistance to serum-mediated destruction and phagocytosis (Blaser and Pei, 1993) and enhances survival in the genital tract. Virulence factors attributed to *C. jejuni* include soluble components with enterotoxin-like activity and poorly defined mechanisms for attaching to and invading host enterocytes. The contribution of heat-stable endotoxin to the pathogenesis of *Campylobacter*iosis is uncertain.

Epidemiology and Transmission

Transmission of *C fetus* subsp *venerealis* is strictly venereal. The infection is most commonly introduced to a herd by a persistently infected bull, and less frequently by a persistently infected female. After a bull becomes infected by serving a carrier female, it may remain persistently infected, disseminating the infection during breeding. Factors influencing the establishment of persistent infection probably relate to the genetic changes of the infecting strain, as it attempts to evade the immune system (Wesley and Bryner, 1989). This antigenic drift has not been well characterised, and bulls vary considerably in both their ability to harbour *C. fetus* and the length of time they may remain as carriers (Dufty *et al.*, 1975). There is little published information on the frequency of the carrier stage in females, but it appears that persistent infection is less frequent in this sex. This is thought to be due to a vigorous IgG-dominated immune response to bacterial colonization of the cervix and uterus (Coebeil and Winter, 1978). Following the introduction of the infection into a herd, the extent of the subsequent infertility episode largely depends on management practices. In susceptible herds, infertility in individual breeding units (a single sire mating with an infected bull) is always dramatic, compared with multiple sire mating practices, where infected and non-infected bulls are available. In herds in which the disease is endemic, pregnancy rates are generally higher and may appear to be satisfactory. This is mainly because fertility is not usually impaired in previously infected females due to acquired immunity. The degree of infertility will largely depend on the proportion and the number of susceptible cows or replacement virgin heifers being introduced to the endemically infected breeding unit.

Ovine genital *Campylobacter*iosis in ewes may be caused by either *C. fetus* subsp. *fetus* or *C. jejuni*. The disease is worldwide in distribution and is one of the most common cause of ovine abortion in some countries (Anon., 1997).

In the US, it has been estimated that food-borne *Campylobacter*s infect around 2.5 million people each year (Mead *et al.*, 1999). In England and Wales, estimates show that there were approximately 3, 60,000 cases of food-borne *Campylobacter* infection in 2000, accounting for 27% of all food-borne disease (Adak *et al.*, 2002).

Range and severity of symptoms and chronic effects

Campylobacter fetus subspecies *venerealis*, the principal cause of bovine genital *Campylobacter*iosis, is transmitted during coitus to susceptible cows by asymptomatic carrier bulls. The bacteria survive in the glandular crypts of the prepuce and bulls may remain infected indefinitely. The disease is characterized by temporary infertility associated with early embryonic death, return to oestrus at irregular periods and occasionally, by sporadic abortion. About one-third of infected cows become carriers. *Campylobacter fetus* subsp. *Venerealis* persists in the vagina of carrier cows, a feature attributed to antigenic shifts in the immunodominant antigens of the S layer proteins. Extension of infection to the uterus with the development of endometritis and salpingitis can occur during the progestational phase of the oestrus cycle when both the numbers and the activity of neutrophils decline. The infertile period following uterine invasion can last for 3-5 months, after which natural immunity may develop. IgA antibodies, which predominate in the vagina, limit spread of infection. IgG antibodies produced in the uterus opsonize the pathogens, facilitating phagocytosis by neutrophils and mononuclear cells. This natural immunity may last for upto 4 years. *Campylobacter fetus* subsp. *fetus*, an enteric organism acquired by ingestion, can cause sporadic abortions in cows.

Classic symptoms of thermophilic *Campylobacter* infection in human beings include diarrhoea (frequently bloody), abdominal pain, fever, malaise, nausea and, rarely vomiting. Complications of acute infection include intestinal hemorrhages, toxic megacolon and haemolytic uraemic syndrome. Mesenteric adenitis (inflammation of abdominal lymph nodes) can mimic acute appendicitis. The duration of illness is usually not longer than 10 days. Patients should be excluded from working as food handlers until they have been symptom-free for 48 hrs but once this period is over there are no public health reasons to restrict them from working. However, some food businesses may ask infected employees to submit stool samples for testing in line with their own occupational health requirements. In the longer term infection with *Campylobacters* may lead to neurological and rheumatological sequel. GBS is considered to be the most common cause of flaccid paralysis worldwide (Nachamkin, 2002). GBS and the non-paralytic variant Miller Fisher Syndrome are recognised sequelae of *Campylobacter* infection (Nachamkin, 2002). It is estimated that around 1 in 1000 infections leads to GBS, the risk increasing to around 1 in 200 for patients infected with a particular *C. jejuni*, Penner type HS:19 (Nachamkin, 2002).

Diagnosis

Isolation and identification of the *Campylobacter fetus* subsp. *venerealis*

a) Collection of samples

i) Bulls: Preputial smegma and semen

ii) Females: Vaginal mucus

iii) Aborted *fetus* and placenta

Transport and enrichment media

1. Clark's Australian transport and enrichment medium
2. Lander's medium of United kingdom
3. Modified SBL medium

Media for isolation of *Campylobacter* spp.

1. Skirrow's medium
2. Clark's selective medium
3. Park and Sanders medium for isolation of thermophilic *Campylobacter* spp.
4. Doyle's medium
5. Preston's selective medium

Colony characteristics

The colonies of *Campylobacter* appear within 2-5 days of incubation on a selective medium under favorable conditions. Growth may be at slower rate if other contaminating flora is present on the plates. The colonies of C. *fetus* are 1-3 mm after3-5 days of incubation. The colonies appear slightly pink, round, convex, smooth and shiny, translucent with a regular edge. *C. jejuni* produce watery dew drop like colonies which swarming along the streaking lines. Circular convex mucoid type colonies may also be seen. *C. coli* mature colonies may show metallic sheen after one week.

Identification of the isolates

Presumptive colonies are tested for oxidase, catalase, morphology by gram's staining, motility, urease, nitrate test, hippurate hydrolysis etc. and then further tested for species differentiation and confirmation. Suspected colonies may be reinoculated in broth and subcultured to get pure cultures which are further tested. Microscopic examination after gram's staining reveals curved, comma, S shaped, long helical shape with spirals may be observed.

Identifying characteristics for genus *Campylobacter*

Characteristics	Reaction
Motility	+
Nitrate reduction	+*
Growth in 3.5% NaCl	-
Growth in 1% glycine	+
H_2S lead paper strip	+**
Glucose utilization	-

*Except *C. doylei*, ** Small amount of H_2S may be produced by *C. hyointestinalis* and some strains of *C. coli*

Differentiation of *Campylobacter* upto species level

Species characteristics	*C. fetus*	*C. jejuni*	*C. coli*	*C. lari*
Growth at 25° C	+	–	–	–
Growth at 30.5° C	NR	–	+	+
Growth at 42° C	–	+	+	+
Cephalothin (30 µg disc)	S	R	R	R
Hippurate hydrolysis		+	–	–
2,3,5,- triphenyltetrazolium chloride	NR	S	R	R
Nalidixic acid	NR	S	S	R

R= Resistant, S=Sensitive, NR= Not required

Molecular diagnosis

Routine diagnostic laboratories would be served best by a simple PCR. Several PCRs have been claimed to be subspecies specific including those developed by Hum *et al.* (1997).

The multiplex PCR described by Hum *et al.* (1997) is currently the most cited PCR. It enables the amplification of a *C. fetus*-specific DNA fragment (approximately 200 bp smaller than the 960 bp described in the original publication), as well as a *C. fetus* subsp. *venerealis*-specific fragment. Thus, performance of this multiplex PCR allows differentiation of the two subspecies (*C. fetus* = one amplification product vs *C. fetus* subsp. *venerealis* = two amplification products). *Campylobacter fetus* subsp. *venerealis* biovar intermedius strains have not been evaluated in Hum's study, but isolates identified as belonging to biovar intermedius with AFLP, classify in the PCR of Hum as either *C. fetus* subsp. *fetus* or *C. fetus* subsp. *venerealis* (Van Bergen *et al.*, 2005). Comparison of this PCR against AFLP and MLST (Van Bergen *et al.*, 2005) and against the glycine test confirms that PCR can give false positive and negative reactions. Also a DNA probe and PCR based identification assays have been described for *C. fetus* (Ezaki *et al.*, 1988; Wesley *et al.*, 1991; Chevrier *et al.*, 1989; Blom *et al.*, 1995; Bastyns *et al.*, 1994; Eaglesome *et al.*, 1995; Hum *et al.*, 1997).

For the detection of the genus *Campylobacter* a highly conserved region such as the 16S rRNA is the target for the PCR, while more specific loci are used for the detection of particular species. One example is the hippurate gene for *C. jejuni* (Bang *et al.*, 2002). A multiplex PCR assay to identify and discriminate between isolates of *Campylobacter coli*, *Campylobacter jejuni*, *Campylobacter lari* and *Campylobacter upsaliensis* by targeting nucleotide Sequence of the Lipid A Gene *lpxA*.

Serological tests/antibody detection

An ELISA is available to detect antigen-specific secretory IgA antibodies in the vaginal mucus following abortion due to *C. fetus* subsp. *venerealis*. These antibodies are long lasting, and their concentration remains constant in the vaginal mucus for several months (Hum *et al.*, 1991). Initial sampling can be done after the early involution period (usually 1 week after abortion) when mucus becomes clear.

Immuno?uorescence antibody test (IFAT) also been used for detection of *C. fetus* In this study samples of CVM previously enriched on MBB (Cipolla *et al.*, 1995a) and on preputial samples (Dufty, 1967). C. *fetus* subsp. *venerealis* and *C. fetus* subsp. *fetus* reference and regional ?eld strains were used as positive control, and local strains of several species of bacteria di?erent from C. *fetus* subsp. were used as negative control, according to Cipolla et al. (1998).

Western blotting: Capsulated strains of C. *fetus* subsp. *fetus*, C. *fetus* subsp. *venerealis* biotype intermedius and C. *fetus* subsp. *venerealis* were subjected to sodium dodecyl sulphate (SDS) - polyacryl amide gel electrophoresis (PAGE) (10% polyacrylamide) with 2-mercaptoethanol in the sample bu?er, followed by Western blotting by Cobo *et al.* (2003).

Treatment and control of BGC

- Dihydrostreptomycin, administered either systematically or topically into prepuce, is used for treating bulls.
- Intrauterine administration of dihydrostreptomycin can be used therapeutically.
- The proposed treatment includes gentamicin and a second antibiotic, e.g. amoxicillin or Augmentin® or ciprofloxacin or imipenem, according to the location and the susceptibility profile.
- Vaccination with bacterins in and oil emulsion adjuvant is used therapeutically and prophylactically in problem herds. Berg and Firehammer (1978) recommend that breeding herd be vaccinated twice prior to the breeding season in order to achieve a high serum IgG titer. However, since bulls can still passively transmit the disease under conditions of intensive sexual activity (Fivaz *et al.*, 1978), but both males and females require immunization.
- The use of artificial insemination that is successful in dairy herds and small farm beef herds is impractical on larger ranches. Maintaining a clean, unexposed herd is possible only if virgin bulls are used and if only clean uninfected females are introduced.
- Cure of female cattle with venereal *Campylobacter*iosis is by systemic immunization of heifers with killed *C. fetus* is sufficient to cure the cervico-vaginal carrier state (Schurig *et al.*, 1975).

References

Adak, G. K., Long, S. M., O'Brien, S. J. (2002). Trends in indigenous foodborne disease and deaths, England and Wales: 1992 to 2000. Gut., **51:** 832–841.

Aldomy, F. M. M. A. (1992). A study of perinatal mortality in small ruminants in Jordan. Ph.D. thesis, University of London, London, England.

Allos, B. M. (2001). *Campylobacter* jejuni infections: update on emerging issues and trends. Clin. Infect. Dis., **32:** 1201-1206.

Amare, L.B., Saleha, A. A., Zunita, Z.,. Jalila, A. and Hassan, L. (2011). Prevalence of *Arcobacter* spp. on chicken meat at retail markets and in farm chickens in Selangor, Malaysia. Food Control., **22:** 732-736.

Anon, (1997). Sheep abortions; analysis of trends in 1996/97.

Bang, D. D.,Wedderkop, A., Pedersen, K., Madsen, M. (2002). Rapid PCR using nested primers of the 16S rRNA and the hippuricase (hip O) genes to detect *Campylobacter* jejuni and *Campylobacter* coli in environmental samples. Molecular and Cellular Probes., **16:** 359–369.

Berg, A.L. and Firehammer, B.D. (1978). Effect of interval between booster vaccination and time of breeding on protection against *Campylobacter*iosis (vibriosis) in cattle. *J.* Am. vet. med. Ass., **173:** 467-471.

Blaser, M. J. (1998). *Campylobacter fetus*-emerging infection and model system for bacterial pathogenesis at mucosal surfaces. Clin. Infect. Dis., **27:** 256–258.

Blaser, M. J. and Pei, Z. (1993). Pathogenesis of *Campylobacter fetus* infections; critical role of high- molecular -weight S- layer proteins in virulence. Journal of Infectious Diseases., **167:** 372-377.

Buzby, J.C., Roberts, T. (1997). Economic costs and trade impacts of microbial foodborne illness. World Health Statistics Quarterly **50:** 57–66.

Cipolla, A., Campero, C. M., Medina, D., Morsella, C., Cosentino, B., Caracino, M., Marcone, J. and Spath, E. (1995a). Un metodo mejorado para el diagnostico de la *Campylobacter*iosis genital en vacas. XIV Annual Meeting A.L.P.A., p. 742.

Cipolla, A., Paolicchi, F., Poso, M., Morsella, C., Casaro, A., Massone, A., Villegas, R., Callejas, S. and Gimeno, E. (1998). Lectin-bindings sites in uterus an oviduct of normal and *Campylobacter fetus* sub species *venerealis*-infected heifers. Eur. J. Histochem., **42:** 63–70.

Corbeil, L. B., Schurig, G. D., Duncan, J. R., Corbeil, R. R. and Winter, A.J. (1974). Immunoglobulin classes and biological functions of *Campylobacter (Vibrio) fetus* antibodies in serum and cervico-vaginal mucus. Infect Immun., **10:** 422-429.

Doyle, L. P. (1944). A Vibrio associated with swine dysentery. Am. J. Vet. Res., **5:** 3-5.

Dufty, J., (1967). Diagnosis of Vibriosis in the bull. Aust. Vet. J., **43:** 433–437.

Dufty, J. H, Clark, B. L, Monsbourgh, M. J. (1975). The influence of age on the susceptibility of bulls to *Campylobacter fetus* subsp. *venerealis*. Aust. Vet. J., **51:** 294-297.

Ellis, W.A., Neill, S. D., O' Brien, J. J. and Hannna, J. (1978). Isolation of *Spirullum*-like organisms from pig foetuses. Vet. Rec., **102:** 106.

Ellis, W.A., Neill, S. D., O' Brien, J. J., Ferguson, H.W. and Hanna, J.(1977). Isolation of *Spirillum/Vibrio*-like organisms from bovine foetuses. Vet. Record., **100:** 451-452.

Ezaki, T., Takeuchi, N., Liu, S., Kai, A., Yamamoto, H. and Yabuuchi. E. (1988). Small scale DNA preparation for rapid genetic identification of *Campylobacter* species without radioisotope. Microbiol. Immunol., **32:** 141-150.

Fivaz, B.H., Swanepool, R. and McKenzie, R.L. (1978). Passive transfer of *Campylobacter fetus* by immunized bulls. Aust. vet. J., **54:** 531-533.

Frost, J. A. (2001). Current epidemiological issues in human *Campylobacter*iosis. J. Appl. Microbiol., **90:** 80S-95S.

Garcia M. M., Eaglesome M. D. and Rigby C. (1983). *Campylobacters* important to veterinary medicine. Vet. Bull., **53:** 793–818.

Houf, K., and Stephan, R. (2007). Isolation and characterization of the emerging food-borne pathogen *Arcobacter* from human stool. J. Microbiol. Methods., **68:** 408-413.

Hum S. (1994). Diagnosis and control of Bovine Venereal *Campylobacter*iosis. Veterinarian, 15-16.

Hum, S, Quinn, K., Brunner, J. and On S. L.W. (1997). Evaluation of a PCR assay for identification and differentiation of *Campylobacter fetus* subspecies. Aust. Vet. J., **75:** 827-831.

Hum, S, Stephens, L. R, Quinn, C. (1991). Diagnosis by ELISA of bovine abortion due to identification and differentiation of *Campylobacter fetus* subspecies. Aust Vet J., **75:** 827-831.

Jones, F. S., Orcutt, M. and Little, R. B. (1931). Vibrios (V. jejuni n. sp.) associated with intestinal disorders of cows and calves. J. Exp. Med., **53:** 853-864.

McFadyean, J. and Stockman, S. (1913). Report of the departmental committee appointed by the board of agriculture and fisheries to enquire into epizootic abortion, Part III, London, HMSO.

Mead, P. S., Slutsker, L., Dietz, V., McCaig, L. F., Bresee, J. S., Shapiro, C., Griffin, P. M., Tauxe, R.V., 1999. Food-related illness and death in the United States. Emerging infectious Diseases., **5:** 607–625.

Moore, J. E., Corcoran, D., Dooby, S. G., Lucey, B., Matsuda, M., McDowell, A., Megraud, F., Millar, B., O'Mahony, R., Riordan, L., O; Rourke, M., Rao, J., Rooney, P., Sails, A., Whyte, P. (2005). *Campylobacter*. Vet. Res., **36:** 351-382.

Nachamkin, I. (2002). Chronic effects of *Campylobacter* infection. Microbes and Infection., **4:** 399–403.

OIE, (2008). Bovine genital *Campylobacter*iosis Chapter 2.4.5. OIE Terrestrial Manual 2008.

Orr, M. (1994). Animal health laboratory network. Review of diagnostic cases. Surveillance **21:** 3–6.

Schurig, G. D., Hall, C. E. and Burda, K. (1973). Persistent genital tract infection with *Vibrio fetus intestinalis* associated with serotypic alteration of the infecting strain. Am J Vet Res., **34:** 1399-1403.

Schurig, G.D., Hall, C.E. and Corbeil, L.B. Bovine venereal vibriosis. (1975). Cure of genital infection in females by systemic immunization. Infect. and Immun. **11:** 245-251.

Sebald M. & Veron M. (1963). Base DNA Content and Classification of *Vibrios*. Ann. Inst. Pasteur, Paris., **105:** 897–910.

Skirrow, M. B. (1994). Disease due to *Campylobacter*, Helicobacter and related bacteria. J. Comp. Pathol., **111:** 113-149.

Smibert, R. M. (1965). *Vibrio fetus var intestinalis* isolated from fecal and intestinal contents of clinically normal sheep: isolation of microaerophilic *Vibrios*. Am. J. Vet. Res., **26:** 315–319.

Smith, T. (1918). Spirilla associated with disease of the fetal membranes in cattle (Infectious abortion). J. Exp. Med., **28:** 701.

Smith, T. and Taylor, M. S. (1919). Some morphological and biological characters of spirilla (Vibrio *fetus* n. sp.) associated with disease of the fetal membranes in cattle. J. Exp. Med., **30:** 299-311.

Stanford, T. D. and Tenkate, R. J. (2001). Risk factors for *Campylobacter* infection in infants and young children: A matched case control study. Epidemiol. Infect., **127:** 399-404.

Stern, N. D. and Line, J. E. (2000). *Campylobacter*. In: The microbiological safety and quality of food. 1040-1056.

Tauxe, R. V. (2002). Emerging foodborne pathogens. Int. J. Food Microbiol., **78:** 31-34.

Van Bergen, M. A., Dingle, K. E. and Maiden, M. C. (2005). Clonal nature of *Campylobacter fetus* as defined by multilocus sequence typing. J Clin Microbiol., **43:** 5888-5898.

Vandamme, P., and De ley, J. (1991). Proposal for a new family *Campylobacteraceae*. Int. J. Syst. Bacteriol., **41:** 451-455.

Véron, M. & Chatelain, R. (1973). Taxonomic study of the genus *Campylobacter* Sebald and Véron and designation of the neotype strain for the type species *Campylobacter fetus* (Smith and Taylor) Sebald and Véron. Int. J. Syst. Bacteriol., **23:** 122–134.

Wesley, I. V, Bryner, J. H. (1989). Antigenic and restriction enzyme analysis of isolates of *Campylobacter fetus* subsp *venerealis* recovered from persistently infected cattle. Am J Vet Res., **50:** 807-813.

Wesley, I. V., Bryner, J. H. (1989). Antigenic and restriction enzyme analysis of isolates of *Campylobacter fetus* subsp *venerealis* recovered from persistently infected cattle. Am J Vet Res., **50:** 807-813.

Wesley, I. V., Wesley, R. D., Cardella, M. F., Dewhirst, E. and Paster, B. J. (1991). Oligodeoxynucleotide probes for *Campylobacter fetus* and *Campylobacter hyointestinalis* based on 16S rRNA sequences. J. Clin. Microbiol., **29:** 1812-1817.

WHO, (2002). Increasing incidence of human *Campylobacter*iosis.

□□□

Chapter 26

Salmonella

R.K. AGARWAL
IVRI, Izatnagar, Bareilly

Introduction

Salmonella were first described at the end of the nineteenth century and was named after D.E. Salmon, who isolated *Salmonella* Choleraesuis, from pigs in 1885 (Le Minor, 1994). The nomenclature of *Salmonella* has gone through a number of historical changes. Currently, there are two recognized species of *Salmonella*: *S. enterica* and *S. bongori*. *Salmonella enterica* is further divided into six subspecies: *enterica* (subspecies I), *salamae* (subspecies II), *arizonae* (subspecies III), *diarizonae* (subspecies IIIb), *houtenae* (subspecies IV), and *indica* (subspecies V) (OIE, 2004). The serotypes of *Salmonella* are based on their O (heat-stabile somatic), Vi (heat-labile capsular), and H (flagellar) antigens (Grimont *et al.*, 2000). The genus *Salmonella* comprises a group of 2610 serovars distributed widely in nature (Guibourdenche *et al.*, 2010). *Salmonella* serotypes differ in their pathogenic potential and serotype distributions often vary vastly between human and animal populations as well as among different animal populations in the same geographic area. *Salmonella* serotypes can be divided into host restricted, host specific, and generalists serotypes (Uzzau *et al.*, 2000).

Host specific serotypes only cause disease in one host species (eg. Paratyphi A and Typhi in human; Gallinarum biovars Gallinarum and Pullorum in poultry). Host restricted serotypes are predominantly associated with one host species, but can cause disease in other species as well (Baumler *et al.*, 1998, Uzzau *et al.*, 2000). For example *S.* Dublin is adapted to cattle but also causes infections in small ruminants, pigs and humans. Similarly, Choleraesuis is adapted to swine but has also been isolated from a range of other host species (Olsen and Skov, 1994). Infections with host adapted or restricted serotypes are typically characterized by low morbidity and high mortality, and systemic disease is common. Generalist serotypes viz., *S. Typhimurium* and *S. Enteritidis* usually induce a self-limiting gastroenteritis and are also capable of inducing systemic disease in a wide range of host animals, have called the un-restricted or broad host-range serotypes (Uzzau *et al.*, 2000). Infections with generalist serotypes are often characterized by high morbidity but low mortality.

Salmonella infection in cattle is typically manifested as watery or bloody diarrhea, and often associated with fever, depression, anorexia, dehydration and endotoxemia. In some cases it may cause abortion and respiratory disease. Mortality rates can be high. Particularly in adult animals *Salmonella* frequently causes subclinical disease, and is known to persist on infected farms for months or years (Vanselow *et al.*, 2007, Wray *et al.*, 1989).

In small ruminants the severity and clinical manifestation of *Salmonella* infection differs by age group and serotype (Uzzau *et al.*, 2001). Acute enteric salmonellosis is common in adult sheep, while septicemia is common in young animals (Sharma *et al.*, 2001, Kusiluka and Kambarag, 1996). Asymptomatic carriage, chronic gastro-enteritis, and abortion have also been described (Kusiluka and Kambarag, 1996, Kumar *et al.*, 1973). *Salmonella* abortion is economically one of the most important diseases of small ruminants (Rushton, 2009). Neonatal mortality in affected herds is usually high. Lambs carried to term frequently die of septicemia (Uzzau *et al.*, 2001).

Pigs infected by *Salmonella* shows variety of conditions, ranging from asymptomatic to peracute disease. All age groups are susceptible to *Salmonella* infection, but disease is most commonly observed among weaned pigs more than eight weeks of age. Infection with host adapted serotype Choleraesuis generally causes severe systemic disease with high mortality. In contrast, infection with generalist serotypes such as Typhimurium usually cause mild or no disease. Clinical manifestations among *Salmonella* infected pigs, including enteritis, septicemia, pneumonia, meningitis, and arthritis. Fever, diarrhea, inappetence, depression, respiratory distress, lameness, edema, and hypoxia in the extremities are common symptoms in clinically sick pigs.

Salmonellosis is an important disease of horses. Equine mortality rates vary depending on host age, predisposing factors and the *Salmonella* serotype involved (Wenkoff, 1973). In general, mortality appears to be considerably lower, but mortalities as high as 40 to 60% have been reported (Begg *et al.*, 1988, Smith *et al.*, 1980). In most cases, animals present with profuse, watery and malodorous diarrhea, frequently associated with abdominal pain and endotoxemia. Both peracute and chronic forms of disease are common, and convalescent carriers may shed *Salmonella* for months (Smith *et al.*, 1980, Morse *et al.*, 1976, McCain and Powell, 1990). Disease may also manifest without gastrointestinal signs. Respiratory forms are comparably frequent, and systemic forms of infection are commonly associated with arthritis, osteomyelitis, or soft tissue abscesses (Blikslager *et al.*, 1991, Platt, 1973). Abortions due to *Salmonella* cause important economic losses on stud farms (Donahue, 1986; Kumar and Gupta, 1972).

Pathogenesis

Salmonella are enteric pathogens that infect a variety of hosts including human and animals. There are a large number of *Salmonella* species and serotypes that can cause a variety of diseases, ranging from localized gastroenteritis to more severe systemic, host specific illness such as fowl typhoid. The outcome of *Salmonella* infections depends not only on the infecting serotype but also on the infected host. An important virulence attribute common to all *Salmonella* is their ability to cross the intestinal epithelial barrier (Falkow, 1992). This process is thought to be essential for the pathogenicity of *Salmonella* and entails entry into several types of cells, including enterocytes, M cells and macrophages. Gaining access to an intracellular compartment may allow these organisms to evade host cell defenses and reach deeper tissues.

Understanding the *Salmonella* strategy for survival is to invade and multiply in gut associated lymphoid tissue (GALT) from the infected intestinal tissues, the pathogens are drained to the regional lymph nodes where the macrophages that line the lymphatic sinuses form the first effective barrier to prevent further spread. If this host defense mechanism successfully limits bacterial expansion, the infection remains localized to intestine and the GALT. On the other hand, if the macrophages located in the draining lymph nodes are unable to limit spread of *Salmonella* then it can cause systemic disease. During systemic infection the pathogen spread from GALT via efferent lymphatics draining into the thoracic duct and finally into the venacava and then spread to whole body.

Several distinct loci necessary for *Salmonella* to enter mammalian cells have been identified (Altmeyer *et al.*, 1993; Finlay and Falkow, 1988). The majority of these loci appear to be located between 58 and 60 minutes on the *Salmonella* chromosome, and it is now estimated that perhaps as much as 100 kb of DNA may be necessary for entry of *Salmonella* into mammalian cells. The *Salmonella* virulent determinants are often clustered on plasmids or on chromosomal pathogenecity islands (SPI) and pathogenecity islets (PI).

Salmonella possesses both a large virulence plasmids and a variety of chromosome encoded Pls. Barrow *et al.* (1987) demonstrated the 85 kb large plasmid of *Salmonella* Gallinarum contribute towards virulence in fowl typhoid and also reported that elimination of 2.5 kb small plasmid has no effect on virulence. Non-typhoid *Salmonella* strains associated with extra-intestinal infections in humans and animals carry an additional locus termed *Salmonella* plasmid virulence (spv). It is not present in typhoid strains. The spv genes are located within a highly homologous region contained on virulence plasmids found in the subspecies 1 lineage of *S. enterica*. The spv genes are located in the chromosome in certain other *S. enterica* lineages. Spv-carrying serovars associated with human disease include Typhimurium, Enteritidis, Choleraesuis, Dublin, and Arizona. Certain host-adapted animal pathogens, such as Gallinarum/Pullorum and Abortusovis, also contain the spv locus. The plasmid spvABCD genes are arranged in an operon positively regulated by the upstream spvR gene. SpvB and SpvC are translocated into the host cell by the *Salmonella* pathogenicity island-2 type-three secretion system. SpvB prevents actin polymerization by ADP-ribosylation of actin monomers, while SpvC has phosphothreonine lyase activity and has been shown to inhibit MAP kinase signaling. The exact mechanisms by which SpvB and SpvC act in concert to enhance virulence are still unclear. SpvB exhibits a cytotoxic effect on host cells and is required for delayed cell death by apoptosis following intracellular infection (Guiney and Fierer, 2011).

Two pathogenicity islands, *Salmonella* pathogenicity island I (SPI-I) and SPI-2 play key roles in mediating disease by *Salmonella enterica* through their respective type III secretary system (TTSS) (Hueck, 1998). The TTSS mediate the translocation of various virulence associated effector proteins from the bacteria into the host cells (Hensel, 2000).

Salmonella possesses at least two TTSS secreting virulence associated effector protein, TTSS-1 and TTSS-2. TTSS-1 is responsible mainly for enteropathogenesis whereas, TTSS-2 influences net intracellular growth (Hensel *et al.*, 1998) and does not influence enteropathogenesis (Tsolis *et al.*, 1999). Jones *et al.* (2001) reported that a function SPI-1 TTSS is not required for serovar Gallinarum to cause fowl typhoid, the SPI2 TTSS is required for the development of fowl typhoid, primarily at the level of macrophage interaction.

Immunity to Salmonella Infection

Immunity against *Salmonella* infection includes both innate and acquired immunity. Initial interaction of *Salmonella* with host cells leads to the activation of innate immune cells. *Salmonella* specific acquired immunity development follows innate immunity. The innate immunity is the first line of defense against invading pathogens. It includes inflammatory reactions, phagocytosis, acute phase reaction, complement proteins, etc. that are constitutional nonspecific defence reactions (Roitt, 1993). *Salmonella*, once engulfed by host macrophages, can escape from variety of antibacterial activities of macrophages through mechanisms involving tolerance to acid stress, resistance to a variety of antimicrobial peptides called defensins (Foster and Spector, 1995), and interference with the fusion of phagosomes with lysosomes (Uchiya *et al.*, 1999) or blocking the formation of phagolysosomes (Mukherjee *et al.*, 2000). Phagocytes and natural killer cells are the main components of early cellular immune response and primary defense mechanism in *Salmonella* infection. The role of gut mucosal immunity especially iELS in protection against enteric pathogens has been well documented. Nencioni *et al.* (1983) reported the natural bactericidal activity of iELS against *Salmonella* Typhimurium in mice. In vitro bactericidal activity of NK cells has been observed against *Salmonella* (Garcia *et al.*, 1989).

Acquired immune response mainly operate through communications of the APC, T cells and B cells by direct cell-to-cell contact using MHC, TCR and immunoglobulins and/or by secreted proteins such as cytokines in a paracrine way (Roitt, 1993). Since *Salmonella* is a facultative intracellular parasite, activation of specific cell mediated immune response is critical for its control and clearance from a host. Hence, protection is mostly dependent on T cell mediated immunity. It has been shown that CD_4 and CD_8 T lymphocytes act synergistically to control infection with virulent *Salmonella* species (Mastroeni *et al.*, 1993). However, induction of strong humoral response, especially antibodies blocking the adherence and entry of bacteria into the host cells, also seems to be important in mediating immunity to *Salmonella* (Mastroeni *et al.*, 2000).

The characteristic dissemination of *Salmonella* on mucosal surface and to systemic sites induces broad based immune responses including cell mediated immune response (CMI), local secretory IgA antibody response and systemic humoral response (Vancott *et al.*, 1996). Cell mediated immunity (CMI) plays a major role in protection against *Salmonella* infection, which has been demonstrated experimentally by several investigators (Babu *et al.*, 2004; Okamura *et al.*, 2004). *Salmonella* Typhimurium like other intracellular microbes has been shown to induce Th_1 dependent immune responses mediated by IFN-α, IL-2 and TNF-β (Vancott *et al.*, 1996). Briles *et al.* (1986) observed that the T lymphocytes of *S.* Typhimurium immune chickens are activated following infection and secreted cytokines that inturn activated macrophage to kill invading bacteria. The chicken CD_8 T lymphocytes mediated cytolysis of *Salmonella* infected target cells via an interferon dependent mechanism have also been demonstrated (Kauffman, 1995). IFN-ã which is best characterized as a component of CMI plays an important role in protection against *Salmonella* infection in avian hosts (Farnell *et al.*, 2001).

Diagnosis

The conventional diagnosis is based on the isolation of the organism either from tissues collected aseptically at necropsy or from faeces, rectal swabs or environmental samples, food products and feedstuffs. Preferably clinical samples are collected during the acute phase of the disease or as soon as possible after death (Caldwell *et al.*, 1998; Kinde *et al.*, 2004).

There are numerous methods for isolation of *Salmonella* in use worldwide (Fricker, 1987; Reissbrodt, 1995). *Salmonella* may be isolated using a variety of techniques, which may include pre-enrichment in non-selective broth to resuscitate sub lethally damaged *Salmonella*e, enrichment media that contain inhibitory substances to suppress competing organisms and selective plating agars to differentiate *Salmonella*e from other enterobacteria. The core of the standard method is pre-enrichment in buffered peptone water, enrichment on modified semi-solid Rappaport–Vassiliadis (MSRV) and isolation on xylose-lysine-deoxycholate (XLD) and an additional plate medium of choice. Various biochemical, serological and molecular tests can be applied to the pure culture to provide a definitive confirmation of an isolated strain.

A number of serological tests have been developed for the diagnosis of *Salmonella* infections in animals. In poultry, the whole blood test which uses a stained antigen and the serum agglutination test have been used successfully for over 50 years for the identification of flocks infected with *S. Pullorum* and *S. Gallinarum*. In the laboratory, the tube agglutination test is the method of choice for export and diagnostic purposes for samples from all species of farm animals. Enzyme linked immunosorbent assays (ELISA) are available for some serovars and may be used for serological diagnosis and surveillance (OIE, 2008).

Different types of ELISA, particularly indirect or double antibody-blocking assays using a variety of antigens such as lipopolysaccharide (LPS), flagella and SEF14 fimbrial antigen have been developed (van Zijderveld *et al.*, 1992; Barrow, 1994; Thorns *et al.*, 1996). ELISA is also helpful in detecting infection in subjects where there is only intermittent faecal excretion of *Salmonella*, because high concentrations of circulating IgG persist for several months following infection with *Salmonella* spp. (Nicholas and Cullen, 1991). It provides information about the *Salmonella* infection status of an animal 30-120 days prior to sample collection (Galland *et al.*, 2000).

Nielsen *et al.* (1995) reported ELISA as a suitable screening test for the presence of infection with S. Typhimurium or S. *Infantis* on a swine herd basis. The mix-ELISA is used in Denmark on serum or tissue fluid released by freezing and thawing muscle samples to detect *Salmonella* infections in pigs (Nielsen *et al.*, 1998). Chow *et al.* (2004) evaluated a commercial *Salmonella* covalent mix-ELISA for serological detection in swine and found that the assay was useful for the screening of the herds as it agrees with bacterial cultures as well as is reproducible, sensitive, specific, repeatable and suitable for automation. Funk *et al.* (2005) compared traditional faecal culture and Danish Mix-ELISA for determination of *S. enterica* prevalence in growing swine. An ELISA based on *S. Typhimurium* LPS was developed by Kich *et al.* (2007) to assess the prevalence of infection in swine herds, in order to implement rapid and cost-effective control programmes in Brazil (Kich *et al.*, 2007).

Several molecular diagnostic tools have been developed for improving the detection of *Salmonella* serotypes and are commercially available (Swaminathan and Feng, 1994; Ricke *et al.*, 1998). A number of molecular typing methods have also been used to differentiate strains below the level of serotypes. These DNA related techniques includes polymerase chain reaction (PCR) tests, multiplex PCR, RT-PCR, real time PCR, quantitative PCR, pulse field gel electrophoresis, random amplified polymorphic DNA assay, restriction fragment length polymorphism, PCR-ribotyping, IS200 finger printing, DNA hybridisation, gene probes, including nucleic acid sequence based amplification (Bailey *et al.*, 1991; Stone *et al.*, 1995; Shaw *et al.*, 1998; Gooding and Choudary, 1999; Cook, 2003; Malorny *et al.*, 2004; Perelle *et al.*, 2004).

Several polymerase chain reaction (PCR) methods for detecting *Salmonella* have been developed utilizing specific gene sequences targeting replicons, gene coding for DNA binding protein, gene coding for abequose and paratose synthase, gene coding for their aggregative fimbriae, agfA, rRNA operon, random genomic fragment, genes from spvR of the virulence plasmid, H-li and H-in flagellin genes, 16S DNA, invA and ompC genes (Agarwal *et al.*, 2009). Schrank *et al.* (2001) used an enrichment culture procedure with PCR amplification of the genus-specific invE/invA genes to distinguish *Salmonella* spp. from other enteric bacteria present in samples from the poultry industry. PCR-based commercial systems are also available. In these systems, PCR may be performed on the pre-enrichment medium after 16-20 hours of incubation. Real time PCR modifications for *Salmonella* detection (Eyigor and Carli, 2003; Perelle *et al.*, 2004; Hein *et al.*, 2006) have been good alternatives to conventional PCR in solving the sensitivity and sample size problems.

Control

Prevalence of *Salmonella* serotypes may vary considerably between localities, districts, regions and countries and therefore, surveillance and identification of the prevalent *Salmonella* serotypes should be carried out in order to develop a control programme for that area (OIE, 2009). *Salmonella* prevention and control may be achieved by adopting general hygiene and management measures in combination with the additional measures such as vaccination and competitive exclusion. No single measure used alone will achieve effective *Salmonella* control.

Strategies for the control of *Salmonella* in animals and poultry can be broadly classified as follows

Measures for excluding Salmonella from a herd or flock free of salmonellosis

- A closed herd policy should be implemented where ever possible
- Animals or birds used to stock a farm should be obtained from breeding herds / flocks that are free from *Salmonella* and remain isolated until negative for *Salmonella* on three consecutive samplings (Quinn *et al.*, 2001).
- ALL IN/ALL OUT POLICY- Another key element of *Salmonella* control though it is not possible in all farms due to capacity issues.
- Rodent control in farms is an essential element since they frequently act as carriers of *Salmonella.*
- A systematic control programme for other mechanical carriers of *Salmonella* (Flies, wild birds and other vermin/animals including dogs and cats) must operate in all areas of the unit.
- Steps should be taken to prevent contamination of feed and water.
- Protective clothing and foot wear should be worn by personnel entering farms. Rajic *et al.* (2006) reported the unusual finding that if boots were disinfected prior to entry, there was a decreased prevalence of *Salmonella.* Therefore foot baths containing suitable disinfectants such as 3 % iodophor should be placed at strategic locations.

Measures for reducing environmental contamination

- Effective routine cleaning and disinfection of buildings and equipments.
- Stress reduction is particularly important since stress on animals will induce carrier state to start shedding *Salmonellas*, leading to increased environment contamination.
- Slurry should be spread on arable land where possible. An interval of at least 2 months should elapse before grazing commences on pastures following application of slurry (Quinn *et al.*, 2001).

- The continuous use of paddocks for susceptible animals should be avoided (Quinn *et al.*, 2001).

Strategies for enhancing resistance and reducing the likelihood of clinical disease

- *Vaccination* : Vaccination can be used as part of an overall *Salmonella* control programme but not as the sole control measure. When the status of the breeding farm from which the replacement stock originates is not known and when moving animals to a previously contaminated shed, vaccination should be considered. Though vaccination against host-specific *Salmonella* serotypes (e.g. S. Gallinarum in poultry) induces a strong serotype-specific protective immunity (Smith, 1956; Barrow and Wallis, 2000), vaccination against non host-specific *Salmonella* serotypes has yielded variable success rates (Barrow, 2007).

  Vaccination is practiced in cattle, sheep, poultry, equines and pigs. Vaccines can be divided into two broad categories: active and passive. An active vaccine is intended to stimulate the body's immune system to produce specific antibodies (humoral response), cellular immune responses (e.g. cytotoxic T-lymphocytes), or both, with the aim of protecting against or eliminating a pathogen. A passive vaccine is a preparation of antibodies that is protective against a pathogen or disease and is administered before, at or around the time of known or potential exposure. Active vaccines can in turn be divided in three main categories, killed vaccines, live attenuated vaccines and subunit vaccines.

  Live attenuated vaccines are generally accepted to be more efficacious in controlling salmonellosis than killed bacterins (Lillehoj *et al.*, 2000). Killed vaccines have been found ineffective because of the following three reasons (Lax *et al.*, 1995). Firstly, they only contain surface antigens, which give an incomplete antibody response. Secondly, they fail to elicit cell-mediated immune response, which is important for long-term protection. Thirdly, they fail to elicit secretory IgA responses, which are potentially important in protecting mucosal surfaces. Though live attenuated vaccines are being worked upon most seriously and are being claimed as the most effective measures of immunoprophylaxis against *Salmonella*, they too have some drawbacks. They cause shedding of the vaccine strain on vaccination making it difficult to differentiate vaccinated and infected animals. Also, the possibility of reversal of attenuated forms to virulent forms cannot be ruled out (Miller and Mekalarz, 1990). These vaccines give protection against the homologues *Salmonella* strains from which the vaccine has been prepared thus leaving the animal exposed to the rest of *Salmonella* serovars (Curtiss *et al.*, 1993).

It has been found that live attenuated *Salmonella* vaccines while protecting against virulent *Salmonella*, paradoxically induced profound immunosuppression against non-*Salmonella* antigens and suppress lymphoproliferative response to mitogen (Al-Ramadi *et al.*, 1992). Thus, development of vaccine based on defined non-toxic components has led researchers to extensively study the complex antigens of *Salmonella*. Subunit vaccines take advantage of the possibility of using only part of the infectious micro-organism to raise a protective immune response, and since subunit vaccines cannot replicate in the host, there is no risk of pathogenicity. The composition of a subunit vaccine can normally be clearly defined, which is a significant advantage in terms of safety considerations and minimization of side-effects. In order to elicit a vigorous immune response, subunit vaccines often require multiple doses, as well as the use of adjuvant. Subunit vaccines can be based on peptides, proteins or polysaccharides that have been shown to contain protective epitopes.

- *Competitive exclusion (CE)* : The phenomenon by which *Salmonella* is suppressed by the early establishment of an adult intestinal microflora in young ones is known as 'competitive exclusion' (CE) and is sometimes described as the 'Nurmi concept', when referring to poultry (Pivnick and Nurmi, 1982). *L. reuteri* cultures (Dunham *et al.*, 1994) and *Saccharomyces boulardii* (Line *et al.*, 1997) are reported to reduce *Salmonella* infection of chicks when administered *in ovo* or via the feed.

Further recommendations for control

Improved genetically defined attenuated DIVA vaccines need to be developed. Vaccines giving cross-protection between *Salmonella* serovars needs to be developed. The genetic improvement of farm animals, including resistance to salmonellosis, is desirable, and research in this area should continue.

References

Agarwal, R.K., Bhilegaonkar, K.N., Biswas, R., John, J.M. and Sailo, B. (2009). Application of molecular tools for detection of *Salmonellosis* in human and animal. In: Practical manual on serological and PCR based diagnosis of economically important infectious diseases of domestic animals. CADRAD, I.V.R.I., U.P., India, pp. 107-112.

Al-Ramdai, B.K., Brodkin, M.A., Greene, J.M., Meissler, J.J. and Eisensteins, T.K. (1992). Immunosuppression induced by attenuated *Salmonella*: Effect of LPS responsiveness on development of suppression. Microbiol. Pathol., **12** : 267-278.

Altmeyer, R.M., McNern, J.K., Bossio, J.C., Rosenshine, I., Finlay, B.B. and Galán, J.E. (1993), Cloning and molecular characterization of a gene involved in *Salmonella* adherence and invasion of cultured epithelial cells. Mol. Microbiol., **7:** 89–98.

Babu, U., Dalloul, R.A., Okamura, M., Lillehoj, H.S., Xie, H., Raybourne, R.B., (2004). *Salmonella* Enteritidis clearance and immune responses in chickens following *Salmonella* vaccination and challenge. Vet. Immunol. Immunopathol. **101:** 251–257

Bailey, J.S., Cox, N.A. and Blankenship, L.C. (1991). A comparison of an enzyme immunoassay, DNA hybridization, antibody immobilization and conventional methods for recovery of naturally occurring *Salmonella* from processed broiler carcasses. J. Food Protect., **54:** 354-356.

Barrow P.A. (1994). Serological diagnosis of *Salmonella* serotype Enteritidis infections in poultry by ELISA and other tests. Int. J. Food Microbiol., **21:** 55–68.

Barrow, P.A. (2007). *Salmonella* infection: immune and non-immune protection with vaccines. Avian Pathology, **36:** 1-13.

Barrow, P. A., Tucker, J. F. and Simpson. J.M. (1987). Inhibition of colonization of the chicken alimentary tract with *Salmonella* Typhimurium Gram-negative facultative anaerobic bacteria. Epidemiol. Infect. **98:** 311–322.

Barrow, P.A. and Wallis, T.S. (2000). Vaccination against *Salmonella* infections in food animals: rationale theoretical basis and practical applications In: Wray C, Wray A, editors. *Salmonella* in domestic animals. New York: CABI Publishing. pp. 323-339.

Baumler, A.J., Tsolis, R.M., Ficht, T.A. and Adams, L.G. (1998). Evolution of host adaptation in *Salmonella* enterica. Infect. Immun. **66:** 4579-4587.

Begg, A.P., Johnston, K.G., Hutchins, D.R. and Edwards, D.J. (1988). Some aspects of the epidemiology of equine *Salmonellosis*. Australian Vet. J. **65:** 221-223.

Blikslager, A.T., Wilson, D.A., Taylor, D.S., MacFadden, K.E., Fischer, J.R. and Fales, W.H. (1991). *Salmonella typhimurium* abscess as a postoperative complication in a horse with colic. J American Vet. Med. Assoc. **199:** 1757-1759.

Briles, D. E., Benjamin, W., Posey, B., Michalek, S.M. and McGhee, J.R. (1986). Independence of macrophage activation and expression of the alleles of the Ity (Immunity to Typhimurium) locus. Microbial. Pathogenesis. **1:** 33-41

Caldwell D.J., Hargis, B.M., Corrier, D.E. and Deloach, J.R. (1998). Frequency of isolation of *Salmonella* from protective foot covers worn in broiler houses as compared with diagnostic sampling. Avian Dis., **42:** 381–384.

Chow, E.Y.W., Wu, J.T.Y., Jauho, E.S., Heegaard, P.M.H., Nilsson, E., Harris, I.T. and Manninen, K. (2004). Evaluation of a covalent mix-ELISA for screening of *Salmonella* antibodies in pig serum. Canadian J. Vet. Res., **68:** 134-139.

Cook, N. (2003). The use of NASBA for the detection of microbial pathogens in food and environmental samples. J. Appl. Microbiol., **53:** 165–174.

Curtiss, R., Kelly, S.M. and Hassan, J.O. (1993). Live oral avirulent *Salmonella* vaccines. Vet. Microbiol. **37:** 397-405.

Donahue, J.M. (1986). Emergence of antibiotic-resistant *Salmonella* Agona in horses in Kentucky. J. American Vet. Med. Assoc. **188:** 592-594.

Eyigor, A. and Carli, K.T. (2003). Rapid detection of *Salmonella* from poultry by real-time polymerase chain reaction with fluorescent hybridization probes. Avian Dis., **47:** 380-386.

Falkow, S., Isberg, R.R. and Portnoy, D.A. (1992). The interaction of bacteria with mammalian cells. Annu. Rev. Cell Biol. **8:** 333-363.

Farnell, M. B., El Halawani, M., You, S., McElroy, A. P., Hargis, B. M. and Caldwell, D. J. (2001). In vivo biologic effects of recombinant turkey interferon gamma in neonatal leghorn chicks protection against *Salmonella* Enteritidis organ invasion. Avian Dis. **45:** 473-478

Finlay, B.B. and Falkow, S. (1988). Comparison of the invasion strategies used by *Salmonella* cholerae-suis, Shigella flexneri and Yersinia enterocolitica to enter cultured animal cells: endosome acidification is not required for bacterial invasion or intracellular replication. Biochimie **70:** 1089-1099.

Foster, J.W. and Spector, M.P. (1995). How *Salmonella* survive against the odds. Annual Rev. Microbiol. **49:** 145-174

Fricker, C.R. (1987). Isolation of *Salmonella* and Campylobacter. J. Appl. Bacteriol., **63:** 99-116.

Funk, J.A., Harris, I.T. and Davies, P.R. (2005). Comparison of faecal culture and Danish Mix-ELISA for determination of S. enterica subsp. enterica prevalence in growing swine. Vet. Microbiol., **107:** 115-126.

Galland, J.C., House, J.K., Hyatt, D.R., Hawkins, L.L., Anderson, N.V., Irwin, C.K. and Smith, B.P. (2000). Prevalence of *Salmonella* in beef feeder steers as determined by bacterial culture and ELISA serology. Vet. Microbiol., **76:** 143-151.

Garcia, P.P., Koster, F.T., Kelley, R.O., McDowels, T.O. and Bankhurst, A.D. (1989). Antibacterial activity of human natural killer cells. J. Exp. Med. **169:** 99-113

Gooding, C.M. and Choudary, P.V. (1999) Comparison of different primers for rapid detection of *Salmonella* using the polymerse chain reaction. Mol. Cell. Probes, **13:** 341–347.

Grimont, P.A.D., Grimont, F. and Bouvet, P. (2000). Taxonomy of the genus *Salmonella*. In : Wray, A. and Wray, C. (eds.) *Salmonella* in domestic animals. CAB International, Oxford, England, p. 1-17

Guibourdenche, M., Roggentin, P., Mikoleit, M., Fields, P.I., Bockemuhl, J., Grimont, P.A.D. and Weill, F. (2010). Supplement 2003-2007 (No. 47) to the White-Kauffmann-Le minor scheme. Res. Microbiol., **161:** 26-29.

Guiney, D.G. and Fierer, J. (2011). The role of the spv genes in *Salmonella* pathogenesis. Front Microbiol. **2:** 129. doi: 10.3389/fmicb.2011.00129

Hein, I., Flekna, G., Krassnig, M. and Wagner, M. (2006). Real-time PCR for the detection of *Salmonella* spp. in food: an alternative approach to a conventional PCR system suggested by the food-PCR project. J. Microbiol. Methods, **66:** 538-547.

Hensel, M., (2000). *Salmonella* pathogenicity island 2. Mol. Microbiol. **36:** 1015-1023.

Hensel, M., Shea, J.E., Waterman, S.R., Mundy, R., Nikolaus, T., Banks, G., Vazquez-Torres, A., Gleeson, C., Fang, F.C. and Holden, D.W. (1998) Genes encoding putative effector proteins of the type III secretion system of *Salmonella* pathogenicity island 2 are required for bacterial virulence and proliferation in macrophages. Mol. Microbiol, **30:** 163–174.

Hueck, C.J. (1998). Type III protein secretion systems in bacterial pathogens of animals and plants. Microbiol. Mol. Biol. Rev., **62:** 379–433.

Jones, M.A.,Wigley, P., Page, K.L., Hulme, S.D. and Barrow, P.A. (2001). *Salmonella enterica* serovar Gallinarum requires the *Salmonella* pathogenicity island 2 type III secretion system but not the *Salmonella* pathogenicity island 1 type III secretion system for virulence in chickens. Infect. Immun. **69:** 5471–5476

Kauffman, S.H. (1995). Immunity to intracellular microbial pathogens. Immunol. Today **16:** 338-342

Kich, J.D., Schwarz, P., Silva, L.E., Coldebella, A., Piffer, I.A., Vizzoto, R. and Cardoso, M.R.I. (2007). Development and application of an enzyme linked immunosorbent assay to detect antibodies against prevalent *Salmonella* serovars in swine in southern Brazil. J. Vet. Diagnostic Invest., **19:** 510-517.

Kinde, H., Castellan, D.M., Kass, P.H., Ardans, A., Cutler, G., Breitmeyer, R.E., Bell, D.D., Ernst, R.A., Kerr, D.C., Little, H.E., Willoughby, D., Riemann, H.P., Snowdon, J.A. and Kuney, D.R. (2004). The occurrence and distribution of *Salmonella* Enteritidis and other serovars on California egg laying premises: a comparison of two sampling methods and two culturing techniques. Avian Dis., **48:** 590–594.

Kumar, S. and Gupta, B.K. (1972). *Salmonella* Anatum from an aborted foal. British Vet. J. 128: lxiv.

Kumar, S., Saxena, S.P. and Gupta, B.K. (1973). Carrier rate of *salmonellas* in sheep and goats and its public health significance. J. Hyg (Lond). **71:** 43-47.

Kusiluka, L. and Kambarag, D. (1996). Diseases of small ruminants: a handbook. In Common Diseases of sheep and goats in Sub-Saharan Africa Edited by: VETAID. Overseas Development Administration Animal Health Program.

Lax, A. J., Baarrow, P. A., Jones, P. W. and Wallis, T. S. (1995). Current perspectives in salmonellosis. Br. Vet. J., **151:** 351-377.

Le Minor, L. (1994). The genus *Salmonella*. In : Ballows, A., Trüper, H.G., Dworkin, M., Harber, W. and Scheiffer, K.H. (eds.). The prokaryotes. Springer, New York, p. 2760-2774

Lillehoj, E.P., Yun, C.H. and Lillehoj, H.S. (2000). Vaccines against the avian enteropathogens *Eimeria, Cryptosporidium* and *Salmonella*. Anim. Health Res. Rev. **1:** 47–65.

Line, J.E., Bailey, J.S., Nelson, A., Cox. and Stern, N.J. (1997). Yeast treatment to reduce *Salmonella* and *Campylobacter* populations associated with broiler chickens subjected to transport stress. Poultry Sci., **76:** 1227–1231.

Malorny, B., Paccassoni, E., Fach, P., Bunge, C., Martin, A. and Helmuth, R. (2004). Diagnostic real-time PCR for detection of *Salmonella* in food. Appl. Environ. Microbiol., **70:** 7046–7052.

Mastroeni, P., Simmons, C., Fowler, R., Hormaeche, C. E. and Dougan, G. (2000). B cell deficient mice fail to mount solid acquired resistanceto oral challenge with virulent *Salmonella* enterica serovar *Typhimurium* and show impaired Th1 T cell responses to *Salmonella* antigens. Infect. Immun. **68:** 46-53.

Mastroeni, P., Villarreal, R. B. and Hormaeche, C. E. (1993). Adaptive transfer of immunity to oral challenge with virulent *Salmonella*e in innately susceptible BALB/C mice requires both immune serum and T-cells. Infect. Immun. **61:** 3981-3984.

McCain, C.S. and Powell, K.C. (1990). Asymptomatic salmonellosis in healthy adult horses. J Vet. Diagn Invest. **2:** 236-237.

Miller, S. I. and Mekalanos, J. J. (1990). Constitutive expression of the phoP regulon attenuates *Salmonella* virulence and survival within macrophages. J. Bacteriol. **172:** 2485-2490

Morse, E.V., Duncan, M.A., Page, E.A. and Fessler, J.F. (1976). Salmonellosis in Equidae: a study of 23 cases. Cornell Vet. **66:** 198-213.

Mukherjee, K., Siddiqi, S. A., Hashim, S., Raje, M., Basu, S. K. and Mukhopadhyay, A. (2000). Live *Salmonella* recruits N-ethylmaleimide-sensitive fusion protein on phagosomal membrane promotes fusion with early endosome. J. Cell Biol. **148:** 741-753

Nencioni, L., Villa, L., Boraschi, D., Berti, B. and Tagliabue, A. (1983).Natural killer and antibody dependent cell mediated activity against *Salmonella* Typhimurium by peripheral and intestinal lymphoid cells in mice. J. Immunol. **130:** 903-907.

Nicholas, R.A.J. and Cullen, G.A. (1991). Development and application of an ELISA for detecting antibodies to *S.* Enteriditis in chicken flocks. Vet. Rec., **128:** 74-76.

Nielsen, B., Baggesen, D., Bager, F., Haugegaard, J. and Lind, P. (1995). The serological response to *Salmonella* serovars Typhimurium and Infantis in experimentally infected pigs. The time course followed with an indirect anti-LPS ELISA and bacteriological examinations. Vet. Microbiol., **47:** 205-218.

Nielsen B., Ekeroth L., Bager F. and Lind P. (1998). Use of muscle fluid as a source of antibodies for serologic detection of *Salmonella* infection in slaughter pig herds. J. Vet. Diagnost. Invest., **10:** 158-163.

OIE. (2004). Manual of Diagnostic Test and Vaccines for Terrestrial Animals, 5th edn., Paris

OIE. (2008). Salmonellosis. In: Manual of diagnostic tests and vaccines for terrestrial animals. 6th edn., Vol. 2, Paris, pp. 1267-1283.

OIE. (2009). Terrestrial Animal Health Standards Commission Report. Prevention, detection and control of *Salmonella* in poultry. Article 6.5

Okamura, M., Lillehoj, H.S., Raybourne, R.B., Babu, U.S., Heckert, R.A. (2004). Cell mediated immune responses to a killed *Salmonella* Enteritidis vaccine: Lymphocyte proliferation, T-cell changes and interleukin-6 (IL-6), IL- 1, IL-2, and IFN-_ production. Comp. Immunol. Microbiol. Infect. Dis. **27:** 255–272

Olsen, J.E. and Skov, M. (1994). Genomic lineage of *Salmonella* enterica serovar Dublin. Vet. Microbiol. **40:** 271-282.

Perelle, S., Dilasser, F., Malorny, B., Grout, J., Hoorfar, J. and Fach, P. (2004). Comparison of PCR-ELISA and LightCycler real-time PCR assays for detecting *Salmonella* spp. in milk and meat samples. Mol. Cell. Probes, **18:** 409–420.

Pivnick, H., and E. Nurmi. (1982). The Nurmi Concept and its role in the control of *Salmonella* in poultry. Pages 41–70 in: Developments in Food Microbiology. Vol. 1. R. Davies, ed. Applied Science Publishers Ltd, Barking, Essex, UK.

Platt, H. (1973) Septicaemia in the foal. A review of 61 cases. British Vet. J. **129:** 221-229.

Popoff, M. Y. and Minor, L. L. (1997). Antigenic formulas of the *Salmonella* serovars, 7th revision. W.H.O. Collaboratoring Centre for Reference and Research on *Salmonella*. Institute Pasteur, Paris, France.

Quinn, P.J., Markey, B.K., Carter, M.E., Donnelly, W.J.C., Leonard, F.C. (2001). Veterinary Microbiology and Microbial Diesease. Blackwell Publishers. pp. 117-119

Rajic, A., B.P. O'Connor., A.E. Deckert., J. Keenslide., M.E. McFall., R.J. Reid-Smith., C.E. Dewey and S.A. McEwen. (2006). Farm-level risk factors for the presence of *Salmonella* in 89 Alberta swine-finishing farms. Can. J. Vet. Res., **71:** 264-270.

Reissbrodt, R. (1995). Conventional and alternative methods for isolation and identification of *Salmonella* : an overview. Biotest. Bull., **5:** 143-156.

Ricke, S.C., Pillai, S.D., Norton, R.A. and Maciorowski, K.G. (1998). Applicability of rapid methods for detection of *Salmonella* spp. in poultry feeds: a review. J. Rapid Meth. Automat. Microbiol., **6:** 239-258.

Roitt, I. M. (1993). Fundamental Immunology, Raven Press, New York.

Rushton, J. (2009). The economics of animal health and production. Cambridge, MA. CABI International.

Schrank, I.S., Mores, M.A.Z., Costa, J.L.A., Frazzon, A.P.G., Soncini, R., Schrank, A., Vainstein, M.H. and Silva, S.C. (2001). Influence of enrichment media and application of a PCR based method to detect *Salmonella* in poultry industry products and clinical samples. Vet. Microbiol., **82:** 45-53.

Sharma, A.K., Tripathi, B.N., Verma, J.C. and Parihar, N.S. (2001). Experimental *Salmonella enterica* subspecies *enterica* serovar Typhimurium infection in Indian goats: clinical, serological, bacteriological and pathological studies. Small Rum. Res. **42:** 125-134.

Shaw, J.S., Blais, B.W. and Nundy, D.C. (1998). Performance of the Dynabeads anti-*Salmonella* systems in the detection of *Salmonella* species in foods, animal feeds and environmental samples. J. Food Prot., **61:** 1507-1510.

Smith, H.W. (1956). The immunity to *Salmonella* Gallinarum infection in chickens produced by live cultures of members of the *Salmonella* genus. J. Hyg., **554:** 433-439.

Smith, B.P., Timm, K., Jahn, S. and Reina-Guerra, M. (1980). *Salmonellosis* in a group of ponies: failure to identify a chronic active carrier. J. American Vet. Med. Assoc. **176:** 215-216.

Stone, G.G., Oberst, R.D., Hays, M.P., McVey, S. and Chengappa, M.M. (1995). Combined PCR-oligonucleotide ligation assay for rapid detection of *Salmonella* serovars. J. Clin. Microbiol., **33:** 2888-2893.

Swaminathan, B. and Feng, P. (1994). Rapid detection of food-borne pathogenic bacteria. Ann. Rev. Microbiol., **48:** 410–426.

Thorns, C.J., Bell, M.M., Sojka, M.G. and Nicholas, R.A. (1996). Development and application of enzyme-linked immunosorbent assay for specific detection of *Salmonella* Enteritidis infections in chickens based on antibodies to sef14 fimbrial antigen. J. Clin. Microbiol., **34:** 792–797.

Tsolis, R.M., Kingsley, R.A., Townsend, S.M., Ficht, T.A., Adams, L.G. and Baumler, A.J. (1999). Comparison of the mouse typhoid model with other *Salmonella* infections of mice, calves, and men. Adv. Experim. Med. Biol., **473:** 261 - 274.

Uchiya, K., Barbieri, M. A., Funato, K., Shah, A. H., Stahl, P. D. and Groisman, E. A. (1999). A *Salmonella* virulence protein that inhibits cellular trafficking. Embo. J. **18:** 3924-3933.

Uzzau, S., Brown, D.J., Wallis, T., Rubino, S., Leori, G., Bernard, S., Casadesus, J., Platt, D.J., Olsen, J.E. (2000) Host adapted serotypes of *Salmonella* enterica. Epidemiol. Infect. **125:** 229-255.

Uzzau, S, Leori, G.S., Petruzzi, V., Watson, P.R., Schianchi, G., Bacciu, D., Mazzarello, V., Wallis, T.S. and Rubino, S. (2001) *Salmonella* enterica serovar-host specificity does not correlate with the magnitude of intestinal invasion in sheep. Infect. Immun. **69:** 3092-3099.

Van Zijderveld, F.G., van Zijderveld-van Bemmel, A.M. and Anakotta, J. (1992). Comparison of four different enzyme linked immunosorbent assays for serological diagnosis of *Salmonella* Enteritidis infections in experimentally infected chickens. J. Clin. Microbiol., **30:** 2560–2566.

Vancott, J.L., Stauts, H.F., Pascual, D.W., Roberts, M., Chatfield, S.N., Yamamoto, M., Coste, M.J., Carter, P. B., Kiyono, H. and Mc Ghee, J.R. (1996). Regulation of mucosal and systemic antibody responses by T helper cells subsets macrophages and derived cytokines following oral immunization with live recombinant *Salmonella*. J. Immunol. **156:** 1504-1514.

Vanselow, B.A., Hum, S., Hornitzky, M.A., Eamens, G.J. and Quinn, K. (2007). *Salmonella* Typhimurium persistence in a Hunter Valley dairy herd. Australian Vet. J. **85:** 446-450.

Wenkoff, M.S. (1973). A review and case report. *Salmonella* Typhimurium septicemia in foals. Canadian Vet. J., **14:** 284-287.

Wray, C., Wadsworth, Q.C., Richards, D.W. and Morgan, J.H. (1989). A three-year study of *Salmonella* Dublin infection in a closed dairy herd. Vet. Rec. **124:** 532-537.

□□□

Chapter 27

Haemorrhagic Septicaemia (HS)

SATISH SHIVCHANDRA
IVRI, Mukteswar Campus, U.K.

Introduction

India is a major country in Asia as well as in the world with the highest domestic animal population especially cattle (185 million) and buffaloes (98 million), which account for the largest in the world, are reared mainly for use as draught animals as well as milk production in the region. However, in recent times, despite the periodic vaccination schedule, the health scenario of cattle and buffalo population is always at great risk of encountering high mortality due to a major bacterial disease manifestation known as 'Haemorrhagic septicaemia (HS)' an acute, fatal and septicaemic disease caused by Gram negative bacterium-*Pasteurella multocida* (Shivachandra *et al.*, 2011). The different serotypes of *P. multocida* are associated with a variety of disease manifestations generally termed as 'Pasteurellosis', in a wide range of domestic as well as wild animals and birds. The OIE classifies the HS, with a number of other bacterial and parasitic diseases, as a List B disease (OIE, 2008). Following the successful control and eradication of rinderpest and continued low mortality with foot and mouth disease (FMD), HS emerged as a disease of considerable economic importance in India. HS alone, as an endemic major bacterial disease is known to cause a loss of worth more than 22 crore rupees per year in India through reduced milk production, draught power and death of cattle and buffaloes.

Etiological agent

The organism *P. multocida* belongs to the family Pasteurellaceae, which includes a large group of Gram-negative bacteria with three genera namely *Pasteurella, Actinobacillus* and *Haemophilus* that are facultatively anerobic, fermentative and known to cause diseases in mammals, birds and reptiles (Christensen and Bisgaard 2010). The history of *Pasteurella* organism dates back to 1782, when it was first studied by Chabert in France. In 1836, Mailet, first used the term 'fowl cholera' for an outbreak of disease in fowl, however, the causative bacterium was first described in 1878-79 by Revolta and Revolee. About the same time, Bollinger from Germany described a disease in cattle and buffaloes. In 1885, Kitts isolated the causative organism. A *septicaemic* disease in rabbits was described by Gaffky in 1881 and a similar disease in swine by Loeffler in 1886. Later, in 1887, Oreste and Armani from Italy proposed the name *'Bacillus septicaemiae'*. In 1887, Trevisan proposed the name *'Pasteurella'* in recognition of pioneering work done in early 1880s by Louis Pasteur on the etiology of fowl cholera (Pasteur, 1880). Initially, the bacterium was named according to the host species in which it caused the disease. The isolates from cattle were named 'Boviseptica', those from pigs as 'suiseptica; and from poultry as 'aviseptica'. Subsequently, there were several changes in the name until in 1939 Rosenbach and Merchant proposed the name *'Pasteurella multocida'* (L. adj. *multus* - many; L. adj. suf. *cidus* - kill; *multocida* - many killing, referring to pathogenicity for many species of animals). It is further divided into three subspecies; *P. multocida* subsp. *multocida, P. multocida* subsp. *septica* (*septica* - poisoning, infecting) and *P. multocida* subsp. *gallicida* (*gallina* - hen; *cida* - kill; *gallicida* - hen killing, referring to pathogenicity for poultry).

Morphologically, *P. multocida* cells are non-motile, small and coccoid to rod shaped, pleomorphic depending on the growth stage, they occur singly, in pairs, or short chains. Gram's reaction is negative, non acid fast and non-endospore forming. Surface colonies on sheep blood agar plates are smooth round, gryeish or yellowish, glistening translucent, non-haemolytic, and grow nearly 1-2 mm in diameter after 24 h of incubation at 37°C. In nutrient broth, there is a slight clouding after 18 h of incubation at 37°C, however, a good growth is achieved in brain heart infusion (BHI) broth. There is no growth on MacConkey's agar. The fresh cultures, blood smears, exudates and infected animal tissues show bipolar staining of organism with Leishman or Methylene blue or Giemsa stain.

Biochemically, bacterial cells are mesophilic, chemo-organotrophic with both oxidative and fermentative types of metabolism. Oxidase, alkaline phospatase and catalase positive, most species are V-factor (b-nicotinamide adenine dinucleotide) and X-factor (protohemin or proto porphyrin IX) independent, although V-factor requiring species and strains do occur. Members of the genus are always positive for fermentation of D-glucose, D-galactose, D-fructose, D-mannose, and sucrose; acid is produced from L-sorbose, L-rhamnose, m-inositol, or adonitol. No hydrolysis of starch, salicin or aesculin occurs. Arginine di hydrolase, lysine decarboxylase, liquefaction of gelatin and urease test are negative. The genome of *Pasteurella* contains 37.7 to 45.9 mol% G+C, with molecular weight ranging from $1.4x10^9$ to $1.9x10^9$ (Mutters *et al.*, 1985). The phenotypic variability among the strains of *P. multocida* of bovine, avian, caprine, leporine and ovine origin has been well documented by many workers (Ekundayo *et al.*, 2008).

Prevalence

HS, which is a primary pasteurellosis with 100% mortality in infected animals, is endemic in most geographical regions of India which rank HS as one of the most economically important bacterial disease. In many instances, *P. multocida* plays a secondary role in the pathogenesis of the disease or acts in combination with other bacterial, viral or parasitic infections. The distribution and frequency of disease occurrence has been attributed to climatic conditions, husbandry practices and types of animals reared. The incidences of disease outbreaks in India are known to vary considerably in different states and also in each state from year to year. Buffaloes are generally believed to be more susceptible to HS than cattle, and in this species, the disease course is shorter. In endemic areas, most deaths are confined to older calves and young adults. In non endemic areas, massive epizootics may occur. Case fatality approaches to 100% if treatment is not carried at early stage. The presence of naturally acquired immunity is observed among buffaloes. It has been opined that HS morbidity and mortality pattern, in endemic and non-endemic areas in a given population, is largely dependent on the proportion of naturally acquired immune to non-immune animals.

On the basis of distribution, endemic nature and utmost economic importance of HS and other related diseases, India has been included under the Category A (FAO-WHO-OIE, 1994). It was estimated that during the years 1936 to 1944, there were an average of 700 reported outbreaks of HS and 40,000 deaths per year. The average mortality per year ranged from 30,000 to 60,000 until 1960s, however, the death rate started to decline to approximately 4000 per year from 1970s, presumably due to improved control measures in the region (FAO, 2005). It has been reported that during the past four decades HS has accounted for 46-55% of all bovine deaths.

Currently, the conventional methods of identification and characterization of field isolates of *P. multocida* in India is being carried out as per the international standards (OIE, 2008). A large number of *P. multocida* organisms have been isolated in the recent past from various outbreaks of pasteurellosis occurring in different agro-climatic geographical regions. Currently, the most widely used serotype designation system based on Carter and Heddleston system (Carter 1955; Heddleston *et al.* 1972) which recognizes five capsular serogroups (A, B, D, E and F) based on the indirect haemagglutination assay (IHA) and sixteen (1-16) somatic serotypes based on agar gel precipitation test have been employed to classify the Indian HS isolates. The causative agent for HS has been named in different classifications as Robert type-I, Heddleston type 2, Carter type B and Namioka & Carter type 6:B and 6:E. The Asian serotype for HS is designated as B:2 and the African serotype E:2. Typically, *P. multocida* serotype B:2 is involved in cases of HS among cattle and buffalos. However, the recent investigations of Indian field isolates have revealed the presence of other serotypes such as A:1,3, A:3, A:4, F:3, and F:3,4, especially serotype A:1 as next predominant to type B:2. The clinical signs as observed by field veterinarians in many of these animals (serotype A:1 infected), did not suggest typical HS. Considerable variation has also been observed among several HS serotypes with respect to host predilection, pathogenicity, and biochemical, cultural and antigenic specificity.

Despite relatively little information about pasteurellosis among Indian wild animals, the presence of *P. multocida* organisms in different wild species viz., lion, tiger, spotted deer, hippopotamus and leopard have been reported. However, the association of these serotypes with disease conditions has to be ascertained following detailed investigation with respect to disease inducing ability of serotypes in wild species.

Virulence factors

A total of 104 putative virulence associated genes which account for ~7% of coding density of *P. multocida* genome have been predicted indicating a several mechanisms or components involved in evading the host defensive immune systems (Al-Hasani *et al.*, 2007). Among them, capsule is a major virulent component which is known to determine the capsular serogroups namely A, B, D, E and F, whose biosynthetic loci has been identified in the recent past (Adler *et al.*, 1999). Polysaccharides constitute the major part of the capsule. Two genes (*bcbA* and *bcbB*) within region 2 of the B:2 cap locus, were known to catalyze the conversion of UDP-*N*-acetylglucosamine to *N*-acetyl-D-mannosaminuronic acid indicating that the mannose as the major type B capsular component. The variable gene expression gives rise to capsular variability of strains and production of capsular material is affected by sub-minimal inhibitory concentration of antibiotics. Moreover, it has been found that the capsular strains are more virulent than their acapsular variants as the capsule plays a significant role in resistance to phagocytosis. The genetically defined acapsular serotype B mutants were found to be high susceptibility as they were uptake by murine macrophages. Removal of hyaluronic acid from capsule increases both adhessiveness of the organisms to the animal cell surfaces as well as its susceptibility to phagocytosis (Harper *et al.*, 2006).

The presence of type IV fimbriae on *P. multocida* serogroup B:2 isolated from calves nasal and tracheal cells have been identified by electron microscopic studies. Type IV fimbriae (pili), which has several repeated subunits (15-20 kDa) with their highly conserved N-terminal sequences (21aa) and divergent carboxyl terminal, has been isolated and characterized from *P. multocida* serotypes A, B, D and F that are able to adhere to mucosal epithelium (Ruffalo *et al.*, 1997). Comparative sequence analysis of *ptfA* gene from *P. multocida* B:2 (strain p52) indicated 78.4% similarity with that of A:1 strain (Siju *et al.*, 2007). The treatment of the organism with pronase, heat, acidity or homogenisation, confirmed the involvement of the fimbriae in the attachment process. Moreover, the anti-fimbrial antibodies specifically inhibited the adherence capabilities of different serotypes which are known to greatly vary for tracheal epithelial cells from different hosts. Similarly, adhesion such as 'Fibronectin-binding protein ComE1 (12.7 kDa), have also been identified by panning a phage library of *P. multocida,* which was found to interact with integrin-binding fibronectin type III (FnII) repeats as well as involved in bacterial competence and DNA uptake. *P. multocida* Pm70 genome sequence predicted two genes encoding for the filamentous haemagglutinin proteins (FhaB1 and Fhab2) which are supposed to increase the bacterial dispersion and colonization. Mutations in adhesin genes of *P. multocida* resulted in significantly reduced virulence in mice. A putative Tad (tight adherence) locus involved in Tad macromolecular transport system required for biofilm formation and colonization, comprised of genes encoding for several OMPs (TadD, RcpA, RcpB, Flp1) has also been identified (May *et al.*, 2001).

Outer membrane proteins (OMPs) constitue a major surface exposed bacterial components with more than 15-20 protein bands ranging from ~16-90kDa in HS strains. A bioinformatics analysis of *P. multocida* genome predicted >129 proteins as secreted and located in the outer membrane, or lipoproteins with a total of 79 proteins as outer membrane localized. However, extraction of OMPs by sarcosyl method, the protein bands with molecular weights viz., 16 kDa, 27kDa, 34kDa, 39kD, 46kDa and 82-87kDa have been identified in all isolates regardless of serotype during protein electrophoresis (Tomer *et al.*, 2002). Serum from vaccinated animals contained antibodies reacting only with few OMP bands. Among these, proteins of 37-39kDa are presumed to be protective antigens. Some of proteins identified in OMP are OmpH, OmpA, Oma87, Pm1069 and iron related proteins, TbpA (transferrin binding protein A), HgbA (haemoglobin binding protein) (Hatfaludi *et al.*, 2010).

Iron plays a critical role in *P. multocida* survival in side the host as evidenced by *in silico* and whole genome microarray analyses which identified >50 genes involved role in iron acquisition and metabolism. As the organism is known to have several mechanisms to uptake iron from host under varied conditions, cells grown in iron deprivation conditions, were able to secrete a growth enhancing factor that functions as a siderophore (multocidin). Siderophores selectively bind ferric iron and were involved in receptor-specific iron transport into the bacterial cell. Several types of siderophores were synthesized by *P. multocida,* of which, three iron regulated OM proteins (~76, 84 and 96 kDa) were expressed in iron-restricted medium, or *in vivo* which were believed to be involved in Fe-multocidin complex formation. Approximately, 1% of the genome was found to encode large proteins (filamentous hemagglutinins). The organism was also capable of obtaining iron for growth by a non-siderophore mediated mechanism. Such acquisition was associated with the production of a number of high molecular weight, iron-regulated OMP including an 82kDa receptor protein (TbpA) for bovine transferrin-bound iron. Comparison of *P. multocida* grown in iron rich, iron depleted media or *in vivo* has demonstrated that many high mol.wt OMPs are regulated by iron levels and called iron regulated OMPs (IROMPs), which were found to play a significant role in cross protective immunity (Wheeler 2009).

Lipopolysaccharide (LPS), a major component of bacterium known to determine 1-16 somatic serotypes, also plays a critical role in pathogenesis of HS in buffalos as they are absolutely required for *in vivo* replication. The complete LPS structure of strains VP161 and X73 belonging to Heddleston serotype 1 and PM70, a Heddleston serotype-3 strain, have been determined. It has been shown that intravenous inoculation of LPS from serotype B:2 strains could reproduce clinical signs of HS in buffalos and role of LPS in adhesion to bovine neutrophils and transmigration through endothelial cells. LPS was considered to be a protective antigen as it was known to stimulate humoral immunity and its role in generation of bactericidal antibodies. Clinical isolates of *P. multocida* from cattle exhibited serum resistance. Moreover, LPS was found to stimulate the release of many interleukins, TNF-α and other tumour inhibition factors from bovine alveolar macrophages due to mitogenic action of the endotoxins.

A limited number of *P. multocida* serogroup B virulent strains (B:2) isolated from HS cases have found to produce several extracellular enzymes such as lipase, neuraminidase and hyaluronidase. Hence, hyaluronidase activity test was employed to presumptive diagnosis of serogroup B:2 strains causing HS. High neuraminidase production was correlated to higher virulence of strains. A putative *pm1426* gene has been predicted to encode OM phospholipase-A which was involved in hydrolysis of phospholipids on the outer surface membrane. Sialidases (neuraminidases) are known to be involved in scavenging sialic acid from host and increase the virulence by blocking the effectiveness of host defences such as mucin. Two sialidase genes encoding for NanH (80kDa) and NanB (120kDa) proteins and their role in uptake of sialidic acid through the tripartite ATP-independent periplasmic (TRAP) sialate transporter have been recently established.

Pathogenesis

The presence of HS-causing *Pasteurellae* in small proportion in the naso-pharynx of apparently normal healthy cattle and buffaloes and recent exposure to outbreaks of HS has been documented for a long time. Further investigations in the experimentally exposed buffaloes and induced carrier animals, which remained clinically normal, have shown the persistence of *Pasteurellae* in the crypts of tonsils for several months despite treatment with antibiotics, before they appeared actively in the nasopharynx and are shed intermittently in the nasal secretions. The factors, responsible for influencing the latent carriers to become active, are still an enigma.

However, it is presumed that under the influence of various incriminating factors including environmental factors are known to trigger the activation of organism (Harper *et al.*, 2006). Following activation, rapid multiplication of bacteria is found in the blood and leading to various clinical manifestations. The disease is known to occur either in acute/sub acute or chronic forms. A typical clinical case of HS is characterized by initial phase of temperature elevation (often unnoticed), a phase of respiratory involvement, and a terminal phase of septicaemia and recumbence leading to death. The incubation period is usually 1-3 days, and the course of the disease may range from sudden death, with no observable clinical signs, to a protracted course extending up to 5 days. The acute form is manifested by sudden onset and death within 24 hours. The animals show a high rise in body temperature (41-42°C), pulse is thin, rapid and shallow respiration with cyanosis of visible mucus membranes. Restlessness, mild colic pain, muscular tremors, lacrymation, nasal discharge and diarrhoea are also observed. In sub-acute form, known as subcutaneous edematous form, animal survives for 2-3 days with oedematous swelling of throat and brisket region and bronchopneumonia. In chronic form, course of infection is longer with signs of short, rapid painful respiration coupled with mucopurulent or blood stained nasal discharge. At post mortem examination, the first obvious lesion is subcutaneous oedema, particularly in the mandibular and brisket region. Other lesions include petechial to echymotic haemorrhages, congestion and / or consolidation of lungs, fibrinous pneumonia, pleurisy and pericarditis.

Most of the laboratory studies on the pathogenesis of HS have used mice as the host animal for capsular type A or B of *P. multocida*. A very small dose of *P. multocida* organism is known to proliferate and kill the mice inoculated intraperitoneally within 24 h. Similar results have been observed by many workers who reported nearly 85% of Indian field isolates to cause death of mice in 24 h following intraperitoneal inoculation, whereas the remaining isolates took more than 24 h. The pathogenicity of an organism in mice depends upon the virulence characteristics of the organism and genetic makeup of the host and variation in pathogenicity of the isolates. Pathogenicity studies of *P. multocida* in chicken having indicated 90% mortality within 48-72 h, whereas other isolates have been found to be pathogenic between 72-96 h. Recent literature and many reviews reveal no better understanding of the mechanisms of pathogenesis, nor of the determinants of virulence of this organism.

Diagnosis

For diagnosis of HS infection, specimens collected from infected live animals are blood samples and nasal secretions, whereas from dead animals, heart blood, liver, spleen, lung and bone marrow of long bones (OIE, 2008). Moreover, the sudden death seen with peracute and acute form of HS must be differentiated from that due to lightening, snakebites, blackleg, rinderpest and anthrax by both conventional and molecular approaches. Conventionally, the diagnosis is usually carried out based on either clinical (characteristic signs, gross pathological lesions, herd history, morbidity and mortality pattern, species susceptibility, age group affected) or laboratory confirmation involving bacteriological (isolation by culture or mice inoculation, bacterial colony morphology, pathogenicity test, biotyping and antibiogram) or serological methods (Rapid slide agglutination test, Indirect haemagglutination assay, Agar gel immunodiffusion test, Counter immune electrophoresis, Passive haemagglutinations, PMPT and ELISA). Sometimes, non-serological methods such as Acriflavine flocculation test and Hyaluronidase tests could also be employed. Serological tests are for detecting antibodies but are not normally used for diagnosis. However, IHA test with high titres from 1/160 upto 1/ 1280 or higher among in-contact animals surviving in the affected herds, are indicative of recent exposure to HS. Other serological tests like passive haemagglutinations, AGID and ELISA have been used with varying degrees of success in attempts to predict level of immunity. The ease of obtaining definite diagnosis through isolation and identification of organisms precludes the need for serodiagnosis. Non-serological methods such as acriflavine flocculation test and hyaluronidase tests could can be employed. However, all these conventional methods of diagnosis with potential problems limit their application in clinical diagnosis of HS.

Recently, Polymerase Chain Reaction (PCR) assays for the specific identification of *P. multocida* and HS causing serotypes have been developed (Townsend *et al.* 1998), which can be applied directly on bacterial colony, bacterial culture lysate and mixed bacterial culture for the rapid and specific identification within 3-4 hours in comparison to conventional methods. PCR assays have also been employed directly on clinical sample to augment the rapid disease diagnosis. Moreover, nucleic acid based typing tools with or without involving PCR machine could also be effectively employed for routine genotypic differentiation of *P. multocida* isolates.

In India, PCR based molecular assays and typing tools have been introduced in parallel to existing conventional methods for more than a decade for rapid and specific diagnosis of HS at various laboratories in the country. A number of workers have extensively used PM-PCR, HSB-PCR and multiplex capsular typing systems for rapid identification and capsular serotyping of field isolates originated from different animal species. The results of PM-PCR conducted either in single reaction or in multiplex PCR reaction using HSB-PCR assay have shown to produce an amplicon size of ~460bp (PM specific) and ~620bp (HSB specific), which correlated well with the results of conventional identification and capsular serotyping. Similarly, the results of serogroup-A specific PCR and multiplex capsular typing system employed on large number of field isolates revealed the correct identification of conventional capsular serogroups. Moreover, PCR assay is able to identify the acapsular isolates of *P. multocida* which could not be typed based on conventional methods of classification. PCR assays did not cross react with any other bacteria and fungi tested in previous studies revealing high specificity as well as high sensitivity which was observed even with 10 ng of DNA used in the reaction mixture. Moreover, the PCR assay could be directly employed on bacterial colony, bacterial culture lysate or mixed culture lysate, homgenised morbid tissue materials viz., spleen, lung, liver, heart, and bone morrow, without the extraction of purified genomic DNA.

The new capsular typing system based on PCR has been developed by Townsend *et al.* (2001) following identification, sequence determination and analysis of the capsular biosynthetic loci of each capsular serogroups A, B, D, E and F. The targeted gene, amplicon size and primers used in this assay. Multiplex Capsular PCR assay is found to be highly specific and its results, correlated well with conventional serotyping. This assay represents a rapid and reproducible alternative to the serological and non-serological methods, which are currently being used for classification of *P. multocida* capsular types (Carter 1955; Heddleston *et al.* 1972). Following agarose gel electrophoresis, amplicons of size ~1044 bp, ~ 760bp, ~851bp and ~ bp indicative of capsular serogroups, A, B, D, and F are observed respectively. The results of Multiplex Capsular Typing system employed on large number of Indian field isolates of *P.multocida* correlated well with the conventional capsular serogroups (Shivachandra *et al.* 2006a). Conventional methods of serotyping depend mainly on production and maintenance of specific antisera for capsular and somatic identification, which are often laborious and difficult to produce (Rhodes and Rimler 1987). Moreover, discrepancies in serological identification between laboratories are primarily due to differences in antisera as a result of different immunological response between animals and methods used, which cause a problem of standardization. Lack of serotyping facility coupled with inability to identify acapsular isolates (such as serotype -:1), would certainly allow the gene based multiplex capsular serotyping as most reliable assay for simultaneous species detection and capsular serogrouping of isolates.

PCR assays are rapid, specific and highly sensitive for identification and capsular serotyping of *P. multocida* isolates irrespective of the host and geographical region of isolation. The simplicity and versatility of PCR assay would enable the technique to be used on routine basis for diagnosis of HS compared to conventional serotyping. The PCR equipment and experience required to perform these techniques is becoming readily available in most laboratories in the country, providing a marked advantage over the current methods of identification.

Compared with *P. multocida* cultivation, PCR assays are less laborious and results are available within six hours, thereby dramatically reducing the time for diagnosis from a few days to a few hours. However, the sensitivity of the assay may be variable for different tissues. Even a low number of organisms can be detected especially in bone marrow of long bones. The storage studies of morbid materials following detection by PCR has also indicated the possibilities of detecting the organism up to 3 days at 37°C, 40 days at 4°C and even upto 100 days at -20°C especially from bone marrow without *in vitro* cultivation. PCR based detection directly from tissues is of greater advantage in early diagnosis of the disease manifestations.

A relatively large number of *P. multocida* isolates originated from different outbreaks of HS in the country have also been analyzed by many researchers in the past by employing various typing techniques viz., Restriction endonuclease analysis (REA) using *Hpa*II, ribotyping, Repetitive Extragenic Palindromic (REP-PCR), Enterobacterial Repetitive Intergenic Consensus (ERIC-PCR), Randomly amplified polymorphic DNA (RAPD-PCR) and single enzyme AFLP for their discriminative ability. Several genotyping studies have documented the existence of maximum genotypic differences among *P. multocida* isolates especially among the isolates originated from HS outbreaks. Involvement of multiple strains of *P. multocida* in HS outbreaks (Biswas *et al.* 2004) could also be investigated by employing PCR based typing tools to detect and differentiate between isolates which phenotypically appear similar by conventional methods.

Among typing tools, RAPD-PCR, REP-PCR and ERIC-PCR techniques have proved to be a valuable tool for rapid epidemiological analysis and differentiation of outbreak related isolates of *P. multocida* (Townsend *et al.* 1997a; Biswas *et al.* 2004; Shivachandra *et al.* 2005a and 2008). As PCR-based assays do not require high quality DNA preparation and ability to perform directly on colonies/culture lysates without any need for extensive DNA extraction, coupled with good discriminatory power, highlights the time advantage over other DNA-based typing methods for routine typing of isolates (Gunawardana *et al.* 2000; Saxena *et al.* 2006).

Pulsed field gel electrophoresis (PFGE), a specialized form of REA, is often considered a 'gold standard' of molecular typing methods as it generates a few fragments 5-20 of 10 to 800 kb in size, larger than REA fragments (Olive and Bean, 1999). Although, the technique has been proven to be highly discriminatory for *P. multocida* isolates, its applicability in routine diagnostic laboratories is limited due to requirement of high quality DNA and expensive electrophoresis apparatus. There was no report of applicability of this technique to characterize Indian HS isolates. However, if employed, the PFGE patterns enable us to create a reference database for the HS strains to compare with emergence of a new strain from an outbreak.

Treatment

Despite a widely accepted fact that treatment is of little use once visible signs have appeared, antibacterial chemotherapy is still being used extensively for treating clinical cases of HS in India with varying success depending mainly on the kind of drug used. However, in recent times, therapy has been compromised due to emergence of multi-drug resistant strains. The conventional antibiotics had shown more resistance which is posing problems in treating the animals suffering from HS. In the last two decades, shift in antibiotic sensitivity spectrum of *Pasteurellae* is well evident. A number of studies on field isolates of *P. multocida* in India have reported variation in the pattern of sensitivity to different antibacterials (Biswas *et al.*, 2004). The variation in the sensitivity pattern of *P. multocida* may result in high morbidity and mortality. Studies have indicated the rise in multiple drug resistant strains of *P. multocida*. The differences in the antibiogram may be due to extensive and indiscriminate use of antimicrobials for treatment of bacterial infections, which might lead to selection of resistant strains.

Although, a serum therapy using 60-100ml of hyperimmune serum has been suggested in treating animals at varying periods from 6 hours before to 18 hours after infection but is found to be less significant in treatment.

In India, so far there is scanty literature pertaining to the drug resistance against HS as the disease is treated with oxytetracycline, co-trimexazole and with a combination of penicillin and streptomycin or with sulphaquino-xazoline which have proved to be effective. According to earlier reports, most of the strains are resistant to sulpha drug, the drug of choice in HS. The strains were also comparatively resistant to oxytetracycline and sulfamethoxazole + trimethoprim. The injudicious use of the antibiotics is leading to the severe problem of antibiotic resistance, the gene for which is plasmid-borne. This also reflects the fact that Indian strains may have plasmids encoding for drug resistance. Although, there are reports of varied antibiotic sensitivity pattern of isolates from a particular region or outbreak, a comprehensive pattern among different hosts and regions still needs to be studied. In view of these facts, it is necessary to have a check on the indiscriminate use of antibiotics in treatment of HS. Moreover, this warrants the need for pre-testing of antibiotic sensitivity against pasteurellae so as to find out an effective antimicrobial agent to be used by veterinarian/specialists for therapeutic purpose.

Control

A vaccination of susceptible animals has been the major strategy of HS control in endemic areas with various formulations and combinations of available HS vaccines. Initially, plain bacterins of *P. multocida* were advocated for prophylactic vaccination of cattle against HS which offered immunity for 6 months. The basic approach in development of HS vaccine was to kill the *P. multocida* organisms using either physical (heat, UV irradiation) or chemical agents (formalin) which still retain the antigens responsible for inducing the host's immune response. Later, several killed vaccines have been developed with different kind of adjuvants to enhance the immune response. The commonly used vaccines are bacterin, alum precipitated, aluminium hydroxide gel, oil adjuvant vaccines (OAV) and multiple emulsion vaccines (Verma and Jaiswal 1998) with vast variation in their duration of immunity and side effects. Agar-wash heat killed or formalized vaccine using higher concentration of bacterial cells was developed (Rau and Govil, 1950) to avoid the protein shock due to killed broth vaccine. Of several formulations, alum-precipitated HS vaccine has been extensively used in different parts of the world as it is known to protect cattle, sheep and goat against *P. multocida* infection for 6 months (Nikhiporova, 1958). Aluminium hydroxide gel HS vaccine used in Thailand

Laos was known to provide lesser immunity despite the incorporation of vitamin E and levamisole as immunomodulators. Simple HS emulsion vaccines (water-in-oil) were developed to enhance the stability of vaccines by using emulsifying agent such as lanolin, and mannite monooleate (Arlacel-A). Subsequently, oil-adjuvant HS vaccines (OAV) were developed using small quantity of mineral oil (Bain, 1956). In a comparative efficacy study involving OAV and alum vaccine, OAV was found to be superior in terms of storage at room temperature for 1 year without deterioration, fairly withstood high temperature (advantage in tropical developing countries), provided protective immunity against challenge after 1 year of vaccination and found to be safe in all ages of cattle and buffaloes (Dhanda *et al.*, 1958; Iyer and Rao, 1959). However, OAV found to be difficult during injection due to its high viscosity, formation of abscess at the site of injection and post-vaccination reactions have often been reported (Verma and Jaiswal, 1998). In order to overcome the limitations, a multiple emulsion (ME) vaccine was prepared by re-emulsifying the OAV with 2% Tween 80, which was easy to administer and equally effective in protection studies, however, with reduced duration of immunity afforded by multi-emulsion HS vaccine (Verma and Jaiswal, 1998; Mittal *et al.*, 1979). Double emulsion (DE) vaccine has been shown to be equally efficient in generation of immunity in buffalo up to 12 months post-vaccination. Generally, vaccination with killed vaccines is practiced in HS endemic areas and found to reduce the incidences, but due to short duration of immunity, outbreaks still occur. Bacterins are inexpensive to produce and give very limited protection against heterologus serotypes as the immunity generated is serotype specific. Further, the protective potency of different batches of vaccines is always unpredictable due to lack of quality control test for ascertaining their protective potency. A successful aerosol live vaccine (*P. multocida* strain B: 3,4 from fallow deer) developed in Myanmar (Myint and Carter, 1989), had been recommended by FAO for safe use in Asian countries, however, currently, it is not being used in India.

Acellular vaccines comprised of only the antigenic part of *P. multocida,* such as capsule, fimbriae, lipopolysaccharide (LPS), outer membrane proteins (OMPs) or part of the cell wall proteins have also been attempted in developing subunit vaccines. Immunization trials with OMPs from *in vivo / in vitro* grown and iron restricted medium were found to elicit the cross-protective antibodies against different serotypes. Killed and acellular vaccines, despite being safe in animals known to induce less durable immune response requiring a booster dose after every few months. In the past, several adjuvants namely, vegetable like saponin or glucan extract; bacterial components like monophosphoryl lipid-A, trehalose dymicolate, LPS and their derivative; chemicals like aluminium hydroxide gel, surfactants and emulsions have been used for development of HS vaccines. Recently, a new generation of adjuvants comprising mainly cytokines viz., γ-IFN or GM-CSF and many micro/nano-particles, are being incorporated in HS vaccine formulations, which are currently under trial.

Several combinations of vaccine formulations (bivalent, trivalent and polyvalent) incorporating two or more disease causing microbes (bacterial and/or viral) have been attempted in order to reduce the number of vaccine shots, cost of production and to increase protective immunity of animals against multiple infections. For example, with killed HS vaccine, other formulations targeting black quarter, rinderpest, foot-and-mouth disease, black leg, infectious bovine rhinotrachaeitis, adenovirus type-3, para-influenza and other pathogens of respiratory diseases with their antigens were incorporated in development of combined vaccine depending on the target host and disease prevalence in a particular area.

Recently, genetic engineering approaches have resulted in generation of purified subunits, synthetic peptides, chemical conjugation of polysaccharides with recombinant proteins, use of recombinant bacteria or defined mutants and bacterial ghosts as vaccines (Hatfaludi *et al.*, 2010). Candidate/target gene cloning and expression resulted in generation of various recombinant proteins from *P. multocida*, which represent only the part of an organism yet stimulate relatively strong immune response (Hatfaludi *et al.*, 2010). For example, Type 4 fimbriae (ptfA), outer membrane protein-87 (Omp87), porin (OmpH), lipoprotein E (pIpE), adhesin (OmpA) and transferrin binding protein (TbpA) have been considered as a candidate antigens (Hatfaludi *et al.*, 2010; Shivachandra *et al.*, 2005). Recombinant proteins used as subunit vaccines are found to be safe for immuno-compromised animals as they do not cause disease. Based on the fact that bovine strains of *P. multocida* regularly harbored several virulent genes (type 4 fimbrial gene-*ptfA*, and iron acquisition genes-*tbpA, hgbA-B, HasR* and genes for multiple haemoglobin-binding proteins), independent of its capsule type and that are highly expressed in the host, strongly suggest their protein products as potential subunit vaccine candidates.

One vaccine strategy that has been adopted in several other bacterial species is to target the surface proteins involved in acquisition of iron from the host as vaccine antigens (Hatfaludi *et al.*, 2010; Paustian *et al.*, 2001). In particular, the OMPs and IROMPs have been a focus for development of subunit vaccines (Pati *et al.*, 1996; Srivastava 1998). Transferrin binding protein (TbpA), an IROMP from *P. multocida* serogroup B:2 revealed high antigenic index and it could be potentially used as a candidate antigen in development of subunit vaccine against HS (Shivachandra *et al.*, 2005). A surface exposed, highly immunogenic lipoprotein (plpE) of *P. multocida* has been recently found to confer 80-100% protective immunity in mice and also indicated the ability to generate cross-serotype protective immunity (Wu *et al.*, 2007). At present, there is no commercial availability of recombinant HS subunit vaccine. However, the search for identifying cross-protective antigens still remains to be elusive.

Recently, attempts were made to develop synthetic peptides based on amino acid sequences of predicted loop structures to mimic the epitopes of *P. multocida*.. For example, synthetic porin (OmpH) peptides have been shown to provide a limited protection against *P. multocida* (Luo *et al.*, 1999). However, development of synthetic peptides was hampered due to their less immunogenicity and requirement of effective adjuvants. Despite its major lacunae, there is a hope to gather much useful information for construction of multi-epitope cross-protective HS vaccines.

In recent years, genetic technologies have emerged as powerful tools to identify targets for the development of defined live-attenuated vaccines. To name a few, *In vivo* expression technology (IVET), substractive hybridization and signature-tagged mutagenesis (STM) have resulted in identification of innumerable number of genes responsible for virulence and pathogenesis of *P. multocida*. Thus, a number of attenuated mutants containing transposon insertions in genes encoding biosynthetic enzymes, virulence factors, regulatory components and unknown function are currently being evaluated at laboratory level. For example, acapsular *cexA* mutant of *P. multocida* B:2 generated by inactivation of *bcbH* gene, predicted to be involved in polysaccharide biosynthesis was found to elicit protective immunity against wild type challenge. Another report suggests the use of stable, non-reverting *aroA* mutants as live vaccines (Ataei *et al.*, 2009). Dagleish *et al.* (2007) reported the protective efficacy of live *P. multocida* B:2 wild type strain-85020 containing a deletion in the *aroA* gene (strain-JRMT12) following intramuscular vaccination against experimental hemorrhagic septicemia in calves. Nevertheless, the efficacy of attenuated mutants warrants further laboratory investigations before field use. Alternatively, other approaches such as bacterial ghosts, a non-living bacterial cell vaccine system as described by Marchart *et al.* (2003) could also be attempted for development of future HS vaccines.

References

Adler B, Bulach D, Chung J, Doughty S, Hunt M, Rajakumar K, Serrano M, Zanden A, Zhang Y and Ruffolo C (1999). Candidate vaccine antigens and genes in *Pasteurella multocida*. Journal of Biotechnology **73:** 83-90.

Al-Hasani K, Boyce J, McCarl VP, Bottomley S, Wilkie I and Adler B (2007). Identification of novel immunogens in *Pasteurella multocida*. Microbial Cell Factories **6:** 3.

Ataei S, Burchmore R, , Finucane A, Parton R and Coote JG (2009). Identification of immunogenic proteins associated with protection against haemorrhagic septicaemia after vaccination of calves with a live-attenuated *aroA* derivative of *Pasteurella multocida* B:2. Research in Veterinary Science **87**(2): 207-210.

Aucouturier J, Dupuis L and Ganne V (2001). Adjuvants designed for veterinary and human vaccines. Vaccine **19:** 2666-2672.

Benkirane A, De Alwis MCL (2002). Haemorrhagic septicaemia, its significance, prevention and control in Asia. Vet Med Czech **47**(8):234-240.

Biswas A, Shivachandra SB, Saxena MK, Kumar AA, Singh VP and Srivastava SK (2004). Molecular variability among strains of *Pasteurella multocida* isolated from an outbreak of Haemorrhagic Septicaemia in India. Veterinary Research Communications **28**(4): 287-298.

Blackall PJ, Miflin JK (2000). Identification and typing of *Pasteurella multocida*: a review. Avian Pathology **29:** 271-287.

Boyce JD, Chung JY, Adler B. (2000). *Pasteurella multocida* capsule: Composition, function and genetics. J Biotec **83:** 153-160.

Christensen H and Bisgaard M (2010). Molecular classification and its impact on diagnostics and understanding the phylogeny and epidemiology of selected members of Pasteurellaceae of veterinary importance. Berlin Munch Tierarztl Wochenschr **123**(1-2): 20-30.

Confer AW (1993). Immunogens of Pasteurella. Veterinary Microbiology. **37:** 353-368.

De Alwis MCL (1999). Haemorrhagic septicaemia. ACIAR Monograph No. 57.

Dagleish MP, Hodgson JC, Ataei S, Finucane A, Finlayson J, Sales J, Parton R and Coote JG (2007). Safety and protective efficacy of intramuscular vaccination with a live *aroA* derivative of *Pasteurella multocida* B:2 against experimental hemorrhagic septicemia in calves. Infection and Immunity **75**(12): 5837-44.

Dhanda MR, Das MD, Lal JM and Seth RN (1958). Immunological studies on *Pasteurella septica* I. Trials on adjuvant vaccine. Indian Journal of Veterinary Science **156:** 273-283.

Dziva F, Muhairwa A P, Bisgaard M and Christensen H (2008). Diagnostic and typing options for investigating diseases associated with *Pasteurella multocida*. Veterinary Microbiology **128:** 1-22.

Ekundayo SO, Odugbo MO, Olabode AO and Okewole PA (2008). Phenotypic variability among strains of *P. multocida* isolated from avian, bovine, caprine, leporine and ovine origin. African Journal of Biotechnology **7**(9): 1347-1350.

FAO (2005). Production Yearbook 2005, FAO, Statistics Division.

FAO-WHO-OIE (1994) Animal Health Yearbook, 1994.

Harper M, Boyce J D and Adler B (2006). *Pasteurella multocida* pathogenesis: 125 years after Pasteur. FEMS Microbiology Letters **265:** 1-10.

Hatfaludi T, Al-Hasani K, Boyce JD and Adler B (2010). Outer membrane proteins of *Pasteurella multocida*. Veterinary Microbiology **144:** 1-17.

Hunt M L, Adler B and Townsend K M (2000). The molecular biology of *Pasteurella multocida*. Veterinary Microbiology **72:** 3-25.

Iyer SV and Rao DVR (1959). Studies on Haemorrhagic septicaemia vaccines. *Indian* Veterinary Journal **36:** 415-26.

Kuhnert P and Christensen H (2008). Pasteurellaceae: Biology, Genomics and Molecular Aspects. Caister Academic Press Norfolk, UK.

Kumar A A, Shivachandra S B, Biswas A, Singh V P, Singh V P and Srivastava S K (2004). Prevalent serotypes of *Pasteurella multocida* isolated from different Animal and Avian species in India. Veterinary Research Communications **28:** 657-667.

Kumar AA, Shivachandra SB (2004). Frontier areas of research on haemorrhagic septicaemia vaccines. In Proc. of annual conference of IAVR, 24-26 Feb, IVRI, Izatnagar, India.

Marchart J, Dropmann G, Lechleitner S, Schlapp T, Wanner G, Szostak MP and Lubitz, W (2003). *Pasteurella multocida* and *Pasteurella haemolytica*-ghosts: new vaccine candidates. Vaccine **21**(25-26): 3988-3997.

May B J, Zhang Q, Li L L, Paustian M L, Whittam T S and Kapur V (2000). Complete genome sequence of *Pasteurella multocida*, Pm70. Proceedings of National Academy of Sciences, *UAS* **98:** 3460-3465.

Mittal KR, Jiaswal TN and Gupta BK (1979). Studies on haemorrhagic septicaemia and multiple emulsion vaccines. Indian Veterinary Journal **3:** 449-454.

Myint A and Carter GR. (1989). Prevention of haemorrhagic septicaemia in cattle and buffaloes with a live vaccine. Veterinary Record **124:** 508-509.

Nagy LK and Pen CW (1979). Protection of cattle against experimental haemorrhagic septcaemia by the capsular antigens of *Pasteurella multocida* type B and E. Research in Veterinary Science **20:** 249-253.

Namioka S and Murata M (1961). Serological studies on *Pasteurella multocida*: a simplified method of capsular typing of the organism. Cornell Veterinarian **51:** 498-507.

Nikhiporova NM (1958). Pasteurellosis of domestic animals. Bulletin African Institute of Epizootiology **50:** 176.

OIE (2008). Haemorrhagic septicaemia, Chapter 2.4.12. Terrestrial manual 739-750.

Olive DM, Bean P (1999). Principles and applications of methods for DNA based typing of microbial organisms: a mini review. Journal of Clinical Microbiology **37**(6): 1661-1669.

Pasteur L (1880). De l'attenuation du virus du cholera des poules. CR Academy of Science **91:** 673-680.

Pati US, Srivastava SK, Roy SC and More T (1996). Immunogenicity of outer membrane protein of *Pasteurella multocida* in buffalo calves. Veterinary Microbiology **52:** 301-311.

Paustian ML, May BJ and Kapur V (2001). *Pasteurella multocida* gene expression in response to iron limitation. Infection and Immunity **69:** 4109–4115.

Rau G and Govil JL (1950). An improved haemorrhagic septicaemia vaccine. Indian Veterinary Journal **27:** 105.

Ruffalo GC, Tennet JM, Michalski WP and Adler B (1997). Identification, purification and characterization of type-4 fimbriae of *Pasteurella multocida*. Infection and Immunity **65:** 339-343.

Saxena MK, Kumar AA, Chaudhuri P, Shivachandra SB, Singh VP, Singh VP and Sharma B (2005). Ribotyping of Indian isolates of *Pasteurella multocida* based on 16S and 23S rRNA genes. Veterinary Research Communications **29**(6): 527-535.

Shivachandra S B, Viswas K N and Kumar A A (2011). A review of haemorrhagic septicaemia in cattle and buffalo. Animal Health Research Reviews, **12:** 67-82.

Siju J, Kumar AA, Shivachandra SB, Chaudhuri P, Srivastava SK and Singh VP (2007). Cloning and characterization of Type 4 fimbrial gene (*ptfA*) of *Pasteurella multocida* Serogroup B:2 (Strain P_{52}). Veterinary Research Communications **31:** 397-404.

Srivastava NC, Harbola PC and Khera SS (1975). Preliminary observations on combined vaccination against haemorrhagic septicaemia and black quarter. Indian Veterinary Journal **53:** 168-172.

Srivastava SK (1998). Immunogenicity of *Pasteurella multocida* grown in iron restricted medium. Journal of Applied Animal Research **136:** 137-144.

Tomer P, Chaturvedi G C, Minakshi, Malik P and Monga D P (2002). Comparative analysis of the outer membrane protein profiles of isolates of the *Pasteurella multocida* (B:2) associated with haemorrhagic septicaemia. Veterinary Research Communications **26**(7): 513-522.

Townsend K M, Boyce J D, Chung J Y, Frost A J and Adler B (2001). Genetic organization of *Pasteurella multocida* cap loci and development of a multiplex capsular PCR typing system. Journal Clinical Microbiology **39:** 924-929.

Townsend K M, Frost A J, Lee C W, Papadimitrious J M and Dawkins H J (1998). Development of PCR assays for species and type specific identification of *Pasteurella multocida* isolates. Journal Clinical Microbiology **36:** 1096-1100.

Verma R and Jaiswal T N (1998). Haemorrhagic septicaemia vaccines. Vaccines, **16:** 1184-1190.

Wheeler R (2009). Outer membrane proteomics of *Pasteurella multocida* isolates to identify putative host-specificity determinants. Bioscience Horizons **2**(1): 1-12.

Wu JR, Shien JH, Shieh HK, Chen CF and Chang PC (2007). Protective immunity conferred by recombinant *Pasteurella multocida* lipoprotein E (PlpE). Vaccine **25:** 4140–4148.

❑❑❑

Chapter 28

Brucellosis

D.K. SINGH
IVRI, Izatnagar, Bareilly

Introduction

Brucellosis, a direct anthropozoonosis of worldwide distribution, is caused by a Gram-negative facultative intracellular bacterium capable of growth and multiplication inside both phagocytic as well as non-phagocytic cells (Celli *et al.* 2005). The disease has probably accompanied the human civilization for over 2,000 years (Capasso 2002). Though controlled in many developed countries, brucellosis remains endemic in many parts of the world particularly in Mediterranean countries, Latin America, the Middle East, Spain, parts of Africa and western Asia. In the year 1861, J. A. Marston, an Assistant Surgeon, first described brucellosis in Malta as Mediterranean gastric remittent fever (Marston 1861). Sir David Bruce isolated the bacterium from the spleen of a British soldier died due to Malta fever (Bruce 1887) and named it *Micrococcus melitensis*. Later, it was renamed *Brucella melitensis* in his honour. However, the zoonotic link of *Brucella* was recognized by Zammit (1905) who isolated it from milk of healthy goats. In India, the presence of brucellosis was first established early in the 20th century and since then has been reported from almost all parts of the country.

The bacteria

The members of the genus *Brucella* are small, Gram-negative, facultative intracellular coccobacilli belonging to α-2 subdivision of the *Proteobacteria*, alongside *Ochrobactrum, Rhizobium, Rhodobacter, Agrobacterium, Bartonella* and *Rickettsia* (Moreno *et al.* 1990). The genus consists of six species based on the host preference and phenotypic differences (Osterman and Moreno, 2006) namely, *B. abortus* (cattle), *B. melitensis* (sheep and goat), *B. suis* (pigs), *B. ovis* (rams), *B. canis* (dogs) and *B. neotomae* (wood rats). Of late, three new species named *B. microti* (voles), *B. pinnipediae* (doplhins) and *B. cetaceae* (seal) have been identified (Ewalt *et al.* 1994, Ross *et al.* 1996, Scholz *et al.* 2008), of which *B. pinnipediae* and *B. cetaceae* are reported to be zoonotic (Brew *et al.* 1999, Sohn *et al.* 2003, McDonald *et al.* 2006). Additional new or seemingly novel species have also been described more recently (De *et al.* 2008, Scholz *et al.* 2008) indicating an ever expanding *Brucella* epidemiology. All *Brucella* species seem to have arisen from a common ancestor to which *B. suis* biotype 3 shares similarity (Moreno *et al.* 2002). Based on DNA hybridization studies, Verger *et al.* (1985) proposed *Brucella* to be monospecific genus with *B. melitensis* as the nomen species with all other as its biovar. However, on the basis of host specificity, phenotypic characteristics, varying virulence, and available genotyping data (Chain *et al.* 2005, Halling *et al.* 2005) the classic taxonomic scheme for the six *Brucella* species and 17 existing biovars was ultimately reapproved in 2003 (Osterman and Moriyon 2006).

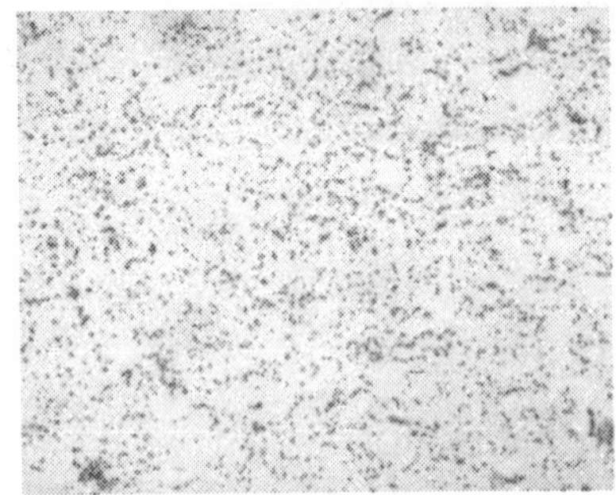

Brucella abortus Gram stained

Brucellae are fairly hardy and the organisms have been recovered from foetal and manure samples that remained in a cool environment for longer than two months. However, exposure to sunlight kills the organism within a few hours (Waring 2005) and the organism is susceptible to many common disinfectants (Anonymous 2006).

Disease occurrence and transmission

Animal brucellosis is endemic worldwide with bovine brucellosis, caused by *B. abortus*, as the most widespread in animals (Corbel 1997). However, in many countries where *B. abortus* infection in bovines was eradicated, *B. melitensis* infection in these species is emerging as a new challenge (Banai 2002). In animals, brucellosis infection is responsible for huge economic losses through reduced productivity, abortions and weak offsprings. It also results in the loss of much needed animal protein for human consumption.

Human brucellosis is mainly caused by *B. melitensis, B. abortus, B. suis* and *B. canis* with *B. melitensis* as the principal cause of human brucellosis worldwide accounting for upto 90% of all cases. *B. melitensis* type 1 predominating in India (Mantur *et al.* 2006) and Spain (Colmenero *et al.* 1996), type 2 in northwestern Greece and type 3 in Turkey (Bodur *et al.* 2003).

Although *B. ovis* is widespread in sheep, it has not been identified in humans. An estimated 5,00,000 human infections occur annually worldwide with great variation in the incidence in the endemic areas ranging from <1/100,000 population in UK, USA and Australia to >20-30/100,000 in southern European countries such as Greece and Spain, and upto >70/100,000 in Middle East countries like Kuwait and Saudi Arabia (Cutler *et al.*, 2005).

Consumption of unpasteurized milk and their products especially soft cheese, yoghurts and ice-cream (Eckman 1975), undercooked traditional delicacies such as liver and spleen are mainly responsible for human brucellosis (Malik 1997). Camel milk is considered to be the most important source of infection in Middle East countries and Mongolia. Rarely, human-to-human transmission takes place through tissue transplantation or sexual contact (Mantur *et al.* 1996) but it is epidemiologically insignificant. The disease can also be caused by contact with vaginal discharge, urine, faeces and blood of infected animals through broken skin and mucous membrane of conjunctiva and through inhalation. The disease is an occupational hazard for livestock owners, abattoir workers, dairy workers, shepherds, farmers, veterinarians and laboratory workers. Brucellosis is one of the most common laboratory acquired infections (Noviello *et al.*; 2004, Fugieret *et al.*, 2007). With the increase in global tourism, brucellosis is emerging as a common travel associated imported disease in the developed world (Memish and Balkhy 2004).

Among cattle and buffaloes, ingestion or inhalation of organisms that are present in foetal fluids or other birth products is the predominant route of natural infection. The herds are typically exposed following the introduction of an infected animal that subsequently aborts or gives birth to an infected foetus contaminating the pasture or water body. However, the transmission of infection through natural services is not important epidemiologically in these species. In contrast, in dogs and sheep, transmission of rough strains of *Brucella* may be more common via the venereal route. Among dogs, the urine of males and vaginal secretions of females are the main sources of infection via the venereal, oral, nasal, or conjunctival routes (Wanke 2004, Hollew 2006).

Global scenario

Brucellosis is major health problem in Mediterranean, Middle East, Latin America, Africa, parts of Mexico, and parts of Asia including India (Refai 2002, Grovel 2008). Syria has the highest annual incidence worldwide (OIE 2005a). The rate of human infection is high in Peru, Kuwait and Saudi Arabia in comparison with sub-Saharan Africa, where the rate is relatively low (McGill 2003).

Only 17 countries claim to be free of brucellosis (Cutler *et al.* 2005). Though it has been eradicated from almost all of Europe, reports still indicate the presence of human brucellosis in Greece, Spain and Turkey. Brucellosis-free status has been granted by the European Union (EU) to Sweden, Denmark, Finland, Germany, the UK (excluding Northern Ireland), Austria, Netherlands, Belgium, and Luxembourg (European Commission 2003). Norway and Switzerland are also considered brucellosis-free countries. France is an example where brucellosis has been successfully eradicated (Anonymous 2005). An increase in the annual number of reported cases in Turkey has been observed, exceeding 15000 cases in 2004 (OIE 2005a) whereas the situation in Iran showed improvement during this period (OIE 2005b). Iraq has high endemicity with the annual incidence of 278.4 cases per million of population (OIE 2005). Brocellosis has shown an increasing trend of incidence in Pakistan particularly in large dairy herds (Jamal *et al.* 2003). Brucellosis is re-emerging in Israel, Kuwait, Saudi Arabia, Brazil and Columbia with an increasing incidence of *B. melitensis* or *B. suis* biovar 1 infection in cattle (Corbel 1997). It has re-emerged in Oman and Malta (Amato Gauci 1995). Serological evidence of brucellosis has been reported in poultry (Choudhary and Narayan 1984, Junaidu *et al.* 2006).

While the occurrence of bovine brucellosis has been reported by 93 countries, the concept of host restriction of different *Brucella* species is gradually eluding with the evidence that *B. suis* biovar 1 has become established in cattle in Brazil and Columbia, thus, becoming a more important reservoir than pigs (Lopez Merino 1989). *B. suis* has the widest host range, with established host-pathogen relationships in reindeer (Tessaro and Forbes 1986) and hares (Vitovec *et al.* 1976) in addition to swine.

B. melitensis infection in cattle is emerging as impending threat in some southern European countries, Israel, Kuwait and Saudi Arabia (McGill 2003). It particularly poses problem as *B. abortus* vaccines does not effectively protect against *B. melitensis* infection and *B. melitensis* Rev.1 vaccine has not been fully evaluated for use in cattle.

Indian perspective

The true incidence of human brucellosis in India is elusive. It has been estimated that the true incidence may be 25 times higher than the reported incidence. Mantur *et al.* (2004) showed a seroprevalence of 1.6% by SAT and isolated *B. melitensis* in 43 of the 93 children during a period of 13 years majority of whom were shepherds habitual of consuming fresh goat milk. They also reported brucellosis in 495 among 26948 adults (1.8%) in Bijapur during a period of 16 years from 1988 to 2004 and isolated *B. melitensis* from 191 cases (Mantur *et al.* 2006). Mathur (1964) reported 8.5% seroprevalence of brucellosis among dairy personnel in contact with infected animals and isolated *Brucella* from 7 cases while Randhawa *et al.* (1974) detected antibodies in 4.2% of abortion cases. In Gujarat, 8.5% prevalence of *Brucella* agglutinins was recorded in human cases (Panjarathinam and Jhala 1986). In Haryana, 34% prevalence of human brucellosis was recorded among veterinarians, attendants and compounders in contact with animals (Chauhan 1999) indicating an occupational association. Thakur and Thapliyal (2002) too observed the disease prevalence in 4.97% persons exposed to animals with a markedly higher prevalence (17.39%) among field veterinarians. Hemashettar and Patil (1991) found 8.2% veterinary workers with *Brucella* specific antibodies. High seroprevalence rate was also noted in specific risk groups such as abattoir workers (Barbuddhe *et al.* 2000, Chadda *et al.* 2004). Kumar *et al.* (1997) too observed high prevalence (25%) among abattoir personnel in Delhi. Handa *et al.* (1998) diagnosed 4 (3.3%) cases of acute brucellosis in 121 patients with fever of unknown origin (FUO). Similarly, Sen *et al.* (2002) detected 28 (6.8%) seropositive cases in a group of 414 patients with FUO, while Kadri *et al.* (2000) reported 28 (0.8%) seropositive cases in 3,532 patients with FUO.

Mudaliar *et al.* (2003) showed the presence of *Brucella* antibodies in 5.33% of the animal handlers of which 4.51% were dairy farm workers and 14.63 % were veterinary doctors. Rana *et al.* (1985) showed a seropositivity of 27.7% among veterinarians in Delhi. Agasthya *et al.* (2007) reported brucellosis in occupationally exposed individuals with high prevalence of 41.23% in veterinary inspectors, 30.92% in veterinary assistants, 12.37% in veterinary officers, 6.18% in veterinary supervisors, 6.18% in group- D workers, 2.06% in shepherds and 1.03% in butchers. Bedi *et al.* (2007 also reported brucellosis in animal handlers in Punjab.

In India, the evidence of brucellosis based on serosurvey has been reported in all domestic animals besides poultry and wild animals (Table 1). The prevalence of brucellosis in animals reportedly varies from as low as 0.13% (Chatterjee *et al.*, 1986) to as high as 44% (Zaki *et al.*, 1975). In general, incidence of brucellosis is reportedly higher in cattle than in buffaloes (Maansi 1999). In a serological survey of brucellosis in cattle and buffalo in 23 states of India, Isloor *et al.* (1998a) demonstrated an overall prevalence of antibodies in 1.9% of cattle and 1.8% of buffaloes in 23 states. They also showed a seropositivity of 4.1% in cattle in 47 organised farms in contrast to 0.7% seropositivity in cattle owned by individual farmers in Karnataka.

The samples predominantly from large herds with a history of abortion and infertility showed a highly variable seroprevalence ranging from 6.6% in Madhya Pradesh (Mehra *et al.*, 2000) to 60% in Assam (Chakraborty *et al.* 2000). Mehra *et al.* (2000) reported 6.5% prevalence in cattle from organized farms compared to 5.1% prevalence in the unorganized sector. National Survey of Bovine Brucellosis (1994-2001) showed national average of brucellosis as 5% in cattle and 3% in buffaloes (Renukaradhya *et al.* 2002). In a similar national survey of sheep and goat brucellosis, Isloor *et al.* (1998b) reported 7.9% cumulative incidence in sheep and 2.2% in goats. In another study, Singh (2008) reported 7.41%, 8.58% and 8.85% seroprevalence of brucellosis in cattle, goat and sheep, respectively.

Serological evidence of *B. ovis* infection in 6 out of 102 rams was reported in Himachal Pradesh (Katoch *et al.* 1996). The seroprevalence of brucellosis in pigs has been recorded as 3.2% in Madhya Pradesh (Soni and Pathak 1969), 11.3% in Tamil Nadu (Kumar and Rao 1980) and 6.3% in Karnataka (Krishnappa *et al.* 1981). In another study, it was estimated as 9.5% in 756 pigs slaughtered in Karnataka (Thoppil 2000). Brucellosis has also been reported in dairy farms in Goa region (Barbuddhe *et al.* 2004). Similarly, Aulakh *et al.* (2008) reported a high prevalence of bovine brucellosis in Punjab. Serological evidence of brucellosis has also been demonstrated in Andaman and Nicobar Islands (Jai-Sunder *et al.* 2005). More recently, the seroprevalence of brucellosis in sheep and goats in 7 states of India has been estimated at 7.58, 11.08, 11.88 and 15.77 per cent on testing by RBPT, STAT, CFT and I-ELISA, respectively (Singh 2009). Brucellosis has also been reported in mithuns (Rajkhowa *et al.* 2005) and yaks (Bandyopadhyay *et al.* 2009).

B. abortus biotypes I and III have been isolated from cattle (Chatterjee *et al.* 1995) besides biotype IV (Batra *et al.* 1989). Though biotype I predominates in cattle in organized farms, biotype III has been usually reported to infect the cattle reared by the village population (Anonymous 1986). Occasionally, *B. melitensis* biotype I has also been isolated from cattle (Hemashettar *et al.* 1987). *B. melitensis* biotypes I, II and III have been isolated from sheep and goats (Sharma *et al.* 1995) besides *B. abortus* biotype I (Panjarathinum and Gulrajani 1974). Of the 3 biotypes of *B. melitensis*, biotype I has been shown to predominate in the sheep and goat population (Sen and Sharma 1972). *B. canis* has been isolated from dogs in Chennai (Pillai *et al.* 1991) while isolation of *B. suis* biotype II from a sow has been reported from Tamil Nadu (Kumar and Rao 1980). Subsequently, isolation of *B. suis* biotype II from an aborted foetus of goat was reported (Reddy and Rao 1984) while *B. suis* biotype I was isolated from dog (Pillai *et al.* 1990). The only report of *B. abortus* and *B. melitensis* isolation from horses is that of Polding (Polding 1947). Isolation of *B. ovis* has not been reported in India. The biotypes of *Brucella* isolated from man and animals in India are shown in Table 2.

Table 1 : Species of *Brucella*, host preference and zoonotic potential

Species	Biotype Potential	Host Preference	First described	Zoonotic
Brucella melitensis	1-3	Sheep, goat	Bruce, 1887	High
Brucella abortus	1-6,7	Cattle	Bang, 1887	Moderate
Brucella suis	1-5	Pig	Traum, 1914	Moderate
Brucella canis	-	Dog	Carmichael and Bruner, 1968	Mild
Brucella ovis	-	Sheep	Van Drimmelen, 1953	Absent
Brucella neotomae	-	Desert Wood rat	Stoenner and Lackman, 1957	Absent
Brucella ceti	-	Cetaceans	Ewalt and Ross, 1994	Mild
Brucella pinnipedoalis	-	Seals	Ewalt and Ross, 1994	Mild

Table 2 : Differential characteristics of the species of the genus *Brucella*

Species	Colony morphology	Lysis by phages[a]				Oxidase	Urease activity
		Tb	Wb	Iz_1	R/C		
B. abortus	smooth	+	+	+	-	+	+[b]
B.melitensis	smooth	-[c]	-	+	-	+	+
B. suis	smooth	-	+	+	-	+	+
B. ovis	rough	-	-	-	+	-	-
B. canis	rough	-	-	-	+	+	+
B. neotomae	smooth	-[c]	+	+	-	-	+

From refs 6, 7 (Alton et. al 1975; OIE manual 2008)

a Phages : Tbilisi (Tb), Weybridge (Wb), Izatnagar1 (Iz1) and R/C

b strain 544 is urease negative

c negative at RTD (Routine Test Dilution)

Bioterrorism potential

B. abortus, B. melitensis, and *B. suis* have been identified as Category B bioterrorism agents (Rotz *et al.* 2002) and as select agents by the US Government (CDC 2005). Also, *B. suis* was one of the earliest agents investigated and developed as a bioweapon in the United States in the 1950s (Christopher *et al.* 2005). In 1954, *Brucella* species became the first agent weaponised by the US offensive biological weapons programme (Sarinas and Chitkara 2003). The propensity of *Brucella* for airborne transmission and ability to induce chronic debilitating disease in man requiring prolonged treatment with a combination of antibiotics, absence of any pathognomonic clinical presentation defying early and rapid diagnosis are some of the important characteristics that make it a potential bioweapon (Pappas *et al.* 2006).

Economic impact

The impact of brucellosis in cattle and buffalo on the national economy of India has been estimated to the tune of Rs. 240 million every year (Schwabe 1984). This amounts to more than half per cent of the total value of all meat and milk products produced in the country. The annual loss due to human brucellosis has been put at 30 million man days. Kunen (1994) estimated that brucellosis costs India at least Rs. 350 million annually in terms of loss of food animals and man days. Earlier to this, the economic loss due to brucellosis among bovines was estimated at Rs. 311.47 million (Mathur and Sharma 1974).

Prevention and control strategies

Brucellosis being a direct zoonosis with no human-to-human transmission, decline in human brucellosis cases is always expected consequent upon the control programmes instituted against animal brucellosis. Indeed, with the fact that there is no human vaccine available for brucellosis, control and eradication programme for animal brucellosis remains a challenge.

Control of animal brucellosis is dependent on two main principles: (a) elimination of infected animals from the herd, and (b) prevention of exposure of animals to infection. Control and eradication of brucellosis in animals may be achieved by test and slaughter of infected animals with or without mass vaccination with approved vaccine depending on the situation with respect to the incidence and prevalence of the disease. In test and slaughter policy, detection of truly infected animals assumes paramount importance and requires a quick, cheap and reasonably sensitive screening test supported with an efficacious confirmatory test. In cattle, Rose Bengal plate agglutination test (RBPT) is recommended as screening test with positive sera tested with complement fixation test (CFT) for confirmation. The milk ring test (MRT) could be used for identifying infected dairy herd with good results followed by sero-testing individual animals. However, this cannot be used on dry animals and its efficacy is doubtful in sheep and goats. However, Mass immunization should be the desired strategy in case of high prevalence of disease. For cattle, *B. abortus* S-19, a live attenuated vaccine, given at the age of 3 to 6 months (in certain cases upto 8 months) is recommended. In spite of certain drawbacks, it has been used with satisfactory results. When used routinely to attain coverage of ³ 80% of population, herd immunity develops with gradual decline in the incidence. If eradication is the target, vaccination should be stopped once the incidence falls below 0.2% and the infected animals must be eliminated. In February 1996, the USDA approved the use of *B. abortus* strain RB51 (RB51) as the official calfhood vaccine for protection against brucellosis (http://www.aphis.usda.gov:80/vs/nahps/Brucellosis/rb51.html). The *Brucella* RB51 strain lacks S-LPS and has much lower pathogenicity in vaccinates. It is considered only mildly abortifacient and presumed to have much lower pathogenicity in humans in response to accidental exposure. In addition, the *B. abortus* RB51 vaccine has a substantial advantage in animal disease control programmes because it does not elicit an antibody response against S-LPS and does not, therefore, interfere with results of serologic testing.

The epidemiology and planning for prevention and control of brucellosis in sheep and goats are similar to that of cattle with minor adjustments. A live attenuated *Brucella* vaccine *B. melitensis* Rev-1 is highly effective and is widely used to vaccinate small ruminants in parts of the world where *B. melitensis* is enzootic. Immunization of young recently weaned rams (weaner rams) with the *B. melitensis* Rev-1 vaccine is also recommended for control of *B. ovis* in some countries (Waring 2005). Like the strain 19 vaccine, this vaccine, too, causes abortions in pregnant animals and short-term shedding of the Rev-1 strain in milk (Banai 2002) leading to human infections with *B. melitensis* Rev-1 as reported in Israel and the Middle East (Refai 2002, Banai 2002, Bardenstein *et al.* 2002). The probability of success in the flocks where contact with other flocks is frequent remains poor. In sheep and goats, allergic test, along with RBPT, could be used to identify infected herd followed by sero-testing of individual animals (Olsen *et al.* 1996).

Control of brucellosis in swine poses particular difficulty because there is neither a satisfactory test to identify infected individual animal nor a satisfactory vaccine. It is, therefore, advisable to slaughter the herd. No effective vaccine against *B. canis* has been identified to date.

Control and eradication of brucellosis in domestic animals, especially bovine brucellosis in India poses particular problem as the cow slaughter is not permitted. Under such situation, it appears prudent to aim control rather than eradication of disease. For this, continued long term vaccination programme with movement control between endemic to non-endemic zone should be instituted so as to achieve vaccination of = 80 per cent animal population to develop herd immunity. Such continued mass vaccination with movement control is expected to bring down the incidence of brucellosis to a level where it may cease to be a cause of worry for animal population. Once the disease is brought under control in animals, the incidence of brucellosis in human population is liable to decline.

Table 3 : Prevalence of brucellosis in man and animals in India

Animal species	Seropositivity	Isolation of *Brucella*
Cattle	+	+
Buffalo	+	+
Sheep	+	+
Goat	+	+
Swine	+	+
Equine	+	+
Camel	+	-
Dog	+	+
Poultry	+	-
Wild animals	+	-
Man	+	+

Table 4 : Biotypes of *Brucella* isolated from man and animals in India

Species	Biotypes	Animal
B. abortus	1,3,4,6	Cattle
	1,3	Buffalo
	1	Sheep
	1	Goat
	1,3	Man
	#	Equine
B. melitensis	1	Cattle
	1,2,3	Sheep
	1,2,3	Goat
	1,2,3	Man
	#	Equine
B. suis	2	Goat
	2	Pig
	1	Dog
B. canis	–	Dog

Future perspective

Brucellosis has always been a challenge to the scientific fraternity. The disease has eluded control and eradication in many parts of the world and has been re-emerging (Seleem *et al.* 2009). Much progress has been made since the identification of brucellosis. A battery of diagnostic tests and vaccines, both live-attenuated and killed, are available. The necessary technical knowhow for control and eradication programmes under different sociocultural and epidemiological situations is available. However, a lot needs to be done. The available vaccines are far from ideal. Vaccine for all species is not available. Prompt reporting of human brucellosis to health authorities is extremely important as there is no vaccine for use in humans. In the areas where brucellosis is enzootic, good animal husbandry is critical to prevent transmission both among animals and between animals and humans. In the management of groups of domestic animals, provision of seperate birthing areas, and implementation of good management practices are important to minimize opportunities for transmission should an infected animal be introduced. Cheeses and other foods made from unpasteurized dairy products from countries where brucellosis is enzootic should be avoided, and meat should not be consumed from animals that appear to be sick at the time of slaughter.

The diagnostic tests, too, are fraught with problems and present many difficulties. It is difficult to differentiate between *Brucella* infection and *Yersinia enterocolitica* O:9 infection; and vaccinated and infected animals. All antigens are not well characterized. The pathogenicity of brucellosis is not clearly elucidated. The mechanism of intracellular survival and elimination of brucellae are yet to be explained. Clearly, until the pathogenicity of the *Brucella* infection is elucidated and the antigens characterized with respect to their virulence properties and immune capability, it would probably not be possible to develop a foolproof diagnostic test or an ideal vaccine. Now that the complete sequence of the *Brucella* genome is available, the days are probably not far off when these shortcomings would be overcome.

Dr Pallab Chaudhury further adds to it;

Brucellosis is a chronic granulomatous infection caused by intracellular bacteria. It is one of the most important zoonotic diseases of livestock worldwide. Brucellosis was described for the first time by Marston in 1860 on the island of Malta. In 1887, Sir David Bruce discovered little coccobacillus in a preparation from a spleen of a soldier who died of brucellosis. It is a devastating infectious disease that causes significant morbidity in animals, and man. In livestock, brucellosis causes severe economic losses as a result of abortion, infertility and decreased milk production. In man, *Brucella* infection is associated with variable symptoms with recurrent fever. Thereby, brucellosis in human is also termed as 'undulent fever'. Human gets infection through consumption of contaminated milk and dairy products. Animal owners, workers and veterinarians are highly prone to get infection due to occupational contact with infected animals. Brucellosis is a true zoonosis, in that virtually all naturally occurring human infections are acquired from animals. It poses a major impediment for international trade of animal and animal products. The severity of this disease, lack of vaccines suitable for use in man and frequent failure of clinical laboratories to correctly identify isolates led to the investigation of *Brucella* as an agent for bioterrorism (1).

Etiological agent

Brucellosis is caused by the members of the bacterial genus, *Brucella*. There are six major species of *Brucella*, namely *Brucella abortus, B. melitensis, B. suis, B. ovis, B. canis* and B. *neotome*, affecting different species of animals. This classification is mainly based on the differences in pathogenicity and host preference (2). Host preference of *Brucella* has been a focus of research because the organisms are very closely related and highly homogeneous at genomic level. The recent isolation of distinctive strains of *Brucella* from marine mammals (*Brucella ceti* and *Brucella pinnipedoalis*) has extended its ecologic range. They belong to the α-proteobacteria group, as many other bacteria that live in close association with a eukaryotic host. Based on cultural and serological properties, *B. abortus, B. melitensis* and *B. suis* are subdivided into several biovars.

The debate of whether the Brucellae should comprise a single monospecific genus or multiple species has been a source of much controversy. Molecular genetic studies have indicated that the genus contains only a single species, *Brucella melitensis*, differentiated into a number of biovars, with certain host preferences (3). This method of taxonomy of Brucellae has not been universally accepted, with many holding the traditional nomenclature of multiple species. The *Brucella* genome consists of two circular chromosomes, suggesting a remarkable difference compared to the single chromosome of many bacteria (3, 4). The recent completion of *B. melitensis* (GenBank NC 003317 and NC 003318) (5), *B. suis* (GenBank NC 002969), and *B. abortus* genome sequence projects has provided tremendous information for understanding the mechanisms of *Brucella* pathogenicity.

Brucellae are a family of Gram-negative coccobacilli with 0.5-0.7 μm width and 0.5-1.5 μm length. They are small, non-motile, non-capsulated and non-spore forming organisms. The organisms grow aerobically or microaerophilically that require enriched medium for primary isolation. In addition, *B.abortus* and *B.ovis* are carboxyphilic and require carbon dioxide (5-10 percent) for growth.

The metabolism of the brucellae is mainly oxidative. Multiplication is slow and the organism grows at an temperature of 37°C. *Brucella* colonies become visible on suitable solid media in 2-3 days. The colonies of smooth strains are small, round and convex but dissociation, with loss of the O chains of the LPS, occurs readily to form rough or mucoid variants. Rough forms are natural in *B canis* and *B ovis* due to lack of O chains in the LPS. The outer cell membrane contains a dominant lipopolysaccharide (LPS) component and three main groups of proteins. No *Brucella* species has been found to harbor plasmids naturally although they readily accept broad-host-range plasmids.

Disease Description

Brucellosis results in serious economic losses due to late term abortion, stillborn and weakly calves. Lesions consist of necrotic placentitis and interstitial mastitis in pregnant cows, and fibrinous pleuritis with interstitial pneumonia in aborted fetuses and newborn calves. In animals, brucellae typically affect the reproductive organs, and abortion is often the only sign of the disorder. Human brucellosis is either an acute febrile disease or a persistent disease with a wide variety of symptoms.

There are so many factors that can affect the prevalence of brucellosis in various species of livestock. Prevalence of brucellosis can vary according to climatic conditions, geography, species, sex, age and diagnostic tests applied.The bacteria are shed from an infected animal at or around the time of calving or abortion. Once exposed, the likelihood of an animal becoming infected is variable, depending on age, pregnancy status, and other intrinsic factors of the animal, as well as the amount of bacteria to which the animal was exposed. The most common clinical signs of cattle infected with *Brucella abortus* are high incidences of abortions, arthritic joints and retained after-birth. There are two main causes for spontaneous abortion in animals. The first is due to erythritol, which can promote infections in the fetus and placenta. The second is due to the lack of anti-*Brucella* activity in the amniotic fluid. Males can also harbor the bacteria in their reproductive tracts, namely seminal vesicles, testicles, and epididymides. Brucellosis is spread from the vaginal discharge of an infected cow or from an aborted fetus. The organism has an affinity for the reproductive tract and abortions, retained placenta, weak calves and infertility frequently occur. Breeding bulls which are infected, can transmit the disease to cows at the time of service by infected semen. Milk produced from an infected cow may also harbor the organism. The infected milk creates a public health hazard as this is the organism that causes undulant fever in humans.

Pathogenesis

Virulence factors associated with brucellae are poorly defined. Pathogenicity islands, specialized secretion systems, virulence plasmids, fimbriae, pili, adhesins, and toxins are all classical bacterial virulence factors. However, many of these factors, though widespread among bacterial pathogens, are not necessarily found among bacteria that colonize eukaryotic cells in a pathogenic/symbiotic relationship. Bacteria that form these relationships have developed other strategies to infect and grow in their hosts. This is particularly true for *Brucella* and other members of the class Proteobacteria.

To be successful infectious agent pathogenic bacteria often depends on their ability to survive and multiply within the host cells. To do so, they alter or adapt to the host cell environment. *Brucella* spp are facultative intracellular bacteria that have the ability to avoid the killing mechanism and proliferate within the macrophages, similar to other intracellular pathogens. To establish infection inside the host cell, *Brucella* requires four steps: adherence, invasion, establishment, and dissemination within the host. *Brucella* can infect both phagocytic and nonphagocytic cells in vivo and in vitro. In addition to direct contact with host cells, antibody or complement mediated phagocytosis facilitates entry of *Brucella* in macrophages. *Brucella* cells can replicate and survive inside macrophages inhibiting phogo-lysosome formation. After infecting the host, the pathogen becomes sequestered within the cells of the reticuloendothelial system. The mechanism by which *Brucella* evades intracellular killing and the host immune system is not fully understood. Lot of research findings attempts to describe possible mechanism of pathogenesis.

The organisms may gain entry into the body through a variety of portals. Because the infection is systemic it is often not possible to determine which portal was involved in a particular case. Once infection is established the organisms are carried from the point of entry to the regional lymph nodes, leading to acute lymphadenitis. Bacteria multiply inside phagocytes and disseminate via systemic circulation to other organs or tissues such as the spleen, lymph nodes, uterus and the mammary gland. In males, *B. abortus* can be found mostly in the testicles where the organisms cause orchitis, and accessory sex glands as well as lymphoid tissue. The bacteremia can last for months, and in cases of chronic disease it can be intermittent, recurring mostly around parturition. The bacteria localize in the uterus during gestation and cause ulceration of the endometrium. The initial lesions are seen in the wall of the uterus, but the organism quickly spreads to the placental cotyledons and destroys the villi. Depending on the severity of the lesions potential sequelae include: abortion, especially in the last trimester, stillbirths, and premature or weak calves. Following abortion or parturition the organism is shed by the uterus for weeks, and the animal remains infected for life.

Brucella can infect both phagocytic and nonphagocytic cells *in vivo* and *in vitro* (8,9). Major target cells for brucellae are macrophages, dendritic cells, and trophoblasts. In order to reach its target cells, *Brucella* needs to cross mucosal barriers of the respiratory, genitourinary or digestive tract, where it undergoes phagocytosis by resident macrophages and dendritic cells, resulting in dissemination of the organism to lymphoid and reproductive organs [10,11]. In the gastro-intestinal tract, the organism invade through M cells. In macrophages, *Brucella* is internalized by phagocytosis that requires a moderate recruitment of actin filaments upon activation during interaction of *Brucella* and receptors on the surface of the macrophage cell membrane. Opsonized *Brucella* is internalized *via* FC or complement receptors whereas non-opsonized bacteria interact with lectin and fibronectin receptors [12]. Cholesterol-rich microdomains (lipids rafts) of macrophage cell membrane also helps in internalization and intracellular trafficking of bacteria [13,14]. Soon after internalization, the *Brucella*-containing phagosome interacts with early and late endosomes. The majority of phagocytosed *Brucella* is destroyed by bactericidal action of free radicals of oxygen, nitric oxide and enzymes inside phagolysosomes. However, a certain number of bacteria resists these bactericidal mechanisms, and after transient fusion with the lysosome can actively exclude lysosomal proteins and redirect the Brucella containing vesicles (BCV) to the endoplasmic reticulum, where the organism is capable of replicating. Importantly, acidification of the *Brucella*-containing phagosome does not injure the bacteria, but it triggers expression of bacterial genes that are essential for intracellular survival during the early stages of infection [15]. *Brucella* has a marked tropism for dendritic cells and able to survive and replicate in the cells more efficiently than macrophages. The behavior of *Brucella* in non-phagocytic cells has been better investigated in epithelial cell lines. Although *Brucella* is capable of invading epithelial and trophoblatic cells, it is much less invasive than other facultative intracellular bacterial pathogens such as *Salmonella enterica*. No specific receptors for *Brucella* have been identified in non-phagocytic cells, but there is evidence that some *Brucella* molecules can contribute to cellular adhesion and invasion [16]. *Brucella* invades epithelial cells *via* recruitment of actin filaments and rearrangement of the host cell membrane. Intracellular trafficking of *Brucella* in epithelial cells is similar to that observed in phagocytes. *Brucella* traffics initially in early phagosome, progressing towards autophagosomes containing the lysosome associated membrane glycoprotein 1 (LAMP1) and then to the a vacuole composed by membranes of the rough endoplasmic reticulum, which is the optimal site for its replicatiorough endoplasmic reticulum [17]. Trophoblastic cells are key target cell of *Brucella* infection during late phase of gestation in ruminants.

Growth of *Brucella* inside trophoblasts is apparently enhanced in the presence of high concentrations of steroid hormones and erythritol during the final third of gestation. The capacity to replicate rapidly and extensively in trophoblasts can compromise the integrity of the placenta and infection of fetus, resulting in abortion or birth of weak offspring.

References

Ackermann MR, Cheville NF, Deyeoe BL. Bovine ileal dome lymphoepithelial cell: endocytosis and transport of *Brucella abortus* strain 19. Vet Pathol 1988; **25:** 28-35.

Agasthya AS, Isloor S, Prabhudas K (2007) Brucellosis in high risk group individuals. Indian J Med Microbiol **25:** 28-31.

Alton G.G., Jones L.M., Angus R.D. and Verger J.M. 1988. Techniques for the Brucellosis laboratory. Institut National de la Recherche Agronomique, Paris. France.

Amato Gauci AJ (1995) The return of brucellosis. Maltese Med J **7:** 7-8.

Anderson TD, Meador VP, Cheville NF. Pathogenesis of placentitis in the goat inoculated with *Brucella abortus*. I. Gross and histologic lesions. Vet Pathol 1986; **23:** 219-216.

Anonymous (1986) Joint FAO/WHO expert committee on brucellosis. VI Report. WHO TRS No. 740, World Health Organization, Geneva.

Anonymous (2005) Brucellose. http://www.invs.sante.fr/surveillance/brucellose/default.htm. Accessed 24 December 2005.

Anonymous (2006) Material safety data sheet - infectious substances, *Brucella* spp. www.phac-aspc.gc.ca/msds-ftss/msds23e.html. Accessed 5 March 2008.

Anonymous, 2000. Brucellosis. Iowa State Department of Public Health. http://idph.state.ia.us/adper/common/pdf/epi_manual/brucellosis.pdf accessed on May 16, 2007.

Aulakh HK, Patil PK, Sharma S *et al.* (2008) A study on the epidemiology of bovine brucellosis in Punjab (India) using milk-ELISA. Acta Vet Brno **77:** 393-399.

Banai M (2002) Control of small ruminant brucellosis by use of *Brucella melitensis* Rev. 1 vaccine: laboratory aspects and field observations. Vet Microbiol **90:** 497-519.

Bandyopadhyay S, Sasmal D, Dutta TK *et al.* (2009) Seroprevalence of brucellosis in yaks (*Poephagus grunniens*) in India and evaluation of protective immunity to S19 vaccine. Trop Anim Hlth Prod **41:** 587-592.

Barbuddhe SB, Chakurkar EB, Bale MA *et al* (2004) Prevalence of brucellosis in organized dairy farms in Goa region. Indian J Anim Sci **74:** 1030-1031.

Barbuddhe SB, Kumar P, Malik SV *et al* (2000) Seropositivity for intracellular bacterial infections among abattoir associated personnels. J Com Dis **32:** 295-299.

Bardenstein S, Mandelboim M, Ficht TA *et al* (2002) Identification of the *Brucella melitensis* vaccine strain Rev.1 in animals and humans in Israel by PCR analysis of the *Pst*I site polymorphism of its omp2 gene. J Clin Microbiol **40:** 1475–1480.

Batra HV, Chand P, Ganju L, Mukherjee R *et al* (1989) Dot-enzyme linked immunosorbent assay for the detection of antibodies in bovine brucellosis. Res Vet Sci **46:** 143-146.

Bedi JS, Sharma JK, Gill JPS *et al* (2007) Seroepidemiological survey of *Brucella* agglutinins in animal handlers in Punjab, India. Indian J Anim Sci **77:** 1283-1285.

Bodur H, Balaban N, Aksaray S *et al* (2003) Biotypes and antimicrobial susceptibilities of *Brucella* isolates. Scand J Infect Dis **35:** 337-338.

Brew SD, Perret LL, Stack JA *et al* (1999) Vet Rec **144:** 483.

Campbell GA, Adams LG, Sowa BA. Mechanism of binding of *Brucella abortus* to mononuclear phagocytes from cows naturally resistant or susceptible to brucellosis. Vet Immunol Immunopathol 1994; **41:** 295-306.

Capasso L (2002) Bacteria in two millennia old cheese, and related epizoonoses in Roman populations. J Infect **45:** 122-127.

Castañeda-Roldan OU, Ahrani-Bettache S, Saldaña Z, *et al*. Characterization of SP41, a surface protein of *Brucella* associated with adherence and invasion of host epithelial cells. Cell Microbiol 2006; **8:** 1877-87.

CDC (2005) Office of Inspector General, Department of Health and Human Services. Possession, use, and transfer of select agents and toxins. Final rule. Fed Register **70:** 13293–13325.

Celli J. Surviving inside a macrophage: the many ways of *Brucella*. Res Microbiol 2006; **157:** 93-8.

Celli SP, Salcedo SP, Grovel JP (2005) N Brucella cooptsthesmall GTPase SarI for intrcellular replication. PNAS **102:** 1673-1678.

Chadda VS, Soni PK, Gupta A *et al* (2004) Incidence of brucellosis in arthritis and chronic low back pain in high risk group. J Assoc Phy India **52:** 338.

Chain PSG, Comerci DJ, Tolmasky ME *et al* (2005) Whole genome analyses of speciation events in pathogenic *Brucellae*. Infect Immun **73:** 8353-8361.

Chakraborty M, Patgiri GP, Barman NN (2000) Application of delayed-type hypersensitivity test (DTH) for the diagnosis of bovine *brucellosis*. Indian Vet J **77:** 849-851.

Chatterjee A, De BN, Mondol P *et al* (1986) Studies on seroprevalence of bovine *brucellosis* in rural areas of West Bengal. Indian Vet J **63:** 95-100.

Chatterjee A, Mondol P, De BN *et al* (1995) Cultural ısolation of *Brucella* in relation to serum agglutinin level. Indian Vet J **72:** 211-215.

Chauhan RS (1999) Brucellosis in India and its impact on export of buffalo meat. J Anim Prod **31:** 316-317.

Choudhary SP, Narayan KG (1984) Prevalence of *Brucella* agglutinin in poultry flocks. Indian J Anim Sci **54:** 289-290.

Christopher GW, Agan MB, Cieslak TJ *et al.* (2005) History of US military contributions to the study of bacterial zoonoses. Military Med **170:** 39-48.

Cloeckaert A, Vizcaino N, Paquet JY *et al.* (2002) Major outer membrane proteins of *Brucella* spp. past, present and future. Vet Microbiol **90:** 229-247.

Colmenero JD, Reguera JM, Martos F *et al.* (1996) Complications associated with *Brucella melitensis* infection: A study of 530 cases. Medicine **75:** 195-211.

Corbel and Brinley-Morgan, 1984.

Corbel MJ (1997) Brucellosis: an overview. Emerg Infect Dis **3:** 213-221.

Cutler SJ, Whatmore AM, Commander NJ (2005) Brucellosis-new aspects of an old disease. J Appl Microbiol **98:** 1270-1281.

De BK, Stauffer L, Koylass MS *et al* (2008) Novel *Brucella* strain (BO1) associated with a prosthetic breast implant infection. J Clin Microbiol **46:** 43-49.

DelVecchio, V. G., V. Kapatral, R. J. Redkar, G. Patra, C. Mujer, T. Los, N. Ivanova, I. Anderson, A. Bhattacharyya, A. Lykidis, G. Reznik, L. Jablonski, N. Larsen, M. D'Souza, A. Bernal, M. Mazur, E. Goltsman, E. Selkoy, P. H. Elzer, S. Hagius, D. O'Callaghan, J. J. Letesson, R. Haselkorn, N. Kyrpides, and R. Overbeek. 2002. The genome sequence of the facultative intracellular pathogen *Brucella melitensis*. Proc. Natl. Acad. Sci. USA **99:** 443-448.

Eckman MR (1975) Brucellosis linked to Mexican cheese. JAMA **232:** 636-637.

European Commission (2003) Report on trends and sources of zoonotic agents in the European Union and Norway. European Commission.

Ewalt DR, Payeur JB, Martin BM *et al* (1994) Characteristics of a *Brucella* species from a bottlenose dolphin (*Tursiops truncates*). J Vet Diagn Invest **6:** 448-452.

Fugier E, Pappas G, Grovel JP (2007) Virulence factors in *brucellosis*: implications for aetiopathogenesis and treatment. Expert Rev Mol Med **9:** 1-10.

Halling SM, Peterson-Burch BD, Bricker BJ *et al* (2005) Completion of the genome sequence of *Brucella abortus* and comparison of the highly similar genomes of *Brucella melitensis* and *Brucella suis*. J Bacteriol **187:** 2715-2726.

Handa R, Singh S, Singh N *et al* (1998) *Brucellosis* in North India: results of a prospective study. J Com Dis **30:** 85-87.

Hemashettar BM, Patil CS (1991) *Brucellosis* among practicing veterinarians. Indian J Med Microbiol **9:** 45-47

Hemashettar BM, Patil CS, Jaikumar K *et al* (1987) Isolation of *Brucella melitensis* biotype I from a cow and two of its attendants. Indian Vet J **64:** 822-825.

Hollett RB (2006) Canine *brucellosis*: outbreaks and compliance. Theriogenol **66:** 575-587.

Isloor S, Renukaradhya GJ, Rajasekhar M (1998a) A serological survey of bovine *brucellosis* in India. Rev Sci Tech Off Int Epi **17:** 781-785.

Isloor S, Renukaradhya GJ, Rajasekhar M (1998b) *Brucellosis* research. In: Annual report (1997–1998) of AICRP on Animal Disease Monitoring and Surveillance (ADMAS), Bangalore, India, 13-18.

Jai-Sunder, Rai RB, Kundu A *et al* (2005) Incidence and prevalence of livestock diseases of Andaman and Nicobar Islands. Indian J Anim Sci **75:** 1041-1043.

Junaidu AU, Ahmed F, Ambursa MA *et al* (2006) *Brucellosis* in local chickens in North Western Nigeria. Int J Poultry Sci **5:** 547-549.

Kadri SM, Rukhsana A, Laharwal MA *et al* (2000) Seroprevalence of brucellosis in Kashmir (India) among patients with pyrexia of unknown origin. J Indian Med Assoc **98:** 170-171.

Katoch RC, Joshi VB, Sharma M (1996) Seroprevalence of *Brucella ovis, Brucella melitensis* and *Chlamydia psittaci* in rams. Indian J Anim Sci **66:** 1130-1131.

Kim S, Watarai M, Suzuki H, *et al.* Lipid raft microdomains mediate class A scavenger receptor-dependent infection of *Brucella abortus*. Microb Pathog 2004; **37:** 11-9.

Krishnappa G, Zaki S, Keshavamurthy BSK (1981). Serological evidence of swine *brucellosis* in and around Bangalore. Mysore J Agri Sci **15:** 77-80.

Kumar P, Singh DK, Barbuddhe SB (1997) Seroprevalence of *brucellosis* among abattoir personnel of Delhi. J Malaria Com Dis **29:** 131-138.

Kumar R, Rao CVN (1980) Porcine *brucellosis* in Tamil Nadu. Indian Vet J **57:** 1-4.

Kunen AV (1994) *Brucellosis* In: *Infectious diseases, diagnosis and management in clinical practice.* CBS Publishers, New Delhi. 448-449.

Lapaque N, Forquet F, de Chastellier C, *et al.* Characterization of *Brucella abortus* lipopolysaccharide macrodomains as mega rafts. Cell Microbiol 2006; **8:** 197-206.

Lopez Merino A (1989) *Brucellosis* in Latin America. In: Young J and Corbel MJ (Eds.). Brucellosis: Clinical and Laboratory aspects, CRC Press Inc: Boca Raton. 151-161.

Maansi (1999) Seroepidemiology of *brucellosis* in animals and man in tarai region. MVSc Thesis GBPUAT, Pantnagar.

Malik GM (1997) A clinical study of brucellosis in adults in the Asir region of southern Saudi Arabia. Am J Trop Med Hyg **56:** 375-377.

Mantur BG, Akki AS, Mangalgi SS *et al* (2004) Childhood brucellosis - a microbiological, epidemiological and clinical study. J Trop Pediatr **50:** 153-157.

Mantur BG, Biradar MS, Bidri RC (2006) Protean clinical manifestations and diagnostic challenges of human brucellosis in adults: 16 years' experience in an endemic area. J Med Microbiol **55:** 897-903.

Mantur BG, Mangalgi SS, Mulimani B (1996) *Brucella melitensis:* A sexually transmissible agent? Lancet **347:** 1763.

Marston JA (1861) Report on fever (Malta). Great Britain Army Med Dept Repor **3:** 486.

Mathur AC, Sharma GL (1974) Studies on the estimates of the economic losses caused *brucellosis* among bovines and its control in India. Indian J Anim Sci **44:** 654-661.

Mathur TN (1964) *Brucella* strains isolated from cows, buffaloes, goats, sheep and human beings at Karnal: Their significance with regard to the epidemiology of *brucellosis*. Indian J Med Res **52:** 1231-1240.

McDonald WL, Jamaludin R, Mackereth G *et al* (2006) Characterisation of a *Brucella* sp. strain as a marine mammal type despite isolation from a patient with spinal osteomyelitis in New Zealand. J Clin Microbiol **44:** 4363-4370.

McGill PE (2003) Geographically specific infections and arthritis, including rheumatic syndromes associated with certain fungi and parasites, *Brucella* species and *Mycobacterium leprae*. Best Practice Res Clin Rheumatol **17:** 289-307.

Mehra KN, Dhanesar NS, Chaturvedi VK (2000) Seroprevalence of *brucellosis* in bovines in Madhya Pradesh. Indian Vet J **77:** 571-573.

Memish ZA, Balkhy HH (2004) Brucellosis and International Travel. J Travel Med **11:** 49-55.

Michaux, S., J. Paillisson, M. J. Carles-Nurit, G. Bourg, A. Allardet-Servent, and M. Ramuz. 1993. Presence of two independent chromosomes in the *Brucella melitensis* 16M genome. J. Bacteriol. **175:** 701-705.

Michaux-Charachon, S., G. Bourg, E. Jumas-Bilak, P. Guigue-Talet, A. Allardet-Servent, D. O'Callaghan, and M. Ramuz. 1997. Genome structure and phylogeny in the genus *Brucella*. J. Bacteriol. **179:** 3244-3249.

Moreno E, Cloeckaert A, Moriyon I (2002) *Brucella* evolution and taxonomy. Vet Microbiol **90:** 209-227.

Moreno E, Stackebrandt E, Dorsch M *et al* (1990) *Brucella Abortus* 16S rRNA and lipid A reveal a phylogenetic relationship with members of the alpha-2 subdivision of the class Proteobacteria. J Bacteriol **172:** 3569-3576.

Mudaliar S, Bhore A, Pandit D (2003) Detection of antibodies to *Brucella abortus* in animal handlers. Indian J Med Sci **57:** 181-186.

Noviello S, Gallo R, Kelly M *et al* (2004) Laboratory-acquired brucellosis. Emerg Infect Dis **10:** 1848-1850.

OIE (World Organisation for Animal Health) (2005a) Handistatus II: zoonoses (human cases): global cases of brucellosis in 2004. http://www.oie.int/hs2/gi_zoon_masld.asp?c_cont=6&c_mald=172&annee=2004 Accessed 13 December 2005.

OIE Manual for diagnositic tests and vaccines for terrestrial animals. Sixth Edition 2008. Paris. France.

Olsen SC, Evans D, Hennager SG *et al* (1996) Serologic responses of *Brucella abortus* strain 19 calfhood-vaccinated cattle following adult vaccination with strain RB51. J Vet Diagn Invest **8:** 451-454.

Olsen SC, Fach SJ, Palmer MV *et al* (2006) Immune responses of elk to initial and booster vaccinations with *Brucella abortus* strain RB51 or 19. Clin Vaccine Immunol **13:** 1098-1103.

Osterman B, Moriyon I (2006) International Committee on Systematics of Prokaryotes: Subcommittee on the taxonomy of *Brucella.* Int J Syst Evol Microbiol **56:** 1173-1175.

Panjarathinam R, Jhala CI (1986) *Brucellosis* in Gujrat state. J Pathol Microbiol **29:** 53-60.

Panjarathinum R, Gulrajani TS (1974) Studies on *brucellosis.* II. Isolation of *Brucella* organism in milk of cows, sheep and goats. Indian J Anim Hlth **13:** 29-35.

Pappas G, Panagopoulou P, Christou L *et al* (2006) *Brucella* as a biological weapon. Cell Mol Life Sci **63:** 2229-2236.

Pillai MT, Nendunchelliyan S, Raghvan N (1990) *Brucellosis* in a dog caused by *B. suis* biovar I in Madras. Cherion **19:** 97-98.

Pillai MT, Nendunchelliyan S, Raghvan N (1991) Serological and bacteriological detection of *Brucella canis* infection of dogs in Madras. Indian Vet J **68:** 399-401.

Pizarro-Cerda J, Méresse S, Parton RG, *et al. Brucella abortus* transits through the autophagic pathway and replicates in the endoplasmic reticulum of nonprofessional phagocytes. Infect Immun 1998; **66:** 5711-24.

Pizarro-Cerda J, Moreno E, Gorvel JP. Invasion and intracellular trafficking of *Brucella abortus* in non phagocytic cells. Rev Microbe Infect 2000; **2:** 829-35.

Polding JB (1947) *Brucellosis* in India. Indian J Vet Sci 147-155.

Porte F, Liautard JP, Kohler S. Early acidification of phagosomes containing *Brucella suis* is essential for intracellular survival in murine macrophages. Infect Immun 1999; **67:** 4041-4047.

Rajkhowa S, Rahman H, Rajkhowa *et al* (2005) Seroprevalence of *brucellosis* in mithuns (*Bos frontalis*) in India. Prev Vet Med **69:** 145-151.

Rana UVS, Sehgal S, Bhardwaj AM (1985) A seroepidemiological study of *brucellosis* among workers of veterinary hospital and slaughter house of Delhi. Int J Zoon **12:** 74-79.

Randhawa AS, Kalra DS, Kapur MP (1974) Some seroepidemiologic observations on brucellosis in humans and animals. Indian J Med Sci **28:** 133-138.

Reddy PRC, Rao PVRC (1984) A note on isolation of *Brucella suis* from foetus of a she-goat. Kerala J Vet Sci **15:** 173-174.

Refai M (2002) Incidence and control of *brucellosis* in the Near East region. Vet Microbiol **90:** 81-110.

Renukaradhya GJ, Isloor S, Rajasekhar M (2002) Epidemiology, zoonotic aspects, vaccination and control/eradication of brucellosis in India. Vet Microbiol **90:** 183-195.

Ross HM, Jahans KL, MacMillan AP (1996) *Brucella* species infection in North Sea seal and cetacean populations. Vet Rec **138:** 647-648.

Rotz LD, Khan AS, Lillibridge SR (2002) Public health assessment of potential biological terrorism agents. Emerg Infect Dis **8:** 225-230.

Sarinas PSA, Chitkara RK (2003) *Brucellosis.* Seminars Resp Infect **18:** 168-182.

Scholz HC, Hubalek A, Sedlacek I (2008) *Brucella microti* sp. nov., isolated from the common vole *Microtus arvalis.* International J Syst Evol Microbiol **58:** 375-382.

Schwabe CW (1984). Veterinary Medicine and Human Health. Waverly Press Inc. Mount Royal Guilford Avenues, Baltimore, MD 21202 US. 16-39

Seleem MN, Boyle SM, Sriranganathan N (2009) *Brucellosis*: a re-emerging zoonosis. Vet Microbiol. Doi: 10.1016/j.vetmic.2009.06.021

Sen GP, Sharma GL (1972) Speciation of seventy eight Indian strains of *Brucella,* an epidemiological study. Indian J Anim Sci **45:** 537.

Sen MR, Shukla BN, Goyal RK (2002) Seroprevalence of *brucellosis* in and around Varanasi. J Com Dis **34:** 226-227.

Sharma M, Batta MK, Asrani RK *et al* (1995) *Brucella melitensis* abortions among organized sheep farms in north-west states in India. Indian J Anim Sci **65:** 874-875.

Singh M (2009) Comparison of ELISA with other serological tests in diagnosis of brucellosis in small ruminants. MVSc Thesis, Deemed University, IVRI, Izatnagar, India.

Singh RK (2008) Prevalence of *brucellosis* among ruminants and comparision of serological test. MVSc Thesis, Deemed University, IVRI, Izatnagar, India.

Sohn AH, Probert WS, Glaser CA *et al* (2003) Human neurobrucellosis with intracerebral granuloma caused by a marine mammal *Brucella* spp. Emerg Infect Dis **9:** 485-488.

Soni JL, Pathak PN (1969) Serological investigations into porcine brucellosis. Indian Vet J **46:** 191-195.

Tessaro SV, Forbes LB (1986) *Brucella suis* biotype 4: a case of granulomatous nephritis in a barren ground caribou (*Rangifer tarandus groenlandicus* L.) with a review of the distribution of rangiferine *brucellosis* in Canada. J Wildlife Dis **22:** 479-483.

Thakur SD, Thapliyal DC (2002) Seroprevalence of *brucellosis* in man. J Com Dis **34:** 106-109.

Thoppil ST (2000) Serodiagnosis of brucellosis in pigs and man and differentiation of cross reactions due to *Yersinia enterocolitica* O:9. MVSc thesis, University of Agricultural Sciences, Bangalore, India.

Vitovec J, Vladik P, Zahor Z *et al.* (1976) Morphological study of 70 cases of brucellosis in rabbits caused by *Brucella suis.* Vet Med (Praha) **21:** 359-368.

Wanke MM (2004) Canine *brucellosis.* Anim Reprod Sci **82-83:** 195-207.

Waring SC (2005). Brucellosis. In: Kahn CM and Line S (Eds.). Merck Veterinary Manual, 9th ed. Whitehouse Station, NJ: Merck. 2546.

Zaki S, Murty BSK, Rao S *et al* (1975) Serological incidence of brucellosis in sheep and goats in Karnataka. Cur Res **4:** 196-197.

Zammit T (1905) A preliminary note on the examination of the blood of goats suffering from Mediterranean fever, reports of the Commission on Mediterranean fever, Part-III, Harrison and Sons, London, 1905, pp 83.

□□□

Chapter 29

Bovine Tuberculosis

CHANDAN PRAKASH GUPTA
IVRI, Izatnagar, Bareilly

Introduction

Bovine TB (bovine tuberculosis) is an infectious and chronic disease of affects cattle and other domesticated animals as well as certain free or captive wildlife species. It is caused by Mycobacterium bovis (*M. bovis*) characterized by the progressive development of specific granulomatous lesions of tubercles in affected tissues. it can affect any body tissue but generally first it affect head and thorax lymph node followed by lung tissue. Distribution of pathological lesion in body is variable depanding upon route of infection, dose inoculam, host species and enviormental conditions. Infectious agent are usually transmiited through aerosol route followed by oral route. Initially innate immunity(macrophage, neutrophill, natural killer cell and gamma delta T cell) try to contain and destroy mycobacterium organism , followed by Th1 mediated cell immune response destroy mycobacteria laden macrophage either by CD4+ mediated activation of macrophage or CD8+ mediated lysis of infected macrophages. When this cell mediated immune response wanes, antibody mediated immune response progress, usually it is associated with disease progression.

Bovine tuberculosis is usually diagnosed by delayed type hypersensitivity after injection of bovine PPD antigen intradermally into infected animal. Specificity of tuberculin skin testing is low due to sharing of mycobacterial antigen among pathogenic and nonpathogenic enviormental mycobacteria giving false positive. Lymphocyte proliferation test and interferon gamma test offer higher sensitivity to detect CMI and these test are able to detect infection at early stage of disease. Serological based assay are not so sensitive and specific for bovine tuberculosis diagnosis but their simplicity, inexpensiveness and ability to develop some pan side diagnostic test made them an alternative of CMI based test. Diagnostic test specificity may be increased by using more specific and refined antigen such as ESAT-6, CFP-10, MPB-70.

Molecular diagnostic test has opened a new era in bovine tuberculosis diagnosis. These are rapid, precise with high sensitivity and specificity but these test require sophisticated equipment and costly molecular reagent.

There is much needed to progress in immunoprophylaxis area of bovine tuberculosis. BCG vaccination is only available vaccine but its efficacy has been debatable. This vaccine can reduce severity of disease but it can not prevent infection, shedding of organism so vaccinated animal may also be a potent source of infection. Moreover BCG vaccinated animal will be positive in bovine PPD tuberculin skin testing. current diagnostic test are not able to differentiate between natural infected and BCG vaccinated animal there in present situation vaccination cannot be recommended in animals.

Mycobacterium bovis present a significant threat to human health. It causes human tuberculosis usually by consumption of raw or unpasteurized milk or inhalation of infected aerosol from infected meat or carcass. Human tuberculosis due to m. bovis has caused a recent concern due to increased incidence of emergence of muti drug resistant tuberculosis, increased HIV epidemics and close association of HIV and TB epidemics.

Host species

Although cattle are considered to be the true hosts of M. bovis, the disease has been reported in many domesticated and wild life animals. Tuberculosis have been recorded from buffaloes, bison, sheep, goats, equines, camels, pigs, wild boars, deer, antelopes, dogs, cats, foxes, mink, badgers, ferrets, rats, primates, South American camelids, kudus, elands, tapirs, elks, elephants, sitatungas, oryxes, addaxes, rhinoceroses, possums, ground squirrels, otters, seals, hares, moles, raccoons, coyotes and several predatory felines including lions, tigers, leopards and lynx (De Lisle *et al.*, 2001; O'Reilly and Doborn., 1995). Birds are usually thought to be resistant to naturally infected with tuberculosis but some bird species like pigeon and crow can be experimental infected with tuberculosis by oral or intratracheal inoculation and after intraperitoneal inoculation respectively .Some avian species, including mallard ducks, appear to be resistant to experimental infection.(Butlaer *et al.*, 2001 and Fitzgerald SD,2005).

Etiology

Bovine TB is an infectious disease caused by Mycobacterium bovis, a member of the Mycobacterium tuberculosis complex (MTC), a closely related group of Mycobacteria including *M. tuberculosis, M. africanum, M. bovis, M. bovis bacilli* Calmette-Guérin (BCG), M. canetti and M. caprae comb. nov. (Van Soolingen *et al.*, 1994; Aranaz *et al.*, 2004; Mostowy *et al.*, 2005). MTC bacteria are 99.9% similar in regard of their DNA, with identical 16S rRNA sequences Brosch *et al.*, 2002. However, there are distinct differences in phenotype, host ranges and pathogenicity (Ayele *et al.*, 2004).

Global distribution / Epidemiology

Although bovine tuberculosis was once found worldwide, control programs have eliminated or nearly eliminated this disease from domesticated animals in many countries. Nations currently classified as tuberculosis-free include Australia, Iceland, Denmark, Sweden, Norway, Finland, Austria, Switzerland, Luxembourg, Latvia, Slovakia, Lithuania, Estonia, the Czech Republic, Canada, Singapore, Jamaica, Barbados and Israel. Eradication programs are in progress in other European countries, Japan, New Zealand, the United States, Mexico, and some countries of Central and South America. Although bovine tuberculosis has been eradicated from the majority of U.S. states but seldom bovine tuberculosis outbreak has been reported from some states of USA. In developed countries wild life reserviour are posisng serious challenge in eradication of bovine tuberculosis particularly white-tailed deer in Michigan (USA), badgers in the U.K. and Ireland, and infected brush-tailed opossums in New Zealand.*(www.cfsph.iastate.edu/Factsheets/pdfs/bovine_tuberculosis.pdf)*.

Bovinc tuberculosis is still widespread in Africa, parts of Asia and some Middle Eastern countries.

Transmission

M. bovis can be transmitted by the inhalation of aerosols, by ingestion, or through breaks in the skin. The importance of these routes varies between species. The respiratory and the alimentary routes are the main transmission pathways. Infectious animals shed M. bovis in a number of ways: in feces, milk, discharging lesions, saliva and urine (Phillips *et al.*, 2003; Neill *et al.*, 2005; Jha *et al.*, 2007). Animal age and behavior, environment, climate and farming practice can modulate the infection [Pollock *et al.*, 1993; Phillips *et al.*, 2003]. Aerosol exposure is considered to be the most important route of infection of cattle. Inhalation of 1 CFU (6-10 bacilli) in an aerosol droplet would be enough to infect an animal and can induce tuberculosis immuno-pathology (Neill *et al.* (1991), Dean *et al.* (2005)). The other managemental and environmental factors are Close contact between animals e.g. intensive farming practice such as common water trough, loose housing system, etc. contributes to effective spread of M. bovis. Ingestion of contaminated products (e.g. carcasses/prey, pastures and water) is considered as a secondary way to spread the disease in cattle [Menzies and Neill, 2000], however it is an important pathway in wildlife (Renwick *et al.*, 2007). Congenital infections, vertical and genital transmission are very rarely observed in cattle [Neill *et al.*, 1994].

Humans get infected either by inhalation of dust-particles and bacteria-containing aerosols shed by infected animals (close contact between humans and animals) or by ingestion of contaminated animal products (e.g. raw milk, raw milk product, and raw meat) (Cosivi *et al.*, 1998; Dankner and Davis, 2000; Guerrero *et al.*, 2000; Wedlock *et al.*, 2002; Smith *et al.*, 2004;, Gibson *et al.*, 2004; Esteban *et al.*, 2005). Ingestion of raw wildlife products or aerosol exposure with infected wildlife have also been described as a source for *M. bovis* infection in humans (Liss *et al.*, 1994; Wei *et al.*, 2004; Wilkins *et al.*, 2008).

M. bovis is considered less virulent in humans than *M. tuberculosis* (Van Soolingen D. 2001) and transmission between humans is rare but has been reported in immunosuppressed HIV patients (Bouvet *et al.*, 1993; Van Soolingen *et al.*, 1994; Grange & Yates , 1994; Gibson *et al.*, 2004).

Incubation Period

The symptoms of bovine tuberculosis usually take months to develop in cattle. Infections can also remain dormant for years and reactivate during periods of stress or in old age. Similarly, severe disease can develop in some deer within a few months of infection, while other deer do not become symptomatic for years. In kittens experimentally infected by the parenteral route, the incubation period is approximately three weeks; it is probably longer under natural conditions. *(www.cfsph.iastate.edu/Factsheets/pdfs/bovine_tuberculosis.pdf)*

Pathogenesis

Cattle become infected with M. bovis by either the oral or respiratory routes (Neill *et al.*, 1994). The oral route is likely most important in calves nursing tuberculous cows, while the respiratory route is most common in cattle in general (Neill *et al.*, 1994). Pulmonary tuberculosis is the most prevalent form of bovine tuberculosis in cattle it is the result of inhalation of bacteria containing aerosols shed by infected animals. In naturally infected cattle, tuberculous lesions are found most frequently in the dorso-caudal, 'apex', region of the lungs, frequently close to the pleural surface (Medlar, 1940; Francis, 1947; Lepper and Pearson, 1973; McIlroy *et al.*, 1986; Dungworth, 1993). Extra pulmonary TB involves predominantly cervical lymph nodes (Kazwala *et al.*, 2001; Gutierrez *et al.*, 1995) but also intestines, liver, spleen, kidneys, pleura and peritoneum together with their associated lymph nodes (Neill, 1994). Outcome of m. bovis infection depends upon several factor such as infective dose, route of infection, immune status of animal, concurrent infection of other bacterial and viral disease, age of animal, stress, envioumental condition such as density of animals, poor ventilation aggravate disease progression.

Containment of the bacteria results in the formation of nonvascular nodular granulomas known as "tubercles". Unlike in man, these primary lesions are rarely contained by the immune system in cattle and bacilli spread by lymphatic.

Granulomatious inflammation and caseous necrosis are central characterstics of bovine tuberculosis pathogenesis as wells as protection of host and has a significant influence on lesion expansion (Fenhalls *et al.*, 2000). Lesions show typically a centre of caseous necrosis with some degree of calcification surrounded by a cell wall of epitheloid cells, lymphocytes and neutrophils (Doherty *et al.*, 1996). Granuloma formation in mycobacterium infection is product of complex interaction of macrophage, neutrophill, (innate immunity), helper T cell and local cytokine mileu within lesion. cell-mediated immunity (CMI) generating T cells capable of both activating and destroying mycobacterial-laden macrophages (Dannenberg, 1999) causes macrophage and T cell apoptosis which makes a significant contribution to caseation of granulomatous lesion. apoptosis have both beneficial and detrimental effects but It depends upon cell type targeted. Macrophage apoptosis is a common defence strategy against intra-cellular pathogens, through removing the intracellular sanctuary macrophages providing shelter for mycobacteria (Keane *et al.*, 1997), the inappropriate apoptosis of particular T-lymphocytes within lesions has the potential to down-regulate the host protective response and could contribute to disease reactivation. Apoptosis have been found more effective than necrosis in controlling mycobacteria and restrict its spread (Das *et al.*, 1999; Seah and Rook, 2001). In addition to above mechanism, innate immunity (Turner *et al.*, 2003), failure of macrophage activation (Orme, 1998) and particular cytokine combinations within developing lesions also contribute to the development of necrosis.

Clinical signs and post mortem lesions

Tuberculosis is usually a chronic debilitating disease in cattle, but it can occasionally be acute and rapidly progressive. It may be either in pulmonary,

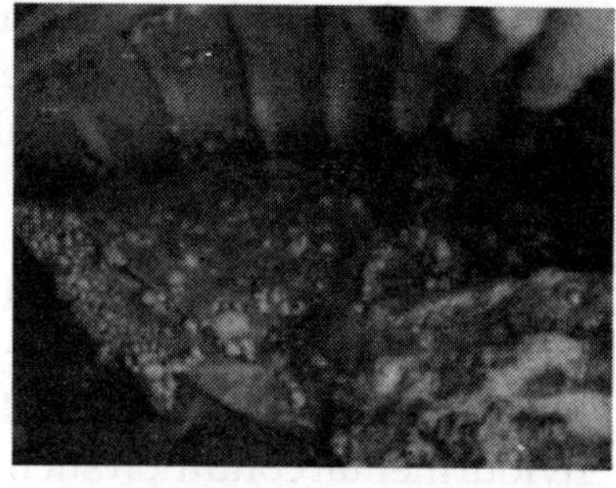

intestinal and disseminated tuberculosis. Early infections are often asymptomatic. In the late stages, common symptoms include progressive emaciation, a low-grade fluctuating fever, weakness and inappetence. Animals with pulmonary involvement usually have a moist cough that is worse in the morning, during cold weather or exercise, and may have dyspnea or tachypnea. In the terminal stages, animals may become extremely emaciated and develop acute respiratory distress. In some animals, the retropharyngeal or other lymph nodes enlarge and may rupture and drain. Greatly enlarged lymph nodes can also obstruct blood vessels, airways, or the digestive tract. In intestinal tuberculosis, intermittent diarrhea and constipation may be seen. In some animals, the only symptom may be abscesses of unknown origin in isolated lymph nodes, and symptoms may not develop for several years. In other cases, the disease may be disseminated, with a rapid, fulminating course.

In cattle, granulomatous tubercles are found in the lymph nodes, particularly those of the head and thorax. They are also common in the lung, spleen, liver and the surfaces of body cavities. In disseminated cases, multiple small granulomas may be found in numerous organs. Lesions are sometimes found on the female genitalia, but are rare on the male genitalia. These granulomas are usually yellowish and either caseous, caseo-calcareous or calcified. They are often encapsulated .(*www.cfsph.iastate.edu/Factsheets/pdfs/bovine_tuberculosis.pdf*)

Immune responses in bovine tuberculosis

Immune response study in natural bovine tuberculosis has been extrapolated either from experimental small animal model or in natural host species and classical studies of human tuberculosis but there may e variation due to difference in host species, enviourment and ecosystem.

Mycobacterium organism first encounter with macrophage after invasion in respiratory epithelial cell, followed by engulfment of organism by macrophage. It is the preferred host cell for the intracellular mycobacteria, but it is also the key effector cell for control and destruction of such pathogens. M. bovis can grow relatively freely in bovine macrophages in vitro (Aldwell *et al.*, 1996; LieÂbana *et al.*, 2000a).

Initially innate immunity including neutrophill, macrophage, natural killer cell (NK cell) and gamma-delta T- cell play active role in destruction of mycobacterium organism through complex interaction between different phogocytic cell and changing local cytokine mileu augmenting destruction of organism. Macrophage try to destroy organism by lysosome pH, lysosomal hydroyses, bactericidal peptides and superoxide (Russell, 1999) but mycobacterium organism also have some inherent quality like inhibition of phagosome-lysosome fusion, prevention of degradation of organism as an apparent mechanism of self-protection (Armstrong & Hart, 1975). There is an initial interplay between macrophage and mycobacteria, the outcome of which will define subsequent events and largely decide the consequencés of the exposure to tubercle bacilli.

Natural killer (NK) cells produce interferon-gamma (IFN-g) and can be cytolytic towards mycobacteria-infected target cells (Yoneda & Ellner, 1998). Furthermore, recent studies of the histopathology of bovine tuberculosis have identified neutrophils as among the earliest cells associated with the developing granuloma (Cassidy *et al.*, 1998).

If, despite the efforts of the battery of innate mechanisms, mycobacteria become established within the macrophage and produce either secreted antigens or breakdown products, these may be presented to T-cells. This interaction begins an acquired immune response, as the responding T-cells will undergo clonal expansion and differentiation, leading to the basis of immunological memory. Experimental infections with M. bovis have demonstrated that all of the main T-cell subsets (gd, CD4 and CD8 T-cells) are involved in the infection progresses (Pollock *et al.*, 1996; Cassidy *et al.*, 2001). Mycobacterial infection triggers a Th1-induced cell-mediated immune response (CMI) which leads to release of cytokines such as tumour necrosis factor-á, Interleukin- 12 (IL-12) and Interferon gamma (IFN-γ). CD4 memory T-cells appear to be the dominant cell population producing IFN-g. CD8 memory T-cells have also been identified as important producers of IFN- g (Hope *et al.*, 2000; Smyth *et al.*, 2001). In the control of mycobacterial growth, CD4 cells contribute to the inhibition of intracellular growth of bacilli, whereas CD8 T-cells lyse M. bovis-infected macrophages (Lie´bana *et al.*, 2000; Skinner *et al.*, 2003). In these models, gd T-cells have been observed to be involved in both the early stages of M. bovis infection and early lesion formation (Pollock *et al.*, 1996; Cassidy *et al.*, 2001), where they may play a significant role in the establishment of bacterial containment through the production of IFN-g (Smyth *et al.*, 2001; Kennedy *et al.*, 2002; Pollock and Welsh, 2002). Following the onset of the CMI response, the development of humoral responses may also be involved in the anti-mycobacterial immune response (Pollock *et al.*, 2001) It is considered that antibodies generally develop in more advanced stages of bovine tuberculosis, and are associated with disease progression . As infection progresses, immune response more biased towards Th2 type including development of antibody responses, reduced CMI responses and a more widespread pattern of disease (Ritacco *et al.*, 1991;Palmer *et al.*, 2000; Welsh *et al.*, 2005). Antibodies are often considered to be unimportant in protective immunity against intracellular mycobacteria, but a recent review has indicated that, under certain circumstances, antibodies may have a role in protection (Glatman-Freedman & Casadevall, 1998).

Diagnosis

Animal usually do not exhibit overt clinical sign unless it has reached in advanced stage of disease. Isolation of mycobacterium bovis from infected animal is considered as standard yard stick for positive cases but it is very tedious, time consuming, high skill demanding procedure. The presence of M. bovis in clinical and post-mortem specimens may be demonstrated by examination of stained smears or tissue sections and confirmed by cultivation of the organism on primary isolation medium.

Isolation of mycobacterium bovis

Mycobacterium bovis is very fastidious and slow growing organism , usually contaminated by rapidly growing enviourmental mycobacteria. Therefore extra precaution should be ensured during collection and shipment of samples to laboratory. Prompt delivery of specimens to the laboratory greatly enhances the chances of cultural recovery of *M. bovis*. If delays in delivery are anticipated, specimens should be refrigerated or frozen to retard the growth of contaminants and to preserve the ycobacteria. In warm ambient conditions, when refrigeration is not possible, boric acid may be added (0.5% [w/v] final concentration) as a bacteriostatic agent, but only for limited periods, no longer than 1 week.

Microscopic examination

Mycobacterium bovis can be demonstrated microscopically on direct smears from clinical samples and on prepared tissue materials. The acid fastness of M. bovis is normally demonstrated with the classic Ziehl–Neelsen stain, but a fluorescent acid-fast stain may also be used. Immunoperoxidase techniques may also give satisfactory results. The presumptive diagnosis of mycobacteriosis can be made if the tissue has characteristic histological lesions (caseous necrosis, mineralisation, epithelioid cells, multinucleated giant cells and macrophages). As lesions are often paucibacillary, the presence of acid-fast organisms in histological sections may not be detected, although *M. bovis* can be isolated in culture. (http://www.oie.int/fileadmin/Home/eng/Health_standards/tahm/2.04.07_BOVINE_TB.pdf)

Culture

Clinical specimen(milk, lymph node aspirate, feces, urine, nasal swab,) are decontaminated for destruction of commonly available enviourmental mycobacteria and other organism ensuring survival of mycobacterium organism.To process specimens for culture, the tissue is first homogenised using a mortar and pestle, cobacterstomacher or blender, followed by decontamination with either detergent (such as 0.375–0.75% hexadecyl-pyridinium chloride [HPC]), an alkali (2-4% sodium hydroxide) or an acid (5% oxalic acid). The alkali or acid mixture is shaken for 10–15 minutes at room temperature and then neutralised. Neutralisation is not required when using HPC. The suspension is centrifuged, the supernatant is discarded, and the sediment is used for culture and microscopic examination. It is recommended that, as a minimum, pooled lymph node samples from the head and thorax be cultured when no visible lesions are detected in tuberculin or interferon test positive animals at post-mortem examination. For primary isolation, the sediment is usually inoculated on to a set of solid egg-based media, such as Lowenstein–Jensen, Coletsos base or Stonebrinks; these media should contain either pyruvate or pyruvate and glycerol. An agar-based medium such as Middlebrook 7H10 or 7H11 or blood based agar medium (Cousins *et al.*, 1998) may also be used. Cultures are incubated for a minimum of 8 weeks (and preferably for 10–12 weeks) at 37°C with or without CO2. The media should be in tightly closed tubes to avoid desiccation. Slopes are examined for macroscopic growth at intervals during the incubation period. When growth is visible, smears are prepared and stained by the Ziehl–Neelsen technique. Growth of M. bovis generally occurs within 3–6 weeks of incubation depending on the media used. Liquid culture systems are used routinely in some hospital and veterinary laboratories; in these systems growth is measured by radiometric or fluorometric means.

Characteristic growth patterns and colonial morphology can provide a presumptive diagnosis of *M. bovis*; however every isolate needs to be confirmed. It is necessary to distinguish *M. bovis* from the other members of the 'tuberculosis complex', *i.e. M. tuberculosis* (the primary cause of tuberculosis in humans), M. africanum (occupies an intermediate phenotypic position between *M. tuberculosis* and M. bovis), *M. microti* (the 'vole bacillus', a rarely encountered organism), *M. pinnipedii* and *M. caprae*. Isolates can be identified by determining traditional cultural and biochemical properties. On a suitable pyruvate-based solid medium, colonies of *M. bovis* are smooth and off-white (buff) in colour. The organism grows slowly at 37°C, but does not grow at 22°C or 45°C. Mycobacterium bovis is sensitive to thiophen-2-carboxylic acid hydrazide (TCH) and to isonicotinic acid hydrazide (INH). This can be tested for by growth on 7H10/7H11 Middlebrook agar medium or on egg-containing media. The egg medium should be prepared without pyruvate because it inhibits INH and could have a similar effect on TCH (which is an analogue of INH) and thus give false-positive (resistant) results. Mycobacterium bovis strains are also sensitive to paraamino salicylic acid and streptomycin. Effective drug concentrations are different for egg-based and agar based media. Results for niacin production and nitrate reduction are negative in M. bovis. In the amidase test, M. bovis is positive for urease and negative for nicotinamidase and pyrazinamidase. It is a microaerophillic and nonchromogenic bacterium. (*http://www.oie.int/fileadmin/Home/eng/Health_standards/tahm/2.04.07_Bovine_TB.pdf*).

Cell mediated immunity based diagnosis

Immune response to M. bovis mainly based on T helper type-1 response as evidenced by IFN-g, interleukin (IL)-12, and tumor necrosis factor (TNF)-a production to pathogen-associated antigen and exacerbation of disease when these cytokine combinations are disrupted. TB diagnosis is mainly based on evaluation of these cell-mediated responses either by skin test (Monaghan *et al.*, 1994) or IFN-g-based assays (Wood and Jones, 2001). Mycobacterial infections also induce antibody responses. In general, specific antibody responses are most easily·detected late in disease and correlate with severe progression of disease (Plackett *et al.*, 1989).

Tuberculin skin testing (the prescribed test for international trade)

The standard method for detection of bovine tuberculosis is the tuberculin test, which involves the intradermal injection of bovine tuberculin purified protein derivative (PPD) and the subsequent detection of swelling (delayed hypersensitivity) at the site of injection 72 hours later. This may be performed using bovine tuberculin alone or as a comparative test using avian and bovine tuberculins. The tuberculin test is usually performed on the mid-neck, but the test can also be performed in the caudal fold of the tail. The skin of the neck is more sensitive to tuberculin than the skin of the caudal fold. To compensate for this difference, higher doses of tuberculin may be used in the caudal fold.

Delayed hypersensitivity may not develop for a period of 3–6 weeks following infection. Thus, if a herd/animal is suspected to have been in contact very recently with infected animals, delaying testing should be considered in order to reduce the probability of false-negatives. As the sensitivity of the test is less than 100%, it is unlikely that eradication of tuberculosis from a herd will be achieved with only a single tuberculin test. It should be recognised that when used in chronically infected animals with severe pathology, the tuberculin test may be unresponsive. However, animals which have been sensitised by non-pathogenic environmental strains of mycobacteria, may react positively to PPD-B, due to the presence of antigens common to virulent and non-virulent mycobacterial strains. Where this occurs, comparison with responses to PPD-A is often used to facilitate discrimination between cattle infected with *M. bovis* and those exposed to environmental strains. (OIE manual, bovine tuberculosis chapter).

The complexity of tuberculins and the presence of cross-reactive components shared by different nonpathogenic enviormental mycobacteria and other organism led to develop diagnostic test based on specific antigen conserved among pathogenic mycobacterium species only. One such antigen, ESAT-6 (Pollock and Andersen, 1997), has been assessed as a diagnostic reagent in different test formats. The specificity of the delayed-type hypersensitivity reaction in cattle has been improved by the introduction of ESAT-6 (Pollock *et al.*, 2003).

Lymphocyte proliferation test

In this method, lymphoblastogenic responses by antigen stimulation is meseaured (Thoen *et al.* (1980)). This type of in-vitro assay compares the reactivity of peripheral blood lymphocytes to tuberculin PPD (PPD-B) and a PPD from Mycobacterium avium (PPD-A). The assay can be performed on whole blood (Buddle *et al.*, 2001) or purified lymphocytes from peripheral blood samples (Griffin *et al.*, 1994). These tests endeavour to increase the specificity of the assay by removing the response of lymphocytes to 'nonspecific' or cross-reactive antigens associated with non-pathogenic species of mycobacteria to which the animal may have been exposed. Results are usually analysed as the value obtained in response to PPD-B minus the value obtained in response to PPD-A. The B–A value must then be above a cut-off point that can be altered in order to maximise either specificity or sensitivity of the diagnosis. The assay has scientific value, but is not used for routine diagnosis because the test is time-consuming and the logistics and laboratory execution are complicated.it requires long incubation times and the use of radio-active nucleotides). Lymphocyte proliferation assay should be performed shortly after blood is collected. The test may be useful in wildlife and zoo animals. The test is relatively expensive and has not yet been subject to inter-laboratory comparisons.

Gamma-interferon assay (the alternative test for international trade)

This test may be an alternative to lymphocyte transformation test. It is based on same principle but in this test lymphoblastogenic activity is indirectly expressed in terms of interferon gamma production by peripheral blood lymphocytes from infected animals following antigenic stimulation.The assay is based on the release of IFN-γ from sensitised lymphocytes during a 16–24-

hour incubation period with specific antigen (PPD-tuberculin) (wood et at., 1990). The test makes use of the comparison of IFN-γ production following stimulation with avian and bovine PPD. The detection of bovine IFN-γ is carried out with a sandwich ELISA that uses two monoclonal antibodies to bovine gamma-interferon. It is recommended that the blood samples be transported to the laboratory and the assay set up as soon as practical, but not later than the day after blood collection (Coad *et al.*, 2007; Ryan *et al.*, 2000). In some areas, especially where 'nonspecificity' is prevalent, some concerns about the accuracy have been expressed. However, because of the IFN-ã test capability of detecting early infections, the use of both tests in parallel allows detection of a greater number of infected animals before they become a source of infection for other animals as well as a source of contamination of the environment (Gormley *et al.*, 2006). The use of defined mycobacterial antigens such as ESAT 6 and CFP-10 enhance specificity . these antigens have been used in many developed countries including United Kingdom and New Zealand for serial testing. The use of such antigens may also offer the ability to differentiate BCG-vaccinated from unvaccinated animals. The other advantage of this test is that animals that are difficult or dangerous to handle, such as excitable cattle or other bovidae, need be captured only once. the IFN-ã test may be used for serial testing (to enhance specificity) and parallel testing (to enhance sensitivity). The test is available as commercial kits for bovine species and primates, however it has been validated in only a few species of these taxa. (OIE manual, bovine TB chapter)

Pollock *et al.* (1994), further developed CMI as a means of identifying tuberculous cattle with the use of proteins and peptides specific to M. bovis. Responses other than cellular proliferation have been used to identify CMI responses to *M. bovis*. O'Nuallain *et al.* (1997) measured the release of soluble IL-2R from antigen-stimulated cells and identified cattle naturally infected with M. bovis. However, perhaps the most significant developments have followed applied diagnostic methods based on the detection of the cytokine IFN-g (Wood and Rothel, 1994).

Serology based diagnosis

Antibody based diagnostic test for bovine tuberculosis are simple, easy to perform, simple interpretation, requiring handling of animal one time only but their sensitivity and specificity are questionable due to inherent nature of mycobacterium bovis immune response. It is well established that cattle infected by *M. bovis* develop early immune responses, dominated by cell-mediated immunity (Dlugovitzky *et al.*, 2000). Therefore, serology is less efficient to identify cattle in the early stages of infection, when antibodies titres are low . Antibodies are often considered to be unimportant in protective immunity against intracellular mycobacteria, but a recent review has indicated that, under certain circumstances, antibodies may have a role in protection (Glatman-Freedman & Casadevall, 1998). Serological test using crude mycobacterial preparations gives generally satisfactory test sensitivity but poor specificity because of broad cross-reactivity with non-TB mycobacteria, such as M. avium (O'Loan *et al.*, 1994; Gaborick *et al.*, 1996). Sensitivity and specificity of serological assay can be successfully increased by using M. bovis specific antigen. Antigen discovery efforts have unveiled numerous seroreactive targets (Fifis *et al.*, 1992; Cataldi *et al.*, 1994;Lyashchenko *et al.*, 1998; Amadori *et al.*, 2002; Koo *et al.*,2005). So far, MPB70 and MPB83 proteins of M. bovis appear to be the major serodominant antigens for detection of tuberculous cattle (Wood *et al.*, 1992; Lightbody *et al.*,1998; McNair *et al.*, 2001; Liu *et al.*, 2007; Wiker, 2009). Various mycobacterial antigens such as ESAT-6, 14 kDa, MPT63, MPT70, MPT51 MPT32 and MPB83 have been shown to contain B-cell epitopes that can be exploited for the serodiagnosis of tuberculosis infections (Lyashchenko *et al.*,1998; McNair *et al.*, 2001).

Recent advances in both antigen discovery and immunoassay technology have facilitated progress in developing novel antibody-based tests for bovine tuberculosis. Nowadays cocktail antigen (using more than one antigen) or multi-epitope fusion proteins is being used to improve sensitivity and specificity of these tests (Waters *et al.*, 2006; Lyashchenko *et al.*, 2008; Whelan *et al.*, 2008).

Apart from the selection of M. bovis specific antigens for antibody detection, the immunoassay format and detection technology are crucial for developing accurate serodiagnostics. Promising recent developments include MAPIA (Waters *et al.*, 2006), a fluorescence polarization assay (FPA) (Jolley *et al.*, 2007), a rapid immunochromatographic test (Lyashchenko *et al.*, 2008), a 96-well plate multiplex system (Whelan *et al.*, 2008), a chemiluminescent platform (Green *et al.*, 2009) which are in developing stage some of these test may be used as a quick animal-side test for field use (Waters *et al.*, 2006; Lyashchenko *et al.*, 2008).

Molecular diagnosis

Molecular diagnosis of bovine tuberculosis is highly sensitive with adequate specificity, rapid, convenient and alternative of conventional diagnosis. Conventional diagnosis relies on isolation and identification of causative organism from clinical specimen. It takes atleast 8 week to grow and 4 week for further biochemical identification. This time gap permit infected animal to excrete organism which infect other susceptible animals and contaminate environment. Non recovery of mycobacterial growth from clinical specimen cannot be considered as tuberculosis free animal because it may be related with destruction of mycobacterium bacilli during decontamination procedure, superseding of environmental mycobacteria over slow growing fastidious pathogenic mycobacteria, latency disease status etc.

Molecular diagnosis rely on amplification of organism specific sequence (DNA, RNA). It is rapid, result can be obtained in a single day, avoiding isolation of organism , usually BSL-3 is required to isolate and handle mycobacterium bovis, safe to laboratory personel.

PCR is universal choice to identify bacterial pathogen and this technique has been used successfully targeting different gene or insertion sequence of mycobacterium tuberculosis complex for diagnosis and epidemiology both. Various mycobacterium tuberculosis complex specific PCR have been developed targeting 16s rRNA, 16S–23S rRNA, the insertion sequences IS6110 and IS1081, and genes coding for M.-tuberculosis-complex-specific proteins such as MPB70 and the 38 kDa antigen. Specific identification of an isolate as M. bovis can be made using PCR targeting a mutation at nucleotide positions 285 in the oxyR gene,169 in the pncA gene, 675/756/1311/1410 and 1450 of the gyrB gene and presence/absence of RDs (Regions of Difference) (Espinosa *et al.*, 1998; Huard *et al.*,2003; Niemann *et al.*, 2000; Parsons *et al.*, 2002) In addition, PCR-based techniques, such as spoligotyping, can be used for identifying M. bovis within the M. tuberculosis complex (lack of spacers 3, 9, 16, and 39–43) (Cousins *et al.*, 1998). A low IS6110 copy number in M. bovis can positively influence the results, with good discriminatory power. Spoligotyping can also improve the discriminatory power of IS6110 restriction length polymorphism (RFLP) typing (Garnier *et al.*, 2003; Zummaragga *et al.*, 1999).

Molecular assays have been primarily used to analyze the epidemiology of bovine tuberculosis; various strains, including laboratory and clinical samples, have been successfully employed . In that regard, PCR-based characterization techniques, such as spoligotyping and mycobacterial interspersed repetitive unit (MIRU) variable number tandem repeat (VNTR) typing, have been adopted due to their various advantages, including faster, simpler, and more cost-effective. It can provide an analysis of organism dispersion due to surveillance of reactive animals to tuberculin tests, characterizing samples, and explaining patterns found in various herds or regions. Furthermore, molecular epidemiology of the disease can be used to monitor and control animal trade,and to assess the efficacy of eradication programs.

Vaccine

Protective immunity against mycobacterium infection is associated with development and maintenance of a strong Th1 biased CMI response having greater capacity to contain the infection. IFN-g producing T-cell clones are important in controlling intracellular growth of *M. bovis,* while CD8+ cells play a crucial role in the lysis of infected cells (Lie´bana *et al.,* 2000; Skinner *et al.,* 2003).

Calmette and Guerin (1911) first used BCG as a vaccine in cattle, thereby preventing the establishment of lesions following challenge with *M. bovis.* The effect of route of administration has been varied ranging from little or no benefits through to significant protection (Rolle and Wiethe, 1956; Berrgren, 1981; Buddle *et al.,* 1995). Recent advances in immunology and the molecular biology of mycobacteria have greatly increased the options for candidate vaccines. The two major groupings are live attenuated vaccines such as BCG and other attenuated mycobacteria of the M. tuberculosis complex, and subunit vaccines based on either mycobacterial protein or DNA. Live attenuated vaccines are advantageous as they promote strong cellular immune responses required for protective immunity against tuberculosis and may only need a single-shot delivery to induce life-long immunity.

The existing BCG vaccine may not be sufficiently effective (e.g., Stuart *et al.,* 1988; Aldwell *et al.,* 1995b; Buddle *et al.,* 1995b; Fine, 1998; Qureshi *et al.* 1999), but has many properties that are desirable for a good vaccine. It is cheap to produce, can be administered via a number of routes, is safe, relatively stable, is derived from *M. bovis,* and has efficacy in reducing haematogenous spread of virulent mycobacteria. The latter observation is an important one for wildlife tuberculosis vaccines since prevention of haematogenous spread of infection might be sufficient to stop the spread of disease to other animals. A minor drawback of BCG or other attenuated strains is their remote potential to 'spill over' into domestic livestock. Cattle exposed to BCG may become sensitized for a positive tuberculin reaction and on this basis, would be scored positive for bovine tuberculosis and be slaughtered. Alternatively, vaccines engineered with an immunological 'tag' or use of diagnostic tests with refined antigens could permit differential diagnosis of bovine tuberculosis from exposure to vaccine (Buddle *et al.,* 1999; Vordermeier *et al.,* 1999).

Recent studies have indicated that not all vaccine candidates identified for M.tuberculosis show equal efficacy for *M. bovis,* and vice versa (Chambers *et al.,* 1999; Williams *et al.,* 1999). For this reason, it is necessary for empirical identification of vaccines with efficacy against M. bovis. Live attenuated strains of *M. bovis* have been made by chemical and transposon mutagenesis and illegitimate recombination (De Lisle *et al.,* 1999) and T cell antigens have been identified by screening M. bovis cosmid libraries expressed in M. smegmatis against blood taken from M. bovis-infected and BCG-vaccinated cattle (Carpenter *et al.,*1995; Hewinson *et al.,* 1995; Gormley *et al.,* 1999).

The successful development of protein subunit vaccines in small animal models has not been repeated in cattle due to the paucity of knowledge relating to protective responses. Gaps in knowledge are currently being addressed and will enhance understanding of bovine immunology and vaccine development.

Zoonotic aspect as human tuberculosis due to *M. bovis*

Bovine tuberculosis is a relevant zoonosis that can spread to humans through inhalation of infectious droplet nuclei and by ingestion of raw milk (Thoen and Barletta, 2005). The global prevalence of human tuberculosis due to M. bovis has been estimated at 3.1% of all human tuberculosis cases, accounting for 2.1% and 9.4% of pulmonary and extra pulmonary TB cases respectively (Cosivi *et al.*, 1998). In developed countries eradication programs have significantly reduced the prevalence of this disease, but reservoirs in wild life make complete eradication difficult. Mycobacterium bovis is classified as a Risk 3 pathogen for public health (OIE, 2005). Historically, M. bovis has been associated with extrapulmonary tuberculosis in infants and children usually occurring due to the consumption of milk which had not been pasteurized or boiled, from infected cattle. digestive route of infection has became less important because of practice of boiling milk or pasteurization. On the other hand, airborne infection continued to be frequent among meat industry and slaughterhouse workers.

There are several possible reasons for under diagnosing M. bovis in humans. In most developing countries, the bacteriological diagnosis of pulmonary tuberculosis usually relies on the acid-fast bacillus (AFB) smear examination due to limited laboratory resources. Use of culture is generally reserved for special situations, such as suspected treatment failures and relapses. In addition, culture is used in special surveys, including those undertaken to measure the prevalence of drug-resistant tuberculosis (Sequeira *et al.*, 2005). There are also limitations in the ability to detect m. bovis from human clinical specimen because they donot use pyruvate containing media , rather they cultivate on glycerol containing media. It is well known fact that glycerol inhibit growth of bovine tubercle bacilli which causes many m. bovis culture undetected. In developed countries laboratories generally use liquid media (e.g., BACTEC 460) for mycobacterial culture and genetic probes (e.g., Accuprobe) for identification (Christie and Callihan, 1995). These genetic probes are able to identify the *M. tuberculosis* complex, but cannot distinguish between *M. tuberculosis* and *M. bovis*. Furthermore, most of clinical laboratories do not uniformly test for pyrazinamide resistance, a possible indicator of M. bovis infection, when performing drug susceptibility testing.

Despite continuing reports of human disease, the global relevance of M. bovis as the cause of humantuberculosis remains low compared to that of M.tuberculosis. In countries where the incidence of human tuberculosis is steadily declining, zoonotic tuberculosis remains essentially stable, at very low levels.(Cotter *et al.*, 1996). However, unexpected causes of immune suppression in humans, as happened with HIV, or transmission from different animal sources, could result in persistence. In developing countries particularly in India, no systematic study of association of m. bovis and human tuberculosis has not been done so far but considering socio-economic condition, close association of animals and humans, sharing niche between animal and human beings, agriculture practices, food practices (consumption of raw/ unpasteurized milk in rural areas), limited diagnostic facilities, poor capability of m. bovis detection from clinical specimen even in referral laboratories clearly underline importance of m. bovis in human tuberculosis.

Food hygiene, sanitary controls, epidemiological surveillance and proper treatment are the main tools to control, eliminate and eventually eradicate human *M. bovis* disease in the industrialized world (Enarson, 2005). The first is to maintain and reinforce the policy of boiling/pasteurization of milk and dairy products, as well as protecting workers in animal related occupations, especially the meat industry, from airborne transmission. The second is to strengthen directly observed therapy, short course (DOTS) in tuberculosis control programs. DOTS has proved to be feasible in low-income, high-burden countries.

Prevention and control

Bovine tuberculosis can be controlled effectively by test-and-slaughter policy but in india, where TB is endemic and a significant proportion of animals are infected test-and-segregation methods are usually followed. Affected herds are re-tested periodically to eliminate cattle that may shed the organism; the tuberculin test is generally used. Infected herds are usually quarantined, and animals that have been in contact with reactors are traced.

Managemental practices can reduce spread of infection from infected to other susceptible animals such as animal handlers must be healthy(TB free), avoiding nursing of calves on tuberculous dam, disinfection of infected fomites, providing balanced feed to animals etc. Sanitation and disinfection may reduce the spread of the agent within the herd. *M. bovis* is relatively resistant to disinfectants and requires long contact times for inactivation. Effective disinfectants include 5% phenol, iodine solutions with a high concentration of available iodine, glutaraldehyde and formaldehyde. In environments with low concentrations of organic material, 1% sodium hypochlorite with a long contact time is also effective. In addition, biosecurity measures on farms decrease interactions between wildlife and domesticated animals. Effective bovine tuberculosis vaccines are not currently available for cattle. New vaccines are being developed and tested, particularly for wildlife reservoirs. (*www.cfsph.iastate.edu/Factsheets/pdfs/bovine_tuberculosis.pdf*)

Antimicrobial treatment in bovine tuberculosis is generally not recommended because it will reduce severity of disease but risk of shedding organisms, hazards to humans, and potential for drug resistance make treatment controversial. (*http://www.oie.int/fileadmin/Home/eng/Health_standards/tahm/2.04.07_Bovine_TB.pdf*)

Future prospects

Bovine tuberculosis remains a major problem and new strategies are clearly needed. In order to address this challenge, improved models are needed with enhanced relevance to the disease as encountered under natural conditions. There is much needed to know tuberculous immunopathology for better understanding of virulence factor and immunodiagnostic antigen. For disease control, obvious benefits will be derived from the development of tests to differentially identify the most severely diseased cattle, which are usually considered to pose the greatest threat of spreading infection. In relation to vaccine development, studies that lead to better characterization of the immune responses of cattle that have been exposed to *M. bovis*, without developing disease will provide important knowledge. There is need to develop a safe, reliable, highly protective tuberculosis vaccine to prevent disease without compromising diagnostic capabilities of diagnostic tests. There is need to develop inexpensive diagnostic test with high sensitivity and specificity having ability to discriminate closely related mycobacterial species including non pathogenic environmental mycobacteria. Diagnostic test must be devised to discriminate between naturally infected and vaccinated animal to prevent false positive and culling of healthy animals.

References

Aldwell, F.E., 1995b. Protection of cattle from bovine tuberculosis by vaccination with BCG by the respiratory or subcutaneous route, but not by vaccination with killed Mycobacterium vaccae. Res. Vet. Sci. **59:** 10-16.

Aldwell, F. E., Wedlock, D. N. and Buddle, B M. (1996).Bacterial metabolism, cytokine mRNA transcription and viability of bovine alveolar macrophages infected with Mycobacterium bovis BCG or virulent M. bovis. Immunology and Cell Biology **74:** 45-51.

Amadori, M., K.P. Lyashchenko, M.L. Gennaro, J.M. Pollock, and I. Zerbini, 2002: Use of recombinant proteins in antibody tests for bovine tuberculosis. Vet. Microbiol. **85:** 379–389.

Aranaz A., deJuan L., Montero N., Sanchez C., Galka M., Delso C., Alvarez J., Romero B., Bezos J., Vela A., Briones V., Mateos A. & Dominguez L. 2004. Bovine tuberculosis (Mycobacterium bovis) in wildlife in Spain. Journal of Clinical Microbiology, June: 2602-2608.

Armstrong, J. A. and Hart, P. D. (1975). Phagosome-lysosome interactions in cultured macrophages infected with virulent tubercle bacilli. Reversal of the unusual nonfusion pattern and observations on bacterial survival. Journal of Experimental Medicine **142:** 1-16.

Ayele W.Y., Neill S.D., Zinsstag J., Weiss M.G. & Pavlik I. 2004. Bovine tuberculosis, an old disease but new threat to Africa. Int.J.Tuberc.Lung Dis. **8**(8): 924-937.

Berrgren, S.A., 1981. Field experiment with BCG vaccine in Malawi. Br. Vet. J. **137:** 88–96.

Bouvet E., Casalino E., Mendoza-Sassi G., Lariven S., Vallee E., Pernet M *et al.* 1993. A nosocomial outbreak of multi-drug resistance Mycobacterium bovis among HIV infected patients. A case-control study. AIDS, **7:** 1453-60.

Brosch R., Gordon S.V., Marmiesse M. *et al.* 2002; A new evolutionary scenario for the Mycobacterium tuberculosis complex. Proc.Natl.Acad.Sci.U.S.A **99:** 3684-3689.

Buddle B.M., Ryan T.J., Pollock J.M., Anderson P. & De Lisle G.W. (2001). Use of ESAT-6 in the interferon-gamma test for diagnosis of bovine tuberculosis following skin testing. Vet. Microbiol., **80:** 37–46.

Buddle, B.M., Keen, D., Thomson, A., Jowett, G., Heslop, J., deLisle, G.W., Stanford, J.L., 1995. Protection of cattle from bovine tuberculosis by vaccination with BCG by the respiratory or subcutaneous route, but not by vaccination with killed Mycobacterium vaccae. Res. Vet. Sci. **59:** 10–16.

Buddle, B.M., Keen, D., Thomson, A., Jowett, G., McCarthy, A.R., Heslop, J., De Lisle, G.W., Stanford, J.L., 1995b. Effectiveness of BCG vaccination in protecting possums against bovine tuberculosis. Res. Vet. Sci. **58:** 90- 95.

Buddle, B.M., Parlane, N.A., Keen, D.L., Aldwell, F.E., Pollock, J.M., Lightbody, K., Andersen, P., 1999. Differentiation between Mycobacterium bovis BCG-vaccinated and M. bovis-infected cattle by using recombinant mycobacterial antigens. Clin. Diag. Lab. Immunol. **6:** 1-5.

Butler KL, Fitzgerald SD, Berry DE, Church SV, Reed WM, Kaneene JB. Experimental inoculation of European starlings (Sturnus vulgaris) and American crows (Corvus brachyrhynchos) with Mycobacterium bovis. Avian Dis. 2001; **45:** 709-18.

Calmette, A., Guerin, C., 1911. Recherches experimentales sur la defense del'orgganisme contre l'infection tuberculose. Ann. Inst. Pasteur **25:** 625–641.

Carpenter, E., Fray, L.M., Sandall, L.J., Kawakami, R.P., Collins, D.M., Gormley, E.P., 1995. Identification of bovine T cell stimulatory antigens using a cosmid library of Mycobacterium bovis in Mycobacterium smegmatis. NZ Vet. J. **43:** 360- 364.

Cassidy, J.P., Bryson, D.G., Cancela, M.M.G., Forster, F., Pollock, J.M., Neill, S.D., 2001. Lymphocyte subtypes in experimentally induced early-stage bovine tuberculous lesions. J. Comp. Pathol. **124:** 46–51.

Cassidy, J.P., Bryson, T.D., Pollock, J.M., Forster, F., Evans, R.T., Neill, S.D., 1998. Early lesion formation in cattle experimentally infected with Mycobacterium bovis. J. Comp. Pathol. **119:** 27–44.

Cataldi, A., M.I. Romano, and F. Bigi, 1994: A western blot characterization of Mycobacterium bovis antigens recognized by cattle sera. Res. Microbiol. **145:** 689–698.

Chambers, M.A., Gavier-Widen, D., Tascon, R., Colston, M.J., Lowrie, D., Williams, A., Marsh, P.D., Hewinson, R.G., 1999. The evaluation of DNA vaccines for Mycobacterium bovis in small animal challenge models. In: Fourth International Conference on the Pathogenesis of Mycobacterial Infections, Stockholm Sweden.

Christie, J.D., Callihan, D.R., 1995. The laboratory diagnosis of mycobacterial diseases. Clin. Lab. Med. **15:** 279–306.

Coad M., Hewinson R.G., Clifford D., Vordermeier H.M. and Whelan A.O. (2007). Influence of skin testing and blood storage on interferon-gamma production in cattle affected naturally with Mycobacterium bovis. Vet. Rec., **160**(19): 660–662.

Cosivi O., Grange J.M. Daborn C.J. *et al.*, 1998; Zoonotic tuberculosis due to Mycobacterium bovis in developing countries. Emerg.Infect.Dis. **4:** 59-70.

Cosivi, O., Grange, J.M., Daborn, C.J., Raviglione, M.C., Fujikura, T., Cousins, D., Robinson, R.A., Huchzermeyer, H.F.A.K., deKantor, I., Meslin, F.-X., 1998. Zoonotic tuberculosis due to M. bovis in developing countries. Emerg. Infect. Dis **4:** 59–70.

Cotter, T.P., Sheehan, S., Cryan, B., O'Shaughnessy, E., Cummins, H., Bredin, C.P., 1996. Tuberculosis due to Mycobacterium bovis in humans in the south-west region of Ireland: is there a relationship with infection prevalence in cattle? Tubercle Lung Dis. **77:** 545–548.

Cousins D.V., Francis B.R. and Gow B.L. (1989). Advantages of a new agar medium in the primary isolation of Mycobacterium bovis. Vet. Microbiol., **20:** 89–95.

Cousins D.V., Skuce R.A., Kazwala R.R. and Van embden J.D.A. (1998). Towards a standardized approach to DNA fingerprinting of Mycobacterium bovis. Int. J. Tuberc. Lung Dis., **2:** 471–478.

Dankner M., and Davis C.E., 2000. Mycobacterium bovis as a significant cause of tuberculosis in children residing along the United-States-Mexico border in the Baja California region. Pediatrics, 105(6).

Dannenberg Jr., A.M., 1999. Pathophysiology: basic aspects. In: Schlossberg, D. (Ed.), Tuberculosis and Nontuberculous Mycobacterial Infections. Fourth Edition. W.B. Saunders, Philadelphia, pp. 17–47.

Das, G., Vohra, H., Saha, B., Agrewala, J.N., Mishra, G.C., 1999. Apoptosis of Th1-like cells in experimental tuberculosis (TB). Clin. Exp. Immunol. **115:** 324–328.

De Lisle G.W., Mackintosh C.G. and Bengis R.G. (2001). Mycobacterium bovis in free-living and captive wildlife, including farmed deer. Rev. sci. tech. Off. int. Epiz., **20:** 86–111.

De Lisle, G.W., Wilson, T., Collins, D.M., Buddle, B.M., 1999. Vaccination of guinea pigs with nutritionally impaired avirulent mutants of *Mycobacterium bovis* protects against tuberculosis. Infect. Immun. **67:** 2624-26.

Dlugovitzky D., Bay M.L., Rateni L., Fiorenza G., Vietti L., Farroni M.A., Bottasso O.A. 2000. Influence of disease severity on nitrite and cytokine production by peripheral blood mononuclear cells (PBMC) from patients with pulmonary tuberculosis (TB). Clin Exp Immunol; **122:** 343–349.

Doherty M.L., Basset H.F., Quinn P.J., Davis W.C., Kelly A.P., Monaghan M.L. 1996. A sequential study of the bovine tuberculin reaction. Immunology. **87:** 9-14

Dungworth, D.L., 1993. The respiratory system. In: Jubb, K.V.F.,Kennedy, P.C., Palmer, N. (Eds.), Pathology of Domestic Animals. fourth ed. Academic Press, San Diego, pp. 641–652.

Enarson, D., 2005. Introduction to M. bovis infections in animals and humans. In: Mycobacterium bovis Infections in Animals and Humans, Blackwell Publishing, Ames, IA.

Espinosa L.E., Galan J.C., Gutierrez M., Samper S., Garcia J.F., Martin C., Dominguez L., De Rafael L., Baquero F., Gomez,E. and Blazquez J. (1998). Allele-specific PCR method based on pncA and oxyR sequences for distinguishing Mycobacterium bovis from *M. tuberculosis*: intraspecific M. bovis pncA sequence polymorphism. J. Clin. Microbiol., **36:** 239–242.

Esteban J., Robles P., Soledad Jime´nez M., Ferna´ndez Guerrero M.L. 2005. Pleuropulmonary infections caused by *Mycobacterium bovis*: a re-emerging disease. Clinical Microbiology and Infection. **11**(10): 840-843

Fenhalls, G., Wong, A., Bezuidenhout, J., van Helden, P., Bardin, P., Lukey, P.T., 2000. In situ production of gamma interferon, interleukin-4, and tumor necrosis factor alpha mRNA in human lung tuberculous granulomas. Infect. Immun. **68:** 2827–2836.

Fifis, T., C. Costopoulos, L.A. Corner, and P.R. Wood, 1992: Serological reactivity to *Mycobacterium bovis* protein antigens in cattle. Vet. Microbiol. **30:** 343–354.

Fine, P.E., 1998. Vaccines, genes and trials. Novartis Found. Symp. **217:** 57-69.

Fitzgerald SD, Boland KG, Clarke KR, Wismer A, Kaneene JB, Berry DE, Church SV, Hattey JA, Bolin CA. Resistance of Mallard ducks (Anas platyrhynchos) to experimental inoculation with *Mycobacterium bovis*. Avian Dis. 2005; **49:** 144-146.

Francis, J., 1947. Bovine Tuberculosis. Staples Press, London.

Gaborick, C.M., M.D. Salman, R.P. Ellis, and J. Triantis, 1996: Evaluation of a five-antigen ELISA for diagnosis of tuberculosis in cattle and Cervidae. J. Am. Vet. Med. Assoc. **209:** 962–966.

Garnier T., Eiglmeier K., Camus j.C., Medina N., Mansoor H., Pryor M., Duthoy S., Grondin S., Lacroix C., Monsempe C., Simon S., Harris B., Atkin R., Doggett J., Mayes R.,

Keating L., Wheeler P.R., Parkhill J., Barrell B.G., Cole S.T., Gordon S.V., Hewinson R.G. (2003). The complete genome sequence of *Mycobacterium bovis*. Proc. Natl Acad. Sci. USA, **100**(13): 7877–7882.

Gibson A.L., Hewinson G., Goodchild T., Watt B., Story A., Inwald J., Drobniewski F.A. 2004. Molecular epidemiology of disease due to Mycobacterium bovis in humans in the United Kingdom. Journal of Clinical Microbiology, **42**(1): 431-434.

Glatman-Freedman, A. & Casadevall, A. (1998). Serum therapy for tuberculosis revisited: reappraisal of the role of antibody-mediated immunity against Mycobacterium tuberculosis. Clinical Microbiology Reviews **11:** 514-32.

GORMLEY E., DOYLE M.B., FITZSIMONS T., MCGILL K. & COLLINS J.D. (2006). Diagnosis of Mycobacterium bovis infection in cattle by use of the gamma-interferon (Bovigam) assay. Vet. Microbiol., **112**(2–4): 171–179.

Gormley, E., Fray, L., Sandall, L., Ke, G., Dupont, C., Carpenter, E., 1999. Detection of Mycobacterium bovis lymphocyte stimulating antigens in culture filtrates of a recombinant Mycobacterium smegmatis cosmid library. Vaccine **17:** 2792- 2801.

Grange J.M., & Yates M.D., 1994. Zoonotic aspects of *M. bovis* infection. Vet.Microbiol. **40:** 137-151.

Green, L.R., C.C. Jones, A.L. Sherwood, I. Garkavi, G.A. Cangelosi, T.C. Thacker, M.V. Palmer, W.R. Waters, and C.R. Rathe, 2009: Single-antigen serological testing for bovine tuberculosis. Clin. Vaccine Immunol, **16:** 1309–1313.

Griffin J.F.T., Cross J.P., Chinn D.N., Rogers C.R. & Buchan G.S. (1994). Diagnosis of tuberculosis due to M. bovis in New Zealand red deer (Cervus elaphus) using a composite blood test (BTB) and antibody (ELISA) assays. N. Z. Vet. J., **42:** 173–179.

Guerrero A., Cobo J., Fortün J., Navas E., Quereda C., Asensio A., *et al.* 2000. Nosocomial transmission of *Mycobacterium bovis* resistant to 11 drugs in people with advanced HIV infection. The Lancet, Vol.350; issue 9093, Dec: 1738-1742.

Gutierrez M., Samper S., Gavigan J.A., Garcia Marin J.F., Martin C. 1995. Differentiation by Molecular Typing of *Mycobacterium bovis* Strains Causing Tuberculosis in Cattle and Goats. Journal of Clinical Microbiology.

Hewinson, R.G., Russell, W.P., Pollock, J.M., Jacobs, W.R.J., 1995. The use of shuttle cosmid libraries to detect novel antigens of *Mycobacterium bovis*. In: Griffin, J.F. (Ed.), Tuberculosis in Wildlife and Domestic Animals, Dunedin, University of Otago Press, pp. 40-43.

Hope, J.C., Kwong, L.S., Sopp, P., Collins, R.A., Howard, C.J.,2000. Dendritic cells induce CD4(+) and CD8(+) T-cell responses to *Mycobacterium bovis* and M. avium antigens in Bacille Calmette Guerin vaccinated and nonvaccinated cattle.Scand. J. Immunol. **52:** 285–291.

http://www.oie.int/fileadmin/Home/eng/Health_standards/tahm/2.04.07_BOVINE_TB.pdf

Huard R.C., De Oliveira Lazzarini L.C., Butler W.R., Van Soolingen D. & Ho J.L. (2003). PCR-based method to differentiate the subspecies of the *Mycobacterium tuberculosis* complex on the basis of genomic deletions. J. Clin. Microbiol., **41**(4): 1637–1650.

Jha V.C., Monta Y., Dhakal M., Besnet B., Sato T., Nagai A., Kato M., Kozawa K.,Yamamoto S., Kimura H., 2007. Isolation of *Mycobacterium* spp. In milking buffaloes and cattle in Nepal. J.Vet.Med.Sci. **69**(8): 819-825

Jolley, M.E., M.S. Nasir, O.P. Surujballi, A. Romanowska, T.B. Renteria, M.A. De la, A. Lim, S.R. Bolin, A.L. Michel, M. Kostovic, and E.C. Corrigan, 2007: Fluorescence polarization assay for the detection of antibodies to *Mycobacterium bovis* in bovine sera. Vet. Microbiol. **120:** 113–121.

Kazwala R.R., Daborn C.J., Sharp J.M., Kambarage D.M., Jiwa S.F., Mbembati N.A. 2001. Isolation of *Mycobacterium bovis* from human cases of cervical adenitis in Tanzania: a cause for concern? Int J Tuberc Lung Dis. **5**(1): 87-91

Keane, J., Balcewicz-Sablinska, M.K., Remold, H.G., Chupp, G.L.,Meek, B.B., Fenton, M.J., Kornfeld, H., 1997. Infection by *Mycobacterium tuberculosis* promotes human alveolar macrophage apoptosis. Infect. Immun. **65:** 298–304.

Kennedy, H.E., Welsh, M.D., Bryson, D.G., Cassidy, J.P., Forster,F.I., Howard, C.J., Collins, R.A., Pollock, J.M., 2002. Modulation of immune responses to *Mycobacterium bovis* in cattle depleted of WC1(+) gamma delta T-cells. Infect. Immun. **70:** 1488–1500.

Koo, H.C., Y.H. Park, J. Ahn, W.R. Waters, M.V. Palmer, M.J.Hamilton, G. Barrington, A.A. Mosaad, K.T. Park, W.K.Jung, I.Y. Hwang, S.N. Cho, S.J. Shin, and W.C. Davis,2005: Use of rMPB70 protein and ESAT-6 peptide as antigens for comparison of the enzyme-linked immunosorbent, immunochromatographic, and latex bead agglutination assays for serodiagnosis of bovine tuberculosis. J. Clin.Microbiol. **43:** 4498–4506.

Lepper, A.W.D., Pearson, C.W., 1973. The route of infection in tuberculosis of beef cattle. Aust. Vet. J. **49:** 266–267.

Lie´bana, E., Aranaz, A., Aldwell, F.E., McNair, J., Neill, S.D.,Smyth, A.J., Pollock, J.M., 2000. Cellular interactions in bovine tuberculosis: release of active mycobacteria from infected macrophages by antigen-stimulated T-cells. Immunology **99:** 23–29.

Lieâbana, E., Aranaz, A., Welsh, M., Neill, S. D. and Pollock, J. M. (2000a). In vitro T-cell activation of monocyte-derived macrophages by soluble messengers or cell-to-cell contact in bovine tuberculosis. Immunology **100:** 194- 202.

Lightbody, K.A., R.A. Skuce, S.D. Neill, and J.M. Pollock, 1998: Mycobacterial antigen-specific antibody responses in bovine tuberculosis: an ELISA with potential to confirm disease status. Vet. Rec. **142:** 295–300.

Liss G.M., Wong L., Kittle D.C., Simor A., Naus M., Martiquet P., Misener C.R. 1994. Occupational exposure to *Mycobacterium bovis* infection in deer and elk in Ontario. Can J Public Health. **85**(5): 326-329.

Liu, S., S. Guo, C. Wang, M. Shao, X. Zhang, Y. Guo, and Q.Gong, 2007: A novel fusion protein-based indirect enzymelinked immunosorbent assay for the detection of bovine tuberculosis. Tuberculosis **87:** 212–217.

Lyashchenko, K.P., J.M. Pollock, R. Colangeli, and M.L.Gennaro, 1998: Diversity of antigen recognition by serum antibodies in experimental bovine tuberculosis. Infect. Immun. **66:** 5344–5349.

Lyashchenko, K.P., R. Greenwald, J. Esfandiari, M.A. Chambers, J. Vicente, C. Gortazar, N. Santos, M. Correia-Neves,B.M. Buddle, R. Jackson, D.J. O'Brien, S. Schmitt, M.V. Palmer, R.J. Delahay, and W.R. Waters, 2008: Animal-side serologic assay for rapid detection of *Mycobacterium bovis* infection in multiple species of free-ranging wildlife. Vet. Microbiol. **132:** 283–292.

McIlroy, S.G., Neill, S.D., McCracken, R.M., 1986. Pulmonary lesions and *Mycobacterium bovis* excretion from the respiratory tract of tuberculin reacting cattle. Vet. Rec. **118:** 718–721.

McNair, J., D.M. Corbett, R.M. Girvin, D.P. Mackie, and J.M. Pollock, 2001: Characterization of the early antibody response in bovine tuberculosis: MPB83 is an early target with diagnostic potential. Scand. J. Immunol. **53:** 365–371.

Medlar, E.M., 1940. Pulmonary tuberculosis in cattle. Am. Rev. Tuberc. **41:** 283–306.

Menzies F.D. & Neill S.D. 2000. Cattle to cattle transmission of bovine tuberculosis. Vet.J. **160:** 92-106.

Monaghan, M.L., Doherty, M.L., Collins, J.D., Kazda, J.F., Quinn, P.J., 1994. The tuberculin test. Vet. Microbiol. **40:** 111–124.

Mostowy S., Inwald J., Gordon S., Martin C., Warren R., Kremer K., Cousins D., Behr M.A. 2005. Revisiting the Evolution of *Mycobacterium bovis*. Journal of Bacteriology, **187**(18): 6386-6395

Neill S.D., Pollock J.M., Bryson D.B. & Hanna J. 1994. Pathogenesis of *Mycobacterium bovis infection* in cattle. Vet.Microbiol. **40:** 41-52.

Neill S.D., Skuce R.A., Pollock J.M., 2005. Tuberculosis-new light from an old window. Journal of Applied Microbiology. **98**(6): 1261-1269

Neill, S.D., Pollock, J.M., Bryson, D.B., Hanna, J., 1994. Pathogenesis of Mycobacterium bovis infection in cattle. Vet. Microbiol. **40:** 41–52.

Niemann S., Harmsen D., Rusch-gerdes S. and Richter E. (2000). Differentiation of clinical Mycobacterium tuberculosis complex isolates by gyrB DNA sequence polymorphism analysis. J. Clin. Microbiol., **38**(9): 3231–3234.

O'Loan, C.J., J.M. Pollock, J. Hanna, and S.D. Neill, 1994: Immunoblot analysis of humoral immune responses to Mycobacterium bovis in experimentally infected cattle: early recognition of a 26-kilodalton antigen. Clin. Diagn. Lab. Immunol. **1:** 608–611.

O'Nuallain, E.M., Davis, W.C., Costello, E., Pollock, J.M.,Monaghan, M.L., 1997. Detection of *Mycobacterium bovis* infection in cattle using an immunoassay for bovine soluble interleukin-2 receptor-alpha (sIL-2R-alpha) produced by peripheral blood T-lymphocytes following incubation with tuberculin PPD. Vet. Immunol. Immunopathol. **56:** 65–76.

O'REILLY L.M. & DABORN C.J. (1995). The epidemiology of Mycobacterium bovis infections in animals and man: a review. Tubercle Lung Dis. (Supple. 1), **76:** 1–46.

OIE, 2005.Bovine Tuberculosis, *http://www.cfsph.iastate.edu/Factsheets/pdfs/bovine_tuberculosis.pdf*

Orme, I.M., 1998. The immunopathogenesis of tuberculosis: a new working hypothesis. Trend. Microbiol. **6:** 94–97.

Palmer, M.V., Whipple, D.L., Olsen, S.C., Jacobson, R.H., 2000.Cell mediated and humoral immune responses of white-tailed deer experimentally infected with Mycobacterium bovis. Res.Vet. Sci. **68:** 95–98.

Parsons L.M., Brosch R., Cole S.T., Somoskovi A., Loder A., Bretzel G., Van soolingen D., Hale Y.M. and Salfinger M. (2002). Rapid and simple approach for identification of *Mycobacterium tuberculosis* complex isolates by PCR-based genomic deletion analysis. J. Clin. Microbiol., **40**(7): 2339–2345.

Phillips C.J.C, Foster C.R.W, Morris P.A. & Teverson R. 2003. Review: the transmission of *Mycobacterium bovis* infection to cattle. Research in Veterinary Science **74:** 1-15.

Plackett, P., Ripper, J., Corner, L.A., Small, K., de Witte, K., Melville, L., Hides, S., Wood, P.R., 1989. An ELISA for the detection of anergic tuberculous cattle. Aust. Vet. J. **66:** 15–19.

Pollock J.M., Rowan T.G., Dixon J.B., Carter S.D., Spiller D., & Warenius H. 1993. Alteration of cellular immune responses by nutrition and weaning in calves. Research in Veterinary Science. **55:** 298-305.

Pollock, J. M., Pollock, D. A., Campbell, D. G., Girvin, R. M., Crockard, A. D., Neill, S. D. and Mackie, D. P. (1996). Dynamic changes in circulating and antigen-responsive T cell subpopulations post *Mycobacterium bovis* infection in cattle. Immunology **87:** 236-41.

Pollock, J.M., Douglas, A.J., Mackie, D.P., Neill, S.D., 1994. Identification of bovine T-cell epitopes for three *Mycobacterium bovis* antigens: MPB70, 19,000 MW and MPB57. Immunology **82:** 9–15.

Pollock, J.M., Andersen, P., 1997. The potential of the ESAT-6 antigen secreted by virulent mycobacteria for specific diagnosis of tuberculosis. J. Infect. Dis. **175:** 1251–1254.

Pollock, J.M., McNair, J., Bassett, H., Cassidy, J.P., Costello, E.,Aggerbeck, H., Rosenkrands, I., Andersen, P., 2003. Specific delayed-type hypersensitivity responses to ESAT-6 identify tuberculosis-infected cattle. J. Clin. Microbiol. **41:** 1856–1860.

Pollock, J.M., McNair, J., Welsh, M.D., Girvin, R.M., Kennedy, H.E., Mackie, D.P., Neill, S.D., 2001. Immune responses in bovine tuberculosis. Tuberculosis **81:** 103–107.

Pollock, J.M., Welsh, M.D., 2002. The WC1+ gd T-cell population in cattle: a possible role in resistance to intracellular infection. Vet. Immunol. Immunop. **89:** 105–114.

Qureshi, T., Labes, R.E., Cross, M.L., Grif®n, J.F.T., Mackintosh, C.G., 1999. Partial protection against oral challenge with *Mycobacterium bovis* in ferrets Mustela furo, following oral vaccination with BCG. Int. J. Tuberc. Lung. Dis. **3:** 1025-1033.

Renwick A.R., White P.C.L., Bengis R.G. 2007. *Bovine tuberculosis* in southern African wildlife: a multi-species host-pathogen system. A review. Epidemiol. Infect. **135:** 529-540.

Ritacco, V., Lopez, B., DeKantor, I.N., Barrera, L., Errico, F., Nader,A., 1991. Reciprocal cellular and humoral immune-responses in bovine tuberculosis. Res. Vet. Sci. **50:** 365–367.

Rolle, M., Wiethe, H., 1956. Results of BCG vaccination in cattle in Bavaria. Vet. Bull. **27:** 105.

RUSSELL, D. G. (1999). Mycobacterium and the seduction of the macrophage. In Mycobacteria: Molecular Biology and Virulence, eds C. RATLEDGE & J. DALE, pp. 371-88. Oxford: Blackwell Science Ltd.

Ryan T.J., Buddle B.M. and De Lisle G.W. (2000). An evaluation of the gamma interferon test for detecting bovine tuberculosis in cattle 8 to 28 days after tuberculin skin testing. Res. Vet. Sci., **69:** 57–61.

Seah, T.G., Rook, G.A.W., 2001. IL-4 influences apoptosis of mycobacterium-reactive lymphocytes in the presence of TNF-a. J. Immunol. **167:** 1230–1237.

Sequeira, M.D., Ritacco, V., Kantor, I.N., 2005. In: Thoen, O.,Gilsdorf, M.J., Steele, J. (Eds.), *Mycobacterium bovis* Infection in Animals and Humans. Blackwell Publishing, Ames, IA.

Skinner, M.A., Parlane, N., McCarthy, A., Buddle, B.M., 2003. Cytotoxic T-cell responses to Mycobacterium bovis during experimental infection of cattle with bovine tuberculosis. Immunology **110:** 234–241.

Smith R.M.M., Drobniewski F., Gibson A., Montague J.D.E., Logan M.N., Hunt D., Hewinson G., Salmon R.L., O'Neill B. 2004. *Mycobacterium bovis* Infection, United Kingdom. Emerging Infectious Diseases, **10**(3): 539-541.

Smyth, A.J., Welsh, M.D., Girvin, R.M., Pollock, J.M., 2001. In vitro responsiveness of gd T-cells from *Mycobacterium bovis*-infected cattle to mycobacterial antigens: Predominant involvement of WC1(+) cells. Infect. Immun. **69:** 89–96.

Stuart, F., Mahmood, K.H., Stanford, J.L., Pritchard, D.G., 1988. Development of diagnostic tests for, and vaccination against, and vaccination against, tuberculosis in badgers. Mamm. Rev. **18:** 74- 75.

Thoen, C.O., Barletta, R., 2005. Pathogenes is of *Mycobacterium bovis*. In: *Mycobacterium bovis* Infections in Animals and Humans, Blackwell Publishing, Ames, IA.

Thoen, C.O., Jarnagin, J.L., Muscoplat, C.C., Cram, L.S., Johnson, D.W., Harrington, R., 1980. Potential use of lymphocyte blastogenic responses in diagnosis of bovine tuberculosis. Comp.Immunol. Microbiol. Infect. Dis. **3:** 355–361.

Turner, O.C., Basaraba, R.J., Orme, I.M., 2003. Immunopathogenesis of pulmonary granulomas in the guinea pig after infection with *Mycobacterium tuberculosis*. Infect. Immun. **71:** 864–871.

Van Soolingen D. 2001. Molecular epidemiology of tuberculosis and other mycobacterial infections: main methodologies and achievements. J.Intern.Med. **249:** 1-26.

Van Soolingen D., de Haas P.E., Haağma J., Eger T., Hermans P:W:, Ritacco V., Alito A. & van Embden J.D. 1994; Use of various genetic markers in differentiation of *Mycobacterium bovis* strains from animals and humans and for studying epidemiology of bovine tuberculosis. J.Clin.Microbiol. **32:** 2425-2433.

Vordermeier, H.M., Cockle, P.C., Whelan, A., Rhodes, S., Palmer, N., Bakker, D., Hewinson, R.G., 1999. Development of diagnostic reagents to differentiate between *Mycobacterium bovis* BCG vaccination and M. bovis infection in cattle. Clin. Diagn. Lab. Immunol. **65:** 675-82.

Waters, W.R., M. Palmer, T.C. Thacker, J.P. Bannantine,H.M. Vordermeier, R.G. Hewinson, R. Greenwald, J. Esfandiari, J. McNair, J.M. Pollock, P. Andersen, and K.P. Lyashchenko, 2006: Early antibody responses to experimental Mycobacterium bovis infection of cattle. Clin. Vacc. Immunol. **13:** 648–654.

Wedlock D.N., Skinner M.A., de Lisle G.W., Buddle B.M., 2002. Control of *Mycobacterium bovis* infections and the risk to human populations. Microbes and Infection. **4**(4): 471-480.

Wei C.Y., Hsu Y.H., Chou W.J., Lee C.P., Tsao W.L. 2004. Molecular and histopathologic evidence for systemic infection by *Mycobacterium bovis* in a patient with tuberculous enteritis, peritonitis, and meningitis: a case report. Kaohsiung J Med Sci. **20**(6): 302-307.

Welsh, M.D., Cunningham, R.T., Corbett, D.M., Girvin, R.M., McNair, J., Skuce, R.A., Bryson, D.G., Pollock, J.M., 2005. Influence of pathological progression on the balance between cellular and humoral immune responses in bovine tuberculosis. Immunology **114:** 101–111.

Whelan, C., E. Shuralev, G. O'Keeffe, P. Hyland, H.F. Kwok,P. Snoddy, A. O'Brien, M. Connolly, P. Quinn, M. Groll,T. Watterson, S. Call, K. Kenny, A. Duignan, M.J. Hamilton,B.M. Buddle, J.A. Johnston, W.C. Davis, S.A. Olwill, and J. Clarke, 2008: Multiplex immunoassay for serological diagnosis of *Mycobacterium bovis* infection in cattle. Clin. Vaccine Immunol. **15:** 1834–1838.

Wiker, H.G., 2009: MPB70 and MPB83–major antigens of Mycobacterium bovis. Review. Scand. J. Immunol. **69:** 492–499.

Wilkins M.J., Meyerson J., Bartlett P.C., Spieldenner S.L., Berry D.E., Mosher L.B., Kaneene J.B., Robinson-Dunn B., Stobierski M.G., Boulton M.L. 2008; Human *Mycobacterium bovis* Infection and Bovine Tuberculosis Outbreak, Michigan, 1994–2007. Emerging Infectious Diseases **14**(4): 657-660.

Williams, A., Hall, G.A., Chambers, M.A., Lowrie, D., Huygen, K., Hewinson, R.G., Marsh, P.D., 1999. The evaluation of DNA vaccines against aerosol challenge with *M. tuberculosis* in guinea pigs. In: Proceedings of the Symposium on the Fourth International Conference on the Pathogenesis of Mycobacterial Infections, Stockholm, Sweden.

Wood P.R., Corner L.A. and Plackett P. (1990). Development of a simple, rapid in vitro cellular assay for bovine tuberculosis based on the production of gamma interferon. Res. Vet. Sci., **49:** 46–49.

Wood, P.R., Jones, S.L., 2001. BOVIGAM TM : an in vitro cellular diagnostic test for bovine tuberculosis. Tuberculosis **81:** 147–155.

Wood, P.R., L.A. Corner, J.S. Rothel, J.L. Ripper, T. Fifis, B.S. McCormick, B. Francis, L. Melville, K. Small, and K. de Witte, 1992: A field evaluation of serological and cellular diagnostic tests for bovine tuberculosis. Vet. Microbiol. **31:** 71–79.

Wood, P.R., Rothel, J.S., 1994. In vitro immunodiagnosis assays for bovine tuberculosis. Vet. Micro. **40:** 125–135.

Yoneda, T. and Ellner, J. J. (1998). CD4 (‡) T cell and natural killer cell-dependent killing of *Mycobacterium tuberculosis* by human monocytes. American Journal of Respiratory Critical Care Medicine **158:** 395- 403.

□□□

Chapter 30

Animal Mycoplasmas

RAJNEESH RANA AND V.P. SINGH
IVRI, Izatnagar, Bareilly

Definition : Mycoplasmas are smallest wall-less prokaryotic organisms capable of self-replication. They belong to class Mollicutes; which means "Soft skin". The term came from the Latin *mollis* means 'soft' and *cutis* means 'skin'. The name 'Mollicutes' is now being used interchangeably with 'Mycoplasma'. There are presently about 200 species of mollicutes. Many mollicutes cause significant diseases in man, animals and plants.

The name mycoplasmas were earlier denoted as pleuropneumonia like organisms. Phylogenetic data shows that mycoplasmas apparently evolved from low G+C content "Clostridium". 16S rRNA sequences of mollicutes establish its phylogenetic relationship with Gram +ve bacterium.

They do not possess any flagella or pili. The G+C content of the mollicutes ranges from 24-36 mol%. Most of the species require sterol and Fatty acid for growth. They are facultative anaerobes. Generally, under favourable conditions, they form "Fried egg" appearance colonies on solid medium. Animal mycoplasmas and Ureaplasmas cause significant health problems in animal and humans. Mycoplasmas infection causes diseases of lungs, urogenital tract, joints and other tissues. Acholeplasmas, Mycoplasmas and Ureaplasmas are found to be associated in several disease conditions of animals.

Classification and nomenclature : The name *Mycoplasma,* from the Greek *mykes* (fungus) and *plasma* (formed), was first used by Albert B Frank in 1889. In ancient period, the name of *Mycoplasma* was **Pleuropneumonia-Like**

Organisms (PPLO), which refers to the organisms causing Contagious Bovine Pleuropneumonia (CBPP). The initial characterization of the mollicutes on the basis of 16S rRNA, indicated that it phylogenetically related with gram positive bacteria of low G+C DNA content. Later during evolution, Acholeplasmas were developed as of divergence of mollicutes from Clostridia branch. They use an alternate genetic code where the codon UGA is encoding for the amino acid tryptophan instead of the usual opal stop codon. The characteristic morphology, colony shape and size and its filterability with 450 nm pore size filters distinguish these mycoplasmas from other prokaryotes.

The isolation of L-forms from *Streptobacillus moniliformis* was the initial existence proof of mycoplasmas. Klieneberger consider them as mycoplasma which lives in symbiosis with the bacteria. In 1950s the L-forms were further defined as the bacterium which had partially or completely lost its cell wall.

Mode of reproduction : The principal mode of reproduction in mollicutes is by Binary fission. The characteristic feature is that the cytoplasmic fission is not always follows with the replication of genome, which causes deficit of genetic material in daughter cells.

Growth requirement and media : Due to smaller genome size, mollicutes have limited biosynthetic ability. This causes them to live parasitic mode of life. For improvement in growth, the growth medium is to be richly supplemented with the animal proteins like sterols which can be added 10-20%. The sterol supplies saturated and unsaturated fatty acids. This enhances the cytoplasmic membrane synthesis. The other main ingredients of the medium are Beef heart infusion, yeast extract and peptone. To avoid any growth contamination, thallium acetate (1:2000) and penicillin (500-1000 units per ml) are to be added. The suitable pH requirement for fermentative mollicutes is 7.6-7.8 and for non fermentative it should be 6.0-6.5. The ideal growth temperature for the mollicutes is 36-37^{0}C. The fermentative mycoplasmas utilise glucose for its energy source.

Habitat : The organisms are widely present in nature. They sustain either as a parasite or commensal with various species of animals, humans, plants, reptiles and fish. The organism remains viable in host system and can transmit from one species of living being to another via direct or indirect contacts.

Morphology and staining : The shape and size of mollicutes vary with species to species and are also dependent on stage of growth. The pleomorphic cells ranges from 300-900 nm diameter. The shape varies from coccoid to coccobacillary; dumbbell shape; branching with beaded or segmented filaments. They are gram negative and stain well with Giemsa. Some mycoplasmas species are having specialized structures at either one or both of their ends. In *M. gallisepticum* they were called as "pear-shaped blebs". The mollicutes are having outer triple layered limiting membrane, which is 7.5-10 nm wide. In some mycoplasmas; the outer membrane is surrounded by capsule. In *M. mycoides* subsp. *mycoides* it is named as galactan. The capsule plays role in pathogenicity.

S.No.	Host	Mycoplasma species	Diseases
1	Cattle	*M. mycoides* subsp. *mycoides*	C.B.P.P. and arthritis
		M.bovigenitalium	Mastitis and genital disease
		M. bovis	Calf pneumonia, mastitis, arthritis
		M. bovoculi	Conjunctivitis
		M. alkalescens	Arthritis
		M. bovirhinis	Mastitis
		M. dispar	Calf pneumonia, mastitis
		Mycoplasma bovine gp.7	Calf pneumonia, arthritis
2	Goats	*M. putrefaciens*	Mastitis, arthritis
		M. capricolum subsp. *capripneumoniae*	Contagious caprine pleuropneumonia
3	Sheep	*M. conjunctivae*	Conjunctivitis
		M. ovipneumoniae	Proliferative interstitial pneumonia
4	Sheep and Goats	*M. agalactiae*	Mastitis, arthritis
		M. mycoides subsp. *mycoides*	Pleuropneumonia & arthritis
5	Swine	*M. hyorhinis*	Pneumonia, arthritis
		M. hyosynoviae	Arthritis
		M. hyopneumoniae	Enzootic pneumonia

***Pathogenesis/Pathogenicity*:** Mycoplasmas adhere firmly to the epithelial cells. The molecular biology of adhesion is known for human mycoplasmas. For animal mycoplasmas it is known for *M. gallisepticum, M. hyopneumoniae* and *M. pulmonis* where evidence of adhesion structures are established. Adhesion is a prerequisite for colonisation which leads to infection. It has been found that the by-products of mycoplasmal metabolism like hydrogen superoxide and superoxide radicals are toxic to the host cell membranes. The activation of the host immune system plays significant role in the pathogenesis of mycoplasmas. Mitogenic stimulation of lymphocytes, immunosuppressive effects and auto-immune reactions in the host has been observed in animals. Recent studies indicate that the interaction of organism with macrophages and monocytes induces the production of proinflammatory cytokines like interferon γ, tumour necrosis factor and interleukins. The mycoplasma membrane lipoproteins and certain lipids induce cytokine secretion in the host.

Cattle and Buffalo

In recent years, more than 20 species of *Mycoplasma, Ureaplasma and Acholeplasma* have been isolated from cattle with different diseases. All of the 20 aforementioned species have been referred to as the Mycoplasmas. It is generally believed that Mycoplasmas play a secondary role in infections, most often exacerbating pre-existing disease; but it has been shown that *Mycoplasma bovis (M. bovis)* can play a primary role. *M. bovis* is considered one of the more pathogenic species and is the most frequent *Mycoplasma* pathogen of pneumonia, mastitis, and arthritis in cattle. Meningitis, otitis media, kerato-conjunctivitis, decubital abscesses, vaginitis and/or abortion are other conditions which may be caused by *M. bovis.* To detect acute infection, paired serum samples are recommended, since rises in antibody titre occur 10-14 days after acute infection with certain *Mycoplasma spp.* PCR is an extremely sensitive method which can be used to confirm *Mycoplasma* infection.

Pneumonia : Contagious bovine pleuropneumonia is caused by infection with *Mycoplasma mycoides* subsp. *mycoides.* In "calf pneumonia", (enzootic pneumonia), *Mycoplasma spp.* are seldom the only pathogens isolated. Most commonly, there is primary and/or concurrent viral and/or bacterial infection. However, *M. dispar, M. bovis* and *Ureaplasma* may also act as primary pathogens. Several species of *Mycoplasma* may be isolated from calves with pneumonia, but only a few of these species are considered pathogenic. Respiratory pathogenic *Mycoplasma* spp. include *M. dispar, M. bovis, M. bovirhinus, M. bovigenitalium, Ureaplasma diversum. Mycoplasmas* can be introduced in a herd by subclinical *Mycoplasma* carriers. These cattle shed the organism through nasal discharge for months to years without showing clinical signs. Clinical signs observed in cattle with pure *Mycoplasma* pneumonia are coughing, induced by stress or movement, slight tachypnea, low grade fever and mild depression. Due to prominent lymphocytic cuffings, this type of pneumonia is also called "cuffing pneumonia". In addition, fluorescent antibody tests for detection of antigen of distinct *Mycoplasma spp.* can be performed. Intramuscular application of oxytetracycline, erythromycin, or tylosin is recommended. In mixed infections with *Mycoplasma spp.* and bacteria, antibacterial therapy must be also effective against involved bacteria.

Mastitis : *M. canadense, M. bovigenitalium, M. californicum* may cause mastitis, *Mycoplasma bovis* is the most prevalent. The disease spreads rapidly within a herd, thus the usual history in a farm with *Mycoplasma* mastitis is that several cows within a short period of time exhibits acute mastitis in one or more quarters. All quarters are usually affected in lactating animals. In addition, the farm may also have problems with lameness, reproductive problems, calf pneumonia, and adult cow respiratory disease. Cows affected with acute *Mycoplasma* mastitis have a dramatic drop in milk production. Affected quarters will be warm, swollen and light brown. Drawn milk appears normal initially, but separates rapidly in a floccular deposit and a clear supernatant. Cows with subclinical infection can return to normal milk production, but they may continue to shed *Mycoplasma* spp. within milk. *Mycoplasma* spp. and, thus, *Mycoplasma* mastitis can be transmitted mechanically via handling, milking machines, and common udder wash solutions. In subacute stages, macrophages predominate as inflammatory cells. Chronic *Mycoplasma* mastitis is characterized by hyperplasia of alveolar and ductular epithelium. For confirmatory diagnosis of *Mycoplasma* mastitis, culture of milk and/or udder parenchyma may be pursued. PCR performed on milk samples is another method which can be used for diagnosis. *Mycoplasmal* mastitis is difficult to treat.

Sheep and goats

The goat is an important species of small ruminants which is being kept as a source of meat and milk. The animal is commonly called as "poor man's cow," as it is an important economy resource for poor livelihood in Asian continent. Many mycoplasmas have been isolated from goats and sheep.

Contagious agalactia of sheep and goats is a disease caused by *Mycoplasma agalactiae*. The disease is contagious for goats and sheep. Both the sexes are susceptible. In agalactic conditions some more mycoplasma species are found to be involved like, *M. capricolum, Mycoplasma mycoides* subsp. *capri, Mycoplasma mycoides* subsp. *mycoides* LC and *M. putrefaciens*. The disease is of great economic importance due to high morbidity and mortality rates. Clinical manifestations in females are primarily noticed after beginning of lactation. There is in general fever and mastitis which leads to decrease in milk yield followed by agalactia. The organism shed in the milk moreover septicaemia also observes for transit period. Severe kerato-conjunctivitis may develop. The organism settles in joints of the affected animals causing polyarthritis. Suckling kids may acquire the infection by ingestion of infected colostrum or milk.The dam can become infected by the introduction of few organisms into the udder during unsanitary procedures or during milking. Similar infections may also occur through udder via teat canal with *M. capricolum* and *M. putrefaciens. Mycoplasma agalactiae* is also found to be associated with the cases of granular vulvovaginitis in goats. The Lung lesions are also not uncommon in *M. agalactiae* infection as the outbreaks of pleurisy among goats have also been reported.

Mycoplasma arginini in goats and sheep has been isolated from various organs sites of hosts. Generally the organisms considered to be non-pathogenic. However under experimentation, after inoculation in udder it does not produced any mastitis, but persist in sheep udders for about 9 days, exhibiting neutrophilia without alteration in milk consistency. *Mycoplasma arginini* has also been isolated from cases of ovine kerato-conjunctivitis, pneumonic lung, goat arthritis etc.

Mycoplasma capricolum is primarily a goat pathogen. It causes acute disease when inoculated via parenteral or oral route. The organism has also been isolated from sheep and cows. In goats, the organism causes high morbidity and mortality. The clinical signs exhibited are arthritis or polyarthritis affecting almost every diarthrodial joint. Fibrin and neutrophil exudation were present in the joint along with the necrosis of the synovial lining. Pyrexia is a clinical sign in kids, however it goes unnoticed in adults. Due to hot, swollen and painful swelling of joints, the animals become unable to stand. In chronic cases the joints become moderately enlarged and reddened. The affected lungs may show a rubbery consistency and red areas of consolidation with diffused interstitial pneumonia. The fibrinous adhesions between lung lobes may also occur. Conjunctivitis or kerato-conjunctivitis have also been observed in affected animal.

Mycoplasma conjunctivae The organism causes ovine and caprine Conjunctivitis or keratoconjunctivitis and is frequently being isolated from the eye and nasopharynx. The infected animal shows lacrimation, conjunctivitis and keratitis etc. The disease is usually mild. Under experimental inoculation, the animals exhibits kerato-conjunctivitis. The major symptoms are lacrimation, hyperemia of the conjunctiva, and corneal opacity with extensive infiltration of mononuclear cells etc.

Mycoplasma mycoides* subsp. *capri was earlier known to be the etiological agent of contagious caprine pleuropneumonia (CCPP). The organism is widely distributed in Asia and has been reported from the south asian countries like India and Pakistan. *M. mycoides* subsp. *capri* is serologically distinct from *M. mycoides* subsp. *mycoides* LC strains. It causes caprine pleuropneumonia in goats. The information regarding the pathogenicity of the organism is clearly documented. The isolations of the organism have been made in recent years from the caprine or ovine pneumonia cases. The disease is experimentally reproducible. The organism when given endobronchially, initiated pleuropneumonia in goats Infected animals developed high fever 105-106^{0}F, dullness, depression, coughing, redness of conjunctiva and loss of appetite. Gross lesions were confined to the lungs, pleura, and pericardium. Lung lobes exhibited various degrees and stages of hepatization with dilation of interlobular septa. The pleura of the affected lung covers with fibrin and adhered to the diaphragm, chest wall, and pericardium. Thoracic fluid and fibrinous pericarditis are also commonly observed. The lymph nodes like bronchial, and mediastinal are found to be enlarged, edematous, and hemorrhagic. The organisms have also been isolated from natural cases of caprine mastitis which has been experimentally reproduced in goats.

Mycoplasma ovipneumoniae had been isolated frequently from the lung, trachea, nose and eyes of sheep with pneumonia. The organism was also found to be associated with the respiratory tract of healthy sheep. Natural disease caused by *M. ovipneumoniae* has been often reported. *M. ovipneumoniae* and *Pasteurella hemolytica* serotype A jointly produced atypical pneumonia which mainly affects lambs. Mortality usually limited up to 10%. The considerable economic loss are due to unthriftiness in animal.

Reports from goats harbouring the *M. ovipneumoniae* are also evident. The disease is experimentally reproducible with mild pathology. The organism was often recovered from the infected goats. It can be said that the experimental infection of goats and sheep with *M. ovipneumoniae* exhibits similar disease patterns. No clinical signs or gross lesions are visible in lungs and trachea. Histopathology of the affected lungs showed mild pneumonia, thickening of the interalveolar septa with neutrophils and mononuclear cells infiltration. The interstitial pneumonia is clearly visible.

Swine

M. hyosynoviae causes arthritis in pigs of almost all age group. Piglets of pre-weaning stage, growers, gilts and boars are affected. The organism grows best in anaerobic medium. The organism commonly presents in pharyngeal region in 7-8 weeks old pigs. Infection occurs via oronasal route and takes place by 10-12 weeks of age. Septicaemia occurs by 2-4 days of infection and organisms settle in joints producing characteristic arthritis and synovitis.

Clinical signs in affected species are frequent lameness, alteration in gait, acute lameness in one or more limbs followed by complete inability to stand. Rise in rectal temperature up to 40 ^{0}C by 1-2 days of exposure. Affected animals are unable to take their food and water so death occurs.

The disease can be diagnosed on the basis of acute lameness, swollen joints etc. The joint fluid from tarsal and knee may exhibit yellowish brown, may contain flacks of fibrin. Swelling and hyperaemia is seen in synovial membrane of the affected joints. The disease can be confirmed by isolation of the organism.

The animal respond to Taimulin when treated 3-5 days however Tylosin or Lincomycin are also found to be equally good.

M. hynopneumoniae causes enzootic pneumonia in pigs. The organisms grows on the cell lining of trachea, bronchi and bronchioles. The paralysis of cilia causes its loss and resulting in the accumulations of respiratory secretions in lower portion of lung causing pneumonia.

The animals of 3-10 weeks of age are affected. Clinical symptoms are transient diarrhoea and dry cough. Barking cough is commonly seen in the animals which are under stress. Coughing spreads gradually in group within 3-14 weeks. Growth rate reduces by 15-20 %. Severe pneumonia and coughing occurs in pigs of 2-4 months of age. Some other clinical signs are inappetence, fever 105°F, respiratory distress and coughing. Mortality occurs in 50% of piglets.

Enzootic pneumonia can be suspected when coughing spread out in herd. It may be associated with uneven growth rate and poor feed conversion ratio. The disease can be correlated with fever, coughing, respiratory distress and mortality. Serological tests like Indirect hemaglutination, CFT and ELISA can be performed for diagnosis followed by molecular characterization of the organisms by PCR.

The disease can be eradicated by depopulation of infected flock and treatment with suitable antibiotics like tiamulin etc.

Poultry

Avian mycoplasmaosis can be caused by several species of *Mycoplasma* including *Mycoplasma gallisepticum, M. synoviae, M. melagridis* and *M. iowae, M. gallisepticum* is the most important pathogen in poultry. *M. gallisepticum* infections are also known as chronic respiratory disease (CRD) of chickens, turkeys infectious sinusitis and house finch conjunctivitis.

Mycoplasma gallisepticum is the most economically significant mycoplasmal pathogen of poultry. *M. galliseptucum* infections can cause significant economic losses on poultry farms from chronic respiratory disease reduced feed efficiency, decreased growth and decreased egg production.

Mycoplasma gallisepticum causes disease in chickens, turkeys and game birds including pheasants, Japanese quail etc. the organisms have also been isolated from ducks and geese.

The disease is transmitted during close contact between birds. Aerosol spread occurs over short distances and can be responsible for vertically transmission within a flock. *M. gallisepticum* is also transmitted in eggs.

M. gallisepticum infections vary from asymptomatic to severe. More severe infections are seen when the birds are infected concurrently with Newcastle disease virus, infectious bronchitis virus, *Escherichia coli* or other pathogens. Infected chickens usually develop respiratory symptoms that may include rales, coughing, sneezing, nasal discharges and dyspnea. Turkeys typically experience more severe disease. Often accompanied by swelling of the paranasal (infraorbital) sinus. Conjunctivitis with frothy ocular exudates is common in turkeys and occurs occasionally in chickens. Production id developed in infected flocks, with decreased weight gain, feed efficiency and egg production. However, acute respiratory disease sometimes occurs in young birds, particularly turkeys.

The Post Mortem lesions typically include milkd sinusitis, tracheitis and airsacculitis. If the chicken is infected concurrently with *E. coli,* thickening and turbidity of the air sacs, exudative accumulation. Fibrinopurulent percarditis and perihepatitis may be seen. In turkey, severe mucopurulent sinusitis may be found, with variably tracheitis and air-sacculitis,. The eyelids may be swollen and inflamed and a clear to cloudy, thickened ocular discharge may be noted.

The organisms can be endemic in large, multiple-age commercial egg laying flocks. Stressors such as viral infections, vaccination with live viruses, cold weather or crowding can trigger disease outbreaks in infected flocks. In chickens, with uncomplicated infections, the morbidity rate is high and the mortality rate low. Under controlled experimental conditions, house finches exhibited morbidity rates approaching 100%, but low mortality rates of approximately 5% or less.

Canines

The first documented occurrence of mycoplasmas in dogs was in 1934.

The dogs have mycoplasmas in the upper respiratory tract as the normal bacterial flora. Only 20–25% of healthy dogs harbor mycoplasmas in the trachea or lungs. Several studies describe the isolation of mycoplasmas in pure culture from respiratory specimens. *Ureaplasma* spp. has also been isolated from the lungs of dogs with pneumonia. Young dogs with concurrent infection with *Bordetella* or Streptococci in the lower airway were more likely to be infected with mycoplasma, and that the presence of mycoplasma was associated with septic inflammation.

Within last 75 years, 15 known species of mycoplasma species have been isolated from dogs:

- *Acholeplasma laidlawii*
- *Mycoplasma arginini*

- *Mycoplasma bovigenitalium*
- *Mycoplasma canis*
- *Mycoplasma cynos*
- *Mycoplasma edwardii*
- *Mycoplasma feliminutum*
- *Mycoplasma felis*
- *Mycoplasma gateae*
- *Mycoplasma haemocanis*
- *Mycoplasma maculosum*
- *Mycoplasma molare*
- *Mycoplasma opalescens*
- *Mycoplasma spumans*
- *Ureaplasma canigenitalium*

The majority of mycoplasma species form part of the normal canine microflora of the urogenital tract, oral cavity, upper respiratory tract and colon. Lungs In 27% of healthy dogs, were colonized by mycoplasmas. The infection causes infertility in both bitches and stud dogs.

Most canine mycoplasmas grow rapidly on B medium and commercially available media in aerobic conditions at 37°C. Some will also grow anaerobically, or even on blood agar. The majority of canine mycoplasmas form identical fried-egg like colonies on solid medium. Growth inhibition, immunofluorescence, metabolism inhibition and double immunodiffusion have all been used to differentiate canine mycoplasma species successfully. Identification of canine mycoplasmas can be confirmed by serological methods that were dependent upon specific antisera to each individual species or serogroup.

The brown dog tick, *Rhipicephalus sanguineus*, is likely to play a role as a vector and reservoir of canine hemoplasmas.

M. canis, M. cynos and *M. haemocanis* are the most important species, being associated with urogenital tract infections/ infertility, respiratory disease and anaemia, respectively.

Vaccines: The decreasing effectiveness of antibiotics in controlling mycoplasmosis may be due to injudicious use of antibiotics in the field, due to which there is a necessity for reliable vaccines. Currently, the vaccines in use for various mycoplasmal disease conditions in animals are as follows:

S.No.	Disease	Vaccines in use
1.	Contagious caprine Pleuropneumonia	Inactivated *M. capricolum* subsp. *capripneumoniae* saponin vaccine from Kenya
2.	Contagious Bovine Pleuropneumonia	T1/44 live vaccine from Africa
3.	Contagious agalactia	Inactivated or Live attenuated vaccine in Europe and Middle East
4.	Caprine Pleuropneumonia	Inactivated saponin vaccine
5.	Enzootic pneumonia in pigs	Inactivated vaccine
6.	CRD in poultry by *M. gallisepticum*	Live mutant vaccine

There is needed to be work upon DNA vaccine as it minimises the biohazard and shall be superior in stability and transportation.

References

Bergonier, D., Bertholet, X. and Poumarat, F. (1997). Contagious agalactia of small ruminants: current knowledge concerning epidemiology, diagnosis and control. Revue Scientifique et Technique (Office International des E ´pizooties), **16:** 848-873.

Greco, G., Corrente, M., Buonovoglia, D., Aliberti, A. and Fasanella, A. (2002). Inactivated vaccine induces protection against Mycoplasma agalactiae infection in sheep. Microbiologica, **25:** 17-20.

Kahane, I. (ed.). 1993. Mycoplasma cell membranes. Subcell. Biochem. **20:** 1-314.

Razin, S., and J. G. Tully (ed.). 1995. Molecular and diagnostic procedures in mycoplasmology, vol. I. Molecular characterization. Academic Press, Inc., San Diego, Calif.

Ruuth, E., and F. Praz. 1989. Interactions between mycoplasmas and the immune system. Immunol. Rev. **112:** 133-160.

Tully, J. G., and S. Razin (ed.). 1996. Molecular and diagnostic procedures in mycoplasmology, vol. II. Diagnostic procedures. Academic Press, Inc., San Diego, Calif.

Ulmer, J. B., J. J. Donnelly, and M. A. Liu. 1996. DNA vaccines promising: a new approach to inducing protective immunity. ASM News **62:** 476-479.

Weisburg, W. G., J. G. Tully, D. L. Rose, J. P. Petzel, H. Oyaizu, D. Yang, L. Mandelco, J. Sechrest, T. G. Lawrence, J. Van Etten, J. Maniloff, and C. R. Woese. 1989. A phylogenetic analysis of the mycoplasmas: basis for their classification. J. Bacteriol. **170:** 6455-6467.

Whitcomb, R. F., and J. G. Tully (ed.). 1989. The mycoplasmas, vol. V. Spiroplasmas, acholeplasmas, and mycoplasmas of plants and arthropods. Academic Press, Inc., San Diego, Calif.

Wise, K. S., D. Yogev, and R. Rosengarten. 1992. Antigenic variation, p. 473-489. *In* J. Maniloff, R. N. McElhaney, L. R. Finch, and J. B. Baseman (ed.), Mycoplasmas: molecular biology and pathogenesis. American Society for Microbiology, Washington, D.C.

Woese, C. R. 1987. Bacterial evolution. Microbiol. Rev. **51:** 221-271.

□□□

Chapter 31

Escherichia coli

R.K. AGARWAL
IVRI, Izatnagar, Bareilly

Introduction

Escherichia coli, a Gram negative bacillus was first described by Theodar Escherich in 1885 as an enteric pathogen. They are member of genus *Escherichia* under the family Enterobactericeae. They are generally inhabited as the normal bacterial flora in the lower intestine and on favorable conditions undergo a rapid multiplication which results in various disease entities in animals and humans (Sharma and Adlakha, 2005).

E. coli is considered as genetically and phenotypically diverse species and their strains are identified by the presence of somatic (O), flagellar (H) and capsular (K) antigens, which constitutely forms the base to represents particular serotype (Wani *et al.,* 2004). These antigens are determined by the polysaccharide portion of lipopolysaccharide (LPS), capsular polysaccharide, and flagellar proteins, respectively (Scheutz *et al.,* 2004). However, serotyping generally involves determination of O and H antigens. At present, there are 174 O antigens and 53 H antigens in the international typing scheme.

Most of the *E. coli* are commensals and only a few strains among them are pathogenic which allows its classification into categories of pathotypes based on the production of virulence factors and on the mechanisms by which they cause disease. These pathotypes are as follows:

(a) Verocytotoxigenic *E. coli* (STEC)/ shigatoxigenic *E. coli* (STEC), which causes haemolytic uremic syndrome (HUS) and haemorrhagic colitis (HC) by the production of shiga toxins.

(b) Enterotoxigenic *E. coli* (ETEC) which causes diarrhea by producing heat labile enterotoxin (LT) and heat stable enterotoxin (ST).

(c) Enteroinvasive *E. coli* (EIEC) which causes diarrhoeal disease resembles shigellae in the disease they cause (DuPont *et al.*, 1971).

(d) Enteroaggregative *E. coli* (EAggEC) is associated with persistent diarrhea in developing countries (Songer and Post, 2005).

(e) Enteropathogenic *E. coli* (EPEC) a term recently used as a synonym for attaching and effacing is an emerging cause of diarrhea on humans and animals (Beutin *et al*, 2003).

(f) Necrotoxigenic *E. coli* (NTEC) is able to elaborate two types of cytotoxic necrotizing factors; CNF1 and CNF2 (Orden *et al*, 1999).

Escherichia coli in animals

Escherichia coli cause a broad range of enteric and extra intestinal diseases in animals. A summary of diseases caused and major *E. coli* pathotype are listed in Table 1.

Table 1 : Animal diseases caused by *E. coli.*

Animal species	Disease	*E. coli* Pathotype
Calves	Septicemic colibacillosis/ colisepticemia Diarrhea and Dysentry	ETEC STEC/EHEC
Cattles	Mastitis	Mastitic
Sheeps	Enteric colibacillosis, systemic colibacillosis	ETEC
Pigs	Neonatal diarrhea, post weaning diarrhea oedema Septicemia/ Systemic colibacillosis	ETEC EHEC NTEC
Rabbits	Diarrhea	EPEC
Dogs	Diarrhea	EPEC/ETEC
Cats	Diarrhea	EPEC/STEC
Goats	Diarrhea	ETEC/EHEC
Horses	Diarrhea	ETEC/EPEC

1) Verocytotoxigenic *E. coli* (STEC)/ shigatoxigenic *E. coli* (STEC)

E. coli that produce verocytotoxin/Shiga toxin (VT/Stx) (STEC/Shiga toxin producing *E. coli*, STEC) are characterized by the production of cytotoxins that interrupt synthesis of protein within host cells. These toxins are known as verocytotoxins (VT), because of their activity on Vero cells, or Shiga toxins (Stx) because of their resemblance with the toxin produced by *Shigella dysenteriae*.

Pathogenicity of STEC is contributed by the multiple virulence factors. Shiga toxin (Stx) inhibits the protein synthesis leading to cell death and play a key role in inducing vascular injury in the intestinal epithelium. Due to interaction of Shiga toxin with epithelial cells, they may also disturb the cytokine expression patterns (Yamasaki *et al.*, 1999).

Shiga toxin have been classified into two major classes, shiga toxin 1(Stx1) and shiga toxin 2 (Stx2) encoded by stx1 and stx_2 genes, respectively (Wani *et al*, 2004). Stx1 and Stx 2 were revealed to be genetically (55% DNA homology) and immunologically (non-cross reactive) different from others (Karmali, 1989). A single strain of STEC can produce both or individual classes of toxins. In early 1980's it was established that Stx1 and Stx2 were phage encoded toxins. (Paton *et al*, 1998).

Stx1 is almost identical to Stx of *S. dysenteriae* (O'Brien *et al*, 1987). These are compound toxins comprising of a single catalytic 32kDa A-subunit and multimeric B-subunit with 7.7kDa monomers. B subunit is involved in the binding of the toxin to the specific glycolipid receptors on the surface of the target cells (O'Brien *et al*, 1987). The basic A-B subunit structure is conserved across all the members of the shiga I toxin family (Nataro, 1998; Paton, 1998; O'Brien 1992). After binding with target receptor, the Stx toxins are internalized by receptor mediated endocytosis leads formation of vesicles. Internalized vesicles fused within lysosomes and are translocated, first to golgi apparatus and then to the cytosol (Sandvig *et al*, 1992). The A subunit is a N-glycosidase, cleaving a single adenine residue near the 3' end of eukaryotic 28 S rRNA, thus preventing elongation factor 1 dependent binding of aminoacyl transfer RNA and results in complete cessation of protein synthesis leads to cell death (Saxena *et al*, 1989)

Stx2 is considered to be the most important virulence factor associated with human diseases and it is 400 fold more toxic to mice than Stx1. It has also shown to induce foetoplacental reabsorbtion, intrauterine haemotoma, fibrin deposition and neutrophil infiltration (Tesh *et al*, 1993). Stx2 is encoded by at least 10 stx_2 gene variants, viz. stx_2, stx_{2c}, stx_{2d}, stx_{2e}, stx_{2f}, stx_{2vh} and have approximately 55% amino acid similarity to Stx1. (Ramachandran *et al*, 2001). stx_{2c} produced by the *E. coli* E32511 strain which is epidemiologically and clinically most important in humans. Stx2e toxin is produced by *E. coli* type strain E57, S1191 , 412 and associated with oedema disease in weaned piglets (Gyles *et al*, 1988). stx_{2f}, a new variant of Stx2 was recently reorted in STEC isolates from pigeons (Schmidt *et al*, 2000). Although there are minor difference between A subunits amino acid sequences of Stx variants but every varaiants appear to display identical enzymatic activity. However, the differences in B subunit amino acids are more significant and crucial in determining the receptor to which the Stx will bind and thus the type of target cell. The B pentamer units of toxin allows it to bind with a specific glycolipid receptor, globotriosylceramide or Gb3 present on the surface of eukaryotic cells , while for the Stx2 E associated variants Gb4 is the main receptor. (Waddell 1988; Lingwood 1987),

The mechanisms and principles of pathogenesis associated with STEC diseases are the similar for a broad range of clinical syndromes observed in animals. After ingestion of the material contaminated with STEC , it will pass through the stomach and then into the intestine, where they colonize and produce Stx. In LEE - positive STEC, it will form AE lesion which is a major feature of intestinal colonization. In LEE - negative STEC, binding of STEC to the epithelium occurs in a non intimate pattern. The amount of the toxin absorbed into the circulation and cause vascular damage in target organs depends on the concentration of the toxin. The production and absorption of toxin from the intestine generally influenced by the some of unknown factors but induction of Stx phages is likely a significant factor in enhancing toxin production. Other bacterial products, such as LPS, may also aid to pathology by stimulation of cytokines and upregulation of receptors for Stx. The main route of STEC infection is via the faecal-oral route and leads to the symptoms ranging from mild uncomplicated diarrhoea to severe bloody diarrhoea. Hemolytic uremic syndrome (HUS) and thrombotic thrombocytopenic purpura (TTP) can occur in some cases as complications of previous symptoms and both of which can result in death.

The term Enterohaemorrhagic *E. coli* (EHEC) was originally used to denote those strains which causes HC, HUS and A/E lesions on epithelial cells, express Stx toxin and have 60-MDa plasmid (Levine, 1987). Enterohaemorrhagic *E. coli* (EHEC) are a subset of STEC which are considered to be human pathogens. EHEC produce ST and have the ability to form attaching and effacing lesions (A/E lesions) on epithelial cells. EHEC also possess an approximately 60-MDa "EHEC plasmid". The ability of EHEC to form A/E lesions in the intestine is also linked to disease in humans and these A/E lesions are characterized by localized destruction (effacement) of brush border microvilli, attachment of the bacteria to the enterocyte membrane, and formation of a cup like pedestal at the site of bacterial contact. Proteins which are essential for the formation of A/E lesions are encoded by the locus of enterocyte effacement (LEE), located on the chromosome. The most important EHEC serotype in public health terms is *E. coli* O157.

2) *Enterotoxigenic E. coli (ETEC)*

ETEC is most commonly involved in *E. coli* diarrhea in farm animals and characterized by the production of enterotoxins and adhesions. These toxin and adhesions are responsible for adherence to the intestinal epithelium and promote colonization. Two type of enterotoxins are produced by ETEC. Heat stable (STa, STb, or enteroaggregative *E. coli* heat - stable enterotoxin 1 [EAST1]) or heat labile (LT) (Nagy and Fekete, 2005).

The oligomeric toxin LTs are closely related in structure and function to the cholera enterotoxin (CT) which is expressed by *Vibrio cholerae* (Sixma *et al* 1993). LT and CT have many similarities including holotoxin structure, protein sequence (80% identity), primary receptor identity, enzymatic activity, and activity in animal and cell culture assays. There are two major serogroups of LT, LT-I and LT-II, which do not cross-react immunologically. LT-I is expressed by *E. coli* strains that are pathogenic for both humans and animals. LT-II is found primarily in animal *E. coli* isolates and rarely in human isolates. But it has not been associated with disease neither in animals nor in humans.

LT-I

LT-I is an 86 kDa oligomeric toxin composed of one 28-kDa A subunit and five identical 11.5-kDa B subunits (Streatfield *et al* 1992). The B subunits are arranged in a ring or "doughnut" and responsible for binding to the ganglioside GM1 and weakly to GD1b. B subunits is also involved in binding with some intestinal glycoproteins (Teneberg *et al* 1994). The A subunit is accountable for the enzymatic activity of the toxin and it can be proteolytically cleaved to yield A1 and A2 peptides which is joined by a disulfide bond. Two variants of LT-I found to be closely related and exhibit partial antigenic cross-reactivity. Both these variants have been described in literature. These variants are called LTp (LTp-I) and LTh (LTh-I) after their initial discovery in strains isolated from pigs or humans, respectively. The genes encoding LT (*elt* or *etx*) are located on plasmids and these plasmids may also contain genes encoding ST and/or colonization factor antigens (CFAs).

LT-II

The LT-II serogroup shows 55 to 57% identity to LT-I and CT in the A subunit but essentially no homology to LT-I or CT in the B subunits (Fukuta *et al* 1988,Guth *et al* 1997, Pickett *et al* 1989, Sears and Kaper 1996, Spangler 1992). Two antigenic variants, LT-IIa and LT-IIb, have 71 and 66% identity in the predicted A and B subunits, respectively. LT-II is responsible for rise in intracellular cAMP levels by similar mechanisms to those involved with LT-I toxicity, but LT-II uses GD1 as its receptor rather than GM1 (Fukuta *et al*

1988). There is no evidence that LT-II is associated with human or animal disease.

ETEC gains entry in the animal by the oral route, and after multiplication they will increase in sufficient numbers. After attachment by fimbrial adhesions to receptors on the small intestinal epithelium or in the mucus coating the epithelium, they will colonize in the small intestine. The ETEC then proliferate rapidly to attain massive numbers to the order of 10 9 per gram of intestine in the mid - jejunum to the ileum. ETEC adhering closely to the intestinal epithelium produce enterotoxins which stimulate the secretion of water and electrolytes into the intestinal lumen. This leads to diarrhea if the excess fluid from the small intestine is not absorbed in the large intestine. ETEC cause severe watery diarrhea, which may lead to dehydration, listlessness, metabolic acidosis, and death.

In some cases, especially in pigs, the infection may progress so rapidly that death occurs before the development of diarrhea, and is referred to as enteric colibacillosis complicated by shock. This phenomenon is probably due to the rapid release of large amounts of LPS by the colonizing ETEC (Gyles *et al,* 2010).

3) Enteroinvasive *E. coli* (EIEC)

EIEC strains are closely related genetically, biochemically and pathogenetically to *Shigella* spp. EIEC strains are generally lysine nonmotile, decarboxylase negative, and lactose negative (Brenner *et al.*, 1973).

The pathogenic features of EIEC are almost identical to those of *Shigella* spp. Both organisms have been shown to invade the colonic epithelium and elaborate one or more secretory enterotoxins. These enterotoxins may play a crucial roles in pathogenesis of diarrhea (Nataro and Kaper, 1998). The route of transmission is faecal-oral route. The ability of organism to invade epithelial cells and intestinal mucosa is the pathognomic feature of EIEC infection. (DuPont *et al.*, 1971). A 120 to 140 MDa plasmid that encodes genes necessary for invasiveness are also present.(Baudry *et al.*, 1987, Small and Falkow, 1988 and Sasakawa *et al.*, 1992). Following invasions of epithelial cells of the distal ileum and colon Shigella and EIEC lyse phagosomal vacuole and multiply within the cytoplasm leading to the destruction of the cells (Sansonetti, 1992). The bacteria move laterally via polymerization of cellular actin filaments and then invade the neighbouring enterocytes or pass into lamina propia.

4) Enteroaggregative *E. coli* (EAggEC)

EAggEC (also known as EAEC) are linked with acute or persistent diarrhea, especially in developing countries and infection is typically followed by a watery, mucoid, diarrhoeal illness with little or no fever and an absence of vomiting. The exact mechanisms by which EAggEC cause diarrhea and the role of the various virulence factors are poorly understood.

The ability of EAggEC strains to adhere aggregatively with tissue culture cells in a distinctive "stacked, brick-like" manner is the characteristics of the strains and is mediated by either aggregative adherence fimbrae I (AAF/I) or AAF/II. Both are encoded for by *aggR* genes. EAggEC also involve in production of an enteroaggregative heat-stable toxin (EAST1) which is similar to ST. EAST1 is encoded on a plasmid by *astA* genes.

5) Enteropathogenic *E. coli* (EPEC)

The infections caused by the EPEC are characterized by effacement of intestinal microvilli and adherence between bacteria and epithelial cell membranes by the formation of bacterial microcolonies. This adherence is mediated by the intimin, which is encoded by *eae,* and Tir. Eae is a bacterial outer membrane protein and a tir is bacterial protein that is inserted into the enterocyte membrane and serves as the receptor for intimin. The attaching and effacing lesion result from both bacterial attachment to enterocytes and disruption of brush border microvilli. Interaction between bacteria and host cells result in accumulation of highly organized cytoskeletal components (actin, myosin, talin, ezrin) in epithelial cells beneath adherent bacteria and this results in the formation of pedestal like structures. EPEC attachment is also responsible for rise in intra enterocyte calcium ion levels and inhibit sodium and chloride absorption. EPEC strains apparently do not produce toxins (Songer and Karen, 2005).

EPEC attach loosely to the intestinal epithelial cells by specific adhesins such as AF/R1, AF/R2, and Ral in the rabbit, and Bfp in the dog. A signal is then delivered from the bacteria to the epithelial cells via the TTSS and secreted proteins (Viswanathan *et al.*, 2009).

The mechanisms of diarrhea induced by EPEC strains are not well understood. The destruction of absorptive microvilli due to AE lesion could results in diarrhea (Nataro and Kaper, 1998). However, the rapid onset of diarrhea suggests that a more active secretory mechanism is also involved and may result from the effect of EPEC signaling activity on intracellular mediators of intestinal ion transport, such as calcium, inositol phosphates, and tyrosine kinase. Diarrhea may also occur due to an increased permeability of tight junctions between epithelial cells or a localized inflammatory response at the lesion site, or chloride secretion following PMN leukocyte transmigration (Gyles *et al.*, 2010).

6) Necrotoxigenic *E. coli* (NTEC)

NTEC elaborate two major types of cytotoxic necrotizing factors; CNF1 and CNF2 (Orden *et al.*, 1999). Both are demonecrotic protein toxins and induce enlargement and multinucleation of vero and HeLA cells. They also cause necrosis in rabbit skin and are lethal for mice. CNF2 induces moderate fluid accumulation in rabbit ileal loops and CNF1 can trigger entry of non invasive bacteria into HEp-2 cells and gene encoding CNF1 is located on a pathogenecity island which also carries genes for α-hemolysin and P-fimriae. These toxin have necrotic and lethal properties and ability to alter the cytoskeleton (Songer and Post, 2005).

Diagnosis

Escherichia coli, a common occupant of the intestinal tract, is linked with both enteric and extraintestinal infection in animals. The most important barrier is to determine whether an isolate is normal flora or an agent of disease in the case of enteric infections. In extraintestinal infections, isolation of *E. coli* from a suitable sample is often all that is required and quantitave culture is sometimes used to guide in assessing significance of the isolate.

A due care should be taken while collecting specimens as *Escherichia coli* in the intestinal tract invade tissues within hour of death. So only from fresh carcasses samples should be collected. The range of samples which could be collected are aseptic culture of heart blood, bone marrows and parenchymatous organs. The recovery of organism from intestinal, urine, milk and vaginal exudates is easy and they can grow readily on most simple media available in the lab. Tryptose blood agar and MacConkey agar are most commonly and routinely used media for isolation. *E. coli* colonies may be smooth or rough and are usually 2 to 3 mm in diameter, low convex, moist, shiny, entire and gray after 24 hour aerobic incubation at 37°C on blood agar, (Balows *et al.*, 1991). Most isolates (90%) are lactose positive and usually surrounded by zone of precipitated bile. In stool, *E. coli* are most often recovered on MacConkey or eosin methylene-blue agar, which selectively allows to grow the members of the *Enterobacteriaceae* and also the differentiation of enteric organisms on the basis of morphology. The CDC recommends the use of SMAC agar for clinical microbiology laboratories those routinely culturing the stool specimens from persons with bloody diarrhea or HUS for *E. coli* O157:H7 with (CDC, 1993).

Diagnosis of ETEC is depends on detection of the enterotoxins LT and/or ST. ST was initially detected in a rabbit ligated ileal loop assay (Evans *et al.*, 1973). But due to the disbursement and lack of standardization procedures this test was replaced by the suckling mouse assay (Giannella 1976). This test was considered as the standard test for the presence of STa for many years. In suckling-mouse assay test the measurement of intestinal fluid in CD4 infant mice after percutaneous injection of culture supernatants will be determined. A number of immunoassays have been developed for detection of ST like radioimmunoassay and an enzyme-linked immunosorbent assay (Giannella, 1981; Cryan, 1990). The major advantage of using these assays is that they can be correlate well with results of the suckling-mouse assay and require substantially less expertise (Cryan, 1990). The execution of these immunologic assays are easier for clinical laboratories (Honda *et al.*, 1981). The newer immunologic methods such as ELISA, latex agglutination and two commercially available tests are also described for detection of ST the reversed passive latex agglutination test and the staphylococcal coagglutination test and both of these tests are reliable and easy to perform (Yolken *et al.*, 1977; Ito *et al.*, 1983; Scotland *et al.*, 1996; Chapman and Daly, 1989; Speirs *et al.*, 1991).

For the identification of diarrheagenic *E. coli* strains it should always keep in mind that these organisms should be differentiated from nonpathogenic members of the normal flora and for this purpose serotypic markers sometimes correlates very closely with specific categories of diarrheagenic *E. coli*. However, these markers are rarely sufficient in and of themselves to reliably identify a strain as diarrheagenic. An exception may be strains of serotype O157:H7, a serotype that serves as a marker for virulent enterohemorrhagic *E. coli* strains.

One of the most useful phenotypic assays for the diagnosis of diarrheagenic *E. coli* is the HEp-2 adherence assay. This assay was first described in 1979 by Cravioto *et al.* and remains the "gold standard" for the diagnosis of EAEC and diffusely adherent *E. coli* (DAEC) with one or more modification in the test proper like extending the incubation time to 6 h or changing the growth medium during the incubation. The HEp-2 adherence assay consist of inoculation of the test strain on a semiconfluent HEp-2 monolayer and kept it for incubation at least for 3 h at 37°C under 5% CO2 and then the monolayer should be washed, fixed, stained, and examined by oil immersion light microscopy. The three patterns of HEp-2 adherence can be differentiated reliably and grouped as localized adherence (LA), aggregative adherence (AA), and diffuse adherence (DA).

Molecular Detection Methods

Diarrheagenic *E. coli* strains were considered as earliest pathogens for which molecular diagnostic methods were developed and remain the most popular and most reliable techniques for differentiating diarrheagenic strains from nonpathogenic members of the stool flora and distinguishing strains from one category to another. Considerable progress has already been made for the development of nucleic acid-based probe technologies as well as PCR methods.

Nucleic acid probes

The use of DNA probes for detection of heat-labile (LT) and heat-stable (ST) enterotoxins in ETEC has made significant development for the study of these organisms, by replacing bulky and costly animal models which were used earlier for toxin detection (Mosely *et al* 1982). For preparation of nucleic acid probe specimen two general methods are commonly used. The first includes the inoculation of purified cultures on the agar plates to obtain "colony" blots, in which 30 to 50 such cultures are inoculated per plate. After incubation, the bacterial growth is transferred to nitrocellulose or Whatman filter paper for hybridization (alternatively, the cultures can be grown directly on the nitrocellulose overlying an agar plate). The bacterial growth on the paper can be lysed, denatured, and hybridized with the probe in situ, and then a radiographic image is generated by exposure to X-ray film. However, for better interpretation of the results this method requires that the *E. coli* strain first be isolated from the patient's stool, to minimize the possibility of wrong colonies picked from a stool culture which may fail to yield the offending pathogenic strain. If the study entails a large number of asymptomatic patients, so to increased sensitivity of the test , five isolates per specimen may be more appropriate.

An alternative to this colony blots is the stool blot method which consist of spotting of stool samples directly onto nitrocellulose filters that have been overlaid onto an agar plate (Lanata *et al* 1985). After overnight incubation, the filter paper is peeled off the from the plate, air dried, and treated as for colony blots. The reward of this technique include (i) that the *E. coli* colonies need not be isolated from the stool and (ii) that there may be increased sensitivity if the pathogenic strain represents a minority member of the flora. In addition, the use of stool blots alone does not result in a pure culture of the pathogen, which may be required for verification of phenotypes. Synthetic oligonucleotide probesn (at least two probes) are usually used for *stx1* and *stx2* and additional probes specific for *stx2c* and *stx2e* to detect strains containing these genes (Thomas *et al.*, 1993). One oligonucleotide probe that hybridizes to *stx1*, *stx2*, and *stx2c* at low temperatures (45°C) but only to *stx1* at a higher temperature (53°C) has been reported (Brown *et al.*, 1989).

PCR

PCR is a major progress made in the field of molecular diagnostics of pathogenic microorganisms, including *E. coli*. PCR primers have been developed successfully for several of the categories of diarrheagenic *E. coli*

(Table 2). Although there is advantages of using PCR with great sensitivity in *in situ* detection of target organisms but there are some substances responsible decrease sensitivity of this method for detection of *E coli* particularly in stools samples. These substances have been shown to interfere with the PCR.(Stacey-Phipps *et al.*, 1995). Several methods have been used successfully to remove such inhibitors substances like Sepharose spin column chromatography and adsorption of nucleic acids onto glass resin (Lou *et al.*, 1997, Stacey- Phipps *et al.*, 1995). Several PCR assays for detection of ETEC are quite sensitive and specific also, when used directly on clinical samples or on isolated bacterial colonies. Multiplex PCR assay are also used with the aim of detecting one of several different diarrheagenic *E. coli* pathotypes in a single reaction (Stacey-Phipps *et al.*, 1995). The PCR technique has been extensively used to detect *stx* genes and multiplex PCR techniques incorporating primers for *eae, ehx, uidA*, or *fliC* (Schmidt *et al.*, 1995).

Loop mediated isothermal amplification (LAMP) has wider application in diagnosis of *E coli*. This assay has high specificity and many characteristics that make it suitable for the rapid and simple detection of nucleic acid sequences in clinical samples (Mori and Notomi, 2009). It has been demonstrated that the *VT* gene from O-157 or O-26 in enrichment culture can be detected by the LAMP assay kit with similar or superior sensitivity to those of some plating methods using agar media (Hara-Kudo *et al.*, 2008). Yano *et al.* (2007) have developed LAMP primer sets for the rapid and sensitive diagnosis of enterotoxigenic *E. coli* infection. Furthermore, Hill *et al.* (2008) have developed a LAMP assay for detection of common strains of *E. coli* from human urine samples with high sensitivity and specificity.

DNA-fingerprinting methods

The principle of this method is the analysis of total DNA from an isolate or culture. This method mainly based on two basic approaches: either the randomized analysis of whole genome DNA or the analysis of probed or amplified targeted DNA. RFLP-based methods are also commonly used in routine typing. RFLP-based methods are based on pattern recognition of DNA fragments which can be visualized by gel electrophoresis. RFLP analysis has been used to distinguish *stx2c* from *stx2* genes (Russmann *et al.*, 1994).

Pulsed field gel electrophoresis

Pulsed field gel electrophoresis (PFGE) is currently considered as the "gold standard" method for typing of *E. coli* O157. PFGE has been used to explore the molecular epidemiology of O157:H7 infections (Meng *et al.*, 1995). PFGE is a more sensitive than phage typing (Krause *et al.*, 1996). PFGE has successfully been used for typing of EPEC in epidemiological studies and in outbreak investigations, although no international database for comparisons of patterns has been established.

Control

For areas where animal contact is possible, design of the entry and exit points for animal contact areas should be planned to facilitate proper visitor flow through transition areas .These transition areas should include educational information and hand-washing facilities. Fences, gates, or other types of barriers can restrict uncontrolled access to animals and animal contact areas and ensure that visitors enter and exit through transition areas. Animal feed and water should not be accessible to the public. In addition, in buildings where animals live, adequate ventilation is essential for both animals and humans.

Manure and soiled animal bedding should be removed promptly. Animal waste and specific tools for waste removal (e.g., shovels and pitchforks) should be confined to designated areas restricted from public access. Manure and soiled bedding should not be transported or removed through non animal areas or transition areas used by visitors. If this is unavoidable, precautions should be taken to avoid spillage and aerosolization. During events where animal contact is encouraged, periodic disinfection of the venue might reduce the risk for disease transmission during the event *(Annon, 2005).*

Prevention of *E. coli* infection can be achieved by ensuring adequate colostral intake by neonates, improving farm sanitation procedures and husbandry decreasing stocking density. Cross - reacting antibodies against LPS core may be a protective factor in colostrum. Antimicrobial therapy has met with variable success because of multiple resistance in many strains.

Vaccination has played and will continue to play an important role in the prevention of *E. coli* induced diseases in animals. ETEC induced diarrhea has significant economic effects on the production of food animals there has been a strong motivation to understand the disease process (Gyles and Fairbrother, 2010). Currently, licensed vaccine are available for ETEC induced diarrhea and so to lesser extent, $K88^+$ weanling diarrhea. Emphasis is on vaccines that stimulate antitoxic or antiadhesion immunity or both by means of killed antigens or attenuated strains. Promising results have been obtained in preventing neonatal deaths from diarrheal disease in herd animals by use of purified fimbriae as vaccines. Antibodies to surface antigens present in intestinal tract play major role in providing protective immunity to enteric *E. coli* infections. Anti - fimbriae antibodies are the major ones in providing immunity. Antibodies to the polysaccharide capsule (anti – K) of ETEC may also be protective. Both these antibodies function by preventing attachment of the ETEC to enterocytes.

In the early stages of UTI with *E. coli*, immune surveillance through TLRs is active in the bladder and recognition of LPS by TLR - 4 is important (Schilling *et al.*, 2003). The release of proinfl ammatory cytokines, notably IL - 6 and IL - 8. TLR - 4 also appears to be capable of inducing the expulsion of intracellular UPEC. Control of *E. coli* mastitis is based primarily on reducing contamination of the udder, but a bacterin consisting of killed *E. coli* strain J5, a rough mutant of an O111 *E. coli*, also provides protection against severe mastitis. Induction of antibodies against antigens in the core region of LPS, which is common to a large number of *E. coli* may be responsible for protection. Other vaccines based on the core LPS of an Enterobacteriaceae have also been reported to reduce the severity and incidence of bovine *E. coli* mastitis.

Septicemic disease in calves is most commonly the result of of agammaglobulinemia or hypogammaglobulinemia due to a failure in passive transfer of colostral immunoglobulins. It appears that specific antibodies are not required for the protection that derives from adequate immunoglobulin levels in the calf. There is considerable evidence that IgM antibodies are the important class of antibodies that are involved in protection, likely by both antiendotoxic effects and antibacterial effects mediated by complement and antibodies. There are currently no vaccines available to control zoonotic STEC (OIE, 2008).

Table 2 : PCR oligonucleotide primers for diarrheagenic *E. coli* strains

S.No.	Primer	Sequence	Amplicon size	Reference
1	stx1F stx1R	5'-ATAAATCGCCATTCGTTGACTAC-3' 5'-AGAACGCCCACTGAGATCATC-3'	180 bp	Paton and Paton (1998)
2	stx2F stx2R	5'-GGCACTGTCTGAAACTGCTCC-3' 5'-TCGCCAGTTATCTGACATTCTG-3'	255 bp	Paton and Paton (1998)
3	eaeAF eaeAR	5'-GACCCGGCACAAGCATAAGC-3' 5'-CCACCTGCAGCAACAAGAGG-3'	384bp	Paton and Paton (1998)
4	hlyAF hlyAR	5'-GCATCATCAAGCGTACGTTCC-3' 5'-AATGAGCCAAGCTGGTTAAGCT-3'	534bp	Paton and Paton (1998)
5	saaF saaR	5'-CGTGATGAACAGGCTATTGC-3' 5'-ATGGACATGCCTGTGGCAAC-3'	119bp	Paton and Paton, 1998

References

Annon. 2005. Compendium of Measures To Prevent Disease Associated with Animals in Public Settings. National Association of State Public Health Veterinarians, Inc. (NASPHV), USA.

Balows, A., Hausler, W. J., Herrmann, K.L., Isenberg, H.D. and Shadomy, H.J. 1991. Manual of clinical microbiology, 5th ed. American Society for Microbiology, Washington, D.C.

Baudry, B., Maurelli, A. T., Clerc, P., Sadoff, J. C. and P. J. Sansonetti. 1987. Localization of plasmid loci necessary for the entry of *Shigella flexneri* into HeLa cells, and characterization of one locus encoding four immunogenic polypeptides. J. Gen. Microbiol., **133:** 3403–3413.

Beutin, L., Marches, O., Betteheim, K.A., Gleier, K., Zimmermann, S., Schmidt, H. and Oswald, E. 2003. Hep-2 cell adherence, actin aggregation and intimin types of attaching and effacing *Escherichia coli* strains isolated from healthy infants in Germany and Australia. Infect. Immunol., **71:** 3995–4002.

Brenner, D.J., Fanning, G.R., Miklos, G.V. and Steigerwalt, A.G. 1973. Polynucleotide sequence relatedness among *Shigella* species. Int. J. Syst. Bacteriol., **23:** 1–7.

Brown, J.E., Sethabutr, O., Jackson, M. P., Lolekha, S. and Echeverria. P. 1989. Hybridization of *Escherichia coli* producing Shiga-like toxin I, Shigalike toxin II, and a variant of Shiga-like toxin II with synthetic oligonucle-otide probes. Infect. Immun., **57:** 2811–2814.

Centre for Disease Control. 1993. Multistate outbreak of *Escherichia coli* O157:H7 infections from hamburgers- Western United States, 1992-1993. Morb. Mortal. Weekly Rept., **42 (14):** 258-263.

Chapman, P.A. and Daly, C.M. 1989. Comparison of Y1 mouse adrenal cell and coagglutination assays for detection of Escherichia coli heat labile enterotoxin. J. Clin. Pathol., **42:** 755-758.

Cravioto, A., Gross, R.J., Scotland, S.M. and Rowe, B. 1979. An adhesive factor found in strains of *Escherichia coli* belonging to the traditional infantile enteropathogenic serotypes. Curr. Microbiol., **3:** 95–99.

Cryan, B. 1990. Comparison of three assay systems for detection of enterotoxigenic *Escherichia coli* heat-stable enterotoxin. J. Clin. Microbiol., **28:** 792–794.

DuPont, H. L., S.B. Formal, R.B. Hornick, M.J. Snyder, J.P. Libonati, D.G. Sheahan, E.H. LaBrec, and J.P. Kalas. 1971. Pathogenesis of *Escherichia coli* diarrhea. N. Engl. J. Med., **285:** 1–9.

Evans, D.G., Evans, D.J. and Pierce, N.F. 1973. Differences in the response of rabbit small intestine to heat-labile and heat-stable enterotoxin of *Escherichia coli*. Infect. Immun., **7:** 873–880.

Fukuta, S., Magnani, J.L., Twiddy, E.M., Holmes, R.K. and Ginsburg. V. 1988. Comparison of the carbohydrate-binding specificities of cholera toxin and *Escherichia coli* heat-labile enterotoxins LTh-I, LT-IIa, and LT-IIb. Infect. Immun., **56:** 1748–1753.

Gianella, R.A. 1976. Suckling mouse model for detection of heat-stable *Escherichia coli* enterotoxin: characteristics of the model. Infect. Immun., **14:** 95–99.

Giannella, R.A., Drake, K.W. and Luttrell. M. 1981. Development of a radioimmunoassay for *Escherichia coli* heat-stable enterotoxin. Infect. Immun., **33:** 186–192.

Guth, B.E., Twiddy, E.M., Trabulsi, L.R. and Holmes, R.K. 1997. Variation in chemical properties and antigenic determinants among type II heat-labile enterotoxins of *Escherichia coli*. Infect. Immun., **54:** 529–536.

Gyles, C.L., De Grandis, S.A.., MacKenzie, C. and Brunton, J.L. 1988. Cloning and nucleotide sequence analysis of the genes determining verocytotoxin production in a porcine edema disease isolate of *Escherichia coli*. Microb. Pathog., **5:** 419–426.

Gyles, C.L. and Fairbrother, J.M. 2010. *Escherichia coli*. In: Pathogenesis of bacterial infections in animals. Gyles, C.L. Prescott, J.F. Songer, J.G. and Thoen, C.O. (eds). Fourth Edition. Blackwell Publishing.

Gyles, C.L., Prescott, J.F., Songer, G. and Thoen, C.O. 2010. Pathogenesis of bacterial infections in animals. pp. 286-308.

Hara-Kudo Y, Konishi N, Ohtsuka K, Hiramatsu R, Tanaka H, Konuma H, Takatori K. 2008.Detection of Verotoxigenic *Escherichia coli* O157 and O26 in food by plating methods and LAMP method: a collaborative study. Int. J. Food Microbiol., **122:** 156–161.

Hill, J., Beriwal, S., Chandra, I., Paul, V.K., Kapil, A. and Singh, T. 2008. Loop-mediated isothermal amplifi cation assay for rapid detection of common strains of *Escherichia coli*. J. Clin. Microbiol., **46:** 2800–2804.

Honda, T., Taga, S., Takeda, Y. and Miwatani, T. 1981. Modified Elek test for detection of heat-labile enterotoxin of enterotoxigenic *Escherichia coli*. J. Clin. Microbiol., **13:** 1–5.

Ito, T., Kuwahara, S. and Yokota. T. 1983. Automatic and manual latex agglutination tests for measurement of cholera toxin and heat-labile enterotoxin of *Escherichia coli*. J. Clin. Microbiol., **17:** 7–12.

Karmali, M. A. 1989. Infection by verocytotoxin-producing *Escherichia coli*. Clin. Microbiol. Rev., **2:** 15–38.

Krause, U., Thomson-Carter, F.M. and Pennington, T.H. 1996. Molecular epidemiology of Escherichia coli O157:H7 by pulsed-field gel electrophoresis and comparison with that by bacteriophage typing. J Clin Microbiol. **34:** 959–961.

.Lanata, C. F., Kaper, J.B., Baldini, M.M., Black, R.B. and Levine, M.M. 1985. Sensitivity and specificity of DNA probes with the stool blot technique detection of *Escherichia coli* enterotoxins. J. Infect. Dis., **152:** 1087–1090.

Levine, M. M. 1987. *Escherichia coli* that cause diarrhea: enterotoxigenic, enteropathogenic, enteroinvasive, enterohemorrhagic, and enteroadherent. J. Infect. Dis., **155:** 377–389.

Lingwood, C.A,, Law, H., Richardson, S., Petric, M., Brunton, J.L., Grandis, S and Karmali, M. 1987. Glycolipid binding of purified and recombinant *Escherichia coli* produced verotoxin *in vitro*. J. Biologic. Chem., **262:** 8834-8839.

Meng, J., Zhao, S., Zhao, T. and Doyle, M. P. 1995. Molecular characterization of *Escherichia coli* O157:H7 isolates by pulsed-field gel electrophoresis and plasmid DNA analysis. J. Med. Microbiol., **42:** 258–263.

Mori, Y. and Notomi, T. 2009. Loop-mediated isothermal amplification (LAMP): a rapid, accurate, and cost-effective diagnostic method for infectious diseases. J. Infect. Chemother., **15:** 62–69.

Moseley, S. L., Echeverria, P., Seriwatana, J., Tirapat, C., Chaicumpa, W., Sakuldaipeara, T. and Falkow, S. 1982. Identification of enterotoxigenic Escherichia coli by colony hybridization using three enterotoxin gene probes. J. Infect. Dis., **145:** 863-869.

Nagy, B. and Fekete, P.Z. 2005 . Enterotoxigenic *Escherichia coli* in veterinary medicine. Int. J. Med. Microbiol., **295:** 443-454.

Nataro, J.P. and Kaper, J.B. 1998. Diarrheagenic *Escherichia coli*. Clin. Microbial. Rev., **11:** 142-201.

O'Brien, A. D., and R. K. Holmes. 1987. Shiga and Shiga-like toxins. Microbiol. Rev. **51:** 206–220.

O'Brien, A. D.,. Tesh, V. L.,. Donohue-Rolfe, A., Jackson, M. P. ., Olsnes, S. ., Sandvig, K., Lindberg, A. A. and Keusch. G. T. 1992. Shiga toxin: biochemistry, genetics, mode of action, and role in pathogenesis. Curr. Top. Microbiol. Immunol., **180:** 65–94.

OIE. World organization for animal health manual for diagnostic tests and vaccines for terrestrial animals (mammals, birds and bees) sixth edition - volume 2.

Orden, J.A., Ruiz-Santa-Quiteria, J.A., Cid, D., Garcia, S., Sanz, R. and de la Fuente, R. 1999. Prevalence and characteristic of necrotoxigenic *Escherichia coli* (NTEC) strains isolated from diarrhoeic dairy calves. Vet. Microbiol., **66:** 265–273.

Paton, J.C. and Paton, A.W. (1998). Pathogenesis and diagnosis of Shiga toxin-producing *Escherichia coli* infections. Clin. Microbiol. Rev., **11:** 450-479.

Pickett, C.L., Twiddy, E.M., Coker, C. and Holmes. R.K. 1989. Cloning, nucleotide sequence, and hybridization studies of the type IIb heat-labile enterotoxin gene of *Escherichia coli*. J. Bacteriol., **171:** 4945–4952.

Ramachandran, V., Hornitzky, M.A., Bettelheim, K.A., Walker, M.J. and Djordjevic, S.P. 2001. The common ovine higa toxin-2 containing *Escherichia coli* serotypes and human isolates of the same serotypes possess a Stx2d toxin type. J. Clin. Microbiol., **39:** 1932–1937.

Russman,, H., Schmidt, H., Heesemann, J., Caprioli, A., Karch, H. (1994). Variants of shiga like toxin II constitute a major toxin component in Escherichia coli O157 strains from patients with haemolytic uraemic syndrome. J. Med. Microbiol., **40:** 358-343.

Sandvig, K., Garred, O.,. Prydz, K., Kozlov, J. V., Hansen, S. H., and van Deurs. B. 1992. Retrograde transport of endocytosed Shiga toxin to the endoplasmic reticulum. Nature, **358:** 510–512.

Sansonetti, P. J. 1992. Molecular and cellular biology of *Shigella flexneri* invasiveness: from cell assay systems to shigellosis. Curr. Top. Microbiol. Immunol., **180:** 1–19.

Sasakawa, C., Buysse, J.M. and Watanabe, H. 1992. The large virulence plasmid of *Shigella*. Curr. Top. Microbiol. Immunol., **180:** 21–44.

Saxena, S.A., O'Brien, A. D. and Ackerman, E. J. 1989. Shiga toxin, Shiga-like toxin II variant, and ricin are all single-site RNA *N*-glycosidases of 28S RNA when microinjected into *Xenopus* oocytes. J. Biol. Chem., **264:** 596–601.

Scheutz, F., Cheasty, T., Woodward, D.and Smith. H.R. 2004. Designation of 0174 and 0175 to temporary 0 groups 0 X 3 and 0 X 7, and six new *E. coli* 0 groups that include verocytotoxin-producing *E. coli* (VTEC) : 0176, 0177, 0178, 0179, 0180 and 0181. APMIS, **112 :** 569-584.

Schilling, J.D., Martin, S.M., Hung, C.S. Lorenz, R.G. and Hultgren. S.J. 2003. Toll - like receptor 4 on stromal and hematopoietic cells mediates innate resistance to uropathogenic *Escherichia coli*. Proc. Nat. Acad. Sci. *USA,* **100:** 4203-4208.

Schmidt, H., Scheef, J., Morabito, S., Caprioli, A., Wieler, L. H. and Karch, H., 2000. A new Shiga toxin 2 variant (stx2f) from *Escherichia coli* from pigeons. J. Clin. Microbiol., **66:** 1205–1208.

Scotland, S.M., Smith, H.R., Cheasty, T., Said, B., Willshaw, G.A., Stokes, N. and Rowe. B. 1996. Use of gene probes and adhesion tests to characterize *Escherichia coli* belonging to enteropathogenic serogroups isolated in the United Kingdom. J. Med. Microbiol., **44:** 438–443.

Sears, C.L. and Kaper, J.B. 1996. Enteric bacterial toxins: mechanisms of action and linkage to intestinal secretion. Microbiol. Rev., **60:** 167–215.

Sharma, S.N and Adlakha, S.C. 2005. In: Textbook of Veterinary Microbiology, p. 199-203.

Sixma, T.K., Kalk, K.H., van Zanten, B.A., Dauter, Z., Kingma, J., Witholt, B. and Hol. W.G. 1993. Refined structure of *Escherichia coli* heatlabile enterotoxin, a close relative of cholera toxin. J. Mol. Biol., **230:** 890–918.

Small, P.L. and Falkow. S. 1986. Development of a DNA probe for the virulence plasmid of *Shigella* spp. and enteroinvasive *Escherichia coli,* p. 121–124. *In* L. Leive, P. F. Bonventre, J. A. Morello, S. D. Silver, and W. C. Wu (ed.), Microbiology. American Society for Microbiology, Washington, D.C.

Songer, J.G. and Post, K.W. 2005. Veterinary microbiology, bacterial and fungal agents of animal disease. p. 113- 119.

Spangler, B.D. 1992. Structure and function of cholera toxin and the related *Escherichia coli* heat-labile enterotoxin. Microbiol. Rev., **56:** 622–647.

Speirs, J., Stavric, S. and Buchanan. B. 1991. Assessment of two commercial agglutination kits for detecting *Escherichia coli* heat-labile enterotoxin. Canadian J. Microbiol., **37:** 877–880.

Stacy-Phipps, S., Mecca, J.J. and Weiss. J.B. 1995. Multiplex PCR assay and simple preparation method for stool specimens detect enterotoxigenic *Escherichia coli* DNA during the course of infection. J. Clin. Microbiol., **33:** 1054–1059.

Streatfield, S.J., Sandkvist, M., Sixma, T.K., Bagdasarian, M., Hol, W.G.J. and Hirst. T.R. 1992. Intermolecular interactions between the A and B subunits of heat-labile enterotoxin from *Escherichia coli* promote holotoxin assembly and stability *in vivo*. Proc. Natl. Acad. Sci. *USA*, **89:** 12140–12144.

Teneberg, S., Hirst, T.R, Ångstro¨m, J. and Karlsson, K.A. 1994. Comparison of the glycolipid-binding specificities of cholera toxin and porcine *Escherichia coli* heat-labile enterotoxin: identification of a receptor-active non-ganglioside glycolipid for the heat-labile toxin in infant rabbit small intestine. Glycoconjugate J., **11:** 533–540.

Tesh, V. L., Burris, J. A., Owens, J. W., Gordon, V. M., Wadolkowski, E.A., O'Brien, A.D. and. Samuel, J. E 1993. Comparison of the relative toxicities of Shiga-like toxins type I and type II for mice. Infect. Immun., **61:** 3392– 3402.

Thomas, A., Smith, H.R. and Rowe. B. 1993. Use of digoxigenin-labelled oligonucleotide DNA probes for VT2 and VT2 human variant genes to differentiate Vero cytotoxin-producing *Escherichia coli* strains of serogroup O157. J. Clin. Microbiol., **31:** 1700–1703.

Viswanathan, V. K. , Hodges, K. and Hecht. G. 2009. Enteric infection meets intestinal function: how bacterial pathogens cause diarrhoea. Nat. Rev. Microbiol., **7:** 110-119.

Waddell, T., Head, S., Petric, M., Cohen, A. and Lingwood, C.A. 1988. Globotriosyl ceramide is specifically recognized by the *Escherichia coli* Verotoxin 2. Biochem. Biophys. Res. Commun., **152:** 674–679.

Wani, S.A., Bhat, M.A., Samanta, I., Nishikawa, Y. and Buchh, A.S. 2004. *Escherichia coli* O116 associated with an outbreak of calf diarrhoea. Vet. Rec., **154:** 506–508.

Yamasaki, C., Natori, Y., Zeng, X.-T., Omura, M., Yamasaki, S., Takeda, Y. and Natori, Y. 1999. Induction of cytokines in a human colon epithelial cell line by Shiga toxin-1 (Stx1) and Stx2 but not by nontoxic mutant Stx1 which lacks *N*-glycosidase activity. FEBS Lett. **442:** 231-234.

Yano, A., Ishimaru, R., Hujikata R. 2007. Rapid and sensitive detection of heat-labile I and heat-stable I enterotoxin genes of enterotoxigenic *Escherichia coli* by loop-mediated isothermal amplifi cation. J. Microbiol. Methods, **68:** 414–420.

Yolken, R.H., Greenberg, H.B., Merson, M.H., Sack, R.B. and Kapikian. A.Z. 1977. Enzyme-linked immunosorbent assay for detection of *Escherichia coli* heat-labile enterotoxin. J. Clin. Microbiol., **5:** 439–444.

□□□